Lippincott's
Critical
Care
Drug Guide

To my husband, Gary,
whose incredible love and support
for my goals has made this book
a reality. He selflessly spent countless hours
helping prepare this book
in addition to providing superb care
to our sons.

To my sons, Brandon and Nathan,
for their patience and understanding.

Marla De Jong

REVIEWERS

Julie Briggs, RN, BSN, MHA,
Certified Emergency Nurse Specialist, PHN
Administrative Director of Emergency Services
Good Samaritan Community Healthcare
Puyallup, Washington

Mary K. Evans, BSN, MSN, NP
Clinical Nurse II/Charge Nurse
Georgetown University Medical Center
Washington, D.C.

Kevin R. George,
MBA, BSN, RN, C, CCRN, CEN
Education Coordinator, Critical Care/Trauma
Orlando Regional Healthcare System
Orlando, Florida

Janet Gysi, RN, MA, CCRN
Instructor of Nursing
Iowa Wesleyan College
Mount Pleasant, Iowa

Maureen Howard, RN, MSN, CCRN, FNP
Cardiovascular Clinical Specialist
Overlook Hospital, Atlantic Health System
Summit, New Jersey

Renee Lewis, MS, RN, CCRN
Professor of Nursing Science
Rose State College
Midwest City, Oklahoma

Lisa Lorenzo, RN, BSN
Cardiology Educational Coordinator
Orlando Regional Healthcare System
Orlando, Florida

Paula Rapp, BSN, BA
RN-Emergency Room
George Washington University Medical Center
Washington, DC

Cheryl Wraa, RN, BSN
Clinical Nurse
University of California, Davis Medical Center
Sacramento, California

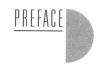
How To Use This Drug Guide

Drug therapy is a crucial component of critical care nursing. Nurses are responsible for delivering safe and appropriate drug therapy while simultaneously managing other dynamic aspects of the patient's care. Critical care and emergency nurses routinely evaluate the appropriateness of a provider's order, decide whether to give or hold a drug, and constantly titrate drug dosages in response to assessment data and in accordance with a provider's orders. In addition, acute care nurse–practitioners are charged with prescribing drug therapy.

The number of new drugs commonly used in critical care and emergency settings increases every year. At the same time, new indications, contraindications, available forms, dosages, and routes available for existing drugs are published. No nurse can memorize all the information required to provide safe and efficacious drug therapy. *Lippincott's Critical Care Drug Guide* features current, state-of-the art facts for drugs regularly used in critical care and emergency department settings.

This book is designed to provide specialized and pertinent information that critical care nurses, emergency nurses, and acute care nurse–practitioners require daily at the bedside. New critical care nurses will relish the dosage titration tables, clear details about intravenous drug preparation and administration, and specific procedures for administering drugs via unique routes. Seasoned critical care nurses and practitioners will appreciate content about the drug's effect on hemodynamic parameters, dosage information for specific indications, and drug interactions. Student nurses in advanced medical-surgical and critical care rotations and their instructors will value the book's easy-to-comprehend facts, formulae for calculation of intravenous doses, and nursing considerations as they gain familiarity with these potent drugs.

Because complex critically ill patients are unstable, critical care and emergency nurses must possess expert assessment skills and flexible time management skills. The book's uncluttered design and larger type makes it easy to use, especially in fast-paced and intense critical care or emergency care arenas. Use of this book will support accurate and effective decision-making and contribute to the delivery of safer and more efficient care.

Part I

Drug information is presented in monograph form, with the monographs arranged alphabetically by generic name. Each page of the book contains guide words at the top, much like a dictionary, to promote easy access to any drug. The right-hand edge of the book contains letter guides, again to facilitate finding a drug as quickly as possible. The spiral binding ensures that the book remains open to the desired page.

Complete Drug Monographs

▸ Each drug monograph is complete in itself—that is, it includes all the clinically important information that nurses need to know to give the drug safely and effectively to critically ill adult patients. Each monograph is organized under standard headings.

▸ The monograph begins with the drug's generic (nonproprietary) name and an alphabetical list of the most common brand names, including common brand names found only in Canada (noted by the designation CAN).

▸ The drug's pregnancy category classification is listed. Appendix E contains more details about each category.

▸ If the drug is a controlled substance, its schedule is identified. Appendix D contains more details about each category.

▸ The commonly accepted pronunciation is provided to help the nurse feel more comfortable discussing the drug with other members of the health care team.

▸ The clinically important drug classes of each drug are indicated, to put the drug in the appropriate context.

▸ Clinical indications for the drug are listed, including important non-FDA approved or "unlabeled" indications, as well as orphan drug uses. To focus the content on "must-know" information, indications that are rarely used in critical care or emergency settings have been omitted.

▸ The therapeutic actions of the drug are described, including (when known) the mechanism(s) by which these therapeutic effects are produced.

▸ When applicable, effects on hemodynamic parameters are listed to guide the nursing assessment and to help nurses anticipate the drug's impact on the patient's condition.

▸ Contraindications to the drug's use and cautions to consider when using the drug are listed.

▸ The available forms are listed to serve as a guide for prescribing or suggesting alternate routes of administration. Note, each facility's pharmacy may or may not carry each form of the drug.

▸ The IV/SC/IM/endotracheal facts section is indispensable as these administration routes are frequently used in critical care and emergency care environments. This section presents "at a glance" all the required information regarding safe drug administration. The preparation section contains specific details about how to reconstitute and/or dilute the drug. Adult dosages and rates of administration are listed according to specific indications. This section contains information about dosage adjustment for certain patient populations, such as the elderly or patients with impaired renal function. As applicable, drug or electrolyte levels are listed. To expedite drug administration of commonly used titratable drugs, the same page also contains an invaluable titration table. These important features eliminate the need to search through the entire monograph or a separate IV handbook for this desired and critical information. In alphabetical order by generic name, other drugs that are Y-site compatible and incompatible with the drug are listed.

▸ Listed next are adult dosages for other routes of administration, such as oral, topical, rectal, and inhalation.

▸ The drug's antidote, if known, and details about treating an overdose of the drug are explained.

▸ The pharmacokinetic profile for each drug is given in table format to ensure easy access to information about the drug's onset, peak, and duration. Facts about the drug's metabolism, half-life, and excretion are listed directly below the table.

▸ Common adverse effects are listed by body system, with potentially life-threatening adverse effects in **bold** and frequently encountered adverse effects in *italics*. Adverse effects that have been reported, but are noted less frequently are also listed to make the drug information as complete as possible.

▸ Clinically important drug interactions are identified and explained to direct the nurse's assessment and follow-up actions.

The last section of each monograph focuses on nursing considerations, which are presented in nursing process format.

▸ The assessment section outlines the information to collect before administering the drug. This section is further divided into two subsections. 1) The section regarding history includes a list of those underlying conditions that constitute contraindications and cautions for use of the drug. 2) The section about physical assessment provides data to collect before beginning drug therapy, both to allow detection of conditions that are contraindications/cautions to use of the drug and to provide baseline data for detecting adverse reactions and therapeutic responses to the drug. Not all assessment parameters may be relevant to every patient; however, these will guide the nurse in performing an individualized patient assessment.

▸ The implementation section lists nursing actions to execute when caring for a patient who is receiving the drug. This includes activities related to drug administration, the provision of safety and comfort measures, and drug storage. Again, not all interventions may be relevant to every patient but these will help the nurse individualize patient care.

▸ Evaluation is usually the last step of the nursing process. In all drug therapy, evaluate the patient for the desired effect of the drug as listed in the Indications, Therapeutic Actions, and Effects on Hemodynamic Parameters sections and the occurrence of adverse effects, as listed in the Adverse Effects section. These points are essential. In some cases, evaluation includes monitoring specific therapeutic serum drug levels; these cases are specifically identified in the Therapeutic Serum Level section.

Appendices
The appendices contain clear-cut information that is useful in nursing practice, but may not lend itself to the monograph format. Appendices include: conversions, formulae for calculation of IV doses, hemodynamic formulae and values relevant to drug administration, DEA schedules of controlled substances, FDA pregnancy categories, peripheral nerve stimulator estimates of neuromuscular blockade; emergency treatment of an acute drug overdose, poisoning, or exposure; emergency treatment of anaphylaxis reactions, commonly used blood products, blood product compatibility, components of common intravenous solutions, procedure for adding drugs to an intravenous solution, procedure for administering multiple solutions or drugs through the same IV line, procedure for administering an IV bolus dose, procedure for administering IV piggyback drugs, procedure for administering IM or SC drugs, procedure for administering drugs through an endotracheal tube, procedure for administering drugs through a nasogastric/orogastric tube, procedure for administering inhaler drugs, procedure for administering nebulized drugs, procedure for administering transdermal drugs, procedure for administering sublingual drugs, management of IV extravasation, selected pharmaceutical web sites, and a suggested bibliography.

Index
The index provides a ready reference to drug information. The generic name of each drug is highlighted in **bold**. If the generic name of a drug is not known, the drug may be found quickly by using whatever name is known. Brand names are listed in *italics*.

Marla J. De Jong, RN, MS, CCRN, CEN, Captain
Amy M. Karch, RN, MS

ACKNOWLEDGMENTS

We would like to thank the many people who have helped to make this book possible: our colleagues, past and present, who helped us learn to apply pharmacology to critical care and emergency care settings; our supervisors for their support and flexibility; our editor, Margaret Zuccarini, who envisioned this project and provided continuous direction and encouragement; and assistant editor, Helen Kogut, who kept us organized, answered our questions, and assisted with the practical aspects of this undertaking.

CONTENTS

Alphabetical Listing of Drugs by Generic Name

A

● **abciximab** *(ab six' ah mab)* ReoPro

Pregnancy Category C

Drug classes
Glycoprotein (GP) IIb/IIIa antagonist
Antiplatelet drug

Indications
❱ Adjunct to percutaneous transluminal coronary angioplasty or atherectomy for the prevention of acute cardiac ischemic complications in patients at high risk for abrupt closure of the treated coronary vessel
❱ Appropriate for patients with unstable angina who do not respond to conventional medical therapy if a percutaneous coronary intervention (PCI) is planned within 24 h
❱ Intended to be used with heparin and aspirin therapy

Therapeutic actions
❱ Is a mouse/human chimeric monoclonal antibody
❱ Has a high affinity and specificity for the platelet's GP IIb/IIIa receptor
❱ Binds to the GP IIb/IIIa receptor on activated platelets and blocks the binding of fibrinogen and von Willebrand's factor to this receptor, thus inhibiting platelet aggregation

Contraindications/cautions
❱ **Contraindications:** abciximab or murine protein allergy, active internal bleeding, recent GI or GU bleeding, cerebrovascular accident within the last 2 y or with significant neurologic deficit, bleeding diathesis, thrombocytopenia, severe uncontrolled hypertension (HTN), recent major surgery or trauma, vasculitis, oral anticoagulant therapy within 7 d (unless the prothrombin time is ≤ 1.2 times control), intravenous (IV) dextran administration either before or during angioplasty, hemostatic disorders, intracranial neoplasm, arteriovenous malformation, or cerebral aneurysm
❱ **Cautions:** patients at risk for bleeding (weight < 75 kg, patients older than 65 y, history of GI disease, patients receiving thrombolytics, heparin anticoagulation, PTCA within 12 h of onset of AMI, prolonged or failed PTCA)

Available form
❱ *Injection:* 2 mg/mL

Adverse effects in *Italics* are most common; those in **Bold** are life-threatening

IV facts
Preparation
▶ Using aseptic technique, withdraw the bolus dose of abciximab into a syringe.
▶ Use a 0.20- or 0.22-mcm filter to filter the drug either when admixing it in 250 mL of D5W or 0.9%NS when administering drug. Filter removes large protein particles that may cause thrombocytopenia.

Dosage
▶ *Adjunct to PCI:* Initiate treatment 10–60 min before the procedure. **Bolus dose:** 0.25 mg/kg IV over at least 1 min. **Maintenance infusion:** 0.125 mcg/kg/min (maximum of 10 mcg/min) IV for 12 h.
▶ *Prior to PCI:* **Bolus dose:** 0.25 mg/kg IV over at least 1 min 18–24 h prior to PCI. **Maintenance infusion:** 0.125 mcg/kg/min IV until 1 h after the intervention. Filter drug as described above.
▶ Administer heparin as ordered; however, do not administer other IV drugs through the line containing abciximab.

Titration Guide

abciximab

7.2 mg in 250 mL

Body Weight									
lb	88	99	110	121	132	143	154	165	176	187
kg	40	45	50	55	60	65	70	75	80	85

Dose ordered in mcg/kg/min	Amounts to Infuse in mL/h								
0.125	10	12	13	14	16	17	18	20	21	21

Body Weight									
lb	198	209	220	231	242	253	264	275	286
kg	90	95	100	105	110	115	120	125	130

Dose ordered in mcg/kg/min	Amounts to Infuse in mL/h								
0.125	21	21	21	21	21	21	21	21	21

Compatibility
Administer in a separate IV line; do not add other drugs to the infusion solution.

Adverse effects in *Italics* are most common; those in **Bold** are life-threatening

TREATMENT OF OVERDOSE/ANTIDOTE
Discontinue drug or decrease dosage. Initiate general supportive and resuscitative measures. A platelet transfusion will reverse the abciximab-induced platelet inhibition and control bleeding.

Pharmacokinetics

Route	Onset	Peak	Duration
IV	Rapid	10 min	Affects platelet function 48 h; in circulation up to 15 d in a platelet-bound state

$T_{1/2}$: <10 min, then 30 min
Excretion: Kidney

Adverse effects

▶ *CNS:* **Hemorrhagic stroke,** *dizziness, abnormal thinking,* confusion, hypesthesia, coma
▶ *CV:* *Hypotension, atrial fibrillation/flutter,* bradycardia, dysrhythmias, intermittent claudication, limb embolism
▶ *Resp:* Pleural effusion, pneumonia
▶ *GI:* **GI bleeding,** nausea, vomiting, diarrhea, constipation, ileus
▶ *GU:* **GU bleeding**
▶ *Allergic:* **Anaphylaxis**
▶ *Hematologic: Bleeding* **(retroperitoneal, venous, and arterial access sites), thrombocytopenia,** anemia, petechiae
▶ *Musc/Skel:* Myopathy, cellulitis, myalgia
▶ *Misc:* *Pain, edema,* pruritus, dysphonia, human antichimeric antibody development, abnormal vision

Clinically important drug–drug interactions

▶ Increased risk of bleeding with anticoagulant, thrombolytic, antithrombotic, aspirin, nonsteroidal anti-inflammatory, or other antiplatelet drugs

● NURSING CONSIDERATIONS

Assessment

▶ *History:* Abciximab or murine protein allergy, active internal bleeding, recent GI or GU bleeding, cerebrovascular accident within the last 2 y or with significant neurologic deficit, bleeding diathesis, thrombocytopenia, severe uncontrolled HTN, recent major surgery or trauma, vasculitis, hemostatic disorders, intracranial neoplasm, arteriovenous malformation, cerebral aneurysm, age, PTCA within 12 h of onset of AMI, prolonged or failed PTCA, GI disease; use of thrombolytics, oral anticoagulants, heparin, or dextran

Adverse effects in *Italics* are most common; those in **Bold** are life-threatening

‣ *Physical:* P, BP, R, ECG, I & O, IV site, weight, arterial and venous access sites, neurologic checks, skin assessment, chest pain assessment, bowel sounds, peripheral perfusion, pain assessment, presence of bleeding, CPK, CPK-MB, cardiac troponin, myoglobin, CBC, liver and renal function tests, APTT, PT, ACT; urine, stool, and emesis guaiac

Implementation

‣ Administer infusion through an IV pump.
‣ Frequently assess potential bleeding sites, paying careful attention to arterial and venous puncture sites and femoral access site.
‣ While the arterial and/or venous sheath is in place, maintain patient on bed rest with head of the bed < 30 degrees. Keep affected extremity flat and straight.
‣ Adhere to strict anticoagulation guidelines per hospital protocol. Administer and titrate weight-adjusted heparin as ordered. Discontinue heparin 2–4 h before sheath removal or according to hospital protocol.
‣ Remove sheaths when APTT is ≤ 45–50 s or the ACT is ≤ 175 to 180 s.
‣ Apply pressure to access site for at least 30 min after sheath removal.
‣ Following initial hemostasis, continue bed rest for 6 to 8 h or according to hospital policy. Apply a pressure dressing to the site.
‣ If bleeding recurs, reapply manual or mechanical compression until hemostasis is achieved.
‣ Mark and measure the size of any hematoma, and monitor it for evidence of enlargement.
‣ After achieving hemostasis, monitor the patient in the hospital for at least 4 h.
‣ Assess for neurovascular compromise of affected leg. Palpate distal pulses, and note extremity's color and warmth. Assess for pain, numbness, tingling of affected leg.
‣ Minimize arterial and venous punctures.
‣ If possible, draw blood from a saline lock.
‣ Do not insert IV access devices into noncompressible sites, such as the subclavian and jugular veins.
‣ Avoid intramuscular injections, urinary catheter insertion, and nasotracheal and nasogastric intubation whenever possible.
‣ Continue aspirin therapy.
‣ Discontinue antiplatelet drug infusions and determine a bleeding time before surgery if the patient requires coronary artery bypass grafting or another surgical procedure.
‣ Check stools, urine, and emesis for occult blood.

Adverse effects in *Italics* are most common; those in **Bold** are life-threatening

▶ Monitor the patient's WBC, Hgb, Hct, APTT, ACT, platelet, and creatinine values; notify provider of abnormal values. Be prepared to transfuse platelets if platelet count is < 50,000 cells/mcL.
▶ Have emergency equipment (defibrillator, drugs, oxygen, intubation equipment) on standby in case anaphylaxis or adverse reaction occurs.
▶ Monitor for evidence of adverse or allergic reactions to the drug. If reaction is suspected, discontinue the drug and initiate resuscitative interventions.
▶ Medicate patient for back or groin pain.
▶ Use a manual blood pressure cuff or ensure that an automatic blood pressure cuff does not apply excessive pressure to the patient's arm.
▶ Use an electric razor to shave patients.
▶ Do not freeze or shake vials. Discard any unused drug left in vial.

⬤ **acebutolol hydrochloride** *(a se byoo' toe lole)*
Monitan (CAN), Rhotral (CAN), Sectral

Pregnancy Category B

Drug classes
Beta-adrenergic blocking agent (β_1 selective)
Antidysrhythmic drug
Antihypertensive drug

Indications
▶ Treatment of hypertension, used alone or with other drugs
▶ Treatment of ventricular dysrhythmias, especially ventricular premature beats

Therapeutic actions
▶ Acts on β_1 (myocardial) receptors to decrease resting heart rate, exercise-induced tachycardia, cardiac output, and BP at rest and after exercise; isoproterenol-induced tachycardia
▶ Delays atrioventricular (AV) conduction time and increases AV node refractoriness without affecting sinus node recovery time, atrial refractory period, or HV conduction time
▶ Inhibits β_2 receptors at higher doses

Effects on hemodynamic parameters
▶ Decreased BP
▶ Decreased CO
▶ Decreased HR

Adverse effects in *Italics* are most common; those in **Bold** are life-threatening

Contraindications/cautions
▸ **Contraindications:** beta-blocker allergy, persistently severe bradycardia, second- or third-degree heart block, overt cardiac failure, cardiogenic shock
▸ **Cautions:** heart failure controlled by digitalis or diuretics, peripheral or mesenteric vascular disease, patients with bronchospastic disease who do not respond to or tolerate other treatments, diabetes, thyrotoxicosis, impaired renal or hepatic function, elderly patients

Available forms
▸ *Capsules:* 200, 400 mg

Oral dosage
▸ *Hypertension:* 400 mg/d or 200 mg bid PO for uncomplicated mild to moderate hypertension. Usual maintenance dosage range is 200–1200 mg/d given twice daily.
▸ *Ventricular dysrhythmias:* 200 mg PO bid. Increase dosage gradually until optimum response is achieved (usually 600–1200 mg/d). Discontinue gradually over 2 wk.
▸ *Elderly:* Because bioavailability doubles, lower doses may be required. Avoid doses > 800 mg/d.
▸ *Renal/hepatic function impairment:* Reduce daily dose by 50% when creatinine clearance is < 50 mL/min/1.73 m^2. Reduce by 75% when creatinine clearance is < 25 mL/min/1.73 m^2. Use caution with hepatic impairment.

TREATMENT OF OVERDOSE/ANTIDOTE
Discontinue drug or decrease dosage. Initiate general supportive and resuscitative measures. Empty stomach by emesis or lavage. Treat bradycardia with IV atropine or isoproterenol. Give vasopressors for hypotension. Treat bronchospasm with aminophylline or terbutaline. Treat cardiac failure with digitalis or diuretics. Acebutolol is dialyzable.

Pharmacokinetics

Route	Onset	Peak	Duration
Oral	1.5 h	3–8 h	24–30 h

Metabolism: Hepatic; T$_{1/2}$: 3–4 h
Excretion: Urine, bile

Adverse effects
▸ *CNS: Headache, fatigue, dizziness,* depression, insomnia, abnormal dreams, anxiety, hyperesthesia, hypoesthesia
▸ *CV:* **Heart failure,** chest pain, edema, hypotension, bradycardia

Adverse effects in *Italics* are most common; those in **Bold** are life-threatening

- ▶ *Resp:* *Dyspnea,* cough, rhinitis, pharyngitis, wheezing
- ▶ *GI:* *Constipation, diarrhea, dyspepsia, nausea,* vomiting, flatulence, abdominal pain, elevated serum transaminases
- ▶ *GU:* Frequency, dysuria, nocturia, dark urine
- ▶ *Derm:* Rash, pruritus
- ▶ *Musc/Skel:* Arthralgia, myalgia, back pain, joint pain
- ▶ *EENT:* Conjunctivitis, dry eyes, eye pain
- ▶ *Misc:* Systemic lupus erythematosus, development of antinuclear antibodies, hypoglycemia

Clinically important drug–drug interactions
- ▶ Increased risk of marked hypotension and bradycardia with prazosin and catecholamine-depleting drugs, such as reserpine
- ▶ Exaggerated hypertensive responses from concurrent use of beta-adrenergic antagonists and alpha-adrenergic stimulants
- ▶ Blunted antihypertensive effects by nonsteroidal anti-inflammatory drugs
- ▶ May potentiate insulin-induced hypoglycemia

⬤ NURSING CONSIDERATIONS

Assessment
- ▶ *History:* Beta-blocker allergy, persistently severe bradycardia, second- or third-degree heart block, overt cardiac failure, cardiogenic shock, heart failure, peripheral or mesenteric vascular disease, bronchospastic disease, diabetes, thyrotoxicosis, impaired renal or hepatic function, age
- ▶ *Physical:* T, P, R, BP, ECG, I & O, weight, neurologic checks, skin assessment, respiratory status, orthostatic BP, peripheral edema, peripheral perfusion, adventitious lung sounds, neck vein distention, abdominal assessment, blood and urine glucose; kidney, liver, and thyroid function tests

Implementation
- ▶ Carefully monitor P, BP, R, and ECG.
- ▶ Minimize orthostatic hypotension by helping the patient change positions slowly.
- ▶ Assess for hypoglycemia; however, its usual manifestations may not be apparent.
- ▶ Assess for early evidence of heart failure as evidenced by increased weight, neck vein distention, oliguria, peripheral edema, crackles over lung fields, dyspnea, decreased SpO_2, cough, decreased activity tolerance, increased respiratory distress when lying flat, S_3 heart sound, tachycardia, hepatomegaly, or confusion.
- ▶ Do not discontinue drug abruptly after chronic therapy. (Hypersensitivity to catecholamines may have developed, causing exacerbation of angina, myocardial infarction, and

Adverse effects in *Italics* are most common; those in **Bold** are life-threatening

ventricular dysrhythmias.) Taper drug gradually over 2 wk with monitoring.
▸ Patients with history of severe anaphylactic reactions may be more reactive on reexposure to the allergen and may be unresponsive to usual doses of epinephrine.
▸ Consult with physician about withdrawing drug if patient is to undergo surgery (withdrawal is controversial).
▸ May give with or without food.

⬤ **acetylcysteine** *(a se teel sis' tay een)* N-acetylcysteine
Mucomyst, Mucosil 10, Mucomyst-10 IV, Mucosil 20, Parvolex (CAN)

Pregnancy Category B

Drug classes
Mucolytic agent
Antidote

Indications
▸ Mucolytic adjuvant therapy for abnormal, viscid, or inspissated mucous secretions in acute and chronic bronchopulmonary disease (chronic emphysema, emphysema with bronchitis, chronic asthmatic bronchitis, tuberculosis, bronchiectasis, primary amyloidosis of lung), acute bronchopulmonary disease (pneumonia, bronchitis, tracheobronchitis), pulmonary complications of cystic fibrosis, tracheostomy care, in pulmonary complications associated with surgery, post-traumatic chest conditions, atelectasis due to mucus obstruction, and diagnostic bronchial studies
▸ Antidote to prevent or lessen hepatic injury that may occur after ingestion of a potentially hepatotoxic dose of acetaminophen; treatment must start as soon as possible and within 24 h of ingestion
▸ Unlabeled uses: as ophthalmic solution to treat keratoconjunctivitis sicca (dry eye); as an enema to treat bowel obstruction due to meconium ileus or its equivalent
▸ Orphan drug: IV use for moderate to severe acetaminophen overdose

Therapeutic actions
▸ Mucolytic activity: splits disulfide links between mucoprotein molecular complexes, resulting in depolymerization and a decrease in mucus viscosity
▸ Antidote to acetaminophen hepatotoxicity: protects liver cells by maintaining or restoring glutathione levels or by acting as an alternate substrate for conjugation and detoxification of acetaminophen's reactive metabolite

Adverse effects in *Italics* are most common; those in **Bold** are life-threatening

A

Contraindications/cautions
▶ **Contraindications: Mucolytic use:** acetylcysteine allergy;
  Antidotal use: none
▶ **Cautions:** asthma, esophageal varices, peptic ulcer

Available forms
▶ *Solution:* 10%, 20%
▶ *Injection:* Orphan drug availability

Dosage
Mucolytic use
▶ *Nebulization (face mask, mouth piece, tracheostomy):* 1–10 mL of 20% solution or 2–20 mL of 10% solution q2–6h; the dose for most patients is 3–5 mL of the 20% solution or 6–10 mL of the 10% solution tid–qid.
▶ *Nebulization (tent, croupette):* Very large volumes are required, occasionally up to 300 mL during a treatment period. The dose is the volume or solution that will maintain a very heavy mist in the tent or croupette for the desired period. Administration for intermittent or continuous prolonged periods, including overnight, may be desirable.

Instillation
▶ *Direct or by tracheostomy:* 1–2 mL of a 10%–20% solution q1–4h; may be introduced into a particular segment of the bronchopulmonary tree by way of a plastic catheter (inserted under local anesthesia and with direct visualization). Instill 2–5 mL of the 20% solution by a syringe connected to the catheter.
▶ *Percutaneous intratracheal catheter:* 1–2 mL of the 20% solution or 2–4 mL of the 10% solution q1–4h by a syringe connected to the catheter.
▶ *Diagnostic bronchogram:* Before the procedure, give 2–3 administrations of 1–2 mL of the 20% solution or 2–4 mL of the 10% solution by nebulization or intratracheal instillation.

Antidotal use
▶ For acetaminophen overdose, administer acetylcysteine immediately if 24 h or less have elapsed since acetaminophen ingestion, using the following protocol:
▶ Empty the stomach by lavage, or induce emesis with syrup of ipecac; repeat dose of ipecac if emesis does not occur in 20 min.
▶ If activated charcoal has been administered, lavage before giving acetylcysteine; charcoal may adsorb acetylcysteine and reduce its effectiveness.

Adverse effects in *Italics* are most common; those in **Bold** are life-threatening

- Draw blood for acetaminophen plasma assay and for baseline AST, ALT, bilirubin, prothrombin time, creatinine, BUN, blood sugar, and electrolytes. If assay cannot be obtained or level is clearly in the toxic range, give full course of acetylcysteine therapy. Monitor hepatic and renal function, fluid balance, and electrolytes.
- Administer acetylcysteine loading dose of 140 mg/kg PO.
- Administer 17 maintenance doses of 70 mg/kg q4h, starting 4 h after loading dose; administer full course of doses unless acetaminophen assay reveals a nontoxic level.
- If patient vomits loading or maintenance dose within 1 h of administration, repeat that dose. An IV form is being studied as an orphan drug.
- If patient persistently vomits the oral dose, administer by duodenal intubation.
- Repeat AST, ALT, bilirubin, prothrombin time, creatinine, BUN, blood sugar, and serum electrolytes daily if acetaminophen level is in the toxic range.

TREATMENT OF OVERDOSE/ANTIDOTE
Discontinue drug or decrease dosage. Initiate general supportive and resuscitative measures.

Pharmacokinetics

Route	Onset	Peak	Duration
Oral	30–60 min	1–2 h	
Instillation/inhalation	1 min	5–10 min	2–3 h

Metabolism: Hepatic; $T_{1/2}$: 6.25 h
Excretion: Urine (30%)

Adverse effects

Mucolytic Use
- **CNS:** Drowsiness, clamminess
- **Resp: Bronchospasm,** chest tightness, tracheal and bronchial tract irritation
- **GI:** *Nausea,* vomiting, stomatitis
- **Allergic:** Urticaria
- **Misc:** Rhinorrhea, fever

Antidotal Use
- **CV:** Tachycardia, hypotension, hypertension
- **Resp: Bronchospasm, angioedema**
- **GI:** *Nausea,* vomiting, other GI symptoms
- **Derm:** Rash, pruritus

Adverse effects in *Italics* are most common; those in **Bold** are life-threatening

A

● NURSING CONSIDERATIONS

Assessment

▶ *History:* Asthma, esophageal varices, peptic ulcer; mucolytic use: acetylcysteine allergy; antidote use: history of acetaminophen ingestion

▶ *Physical:* T, P, R, BP, I & O, SpO$_2$, weight, neurologic checks, skin assessment, adventitious lung sounds, respiratory effort, assessment of respiratory secretions, abdominal assessment, liver palpation, AST, ALT, bilirubin, prothrombin time, creatinine, BUN, blood sugar, serum electrolytes, acetaminophen level

Implementation

Mucolytic Use

▶ Dilute the 20% acetylcysteine solution with either Normal Saline or Sterile Water for Injection or Inhalation; use the 10% solution undiluted. Refrigerate unused, undiluted solution, and use within 96 h. Drug solution in the opened bottle may change color, but this does not alter its safety or efficacy.

▶ Use water to remove residual drug solution on the patient's face after administration by face mask.

▶ Inform patient that nebulization may produce an initial disagreeable odor, but it will soon disappear.

▶ Monitor nebulizer for buildup of drug from evaporation; dilute with Sterile Water for Injection to prevent concentrate from impeding nebulization and drug delivery.

▶ Establish routine for pulmonary toilet; keep suction equipment nearby.

Antidotal Use

▶ Dilute the 20% acetylcysteine solution with cola drinks or other soft drinks to a final concentration of 5%; if administered by gastric tube or Miller-Abbott tube, may dilute with water. Dilution minimizes the risk of vomiting.

▶ Prepare fresh solutions, and use within 1 h; undiluted solution in opened vials may be kept for 96 h.

▶ Administer the following drugs separately because they are incompatible with acetylcysteine solutions: tetracycline, chlortetracycline, oxytetracycline, erythromycin lactobionate, sodium ampicillin, amphotericin B, iodized oil, chymotrypsin, trypsin, hydrogen peroxide.

▶ Maintain fluid and electrolyte balance; treat hypoglycemia.

▶ Give vitamin K$_1$ if prothrombin ratio exceeds 1.5; give fresh-frozen plasma if PT ratio exceeds 3.

▶ Avoid diuretics and forced diuresis.

Adverse effects in *Italics* are most common; those in **Bold** are life-threatening

● **acyclovir** *(ay sye' kloe ver)* acycloguanosine
Alti-Acyclovir (CAN), Avirax (CAN), Zovirax

Pregnancy Category C

Drug class
Antiviral

Indications
- Treatment of initial and recurrent mucosal and cutaneous herpes simplex virus (HSV)-1 and HSV-2 and varicella-zoster (shingles) infections in immunocompromised patients (parenteral)
- Treatment of herpes simplex encephalitis (parenteral)
- Treatment of severe initial clinical episodes of genital herpes in patients who are not immunocompromised (parenteral)
- Treatment of initial episodes and management of recurrent episodes of genital herpes in patients depending on severity of disease, patient's immune status, frequency and duration of episodes, and degree of cutaneous or systemic involvement (oral)
- Acute treatment of herpes zoster (shingles) and chickenpox (varicella) (oral)
- Management of initial episodes of herpes genitalis and non–life-threatening mucocutaneous herpes simplex virus infections in immunocompromised patients (ointment)
- Unlabeled uses: treatment of cytomegalovirus and HSV infection after bone marrow or renal transplantation; herpes simplex-associated erythema multiforme; herpes simplex labialis, ocular infections, proctitis, whitlow; herpes zoster encephalitis; infectious mononucleosis; varicella pneumonia

Therapeutic actions
- Is converted to its active form by HSV-infected cells
- Interferes with HSV DNA polymerase
- Inhibits viral DNA replication

Contraindications/cautions
- **Contraindications:** allergy to acyclovir or its components
- **Cautions:** underlying neurologic abnormalities (lethargy, tremors, confusion, hallucinations, agitation, seizures, coma); renal, hepatic, or electrolyte abnormalities; hypoxia; patients with prior neurologic reactions to cytotoxic drugs; hypovolemia

Available forms
- *Powder for injection:* 500, 1000 mg/vial
- *Tablets:* 400, 800 mg
- *Capsules:* 200 mg

Adverse effects in *Italics* are most common; those in **Bold** are life-threatening

▶ *Oral suspension:* 200 mg/5 mL
▶ *Ointment:* 50 mg/g

IV facts
Preparation
▶ Dissolve contents of 500- or 1000-mg vial in 10 or 20 mL Sterile Water for Injection, respectively, to yield final concentration of 50 mg/mL. Do *not* use bacteriostatic water containing benzyl alcohol or parabens.
▶ Further dilute calculated dose in D5W or 0.9%NS to a concentration of 7 mg/mL or less.
▶ Do not add acyclovir to biologic or colloidal fluids (blood products, protein solutions).

Dosage
▶ Avoid IV bolus or rapid IV administration.
▶ Infuse acyclovir over at least 1 h to prevent renal tubular damage.
▶ *Mucosal and cutaneous HSV infections in immunocompromised patients:* 5 mg/kg IV q8h for 7 d.
▶ *Varicella-zoster infections (shingles) in immunocompromised patients:* 10 mg/kg IV q8h for 7 d.
▶ *Herpes simplex encephalitis:* 10 mg/kg IV q8h for 10 d.
▶ *Renal function impairment:* See following chart for acyclovir dosage:

Creatinine Clearance (mL/min/1.73m^2)	% of Recommended Dose	Dosing Interval (h)
> 50	100%	8
25–50	100%	12
10–25	100%	24
0–10	50%	24

▶ *Hemodialysis patients:* Give acyclovir dose after each hemodialysis.

Compatibility
Acyclovir may be given through the same IV line as allopurinol, amikacin, ampicillin, cefamandole, cefazolin, cefonicid, cefoperazone, cefotaxime, cefoxitin, ceftazidime, ceftizoxime, ceftriaxone, cefuroxime, cephapirin, chloramphenicol, cimetidine, clindamycin, dexamethasone, dimenhydrinate, diphenhydramine, doxycycline, erythromycin, famotidine, filgrastim, fluconazole, gallium, gentamicin, granisetron, heparin, hydrocortisone, hydromorphone, imipenem-cilastatin, lorazepam, magnesium sulfate, melphalan, methylprednisolone, metoclopramide, metronidazole, multivitamins, nafcillin, oxacillin, paclitaxel, penicillin G

potassium, pentobarbital, perphenazine, piperacillin, potassium chloride, propofol, ranitidine, sodium bicarbonate, tacrolimus, teniposide, theophylline, thiotepa, ticarcillin, tobramycin, trimethoprim-sulfamethoxazole, vancomycin, zidovudine.

Incompatibility

Do not administer through the same IV line as amifostine, amsacrine, aztreonam, cefepime, dobutamine, dopamine, fludarabine, foscarnet, idarubicin, ondansetron, piperacillin-tazobactam, sargramostim, vinorelbine.

Oral/topical dosage

- *Initial herpes simplex:* 200 mg PO q4h 5 times a day for 10 d.
- *Chronic suppressive therapy:* 400 mg PO bid for up to 12 mo.
- *Intermittent therapy:* 200 mg PO q4h 5 times a day for 5 d. Initiate at earliest sign or symptom of recurrence.
- *Herpes zoster, acute treatment:* 800 mg PO q4h 5 times a day for 7–10 d.
- *Chickenpox:* 20 mg/kg PO (not to exceed 800 mg) qid for 5 d. Initiate at earliest sign or symptom.
- *Renal function impairment with creatinine clearance ≤ 10 mL/min:* Give same mg dosage but increase dosing interval to q12h.
- *Herpes genitalis/mucocutaneous herpes simplex virus infections:* Use sufficient quantity to cover all lesions q3h 6 times a day for 7 d. Use glove to apply ointment to prevent autoinoculation of other body sites and transmission of infection to other people. Initiate at earliest sign or symptoms.

TREATMENT OF OVERDOSE/ANTIDOTE

Discontinue drug or reduce dosage. Initiate general supportive and resuscitative measures. To prevent renal tubule precipitation, maintain urine output of ≥ 500 mL/g drug infused. Acyclovir can be removed by hemodialysis.

Pharmacokinetics

Route	Onset	Peak	Duration
IV	Immediate	1 h	8 h
Oral	30–120 min	1.5–2 h	

$T_{1/2}$: 2.5–3 h (up to 19.5 h with impaired renal function)
Excretion: Urine

Adverse effects

- *CNS:* Encephalopathic changes (**seizures,** lethargy, obtundation, tremors, confusion, hallucination, agitation, coma), headache, dizziness, fatigue

Adverse effects in *Italics* are most common; those in **Bold** are life-threatening

- *CV:* Edema, chest pain, hypotension
- ▶ *Resp:* **Pulmonary edema with cardiac tamponade**
- *GI:* *Nausea, vomiting, elevation of transaminases,* thirst, diarrhea, medication taste, constipation, flatulence
- *GU:* **Renal failure,** *transiently elevated BUN or creatinine,* crystalluria with rapid IV administration, hematuria, anuria, pressure on urination, abnormal UA (sediment)
- *Derm:* *Inflammation or phlebitis at injection site, transient burning or stinging at site of topical application, rash, hives, itching,* diaphoresis
- *Hematologic:* Anemia, neutropenia, thrombocytopenia, thrombocytosis, leukocytosis, neutrophilia, hemoglobinemia
- *Misc:* Rigors, ischemia of digits, hypokalemia, leg pain, sore throat

Clinically important drug–drug interactions
- Severe drowsiness and lethargy with zidovudine
- Increased effects, increased half-life, and decreased renal clearance with probenecid
- Increased renal impairment with other nephrotoxic drugs

● NURSING CONSIDERATIONS
Assessment
- *History:* Allergy to acyclovir or its components; underlying neurologic abnormalities (lethargy, tremors, confusion, hallucinations, agitation, seizures, coma); renal, hepatic, or electrolyte abnormalities; hypoxia; patients with prior neurologic reactions to cytotoxic drugs; hypovolemia
- *Physical:* T, P, BP, R, ECG, I & O, IV site, weight, neurologic checks, reflexes, skin assessment, cardiac auscultation, peripheral pulses, peripheral perfusion, edema, adventitious lung sounds, hydration status, electrolyte levels, renal function tests, UA, specimens for culture and sensitivity

Implementation
- Always administer IV infusions using an IV infusion pump.
- Ensure patient is adequately hydrated; to prevent precipitation in renal tubules, recommended urine output is ≥ 500 mL/g drug infused, especially during first 2 h following infusion.
- Monitor renal function throughout therapy.
- Carefully assess IV site for phlebitis or infiltration. Rotate infusion site to minimize phlebitis.
- Oral acyclovir absorption is not affected by food.
- Once IV solution is prepared, use within 24 h.
- Refrigeration of reconstituted solutions may result in formation of a precipitate, which will redissolve at room temperature.

Adverse effects in *Italics* are most common; those in **Bold** are life-threatening

⬤ **adenosine** *(a den' oh seen)* Adenocard
Pregnancy Category C

Drug class
Antidysrhythmic

Indication
▸ Conversion of paroxysmal supraventricular tachycardia (PSVT), including dysrhythmias associated with accessory bypass tracts (WPW syndrome), to sinus rhythm; before administration, vagal maneuvers attempted when appropriate

Therapeutic actions
▸ Slows conduction through the AV node
▸ Interrupts the reentry pathways through the AV node
▸ Restores normal sinus rhythm in patients with PSVT, including PSVT associated with WPW syndrome

Effects on hemodynamic parameters
▸ Decreased BP with large doses
▸ Decreased SVR with large doses
▸ Decreased HR

Contraindications/cautions
▸ **Contraindications:** adenosine allergy, sick sinus syndrome (unless functioning pacemaker in place), second- or third-degree heart block (unless functioning pacemaker in place), ventricular tachycardia, atrial fibrillation, atrial flutter
▸ **Caution:** asthma

Available form
▸ *Injection:* 3 mg/mL

IV facts
Preparation
▸ No further preparation needed; adenosine is for rapid bolus IV use only.

Dosage
▸ *Initial dose:* 6 mg IV given over 1–2 s. Administer drug either directly into a vein or into an IV line as close to the patient as possible. Immediately follow dose with rapid saline flush.
▸ *Repeat administration:* If first dose does not eliminate PSVT within 1–2 min, give 12 mg adenosine IV over 1–2 s. May repeat this 12-mg dose a second time if needed. Doses > 12 mg are not recommended.

Adverse effects in *Italics* are most common; those in **Bold** are life-threatening

Compatibility
Do not mix adenosine with other drugs or administer through an IV line containing other drugs.

> **TREATMENT OF OVERDOSE/ANTIDOTE**
> Because adenosine has a short half-life, adverse effects are usually rapidly self-limiting. Initiate interventions aimed at treating any specific prolonged effects. Consider antagonism by methylxanthines, such as caffeine and theophylline.

Pharmacokinetics

Route	Onset	Duration
IV	Immediate	1–2 min

Metabolism: Metabolized to inosine and adenosine monophosphate; $T_{1/2}$: < 10 s

Adverse effects
- *CNS: Headache, lightheadedness,* dizziness, arm tingling and heaviness, numbness, apprehension, blurred vision, burning sensation, neck and back pain
- *CV:* **Asystole, heart block,** *facial flushing, dysrhythmias,* sweating, palpitations, chest pain, hypotension
- *Resp: Dyspnea, chest pressure,* hyperventilation
- *GI: Nausea,* metallic taste, tightness in throat, pressure in groin

Clinically important drug–drug interactions
- Increased degree of heart block with carbamazepine
- Enhanced effects with dipyridamole
- Decreased effects with methylxanthines (caffeine, theophylline)
- Rarely associated with ventricular fibrillation when used with patients receiving digitalis

⬤ NURSING CONSIDERATIONS

Assessment
- *History:* Adenosine allergy, sick sinus syndrome, dysrhythmias, presence of pacemaker, asthma
- *Physical:* P, BP, R, ECG, IV site, neurologic checks, peripheral perfusion, color, adventitious lung sounds, diaphoresis, palpitations, vertigo, chest pain

Implementation
- Exercise extreme caution when calculating and preparing IV dose.
- Monitor HR, R, BP, and ECG continuously during administration. Assess for dysrhythmias.

Adverse effects in *Italics* are most common; those in **Bold** are life-threatening

- Maintain emergency equipment (defibrillator, drugs, oxygen, intubation equipment) on standby during administration.
- Keep theophylline on standby to reverse drug if needed.
- Store drug at room temperature.
- Discard any unused portion of the drug.

● albumin, human *(al byoo' min)*

normal serum albumin
5%: Albuminar-5, Albunex, Albutein 5%, Buminate 5%,
Normal Serum Albumin (Human) 5%, Plasbumin-5
25%: Albuminar-25, Albutein 25%, Buminate 25%,
Normal Serum Albumin (Human) 25%, Plasbumin-25

Pregnancy Category C

Drug classes
- Blood product
- Plasma protein
- Volume expander

Indications
- Supportive treatment of shock due to burns, trauma, surgery, or infection
- Burns: albumin 5% used in conjunction with adequate infusions of crystalloids to prevent hemoconcentration and water and protein losses
- Hypoproteinemia if sodium restriction is not a problem
- Adult respiratory distress syndrome: albumin 25% with a diuretic
- Cardiopulmonary bypass: preoperative blood dilution with 25% albumin
- Acute liver failure
- Sequestration of protein-rich fluids in acute peritonitis, pancreatitis, mediastinitis, extensive cellulitis
- Erythrocyte resuspension: may be required to avoid hypoproteinemia during exchange transfusions or with use of very large volumes of previously frozen or washed red cells
- Acute nephrosis: albumin 25% and loop diuretic to control edema
- Renal dialysis: albumin 25% to treat shock and hypotension
- Hyperbilirubinemia: adjunct in exchange transfusions

Therapeutic actions
- Is a normal blood protein
- Increases plasma colloid osmotic pressure, which mobilizes fluids from interstitial space to intravascular space
- Maintains normal blood volume
- 25 g of albumin is the osmotic equivalent of about 2 U of FFP

Adverse effects in *Italics* are most common; those in **Bold** are life-threatening

- 100 mL of normal serum albumin 25% provides about as much plasma protein as 500 mL plasma or 2 pints whole blood
- Contains 130 to 160 mEq sodium/L

Effects on hemodynamic parameters
- Increased BP
- Increased CVP
- Increased PCWP
- Increased CO
- Decreased HR

Contraindications/cautions
- **Contraindications:** allergy to albumin, severe anemia, cardiac failure, normal or increased intravascular volume, concurrent use of cardiopulmonary bypass
- **Cautions:** hepatic or renal failure, dehydration, low cardiac reserve

Available forms
- *Injection:* 5%, 25%

IV facts
Preparation
- May be given undiluted. May dilute 25% albumin in D5W; D10W; Dextrose-LR combinations; Dextrose-saline combinations; LR; 0.45%NS; 0.9%NS; Ringer's injection; or Sodium Lactate (1/6 Molar) Injection.

Dosage
- Administer by an IV infusion only.
- *Hypovolemic shock:* **5% albumin:** 500 mL IV given as rapidly as possible; additional 500 mL may be given in 30 min. Base therapy on clinical response; if > 1000 mL is required, consider need for packed red blood cells (PRBCs) or whole blood. Give 1–2 mL/min to patients with slightly low or normal blood volume. **25% albumin:** Base therapy on clinical response. Administer IV as rapidly as tolerated. Repeat dose 15–30 min after first dose if initial patient response inadequate. Give 1 mL/min to patients with slightly low or normal blood volume.
- *Hypoproteinemia:* 5% albumin IV for acute replacement of protein; if edema is present, use 25% albumin 50–75 g/d IV. Do not exceed 2 mL/min. May mix 200 mL of 25% albumin with 300 mL of 10% glucose solution; give by continuous drip at 100 mL/h.
- *Burns:* 5% or 25% albumin may maintain colloid osmotic pressure. Maintain plasma albumin level of 2.5 g/100 mL or a total serum protein level of 5.2 g/100 mL.

Adverse effects in *Italics* are most common; those in **Bold** are life-threatening

- *Nephrosis:* 100 mL of 25% albumin IV with a loop diuretic repeated daily for 7–10 d.
- *Renal dialysis:* Usual volume is 100 mL of 25% albumin; avoid fluid overload.
- *Erythrocyte resuspension:* 25 g of albumin per liter of erythrocytes is commonly used. Add albumin 25% to isotonic suspension of washed red cells immediately before transfusion.

Compatibility
Albumin may be given through the same IV line as diltiazem or lorazepam.

Incompatibility
Do not administer through the same IV line as midazolam, vancomycin, verapamil.

> **TREATMENT OF OVERDOSE/ANTIDOTE**
> Discontinue drug or decrease dosage. Initiate general supportive and resuscitative measures.

Pharmacokinetics

Route	Onset
IV	15–30 min

$T_{1/2}$: In patients with depleted blood volume, hemodilution effects last many hours. In patients with normal blood volume, hemodilution effects last only a few hours. Half-life is 15–20 d with a turnover of 15 g/d.

Adverse effects
- *CV:* **Pulmonary edema after rapid infusion,** hypotension, CHF, dyspnea
- *Allergic: Fever, chills,* flushing, urticaria, back pain, headache, nausea, vomiting, tachycardia, rash; changes in P, R, and BP

● NURSING CONSIDERATIONS

Assessment
- *History:* Allergy to albumin, severe anemia, cardiac failure, normal or increased intravascular volume, concurrent use of cardiopulmonary bypass, hepatic or renal failure, dehydration, low cardiac reserve
- *Physical:* T, P, BP, R, I & O, SpO_2, CO, PCWP, CVP, skin assessment, peripheral perfusion, respiratory effort, adventitious lung sounds, edema, JVD, hydration status, presence of

Adverse effects in *Italics* are most common; those in **Bold** are life-threatening

bleeding, liver and renal function tests, CBC, serum electrolytes, albumin and protein levels

Implementation
- No crossmatching required.
- Solutions are heat treated, so albumin will not transmit hepatitis.
- Monitor for evidence of vascular overload (pulmonary edema, crackles, increased CVP and PCWP, JVD, dyspnea).
- Consider using whole blood; infusion provides only symptomatic relief of hypoproteinemia.
- Albumin is not a substitute for whole blood or PRBCs when oxygen carrying capacity is needed.
- Give additional fluids for patients with hypovolemia.
- For postoperative or trauma patients, assess bleeding points that may have failed to bleed at lower blood pressures; new hemorrhage and shock may occur.
- Stop infusion if hypersensitivity reactions occur; treat reaction with antihistamines. If a plasma protein is still needed, try material from a different lot number.
- Do not begin administration more than 4 h after container is entered; product contains no preservatives.
- Check with manufacturer for storage requirements. Some products are stored at room temperature; others are stored in refrigerator.

albuterol *(al byoo' ter ole)* Proventil, Proventil HFA, Ventolin

albuterol sulfate Airet, Asmavent (CAN), Proventil, Proventil Repetabs, Proventil HFA, Ventolin, Ventolin Nebules, Novo-Salmol (CAN), Ventolin Rotacaps, Ventodisk (CAN), Volmax

Pregnancy Category C

Drug classes
Sympathomimetic drug
Bronchodilator

Indications
- Relief of bronchospasm in patients with reversible obstructive airway disease
- Prevention of exercise-induced bronchospasm
- Unlabeled use: adjunct in treating serious hyperkalemia in dialysis patients; seems to lower potassium concentrations when inhaled by patients on hemodialysis

Adverse effects in *Italics* are most common; those in **Bold** are life-threatening

Therapeutic actions

- In low doses, acts relatively selectively at β_2-adrenergic receptors to cause bronchodilation and vasodilation; bronchodilation may facilitate expectoration
- At higher doses, loses β_2-selectivity and acts at β_1 receptors, causing increased myocardial contractility and conduction

Contraindications/cautions
- **Contraindications:** hypersensitivity to albuterol or its components
- **Cautions:** cardiovascular disease, coronary insufficiency, dysrhythmias, hypertension, convulsive disorders, hyperthyroidism, diabetes mellitus, patients who are unusually responsive to sympathomimetic amines, hypokalemia

Available forms

- *Tablets:* 2, 4 mg
- *Extended-release tablets:* 4, 8 mg
- *Syrup:* 2 mg/5 mL
- *Aerosol:* 90 mcg/actuation
- *Solution for inhalation:* 0.083%, 0.5%
- *Capsules for inhalation:* 200 mcg

Oral/inhalation dosage

- *Inhalation solution:* 2.5 mg tid–qid nebulized. Dilute 0.5 mL 0.5% solution with 2.5 mL sterile normal saline. Deliver over 5–15 min.
- *Inhalation aerosol:* Shake canister well before using; 2 inhalations q4–6h. One inhalation q4h may be sufficient.
- *Inhalation capsules:* Contents of 200-mcg capsule inhaled q4–6h using a Rotahaler device. Some patients may need 400 mcg q4–6h.
- *Tablets:* 2 or 4 mg PO tid–qid. Do not exceed 32 mg/d. Use doses > 4 mg qid only if patient fails to respond.
- *Elderly patients and those sensitive to beta-adrenergic stimulants:* Start with 2 mg PO tid–qid. Increase gradually to as much as 8 mg tid–qid.
- *Volmax extended-release:* 8 mg PO q12h; 4 mg PO q12h may be sufficient. Do not exceed 32 mg/d.
- *Proventil Repetabs:* Begin with 4–8 mg PO q12h. Use doses > 8 mg bid when patient fails to respond to this dose. Do not exceed 16 mg bid.
- *Syrup:* 2 or 4 mg (1–2 tsp) PO tid–qid. Increase gradually if indicated. Do not exceed 32 mg/d.

Adverse effects in *Italics* are most common; those in **Bold** are life-threatening

A

Pharmacokinetics

Route	Onset	Peak	Duration
Inhalation	Within 5 min	0.5–2 h	3–6 h
Oral	Within 30 min	2–3 h	4–8 h

Metabolism: Hepatic; $T_{1/2}$: 5–6 h
Excretion: Urine

Adverse effects

- *CNS: Tremors, headache, insomnia, hyperactivity, shakiness, nervousness, dizziness,* weakness, drowsiness, restlessness, CNS stimulation
- *CV:* Palpitations, tachycardia, hypertension, chest tightness, angina
- *Resp:* **Bronchospasm,** dyspnea, cough, wheezing, throat dryness/irritation, bronchitis, nasal congestion
- *GI: Nausea, vomiting,* heartburn, GI distress, diarrhea, dry mouth, anorexia, unusual or bad taste
- *Allergic:* **Angioedema, bronchospasm, oropharyngeal edema,** urticaria, rash
- *Misc:* Flushing, sweating, hypokalemia

Clinically important drug–drug interactions

- Increased sympathomimetic effects with other sympathomimetic drugs
- Increased effects on the vascular system with MAO inhibitors and TCAs
- Beta-blockers and albuterol inhibit the effects of each other
- Lowers potassium levels; use with caution if patient is receiving other drugs with this effect
- Decreased serum levels and therapeutic effects of digoxin

● NURSING CONSIDERATIONS

Assessment

- *History:* Hypersensitivity to albuterol or its components, cardiovascular disease, coronary insufficiency, dysrhythmias, hypertension, convulsive disorders, hyperthyroidism, diabetes mellitus, patients who are unusually responsive to sympathomimetic amines, hypokalemia
- *Physical:* P, R, BP, ECG, SpO_2, neurologic checks, skin assessment, respiratory effort, adventitious lung sounds, serum

Adverse effects in *Italics* are most common; those in **Bold** are life-threatening

electrolytes, serum glucose, ABG, peak flow test, pulmonary function tests

Implementation
- Use minimal doses for minimal periods; drug tolerance may occur with prolonged use.
- Have emergency equipment (defibrillator, drugs, oxygen, intubation equipment) on standby in case an allergic or adverse reaction occurs.
- Initial nasal inhaler priming requires four actuations of the pump. If not used for > 2 wk, reprime with 2 actuations.
- Do not exceed recommended dosage; administer pressurized inhalation drug forms during second half of inspiration, because the airways are open wider, and the aerosol distribution is more extensive.
- Teach patient proper use of inhaler.
- Protect solution from light, and store in refrigerator.

● alteplase, recombinant *(al ti plaze')*
Activase

Pregnancy Category C

Drug class
Thrombolytic enzyme (tissue plasminogen activator)

Indications
- Treatment of acute myocardial infarction (MI) to reduce congestive heart failure, improve ventricular function, and reduce mortality
- Treatment of diagnostically confirmed acute, massive pulmonary embolism in adults with obstruction in blood flow to a lobe or multiple segments of the lungs or when embolis is accompanied by unstable hemodynamics
- Treatment of acute ischemic stroke to improve neurologic recovery and reduce disability
- Unlabeled uses: treatment of unstable angina, clearance of thrombi in central venous catheters, management of peripheral arterial thromboembolism

Therapeutic actions
- Is a human tissue plasminogen activator (tPA) produced by recombinant DNA techniques
- Binds to fibrin in a thrombus and converts the entrapped plasminogen to plasmin, initiating local fibrinolysis with limited systemic proteolysis

Adverse effects in *Italics* are most common; those in **Bold** are life-threatening

Contraindications/cautions

❯ **Contraindications: Acute MI or PE:** tPA allergy; active internal bleeding; recent (within 2 mo) cerebrovascular accident (CVA), intracranial or intraspinal surgery; intracranial neoplasm, arteriovenous malformation, or aneurysm; bleeding diathesis; severe uncontrolled hypertension. **CVA:** evidence of current intracranial hemorrhage; suspicion of subarachnoid hemorrhage; recent intracranial surgery, serious head trauma, or CVA; history of intracranial hemorrhage; uncontrolled hypertension (> 185 mmHg systolic or > 110 mmHg diastolic); seizure at onset of stroke; active internal bleeding; intracranial neoplasm, arteriovenous malformation, or aneurysm; bleeding diathesis

❯ **Cautions:** liver dysfunction; old age (> 75 y: risk of bleeding may be increased); recent (≤ 10 d) major surgery (coronary artery bypass grafting [CABG], organ biopsy, obstetrical delivery; puncture of noncompressible vessels); GI or GU bleeding; trauma; hypertension (≥ 180 mmHg systolic or ≥ 110 mmHg diastolic); left heart thrombus; acute pericarditis; subacute bacterial endocarditis; hemostatic defects secondary to severe hepatic or renal disease; diabetic hemorrhagic retinopathy or other ophthalmic hemorrhaging; septic thrombophlebitis; occluded AV cannula at seriously infected site; current oral anticoagulant therapy; other conditions in which bleeding is a hazard or would be difficult to manage

Available forms

❯ *Powder for injection:* 50, 100 mg/vial

IV facts

Preparation

❯ Reconstitute only with Sterile Water for Injection without preservatives. Do not use Bacteriostatic Water for Injection.

❯ **50-mg vial:** Do not use if vacuum is not present. Reconstitute with an 18-gauge needle, directing the stream of Sterile Water for Injection into the lyophilized cake. Avoid excessive agitation during dilution.

❯ **100-mg vial:** Does not contain a vacuum. Use transfer device provided for reconstitution. Avoid excessive agitation during dilution.

❯ Slight foaming may occur with reconstitution but should dissipate when left undisturbed for several minutes.

❯ Reconstituted solution should be colorless to pale yellow and transparent; contains 1 mg/mL with a pH of 7.3.

• Reconstituted solution is 1 mg/mL. Administer as reconstituted or further dilute with an equal volume of D5W or 0.9%NS to yield 0.5 mg/mL.

Dosage

• *Acute MI (standard dosing):* Give total dose of 100 mg IV as follows: 60 mg the first hour (with 6–10 mg given as a bolus over the first 1–2 min), 20 mg infused over the second hour, and 20 mg infused over the third hour. **Do not use a total dose of 150 mg because of the increased risk of intracranial bleeding.**
• *Acute MI (accelerated dosing):* For patients weighing > 67 kg, give 100 mg IV as follows: 15 mg IV bolus, 50 mg infused over 30 min, 35 mg infused over the next 60 min. For patients weighing ≤ 67 kg, give 15 mg IV bolus, followed by 0.75 mg/kg infused over next 30 min (not to exceed 50 mg), and then 0.5 mg/kg infused over next 60 min (not to exceed 35 mg).
• *Pulmonary embolism:* 100 mg administered by IV infusion over 2 h. Initiate heparin therapy near end of or immediately following alteplase infusion.
• *Acute ischemic stroke:* 0.9 mg/kg (maximum of 90 mg) infused over 60 min with 10% of total dose given as an IV bolus over the first 1 min.

Compatibility

Alteplase may be given through the same IV line as lidocaine, metoprolol, propranolol.

Incompatibility

Do not administer through the same IV line as dobutamine, dopamine, heparin, nitroglycerin.

TREATMENT OF OVERDOSE/ANTIDOTE

Discontinue infusion and any other anticoagulant or antiplatelet drugs if severe bleeding, neurologic changes, or severe hypotension occurs. Initiate general supportive and resuscitative measures. Administer IV fluids, packed red blood cells, fresh frozen plasma, platelets, and cryoprecipitate as indicated. Avoid dextran. Aminocaproic acid may be given as an antidote.

Pharmacokinetics

Route	Onset	Peak	Duration
IV	Immediate	45 min average time to reperfusion	2.5–3 h

Metabolism: Liver; $T_{1/2}$: > 50% drug cleared within 5 min after infusion discontinued; 80% cleared within 10 min

Adverse effects in *Italics* are most common; those in **Bold** are life-threatening

Adverse effects
- *CNS:* **Intracranial hemorrhage, cerebral edema**
- *CV:* **Cardiogenic shock, heart failure, cardiac arrest, re-infarction, myocardial rupture, cardiac tamponade, electromechanical dissociation, cholesterol embolism, dysrhythmias,** *reperfusion dysrhythmias,* pulmonary edema, mitral regurgitation, pericardial effusion, pericarditis, recurrent ischemia, pericarditis, hypotension
- *GI:* **GI bleeding,** nausea, vomiting
- *GU:* **GU bleeding**
- *Hematologic:* **Bleeding** (particularly at venous or arterial access sites), ecchymosis, retroperitoneal and gingival bleeding, epistaxis, venous thrombosis and embolism
- *Allergic:* **Anaphylaxis**
- *Misc:* Urticaria, fever

Clinically important drug–drug interactions
- Increased risk of hemorrhage if used with vitamin K antagonists, heparin, oral anticoagulants, and drugs that alter platelet function (aspirin, dipyridamole, abciximab, tirofiban, eptifibatide, ticlopidine, clopidogrel)

⬤ NURSING CONSIDERATIONS

Assessment
- *History:* tPA allergy; active internal bleeding; recent (within 2 mo) intracranial or intraspinal surgery; intracranial neoplasm, arteriovenous malformation, or aneurysm; bleeding diathesis, severe uncontrolled hypertension; evidence of current intracranial hemorrhage; suspicion of subarachnoid hemorrhage; recent intracranial surgery, serious head trauma, or CVA; history of intracranial hemorrhage; uncontrolled hypertension; seizure at onset of stroke; liver dysfunction; age; recent (≤ 10 d) major surgery (CABG, organ biopsy, obstetrical delivery, puncture of noncompressible vessels); GI or GU bleeding; trauma; hypertension; left heart thrombus; acute pericarditis; subacute bacterial endocarditis; hemostatic defects secondary to severe hepatic or renal disease; diabetic hemorrhagic retinopathy or other ophthalmic hemorrhaging; septic thrombophlebitis; occluded AV cannula at seriously infected site; current oral anticoagulant therapy; other conditions in which bleeding is a hazard or would be difficult to manage
- *Physical:* T, P, R, BP, ECG, I & O, SpO_2, IV site, neurologic checks, skin assessment, ophthalmic exam, peripheral perfusion, presence of bleeding, chest pain assessment, cardiac auscultation, JVD, peripheral perfusion, adventitious lung sounds, liver evaluation, ABG, CBC, CPK, CPK-MB, cardiac

Adverse effects in *Italics* are most common; those in **Bold** are life-threatening

troponin, myoglobin, TT, APTT, PT, INR, FSP, type and cross-match; urine, stool, and emesis guaiac

Implementation

▶ Administer drug as soon as possible after diagnosis. Initiate within 6 h after onset of acute MI symptoms and within 3 h after onset of stroke symptoms.
▶ Administer infusion using IV pump.
▶ Have emergency equipment (defibrillator, drugs, oxygen, intubation equipment) on standby in case anaphylaxis, hemorrhage, or adverse reaction occurs.
▶ Before starting drug, initiate at least two to three peripheral IVs.
▶ Continuously monitor ECG for evidence of reperfusion (decreased chest pain, decreased ST segment elevation, reperfusion dysrhythmias).
▶ Initiate bleeding precautions.
▶ Assess patient for evidence of bleeding and hemorrhage.
▶ Carefully assess recent puncture sites and sites of lines or tubes (catheter insertion sites, cutdown sites, needle puncture sites, recent surgical incisions).
▶ Apply pressure to arterial and venous puncture sites for at least 30 min or until hemostasis is achieved. Apply a pressure dressing to site to prevent bleeding. Assess all puncture sites q15min.
▶ Apply pressure or pressure dressings to control superficial bleeding.
▶ Avoid IM injections before, during, and for 24 h after therapy. Do not attempt central venous access or arterial puncture unless absolutely necessary. If arterial puncture is necessary, use an upper extremity vessel that is accessible to manual pressure.
▶ Guaiac all stools, urine, and emesis for blood.
▶ Handle patient carefully to avoid ecchymosis and bleeding.
▶ If possible, draw blood for laboratory analysis from an existing saline lock.
▶ Take BP with manual BP cuff or ensure that NIBP cuff does not inflate excessively above patient's SBP.
▶ Shave patient with an electric razor.
▶ Heparin is often administered with alteplase.
▶ Type and crossmatch blood in case serious blood loss occurs and blood transfusions are required.
▶ When given for acute MI, assess for chest pain (type, character, location, intensity, radiation), and monitor ECG before, during, and after therapy. Assess for ST segment changes.
▶ When given for PE, assess respiratory effort, SpO_2, ABGs, and chest pain.
▶ Monitor BP, P, R, and neurologic status continuously.

Adverse effects in *Italics* are most common; those in **Bold** are life-threatening

- Initiate other interventions as standard for patients with acute MI, CVA, or PE.
- Reconstituted solution may be used for up to 8 h after reconstitution when stored at 36° to 46°F.

● aminocaproic acid *(a mee noe ka proe' ik)* Amicar
Pregnancy Category C

Drug class
Systemic hemostatic agent

Indications
- To treat excessive bleeding resulting from systemic hyperfibrinolysis and urinary fibrinolysis
- Unlabeled uses: to prevent recurrence of subarachnoid hemorrhage, to decrease need for platelet administration in managing megakaryocytic thrombocytopenia, to abort and treat attacks of hereditary angioneurotic edema, to reduce postsurgical bleeding complications for patients undergoing cardiopulmonary bypass procedures, bladder irrigant to control bleeding following transurethral resection of the prostate and intractable bladder hemorrhage

Therapeutic actions
- Inhibits fibrinolysis and prevents clot dissolution by inhibiting plasminogen activator substances and through antiplasmin activity

Contraindications/cautions
- **Contraindications:** aminocaproic acid allergy, active intravascular clotting, disseminated intravascular coagulation (DIC) without concomitant heparin administration
- **Cautions:** hematuria of upper urinary tract origin; cardiac, renal, or hepatic disease

Available forms
- *IV injection:* 250 mg/mL
- *Tablets:* 500 mg
- *Syrup:* 250 mg/mL

IV facts
Preparation
- Rapid injection of aminocaproic acid undiluted into a vein is not recommended.
- **Initial infusion:** Add 4–5 g to 250 mL of D5W; 0.9%NS; Ringer's solution; or Sterile Water for Injection.

Adverse effects in *Italics* are most common; those in **Bold** are life-threatening

▶ **Maintenance infusion:** Add 5 g to 250 mL of D5W; 0.9%NS; Ringer's solution; or Sterile Water for Injection.

Dosage
▶ 4–5 g in 250 mL IV over 1 h. Follow by continuing infusion at 1–1.25 g/h. Continue treatment for 8 h or until bleeding is controlled. Do not exceed 30 g in 24 h.

Titration Guide

aminocaproic acid					
5g in 250 mL					
g/hr	1	1.05	1.1	1.15	1.2	1.25
mL/hr	50	53	55	58	60	63

Compatibility
Aminocaproic acid may be given through the same IV line as netilmicin sulfate.

Oral dosage
▶ Administer 10 tablets (5 g) or 4 teaspoonfuls of syrup (5 g) PO during the first hour of treatment.
▶ Follow with 2 tablets (1 g) or 1 teaspoonful (1.25 g) PO per hour.
▶ Continue treatment for 8 h or until bleeding is controlled.

> **TREATMENT OF OVERDOSE/ANTIDOTE**
> Decrease infusion rate or temporarily discontinue infusion until patient is stabilized. Initiate resuscitative measures as indicated. Drug is removed by hemodialysis and may be removed by peritoneal dialysis.

Pharmacokinetics

Route	Onset	Peak	Duration
IV	Immediate		2–3 h
Oral	10 min	45–100 min	

$T_{1/2}$: 2 h
Excretion: Urine

Adverse effects
▶ *CNS: Dizziness, tinnitus, headache,* syncope, delirium, **intracranial hypertension**, hallucinations, psychotic reactions, weakness

Adverse effects in *Italics* are most common; those in **Bold** are life-threatening

▶ **CV: Dysrhythmias** (with rapid IV injection), hypotension, bradycardia, ischemia, thrombosis, edema
▶ **Resp: Pulmonary embolism,** dyspnea, nasal stuffiness
▶ *GI: Nausea, cramps, diarrhea,* emesis
▶ *GU:* Renal failure, elevated BUN, intrarenal obstruction, ejaculatory disorder
▶ *Allergic:* **Anaphylaxis**
▶ *Hematologic: Elevated serum CPK,* AST, aldolase, serum potassium; leukopenia, thrombocytopenia
▶ *Musc/Skel: Malaise,* myopathy, symptomatic weakness, fatigue, rhabdomyolysis
▶ *Misc:* Skin rash, thrombophlebitis, fever, conjunctival suffusion

Clinically important drug–drug interactions
▶ Risk of hypercoagulable state with oral contraceptives, estrogens

● NURSING CONSIDERATIONS
Assessment
▶ *History:* Aminocaproic acid allergy, active intravascular clotting, DIC, hematuria of upper urinary tract origin; cardiac, renal, or hepatic disease
▶ *Physical:* T, P, BP, R, ECG, I & O, IV site, bleeding, skin assessment, neurologic checks, peripheral perfusion, liver evaluation, chest or leg pain, Homan's sign, bowel sounds, coagulation studies, platelet count, CPK, UA, potassium level, liver and kidney function tests

Implementation
▶ Always administer an infusion with an IV infusion pump.
▶ Monitor BP, P, R, and neurologic status.
▶ Have emergency equipment (defibrillator, drugs, oxygen, intubation equipment) on standby in case anaphylaxis or adverse reaction occurs.
▶ Monitor coagulation, renal, and electrolyte studies.
▶ Discontinue drug if CPK levels rise.
▶ Monitor patient for signs of clotting.
▶ Assess IV site frequently for evidence of thrombophlebitis.

● **aminophylline** *(am in off' i lin)*
theophylline ethylenediamine
Phyllocontin, Truphylline
Pregnancy Category C
Drug classes
Bronchodilator
Xanthine

Indications

▸ Symptomatic relief or prevention of bronchial asthma and reversible bronchospasm associated with chronic bronchitis and emphysema

Therapeutic actions

▸ Relaxes smooth muscle of the bronchi and pulmonary blood vessels, causing bronchodilation and increasing vital capacity that has been impaired by bronchospasm and air trapping
▸ Affects diaphragmatic contractility; may be capable of reducing fatigue and improving contractility in patients with chronic obstructive airway diseases
▸ Stimulates CNS, induces diuresis, increases gastric acid secretion, reduces lower esophageal sphincter pressure
▸ May inhibit extracellular adenosine, stimulate endogenous catecholamines, antagonize prostaglandins PGE_2 and $FGF_{2\alpha}$, mobilize intracellular calcium causing smooth muscle relaxation, and exert beta-adrenergic agonist activity on the airways
▸ May be mediated by phosphodiesterase inhibition, which increases the concentration of cyclic adenosine monophosphate

Contraindications/cautions

▸ **Contraindications:** hypersensitivity to any xanthine or to ethylenediamine, underlying seizure disorder (unless on anticonvulsant drugs), active peptic ulcer disease or gastritis, status asthmaticus (oral preparations), rectal or colonic irritation or infection (rectal preparations)
▸ **Cautions:** dysrhythmias, cardiac disease, congestive heart failure (CHF), cor pulmonale, acute pulmonary edema, fever, hypertension, hypoxemia, hepatic disease, hypothyroidism, alcoholism, use of tobacco or marijuana, influenza, multiorgan failure, shock, elderly patients (especially men)

Available forms

▸ *Injection:* 250 mg/10 mL
▸ *Tablets:* 100, 200 mg
▸ *Controlled-release tablets:* 225 mg
▸ *Liquid:* 105 mg/5 mL
▸ *Suppositories:* 250, 500 mg

Adverse effects in *Italics* are most common; those in **Bold** are life-threatening

A

IV facts
Preparation
▶ Dilute in 100–1000 mL D5W/0.9%NS; D5W; D10W; D20W; Dextran 6% in Dextrose 5%; Dextrose-LR combinations; Dextrose-Ringer's combinations; Dextrose-Saline combinations; Ionosol products; Invert Sugar 5% in Water or 0.9%NS; LR; 0.45%NS; 0.9%NS; Ringer's injection; or Sodium Lactate (1/6 Molar) Injection.

Dosage
▶ Individualize dosage to patient's needs, response, and tolerance. Calculate dosages by lean body weight and anhydrous theophylline content. Convert to oral therapy as soon as possible.
▶ *Loading dose:* 6 mg/kg IV for patients not already receiving theophylline products. Do not exceed 25 mg/min IV. Each 0.6 mg/kg dose of aminophylline administered IV as a loading dose will result in about a 1 mcg/mL increase in serum theophylline.
▶ *Patients currently receiving theophylline products:* Defer loading dose if serum theophylline concentration can be obtained rapidly. Determine time and amount of last dose. If patient is experiencing respiratory distress that warrants the risk, give aminophylline 3.1 mg/kg IV. This will increase serum theophylline levels by about 5 mcg/mL and is unlikely to cause dangerous adverse effects if the patient is not experiencing theophylline toxicity before this dose. Base further administration on theophylline levels.
▶ *Maintenance dose:* Give by large volume (500–1000 mL) infusion to deliver desired amount of drug each hour. Titrate to maintain therapeutic theophylline level. The following table lists recommended infusion rates:

Patient Group	Infusion Rate First 12 h	Infusion Rate Beyond 12 h
Young adult smokers	1 mg/kg/h	0.8 mg/kg/h
Nonsmoking adults, otherwise healthy	0.7 mg/kg/h	0.5 mg/kg/h
Older patients and patients with cor pulmonale	0.6 mg/kg/h	0.3 mg/kg/h
Patients with CHF, liver disease	0.5 mg/kg/h	0.1–0.2 mg/kg/h

Adverse effects in *Italics* are most common; those in **Bold** are life-threatening

Titration Guide

	aminophylline								
	250 mg in 250 mL								

	Body Weight								
lb	88	99	110	121	132	143	154	165	176	187
kg	40	45	50	55	60	65	70	75	80	85

Dose Ordered in mg/kg/h	Amounts to Infuse in mL/h								
0.1	4	5	5	6	6	7	7	8	8	9
0.2	8	9	10	11	12	13	14	15	16	17
0.3	12	14	15	17	18	20	21	23	24	26
0.5	20	23	25	28	30	33	35	38	40	43
0.6	24	27	30	33	36	39	42	45	48	51
0.7	28	32	35	39	42	46	49	53	56	60
0.8	32	36	40	44	48	52	56	60	64	68
1	40	45	50	55	60	65	70	75	80	85
1.2	48	54	60	66	72	78	84	90	96	102

	Body Weight								
lb	198	209	220	231	242	253	264	275	286
kg	90	95	100	105	110	115	120	125	130

Dose Ordered in mg/kg/h	Amounts to Infuse in mL/h								
0.1	9	10	10	11	11	12	12	13	13
0.2	18	19	20	21	22	23	24	25	26
0.3	27	29	30	32	33	35	36	38	39
0.5	45	48	50	53	55	58	60	63	65
0.6	54	57	60	63	66	69	72	75	78
0.7	63	67	70	74	77	81	84	88	91
0.8	72	76	80	84	88	92	96	100	104
1	90	95	100	105	110	115	120	125	130
1.2	108	114	120	126	132	138	144	150	156

Therapeutic serum level

▸ 10–20 mcg/mL; obtain serum sample 15–30 min after IV loading dose, 1–2 h after giving immediate-release products, and 5–9 h after morning dose for controlled-release formulations.

Compatibility

Theophylline may be given through the same IV line as allopurinol, amifostine, amrinone, aztreonam, ceftazidime, cimetidine, cladribine, enalaprilat, esmolol, famotidine, filgrastim, fluconazole, fludarabine, foscarnet, gallium, granisetron, heparin-hydrocortisone, labetalol, melphalan, meropenem, morphine, netilmicin, paclitaxel, pancuronium, piperacillin-tazobactam, potassium chloride, propofol, ranitidine, sargramostim, tacrolimus, teniposide, thiotepa, tolazoline, vecuronium, vitamin B complex with C.

Incompatibility
Do not administer through the same IV line as amiodarone, ciprofloxacin, dobutamine, hydralazine, ondansetron, vinorelbine.

Oral/rectal dosage
▶ *Acute symptoms requiring rapid theophyllinization in patients not receiving theophylline:* An initial loading dose is required. Dosage recommendations for aminophylline anhydrous are:

Patient Group	Oral Loading	Maintenance
Young adult smokers	5.8 mg/kg	3.5 mg/kg q6h
Nonsmoking adults, otherwise healthy	5.8 mg/kg	3.5 mg/kg q8h
Older patients and patients with cor pulmonale	5.8 mg/kg	2.3 mg/kg q8h
Patients with CHF	5.8 mg/kg	1.2–2.3 mg/kg q12h

▶ *Chronic therapy:* Usual range is 600–1600 mg/d PO in 3–4 divided doses. Adjust as needed to maintain desired drug level.
▶ *Rectal:* 500 mg q6–8h PR.

TREATMENT OF OVERDOSE/ANTIDOTE
Discontinue drug or decrease dosage. Initiate general supportive and resuscitative measures. Do not administer stimulants. If a seizure occurs, establish an airway and administer oxygen. Administer diazepam 0.1–0.3 mg/kg, up to 10 mg. Monitor vital signs, maintain blood pressure, and provide adequate hydration. After seizure, perform intubation and lavage instead of inducing emesis. Administer a cathartic and activated charcoal through a large-bore gastric lavage tube. If activated charcoal is not effective or if serum concentration is > 60 mcg/mL, consider charcoal hemoperfusion or hemodialysis. If a seizure *has not* occurred, induce vomiting, preferably with ipecac syrup, even if emesis has occurred spontaneously. Administer a cathartic and activated charcoal. Prophylactic phenobarbital may increase the seizure threshold. Treat atrial dysrhythmias with verapamil and ventricular
(treatment continued on next page)

Adverse effects in *Italics* are most common; those in **Bold** are life-threatening

dysrhythmias with lidocaine or procainamide. Treat dehydration, acid–base imbalance, and hypotension with IV fluids. Treat hypotension with vasopressors.

Pharmacokinetics

Route	Onset	Peak	Duration
IV	Rapid	End of infusion	6–8 h
Oral	1–6 h	4–6 h	6–8 h

Metabolism: Hepatic; $T_{1/2}$: 3–15h (nonsmokers) or 4–5h (smokers, 1–2 packs/d)
Excretion: Urine

Adverse effects

▸ ***Serum theophylline levels < 20 mcg/mL:*** Adverse effects uncommon
▸ ***Serum theophylline levels > 20 mcg/mL:*** *Nausea, vomiting, diarrhea, headache, insomnia, irritability* (75% of patients)
▸ ***Serum theophylline levels > 35 mcg/mL:*** Hyperglycemia, hypotension, cardiac dysrhythmias, tachycardia, **seizures, brain damage, death**
▸ *CNS:* **Convulsions,** irritability, restlessness, headache, insomnia, reflex hyperexcitability, muscle twitching
▸ *CV:* **Life-threatening ventricular dysrhythmias, circulatory failure,** palpitations, tachycardia, hypotension, extrasystoles
▸ *Resp:* **Respiratory arrest,** tachypnea
▸ *GI:* Hematemesis, epigastric pain, increased AST, gastroesophageal reflux during sleep, rectal bleeding or irritation (suppositories)
▸ *GU:* Proteinuria, increased excretion of renal tubular cells and RBCs; diuresis (dehydration), urinary retention in men with prostate enlargement
▸ *Misc:* Fever, flushing, hyperglycemia, syndrome of inappropriate antidiuretic hormone, rash, alopecia

Clinically important drug–drug interactions

▸ Increased effects and toxicity with allopurinol, nonselective beta-blockers, calcium carbamazepine, calcium channel blockers, cimetidine, corticosteroids, disulfiram, ephedrine, erythromycin, interferon, isoniazid, loop diuretics, macrolides, mexiletine, quinolones, ranitidine, thiabendazole, thyroid hormones
▸ Decreased levels with aminoglutethimide, barbiturates, carbamazepine, charcoal, hydantoins, isoniazid, ketoconazole,

Adverse effects in *Italics* are most common; those in **Bold** are life-threatening

A

loop diuretics, rifampin, sucralfate, sulfinpyrazone, sympathomimetics (beta-agonists), thioamines
▸ Decreased effects in patients who are cigarette smokers (one to two packs a day)
▸ Decreased theophylline and phenytoin levels when used concurrently
▸ Effects of propofol, benzodiazepines counteracted
▸ Neuromuscular blockade possibly reversed
▸ Reduced lithium plasma levels
▸ Enhanced adverse reactions with tetracyclines
▸ Adenosine receptors possibly blocked, decreasing effects of adenosine
▸ Decreased clearance with alcohol, ticlopidine
▸ Increased effects and toxicity of sympathomimetics (especially ephedrine)

Clinically important drug–food interactions
▸ Theophylline elimination is increased by a low-carbohydrate, high-protein diet and by charcoal-broiled beef.
▸ Theophylline elimination is decreased by a high-carbohydrate, low-protein diet.
▸ Food may alter bioavailability, absorption of controlled-release theophylline preparations; these may rapidly release their contents with food and cause toxicity; give controlled-release forms on an empty stomach.

⬤ NURSING CONSIDERATIONS

Assessment
▸ *History:* Hypersensitivity to any xanthine or to ethylenediamine, underlying seizure disorder, active peptic ulcer disease or gastritis, status asthmaticus, rectal or colonic irritation or infection, dysrhythmias, cardiac disease, CHF, cor pulmonale, acute pulmonary edema, fever, hypertension, hypoxemia, hepatic disease, hypothyroidism, alcoholism, use of tobacco or marijuana, influenza, multiorgan failure, shock, age, gender
▸ *Physical:* T, P, BP, R, ECG, I & O, weight, neurologic checks, presence of seizures, skin assessment, respiratory effort, SpO_2, retractions, nasal flaring, adventitious lung sounds, bowel sounds, theophylline level, pumonary function tests, peak flow test, ABG; thyroid, liver, and kidney function tests

Implementation
▸ Administer IV aminophylline using an IV infusion pump.
▸ Give immediate-release, liquid dosage forms with food if GI effects occur.

Adverse effects in *Italics* are most common; those in **Bold** are life-threatening

- Give controlled-release preparations on an empty stomach, 1 h before or 2 h after meals.
- Caution patient not to chew or crush controlled-release preparations.
- Monitor results of serum theophylline level determinations carefully; reduce dosage if serum levels exceed therapeutic range of 10–20 mcg/mL.
- Monitor carefully for clinical signs of adverse effects, particularly if serum theophylline levels are not available.
- Have emergency equipment (defibrillator, drugs, oxygen, intubation equipment) on standby in case of adverse reaction.
- Maintain diazepam on standby to treat seizures.
- Maintain adequate hydration.
- Theophylline products are not necessarily interchangeable; use caution when switching from one brand to another.

◯ **amiodarone hydrochloride**
(a mee o' da rone) Cordarone, Pacerone

Pregnancy Category D

Drug class
Antidysrhythmic

Indications
- Initiation of treatment and prophylaxis of frequently recurring ventricular fibrillation and hemodynamically unstable ventricular tachycardia in patients refractory to other therapy; patients for whom oral amiodarone is indicated but who are unable to take oral drugs (parenteral)
- Treatment of life-threatening recurrent ventricular fibrillation or hemodynamically unstable ventricular tachycardia that does not respond to other antidysrhythmics or when alternative agents are not tolerated (oral)
- Unlabeled uses: treatment of refractory sustained or paroxysmal atrial fibrillation and paroxysmal supraventricular tachycardia; treatment of symptomatic atrial flutter; may produce benefit in left ventricular ejection fraction, exercise tolerance, and ventricular dysrhythmias in patients with CHF
- Orphan drug use: incessant ventricular tachycardia

Therapeutic actions
- Is a type III antidysrhythmic but possesses characteristics of all four antidysrhythmic classes
- Blocks sodium channels at rapid pacing frequencies
- Exerts noncompetitive alpha- and beta-adrenergic inhibition
- Lengthens the cardiac action potential

Adverse effects in *Italics* are most common; those in **Bold** are life-threatening

- Exerts a negative chronotropic effect in nodal tissues
- Blocks myocardial potassium channels, which contributes to slower conduction and longer refractoriness
- Exerts a vasodilatory action that decreases cardiac workload and myocardial oxygen consumption
- Prolongs intranodal conduction and refractoriness of the atrioventricular node
- Acts directly on cardiac cell membrane; prolongs repolarization and refractory period; increases ventricular fibrillation threshold; acts on peripheral smooth muscle to decrease peripheral resistance

Effects on hemodynamic parameters
- Decreased SVR (parenteral)
- Increased CI (parenteral)

Contraindications/cautions
- **Contraindications:** amiodarone allergy; parenteral: marked sinus bradycardia, second- or third-degree heart block (except if functioning pacemaker available), cardiogenic shock; oral: severe sinus node dysfunction, second- or third-degree heart block, severe bradycardia (except if functioning pacemaker available)
- **Cautions:** hypokalemia, hypomagnesemia, elderly patients, hepatic or pulmonary disease

Available forms
- *Injection:* 50 mg/mL
- *Tablets:* 200 mg

IV facts
Preparation
- Mix in a glass or polyolefin bottle. Dilute 150 mg in 100 mL D5W for rapid loading dose (1.5 mg/mL). Dilute 900 mg in 500 mL D5W for slow infusions (1.8 mg/mL). Use a concentration of 1–6 mg/mL for a maintenance infusion.
- Administer through PVC tubing; use an in-line filter.

Dosage
- Begin with 1 g IV over the first 24 h given as below.
- *Loading infusions:* **Rapid:** 150 mg IV over 10 min. **Followed by slow:** 360 mg IV over next 6 h.
- *Maintenance infusion:* 540 mg IV over the remaining 18 h. After the first 24 h, continue infusion at 0.5 mg/min for up to 2–3 wk. If breakthrough ventricular fibrillation or unstable ventricular tachycardia occurs, may give 150 mg supplemental infusions of amiodarone (150 mg in 100 mL D5W IV over 10 min).

Adverse effects in *Italics* are most common; those in **Bold** are life-threatening

Therapeutic serum level
▶ 0.5–2.5 mcg/mL

Compatibility
Amiodarone may be given through the same IV line as amikacin, bretylium, clindamycin, dobutamine, dopamine, doxycycline, erythromycin, esmolol, gentamicin, insulin (regular), isoproterenol, labetalol, lidocaine, metaraminol, metronidazole, midazolam, morphine, nitroglycerin, norepinephrine, penicillin G potassium, phentolamine, phenylephrine, potassium chloride, procainamide, tobramycin, vancomycin.

Incompatibility
Do not administer through the same IV line as aminophylline, cefamandole, heparin, mezlocillin, sodium bicarbonate.

Oral dosage
▶ *Life-threatening ventricular dysrhythmias:* **Loading dose:** 800–1600 mg/d PO in divided doses with meals for 1–3 wk until therapeutic response occurs. Gradually discontinue other antidysrhythmics. When adequate dysrhythmia control is achieved, reduce dose to 600–800 mg/d in divided doses for 1 mo. **Maintenance dose:** 400-600 mg/d in 1–2 divided doses. Titrate to the lowest possible dose to limit side effects.

> **TREATMENT OF OVERDOSE/ANTIDOTE**
> Discontinue drug or decrease dosage. Initiate general supportive and resuscitative measures. Treat bradycardia with a beta-adrenergic agonist or a pacemaker. Use positive inotropic or vasopressor agents, and volume expanders to treat hypotension with inadequate tissue perfusion. Cholestyramine may accelerate the reversal of amiodarone's side effects by enhancing drug elimination.

Pharmacokinetics
Route	Onset	Peak	Duration
IV	Immediate	10 min	30–45 min after stopping infusion
Oral	2–3 d	3–7 h	Weeks–months

Metabolism: Hepatic; $T_{1/2}$: 2.5–10 d, then 26–107 d
Excretion: Bile

Adverse effects
Parenteral
▶ *CV: Hypotension,* **asystole, ventricular tachycardia, ventricular fibrillation, AV block, cardiac arrest, electromechanical dissociation, cardiogenic shock,** CHF, bradycardia, atrial fibrillation, nodal dysrhythmias, prolonged QT interval, sinus bradycardia

Adverse effects in *Italics* are most common; those in **Bold** are life-threatening

- **GI:** Diarrhea, vomiting, increased ALT and AST
- **Misc:** **Stevens-Johnson syndrome, shock, thrombocytopenia,** fever, lung edema, respiratory disorder, peripheral vein phlebitis

Oral

- **CNS:** *Malaise, fatigue, dizziness, tremors, ataxia, paresthesias, lack of coordination,* headache, sleep disturbances, peripheral neuropathy
- **CV:** **Dysrhythmias,** bradycardia, SA node dysfunction, CHF, hypotension
- **Resp:** **Pulmonary toxicity, pulmonary infiltrates or fibrosis, hypersensitivity pneumonitis, interstitial/alveolar pneumonitis**
- **GI:** **Liver toxicity,** *nausea, vomiting, constipation, anorexia, constipation, elevated liver enzymes;* abnormal taste, smell, and salivation
- **Endocrine:** *Hypothyroidism* or *hyperthyroidism*
- **EENT:** Optic neuropathy, optic neuritis, visual impairment, blindness, papilledema, corneal degeneration, photosensitivity, eye discomfort, lens opacities, photophobia, dry eyes, visual halos
- **Misc:** **Thrombocytopenia, angioedema,** edema, coagulation abnormalities, flushing, epididymitis, vasculitis, pseudotumor cerebri

Clinically important drug–drug interactions

- Increased toxicity with digoxin, theophylline
- Increased QT prolongation and dysrhythmias with disopyramide
- Increased hypotension, bradycardia and decreased cardiac output with fentanyl
- Reduced dose of flecainide needed to maintain therapeutic levels
- Impaired metabolism of dextromethorphan, methotrexate with chronic use
- Increased toxicity with quinidine, procainamide
- Increased drug level with cimetidine, ritonavir
- Increased cyclosporin levels even if reduced dose of cyclosporin given
- Increased phenytoin toxicity with phenytoin, ethotoin, mephenytoin
- Increased PT and bleeding tendencies with warfarin
- Sinus arrest, heart block, bradycardia, and hypotension with beta-blockers, calcium channel-blockers
- Decreased drug level, from increased elimination, with cholestyramine

Adverse effects in *Italics* are most common; those in **Bold** are life-threatening

⬤ NURSING CONSIDERATIONS

Assessment

▸ *History:* Amiodarone allergy, marked sinus bradycardia, second- or third-degree heart block, cardiogenic shock, severe sinus node dysfunction, severe bradycardia, hypokalemia, hypomagnesemia, age, hepatic or pulmonary disease
▸ *Physical:* T, P, R, BP, ECG, I & O, SpO$_2$, IV site, neurologic checks, skin assessment, eye exam, adventitious lung sounds, respiratory effort, edema, abdominal assessment, liver evaluation, baseline chest x-ray, liver function tests, serum electrolytes, CBC, ABG, pulmonary function tests, T$_4$ and T$_3$

Implementation

▸ Exercise extreme caution when calculating and preparing IV doses. Amiodarone is a very potent drug; small dosage errors can cause serious adverse effects. Avoid inadvertent bolus of drug.
▸ Always administer IV amiodarone using an infusion pump.
▸ When possible, give IV through a central venous catheter. Do not exceed 2 mg/mL for greater than 1 h unless a central venous catheter is used.
▸ Monitor cardiac rhythm continuously during IV therapy.
▸ Monitor for an extended period when dosage adjustments are made.
▸ Give oral drug with meals to decrease GI upset.
▸ Monitor for evidence of hypothyroidism as evidenced by edema, pale and cool skin, hypothermia, yellow skin tint, stiff and aching muscles, bradycardia, decreased BP, diminished heart sounds, weight gain, constipation, slowed thinking and speech, lethargy, somnolence, anemia, or hypoglycemia.
▸ Monitor for evidence of hyperthyroidism as evidenced by warm and moist skin, perspiration, palmar erythema, rosy complexion, thin skin, increased pigmentation, weakness, fatigue, tachycardia, hypertension, palpitations, dysrhythmias, tachypnea, dyspnea, weight loss, increased appetite, diplopia, eyelid edema, exophthalmos, restlessness, short attention span, hyperglycemia, or fever.
▸ Monitor chest x-ray, SpO$_2$, and ABGs to evaluate pulmonary status.
▸ Monitor liver enzymes, thyroid hormone, and drug levels.
▸ Protect from light during storage.

⬤ **amphotericin B** *(am foe ter' i sin)* Abelcet, Amphotec, AmBisome, Fungizone, Fungizone Intravenous

Pregnancy Category B

Adverse effects in *Italics* are most common; those in **Bold** are life-threatening

Drug class
Antifungal antibiotic

Indications
▶ Amphotericin B deoxycholate: potentially life-threatening invasive fatal infections: cryptococcosis; North American blastomycosis; disseminated moniliasis; candidiasis; coccidioidomycosis; histoplasmosis; zygomycosis, including mucormycosis caused by species of *Mucor, Rhizopus, Absidia;* infections caused by species of *Conidiobolus* and *Basidiobolus;* sporotrichosis; aspergillosis
▶ Lipid-based formulations: fungal infections refractory to conventional amphotericin B deoxycholate therapy (lipid complex), patients with renal impairment or toxicity who cannot use deoxycholate therapy (lipid complex), treatment of invasive aspergillosis (cholesteryl); treatment of infections caused by *Aspergillus, Candida,* or *Cryptococcus* species (liposomal)
▶ Empirical treatment in febrile, neutropenic patients with presumed fungal infection (liposomal)
▶ Adjunct treatment of American mucocutaneous leishmaniasis (not a choice in primary therapy)
▶ Treatment of cutaneous and mucocutaneous mycotic infections caused by *Candida* species (topical application)
▶ Treatment of oral candidiasis caused by *Candida albicans*
▶ Treatment of visceral leishmaniasis (liposomal only)
▶ Unlabeled uses: prophylactic use to prevent fungal infections in bone marrow transplants, treatment of primary amoebic meningoencephalitis caused by *Naegleria fowleri,* treatment of severe meningitis unresponsive to IV therapy (deoxycholate)

Therapeutic actions
▶ Binds to sterols in the fungal cell membrane; changes its membrane permeability, which allows leakage of intracellular components
▶ Is fungicidal or fungistatic depending on concentration and organism
▶ Can bind to the mammalian cell, leading to cytotoxicity

Contraindications/cautions
▶ **Contraindications:** allergy to amphotericin B (except when infection is life-threatening and treatable only with this drug)
▶ **Cautions:** renal dysfunction, dehydration, cardiac disease, uncontrolled diabetes, leukocyte transfusions, pulmonary disease, electrolyte abnormalities

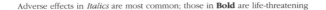

Adverse effects in *Italics* are most common; those in **Bold** are life-threatening

Available forms
▸ *Powder for injection:* 50, 100 mg
▸ *Suspension for injection:* 100 mg/20 mL
▸ *Oral suspension:* 100 mg/mL
▸ *Cream/lotion/ointment:* 3%

IV facts
Preparation
▸ Do not dilute or reconstitute with saline solutions or mix with other drugs or electrolytes.
▸ **Fungizone:** For initial concentration of 5 mg/mL, rapidly inject 10 mL Sterile Water for Injection without a bacteriostatic agent directly into the lyophilized cake using a sterile needle (minimum diameter, 20 gauge). Shake vial until clear. For infusion solution of 0.1 mg/mL, further dilute with D5W with a pH above 4.2. Use strict aseptic technique. Do not use if any precipitation is found. Use solutions prepared for IV infusion promptly. Protect solution from light during administration if not infused within 8 hours of reconstitution. Refrigerate vials; protect from exposure to light; store in dark at room temperature for 24 h or refrigerated for 1 wk. Discard any unused material.
▸ **Abelcet:** Shake vial gently until no yellow sediment is seen. Withdraw dose using an 18-gauge needle. Replace needle with a 5-mcm filter needle; each filter needle may be used to filter the content of ≤ four vials. Inject drug into bag containing D5W to a concentration of 1 mg/mL. Store vials in refrigerator; protect from light. Stable for 48 h once prepared if refrigerated, for 6 h at room temperature.
▸ **Amphotec:** Reconstitute with Sterile Water for Injection: 10 mL to 50 mg vial or 20 mL to 100 mg vial. Shake gently by hand; rotate vial until all solids are dissolved. Further dilute with D5W to 0.6 mg/mL. Refrigerate after reconstitution; use within 24 h.
▸ **AmBisome:** Add 12 mL Sterile Water for Injection to each vial to yield 4 mg/mL. Shake vial vigorously for 30 s to disperse drug completely until a yellow, translucent suspension is formed. Withdraw appropriate amount of solution into a sterile syringe. Attach a 5-mcm filter and inject contents of syringe through filter needle into an appropriate volume of D5W (use only one filter needle per vial) to yield a final concentration of 1–2 mg/mL. Store unopened vials in refrigerator. Store reconstituted product for up to 24 h. Use within 6 h of dilution in D5W.

Dosage
▸ Individualize and adjust dosage based on patient's clinical status.

Adverse effects in *Italics* are most common; those in **Bold** are life-threatening

▶ If administering through an existing IV line, flush with D5W (do not use 0.9%NS or heparin) prior to and following infusion, or use a separate line.
▶ *Systemic fungal infection*
  ▶ *Fungizone:* **Test dose:** 1 mg in 20 mL D5W infused IV over 20–30 min. Initial dose: *0.25–0.3 mg/kg/d prepared as 0.1 mg/mL infusion and given IV over 2–6 h.* **Maintenance dose:** Gradually increase dose by 5–10 mg/d up to total dose of 0.5–0.7 mg/kg/d. Some mycoses may require total doses of 1–1.5 mcg/kg/d. Do not exceed total daily dose of 1.5 mg/kg/d. May use an in-line filter of ≥ 1mcm.
  ▶ *Amphotec:* Test dose is advisable: 1.6–8.3 mg IV over 15–30 min. Then 3–4 mg/kg/d prepared as a 0.6 mg/mL infusion delivered at 1 mg/kg/h. Do not use an in-line filter.
  ▶ *Abelcet:* 5 mg/kg/d prepared as a 1 mg/mL infusion and delivered IV at 2.5 mg/kg/h. May dilute to 2 mg/mL for patients with CV disease. If infusion exceeds 2 h, mix contents of bag by shaking infusion bag q2h. Do not use an in-line filter.
  ▶ *AmBisome:* 3–5 mg/kg/d prepared as a 1–2 mg/mL infusion delivered IV initially over 120 min. May reduce infusion time to 60 min or increase infusion time if patient experiences discomfort. May use an in-line membrane filter of ≥ 1 mcm.
  ▶ *Fungal infection, empirical:* 3 mg/kg/d of liposomal amphotericin B IV over 2 h. May reduce infusion time to 1 h or increase infusion time if patient experiences discomfort.
▶ *Leishmaniasis*
  ▶ *AmBisome:* 3 mg/kg/d IV on days 1–5, 14, and 21 to immunocompetent patients. Repeat therapy may be useful if parasitic clearance is not achieved. Administer 4 mg/kg/d IV on days 1–5, 10, 17, 24, 31, and 38 to immunosuppressed patients.
  ▶ *Fungizone:* 0.5 mg/kg/d IV administered on alternate days for 14 doses.
  ▶ *Meningitis, coccidioidal or cryptococcal:* Give amphotericin B deoxycholate intrathecally at initial doses of 0.025 mg. Gradually increase to maximum tolerable dose. Usual dose is 0.25–1 mg q48–72h.
  ▶ *Paracoccidioidomycosis:* Give 0.4–0.5 mg/kg/d slow IV infusion; treat for 4–12 wk.

Compatibility
Amphotericin B may be given through the same IV line as aldesleukin, diltiazem, famotidine, tacrolimus, teniposide, thiotepa, zidovudine. Do not mix with other drugs or electrolytes.

Incompatibility
Do not administer through the same IV line as allopurinol, amifostine, amsacrine, aztreonam, cefepime, enalaprilat, filgrastim,

Adverse effects in *Italics* are most common; those in **Bold** are life-threatening

fluconazole, fludarabine, foscarnet, granisetron, melphalan, meropenem, ondansetron, paclitaxel, piperacillin-tazobactam, propofol, vinorelbine. Do not use with bacteriostatic agents or with solutions with pH < 4.2.

Oral/topical dosage

▶ *Treatment of oral candidiasis:* 100 mg PO qid.
▶ *Cutaneous and mucocutaneous mycotic infections:* Apply liberally to candidal lesion bid–qid. Treatment ranges from 1–4 wk depending on patient's response.

> **TREATMENT OF OVERDOSE/ANTIDOTE**
> Discontinue drug or decrease dosage. Initiate general supportive and resuscitative measures. May cause cardiorespiratory arrest.

Pharmacokinetics

Route	Onset	Peak	Duration
IV	20–30 min	1–2 h	20–24 h

$T_{1/2}$: 24 h initially, then 15 d; 173.4 h (Abelcet)
Excretion: Urine

Adverse effects

Systemic Administration

▶ *CNS: Confusion, headache, depression, abnormal thinking, insomnia*
▶ *CV:* **Cardiac arrest, cardiac failure, pulmonary edema, acute myocardial infarction, pulmonary embolus, ventricular fibrillation, shock, hemorrhage,** *hypotension, hypertension, tachycardia, tachypnea, dysrhythmias, postural hypotension, cardiomyopathy, syncope, edema*
▶ *Resp:* **Respiratory failure, apnea,** *pneumonia, dyspnea, hypoxia, epistaxis, increased cough, hemoptysis, hyperventilation, pleural effusion, rhinitis*
▶ *GI:* **GI hemorrhage,** *nausea, vomiting, dyspepsia, diarrhea, cramping, epigastric pain, anorexia, gastroenteritis, hematemesis, dyspepsia, hepatomegaly, cholangitis, cholecystitis,* weight loss
▶ *GU:* **Acute renal failure, nephrotoxicity,** *hematuria, hypokalemia, azotemia, hyposthenuria, renal tubular acidosis, nephrocalcinosis*
▶ *Derm: Pain at the injection site with phlebitis and thrombophlebitis*
▶ *Misc:* **Multiple organ failure, sepsis,** infection, rash, sweating, eye hemorrhage, asthenia

Adverse effects in *Italics* are most common; those in **Bold** are life-threatening

▸ *Allergic:* **Anaphylaxis**
▸ *Hematologic:* **Agranulocytosis, thrombocytopenia, leukopenia,** *normochromic, normocytic anemia; coagulation disorder, leukocytosis*

Topical Application
▸ **Derm:** *Drying effect on skin, local irritation* (cream); *pruritus,* allergic contact dermatitis (lotion); local irritation (ointment)

Clinically important drug–drug interactions
▸ Concurrent use with corticosteroids or corticotropin may potentiate hypokalemia and predispose patient to cardiac dysfunction; do not use these unless they are needed to control symptoms
▸ Increased nephrotoxicity, bronchospasm, hypotension with antineoplastics
▸ Increased renal toxicity with other nephrotoxic agents
▸ May induce hypokalemia and lead to digitalis toxicity
▸ Increased nephrotoxic effects with cyclosporine
▸ Increased flucytosine toxicity
▸ Intensified electrolyte depletion when given with thiazides; monitor potassium levels
▸ Enhanced curariform effect of skeletal muscle relaxants through potassium depletion

● NURSING CONSIDERATIONS
Assessment
▸ *History:* Allergy to amphotericin B, renal dysfunction, dehydration, cardiac disease, uncontrolled diabetes, leukocyte transfusions, pulmonary disease, electrolyte abnormalities
▸ *Physical:* T, P, BP, R, ECG, I & O, weight, neurologic checks, adventitious lung sounds, skin assessment, injection site, bowel sounds, liver evaluation, renal and liver function tests, electrolytes, CBC, culture of affected area

Implementation
▸ Always administer infusions using an IV infusion pump. Avoid rapid IV infusions.
▸ Obtain cultures before giving first dose; begin treatment before lab results are returned.
▸ Record the patient's vital signs q30min for 2–4 h after administration.
▸ Have emergency equipment (defibrillator, drugs, oxygen, intubation equipment) on standby in case anaphylaxis or adverse reaction occurs.
▸ Monitor injection sites and veins for signs of phlebitis.
▸ Cleanse affected lesions before applying topical drug; apply liberally to lesions and rub in gently; do not cover with plastic wrap.

Adverse effects in *Italics* are most common; those in **Bold** are life-threatening

- Use soap and water to wash hands, fabrics, and skin that may discolor from topical application.
- Provide aspirin, antihistamines, antiemetics, and maintain sodium balance to ease drug discomfort. Minimal use of IV corticosteroids may decrease febrile reactions. Meperidine has been used to relieve chills and fever.
- Monitor renal function tests weekly; discontinue or decrease dosage of drug at any sign of increased renal toxicity.
- Discontinue topical application if hypersensitivity reaction occurs.

⬤ **ampicillin** *(amp ih sill' in)* Oral: Ampicin (CAN), Apo-Ampi (CAN), Marcillin, Novo-Ampicillin (CAN), Nu-Ampi (CAN), Omnipen, Principen, Totacillin

⬤ **ampicillin sodium** Parenteral: Omnipen-N

Pregnancy Category B

Drug class
Antibiotic: penicillin

Indications
- Treatment of infections caused by susceptible strains of *Shigella, Salmonella, Escherichia coli, Haemophilus influenzae, Proteus mirabilis, Neisseria gonorrhoeae,* and enterococci
- Effective in treatment of meningitis caused by *Neisseria meningitidis*
- Infections caused by susceptible gram-positive organisms: Penicillin G-sensitive staphylococci, streptococci, and pneumococci

Therapeutic actions
- Bactericidal: inhibits biosynthesis of cell wall mucopeptide, causing cell death

Contraindications/cautions
- **Contraindications:** allergy to penicillins or cephalosporins
- **Cautions:** history of multiple allergies, renal function impairment, patients who require sodium restriction

Available forms
- *Powder for injection:* 125, 250, 500 mg; 1, 2, 10 g
- *Capsules:* 250, 500 mg
- *Powder for oral suspension:* 125 mg/5 mL, 250 mg/5 mL when reconstituted

Adverse effects in *Italics* are most common; those in **Bold** are life-threatening

IV/IM facts
Preparation
▶ **Standard vials:** Reconstitute with Sterile Water for Injection or Bacteriostatic Water for Injection. Add 1.2 mL to the 125-mg vial, 1 mL to the 250-mg vial, 1.8 mL to the 500-mg vial, 3.5 mL to the 1-g vial, or 6.8 mL to the 2-g vial. **Direct IV injection:** give without further dilution. Give within 1 h after preparation. **Intermittent IV infusion:** further dilute with D5W/0.45%NS; D5W; Invert Sugar 10%; LR; 0.9%NS; Sodium Lactate (1/6 Molar) Injection; or Sterile Water for Injection to a concentration of ≤ 30 mg/mL. After dilution in a compatible IV solution, drug is stable for 3–72 h when stored at 4°C, depending on diluent and concentration.
▶ **ADD-Vantage vials:** Reconstitute with 0.9%NS. Activate the ADD-Vantage vial by pulling the inner cap from the drug vial. Allow drug and diluent to mix.
▶ **IM use:** Reconstitute with Sterile Water for Injection or Bacteriostatic Water for Injection. See above for diluent amounts. Give within 1 h after preparation.

Dosage
▶ Give by direct IV injection over 3–5 min or infuse volumes of 50–100 mL over 15–30 min. More rapid administration may result in seizures.
▶ Give IM by deep intramuscular injection.
▶ Dose range is 1–12 g/d in divided doses q4–6h.
▶ *Respiratory tract and soft-tissue infections:* Patients ≥ 40 kg: 250–500 mg IV or IM q6h. Patients ≤ 40 kg: 25–50 mg/kg/d IV in divided doses at 6- to 8-h intervals.
▶ *Bacterial meningitis:* 150–200 mg/kg/d in divided dose q3–4h. Initial treatment is usually by IV drip, followed by frequent (q3–4h) IM injections.
▶ *Septicemia:* 150–200 mg/kg/d IV for at least 3 d. Then IM q3–4h.
▶ *N. gonorrhea:* Patients ≥ 40 kg: 500 mg IV or IM q6h.
▶ *Urethritis caused by N. gonorrhea in males:* Males ≥ 40 kg: Two 500-mg doses, IV or IM, at an 8- to 12-h interval. Repeat or extend treatment if needed.
▶ *Prevention of bacterial endocarditis:* 2 g IV or IM 30 min prior to dental, oral, or upper respiratory tract procedures in patients at moderate risk. Or for patients at high-risk, 2 g ampicillin IV or IM plus gentamicin 30 min before the procedure; 6 h later, ampicillin 1 g IV or IM or amoxicillin PO.
▶ *Renal function impairment:* Increase dosing interval to 12–16 h if creatinine clearance ≤ 10 mL/min.

Adverse effects in *Italics* are most common; those in **Bold** are life-threatening

Compatibility

Ampicillin may be given through the same IV line as acyclovir, allopurinol, amifostine, aztreonam, cyclophosphamide, enalaprilat, esmolol, famotidine, filgrastim, fludarabine, foscarnet, granisetron, heparin, heparin with hydrocortisone, insulin (regular), labetalol, magnesium sulfate, melphalan, meperidine, morphine, multivitamins, ofloxacin, perphenazine, phytonadione, potassium chloride, propofol, tacrolimus, teniposide, theophylline, thiotepa, tolazoline, vitamin B complex with C.

Incompatibility

Do not administer through the same IV line as epinephrine, fluconazole, hydralazine, midazolam, ondansetron, sargramostim, verapamil, vinorelbine.

Oral dosage

▸ *Respiratory tract and soft-tissue infections:* Patients ≥ 20 kg: 250 mg PO q6h.
▸ *GI and GU infections other than N. gonorrhea:* Patients ≥ 20 kg: 500 mg PO q6h. Use larger doses for severe or chronic infections, if needed.
▸ *N. gonorrhea:* Single dose of 3.5 g PO given simultaneously with 1 g probenecid.
▸ *Renal function impairment:* Increase dosing interval to 12–16 h if creatinine clearance ≤ 10 mL/min.

> ### TREATMENT OF OVERDOSE/ANTIDOTE
> Discontinue drug or decrease dosage. Initiate general supportive and resuscitative measures. Hemodialysis may remove the drug from the circulation.

Pharmacokinetics

Route	Onset	Peak	Duration
IV	Immediate	End of infusion	6–8 h
IM	Rapid	1 h	6–8 h
PO	30 min	2 h	6–8 h

Metabolism: Liver; $T_{1/2}$: 1–1.4 h
Excretion: Urine, bile

Adverse effects

▸ *CNS:* **Seizures,** lethargy, hallucinations
▸ *CV:* **Cardiac arrest,** hypotension, edema
▸ *GI:* **Pseudomembranous colitis,** *diarrhea,* nausea, vomiting, flatulence, abdominal distention, stomatitis, glossitis

Adverse effects in *Italics* are most common; those in **Bold** are life-threatening

▸ *GU:* **Interstitial nephritis,** dysuria, increased BUN and creatinine; presence of RBCs and casts in urine
▸ *Derm:* *Pain, phlebitis,* thrombosis at injection site (parenteral)
▸ *Allergic:* **Anaphylaxis, angioedema, laryngospasm,** *rash, drug fever, wheezing,* itching, rash
▸ *Hematologic:* **Thrombocytopenia, leukopenia, neutropenia,** anemia, prolonged bleeding time
▸ *Misc:* *Superinfections*

Clinically important drug–drug interactions

▸ Certain parenteral aminoglycosides inactivated; do not mix in the same IV solution
▸ Increased bleeding time and risk of bleeding with anticoagulants, heparin
▸ Reduced bioavailability of atenolol
▸ Reduced efficacy of oral contraceptives and increased breakthrough bleeding
▸ Impaired bactericidal effects with tetracyclines

⬤ NURSING CONSIDERATIONS

Assessment

▸ *History:* Allergy to any penicillin, renal function impairment, history of multiple allergies
▸ *Physical:* T, P, R, BP, I & O, IV or IM site, weight, neurologic checks, skin assessment, respiratory status, abdominal assessment, bowel sounds, culture and sensitivity tests of infected area, renal and liver function tests, serum sodium level, UA, CBC

Implementation

▸ Obtain specimens for culture and sensitivity of infected area before beginning therapy. May begin drug before results are available.
▸ Have emergency equipment (defibrillator, drugs, oxygen, intubation equipment) on standby in case anaphylactic reaction occurs.
▸ Assess for evidence of anaphylaxis; if suspected, discontinue drug immediately and notify provider.
▸ Give aminoglycosides at a separate site.
▸ Monitor renal, hepatic, and hematopoietic function.
▸ Monitor for occurrence of superinfections; treat as appropriate.
▸ Discontinue drug at any sign of colitis; initiate appropriate supportive treatment.
▸ Give orally with 240 mL of water 30 min before or 2 h after meals.

Adverse effects in *Italics* are most common; those in **Bold** are life-threatening

⬤ ampicillin sodium—sulbactam sodium *(amp ih sill' in—sull bak' tam)* Unasyn

Pregnancy Category B

Drug classes
Antibiotic: penicillin

Indications
▸ Skin and skin-structure infections caused by β-lactamase-producing strains of *Staphylococcus aureus, Escherichia coli, Klebsiella* species, *Proteus mirabilis, Bacteroides fragilis, Enterobacter* species, *Acinetobacter calcoaceticus*
▸ Intra-abdominal infections caused by β-lactamase-producing strains of *E. coli, Klebsiella* species, *Bacteroides, Enterobacter* species
▸ Gynecologic infections caused by β-lactamase-producing strains of *E. coli, Bacteroides* species

Therapeutic actions
▸ Bactericidal: inhibits biosynthesis of cell wall mucopeptide, causing cell death; sulbactam component is effective against β-lactamases that are often associated with drug resistance; most effective during stage of active multiplication

Contraindications/cautions
▸ **Contraindications:** allergy to any penicillin, mononucleosis
▸ **Cautions:** history of multiple allergies, patients who require sodium restriction

Available forms
▸ *Powder for injection:* 1.5, 3, 10 g

IV/IM facts
Preparation
▸ **Bottles:** Reconstitute with D5W/0.45%NS; D5W; Invert Sugar 10%; LR; 0.9%NS; Sodium Lactate (1/6 Molar) Injection; or Sterile Water for Injection to yield a solution of 3–45 mg/mL. Allow solution to stand so that any foaming will dissipate.
▸ **Standard vials:** Dilute each 1.5 g with 3.2 mL of Sterile Water for Injection to yield 375 mg/mL (withdrawal volume is 4 mL). Allow solution to stand so that any foaming will dissipate. Then further dilute with D5W/0.45%NS; D5W; Invert Sugar 10%; LR; 0.9%NS; Sodium Lactate (1/6 Molar) Injection; or Sterile Water for Injection to a concentration of 3–45 mg/mL. Solution is stable for 2–8 h at 21°C, depending on diluent and concentration.

Adverse effects in *Italics* are most common; those in **Bold** are life-threatening

◗ **ADD-Vantage vials:** Reconstitute only with 0.9%NS. Activate the ADD-Vantage vial by pulling the inner cap from the drug vial. Allow drug and diluent to mix. Use within 8 h.
◗ **IM use:** Reconstitute using 0.5% or 2% Lidocaine Hydrochloride Injection or Sterile Water for Injection. Give within 1 h after preparation.

Dosage
◗ Give by direct IV injection over 10–15 min, or infuse volumes of 50–100 mL over 15–30 min.
◗ Give IM by deep intramuscular injection.
◗ 1.5 g (1 g ampicillin and 0.5 g sulbactam) to 3 g (2 g ampicillin and 1 g sulbactam) IV or IM q6h.
◗ *Renal function impairment:* Refer to table below for dosages.

Creatinine Clearance (mL/min)	Dosage
≥ 30	1.5–3 g q6–8h
15–29	1.5–3 g q12h
5–14	1.5–3 g q24h

Compatibility
Ampicillin-sulbactam may be given through the same IV line as amifostine, aztreonam, cefepime, enalaprilat, famotidine, filgrastim, fluconazole, fludarabine, gallium, granisetron, heparin, insulin (regular), meperidine, morphine, paclitaxel, tacrolimus, teniposide, theophylline, thiotepa.

Incompatibility
Do not administer through the same IV line as aminoglycosides, ciprofloxacin, idarubicin, ondansetron, sargramostim. Do not admix with aminoglycosides.

> **TREATMENT OF OVERDOSE/ANTIDOTE**
> Discontinue drug or decrease dosage. Initiate general supportive and resuscitative measures. Hemodialysis may remove the drug from the circulation.

Pharmacokinetics

Route	Onset	Peak
IV	Immediate	End of infusion
IM	Rapid	

Metabolism: Liver; $T_{1/2}$: 1 h
Excretion: Urine

Adverse effects in *Italics* are most common; those in **Bold** are life-threatening

Adverse effects
▸ *CNS:* Fatigue, malaise, headache
▸ *CV:* Chest pain, edema
▸ *GI:* **Pseudomembranous colitis,** *diarrhea,* nausea, vomiting, flatulence, abdominal distention, glossitis; increased AST, ALT, alkaline phosphatase, and LDH
▸ *GU:* Urine retention, dysuria, increased BUN and creatinine; presence of RBCs and casts in urine
▸ *Allergic:* **Anaphylaxis,** *rash,* itching, drug fever, rash, tightness in throat
▸ *Hematologic:* Decreased Hgb, Hct, RBC, WBC, neutrophils, lymphocytes, and platelets; increased lymphocytes, monocytes, basophils, eosinophils, and platelets
▸ *Misc:* *Superinfections;* pain or phlebitis at IV or IM injection site, facial swelling, mucosal swelling, erythema, chills; decreased albumin and total proteins

Clinically important drug–drug interactions
▸ Increased and prolonged drug levels related to decreased excretion with probenecid
▸ Rash with allopurinol

⬤ NURSING CONSIDERATIONS

Assessment
▸ *History:* Allergy to any penicillin, mononucleosis, history of multiple allergies
▸ *Physical:* T, P, R, BP, I & O, IV or IM site, weight, neurologic checks, skin assessment, respiratory status, abdominal assessment, bowel sounds, culture and sensitivity tests of infected area, renal and liver function tests, serum sodium level, UA, CBC

Implementation
▸ Obtain specimens for culture and sensitivity of infected area before beginning therapy. May begin drug before results are available.
▸ Have emergency equipment (defibrillator, drugs, oxygen, intubation equipment) on standby in case anaphylactic reaction occurs.
▸ Assess for evidence of anaphylaxis; if suspected, discontinue drug immediately and notify provider.
▸ Give aminoglycosides at a separate site.
▸ Monitor renal, hepatic, and hematopoietic function.
▸ Monitor for occurrence of superinfections; treat as appropriate.
▸ Discontinue drug at any sign of colitis; initiate appropriate supportive treatment.

Adverse effects in *Italics* are most common; those in **Bold** are life-threatening

◗ **amrinone lactate** *(am' ri none)* Inocor

A

Pregnancy Category C

Drug class
Cardiac inotropic agent

Indication
▸ CHF: short-term management of patients who are closely monitored and who have not responded adequately to digitalis, diuretics, or vasodilators

Therapeutic actions
▸ Is a positive inotropic agent that inhibits myocardial cyclic adenosine monophosphate (c-AMP) phosphodiesterase activity and increases cellular levels of c-AMP
▸ Causes vasodilation by a direct relaxant effect on vascular smooth muscle

Effects on hemodynamic parameters
▸ Decreased SVR
▸ Decreased CVP
▸ Increased CO
▸ Decreased PCWP
▸ Decreased BP
▸ Increased or unchanged HR
▸ Unchanged myocardial oxygen consumption

Contraindications/cautions
▸ **Contraindications:** amrinone allergy, hypersensitivity to bisulfites, severe aortic or pulmonic valvular disease
▸ **Cautions:** hypovolemia related to diuretic therapy, supraventricular and ventricular dysrhythmias, thrombocytopenia, acute myocardial infarction (AMI)

Available form
▸ *IV injection:* 5 mg/mL

IV facts
Preparation
▸ For a continuous infusion, add 250 to 750 mg amrinone to 250–500 mL of 0.45%NS or 0.9%NS.

Dosage and titration
▸ *Initial loading dose:* 0.75 mg/kg IV bolus over 2–3 min. A supplemental bolus dose of 0.75 mg/kg IV may be given after 30 min if needed.

Adverse effects in *Italics* are most common; those in **Bold** are life-threatening

‣ *Maintenance infusion:* 5–10 mcg/kg/min IV. Titrate to achieve desired response. Do not exceed a total of 10 mg/kg/d. A few patients have received up to 18 mg/kg/d for short durations of therapy.

Titration Guide

amrinone lactate									
500 mg in 250 mL									

	Body Weight									
lb	**88**	**99**	**110**	**121**	**132**	**143**	**154**	**165**	**176**	**187**
kg	**40**	**45**	**50**	**55**	**60**	**65**	**70**	**75**	**80**	**85**
Dose ordered in mcg/kg/min	**Amounts to Infuse in mL/h**									
5	6	7	8	8	9	10	11	11	12	13
6	7	8	9	10	11	12	13	14	14	15
7	8	9	11	12	13	14	15	16	17	18
8	10	11	12	13	14	16	17	18	19	20
9	11	12	14	15	16	18	19	20	22	23
10	12	14	15	17	18	20	21	23	24	26

	Body Weight								
lb	**198**	**209**	**220**	**231**	**242**	**253**	**264**	**275**	**286**
kg	**90**	**95**	**100**	**105**	**110**	**115**	**120**	**125**	**130**
Dose ordered in mcg/kg/min	**Amounts to Infuse in mL/h**								
5	14	14	15	16	17	17	18	19	20
6	16	17	18	19	20	21	22	23	23
7	19	20	21	22	23	24	25	26	27
8	22	23	24	25	26	28	29	30	31
9	24	26	27	28	30	31	32	34	35
10	27	29	30	32	33	35	36	38	39

Therapeutic serum level
‣ 3.7 mcg/mL

Compatibility
Amrinone may be given through the same IV line as aminophylline, atropine, bretylium, calcium chloride, cimetidine, digoxin, dobutamine, dopamine, epinephrine, famotidine, hydrocortisone, isoproterenol, lidocaine, metaraminol, methylprednisolone, nitroglycerin, nitroprusside sodium, norepinephrine, phenylephrine, potassium chloride, propofol, propranolol, verapamil.

Adverse effects in *Italics* are most common; those in **Bold** are life-threatening

Incompatibility
Do not administer through the same IV line as dextrose solutions, furosemide, sodium bicarbonate.

> **TREATMENT OF OVERDOSE/ANTIDOTE**
> Decrease infusion rate or temporarily discontinue infusion until patient is stabilized. Initiate resuscitative measures as indicated.

Pharmacokinetics

Route	Onset	Peak	Duration
IV	2–5 min	10 min	0.5–2 h

Metabolism: Hepatic; $T_{1/2}$: 3.6–5.8 h
Excretion: Urine, feces

Adverse effects
▶ *CV: Dysrhythmias,* hypotension, chest pain
▶ *GI:* Nausea, vomiting, anorexia, abdominal pain, hepatoxicity
▶ *Allergic:* Pericarditis, pleuritis, ascites, vasculitis, hypoxemia, jaundice, elevated sedimentation rate
▶ *Hematologic: Thrombocytopenia*
▶ *Misc:* Fever, burning at injection site

Clinically important drug–drug interactions
▶ Excessive hypotension when given concurrently with disopyramide
▶ Increased effect when used concurrently with digoxin

⬤ NURSING CONSIDERATIONS

Assessment
▶ *History:* Amrinone or bisulfite allergy, severe aortic or pulmonic valvular disease, AMI, hypovolemia
▶ *Physical:* T, P, BP, R, CO, CVP, PCWP, IV site, I & O, weight, neurologic checks, cardiac auscultation, peripheral edema, adventitious lung sounds, peripheral perfusion/pulses, bowel sounds, liver evaluation, hydration status, serum electrolytes, platelet count, liver function tests

Implementation
▶ Exercise extreme caution when calculating and preparing doses; amrinone is a very potent drug; small dosage errors can cause serious adverse effects.

Adverse effects in *Italics* are most common; those in **Bold** are life-threatening

- Always administer an infusion using an IV infusion pump.
- Administer into large veins of antecubital fossa rather than hand or ankle veins. Use a central line whenever possible.
- Correct hypovolemia before administering amrinone.
- Monitor ECG, BP, CO, and I & O closely during infusion. Adjust dose/rate accordingly.
- Monitor electrolyte levels and liver enzymes; record daily weights.
- Monitor platelet counts if patient is on prolonged therapy. Reduce dose if platelet levels fall.
- Assess IV site; instruct patient to report any burning.
- Use diluted solutions within 24 h.
- Protect amrinone vials from light.
- Amrinone is a clear yellow solution.

● amyl nitrite *(am' il)*
Pregnancy Category X

Drug classes
Antianginal drug
Nitrate
Antidote

Indications
- Relief of angina pectoris
- Cyanide poisoning

Therapeutic actions
- Relaxes vascular smooth muscle
- Dilates postcapillary vessels, including large veins
- Improves blood flow to ischemic myocardium
- Decreases myocardial oxygen consumption
- Converts hemoglobin to methemoglobin, which can bind to cyanide

Effects on hemodynamic parameters
- Decreased SVR/PVR
- Decreased LVEDP
- Decreased BP
- Decreased CVP
- Decreased PCWP
- Possible reflex tachycardia
- Unchanged, increased, or decreased CO

Adverse effects in *Italics* are most common; those in **Bold** are life-threatening

A

Contraindications/cautions
▶ **Contraindications:** allergy to nitrates, severe anemia, angle-closure glaucoma, postural hypotension, head trauma, cerebral hemorrhage
▶ **Cautions:** hypertrophic cardiomyopathy, glaucoma, hypotension

Available forms
▶ *Inhalation capsules:* 0.3 mL

Inhalation dosage
▶ *Angina:* 0.3 mL by inhalation of vapor from crushed capsule; may repeat in 3–5 min for relief of angina. 1–6 inhalations are usually sufficient to produce desired effect.
▶ *Cyanide poisoning:* 0.3 mL by inhalation of vapor from crushed capsule; inhale for 30 s of each minute; replace with fresh capsule q3–4min.

TREATMENT OF OVERDOSE/ANTIDOTE
Discontinue drug or decrease dosage. Initiate general supportive and resuscitative measures.

Pharmacokinetics

Route	Onset	Peak	Duration
Inhalation	30 s	3 min	3–5 min

Metabolism: Hepatic; $T_{1/2}$: 1–4 min
Excretion: Urine

Adverse effects
▶ *CNS: Headache, apprehension, restlessness, weakness,* vertigo, dizziness, faintness, euphoria, malaise
▶ *CV:* **Cardiovascular collapse,** *tachycardia, hypotension,* retrosternal discomfort, palpitations, syncope, collapse, postural hypotension, angina, dysrhythmias, edema
▶ *Resp:* Bronchitis, pneumonia, upper respiratory tract infection
▶ *GI: Nausea,* vomiting, dyspepsia, incontinence of urine and feces, abdominal pain
▶ *Derm: Cutaneous vasodilation with flushing,* rash, exfoliative dermatitis, pruritus
▶ *Drug abuse:* Abused for sexual stimulation and euphoria, effects of inhalation are instantaneous
▶ *Misc:* **Methemoglobinemia,** muscle twitching, arthralgia, pallor, perspiration, cold sweat, hemolytic anemia, blurred vision, rigors

Adverse effects in *Italics* are most common; those in **Bold** are life-threatening

Clinically important drug–drug interactions

▸ Severe hypotension and CV collapse if used with alcohol
▸ Hypotension with antihypertensive drugs, beta-adrenergic blockers

● NURSING CONSIDERATIONS

Assessment

▸ *History:* Allergy to nitrates, severe anemia, angle-closure glaucoma, postural hypotension, head trauma, cerebral hemorrhage, hypertrophic cardiomyopathy, glaucoma, hypotension, cyanide ingestion
▸ *Physical:* BP, P, R, T, ECG, I & O, SpO$_2$, skin color, neurologic checks, ophthalmic exam, skin assessment, orthostatic BP, peripheral perfusion, adventitious lung sounds, pain assessment, cardiac assessment, chest pain assessment, liver evaluation, CBC, ABG, serum lactate level, CPK, CPK-MB, cardiac troponin, myoglobin, cyanide level, methemoglobin level

Implementation

▸ Patient may develop drug tolerance and need more drug for subsequent attacks.
▸ Use drug when patient is lying down. Have patient rest in cool, quiet environment after use.
▸ Aspirin or acetaminophen may relieve headaches associated with amyl nitrite.
▸ Use drug in a well-ventilated room.
▸ Gradually reduce dose if anginal treatment is being terminated; rapid discontinuation can cause withdrawal.
▸ Protect the drug from light; store in a cool place.

● **anistreplase** *(an is tre plaze')*

anisoylated plasminogen streptokinase activator complex (APSAC)
Eminase

Pregnancy Category C

Drug class

Thrombolytic enzyme

Indications

▸ Management of AMI for the lysis of thrombi obstructing coronary arteries to reduce infarct size, improve ventricular function following AMI, and reduce mortality associated with AMI

Therapeutic actions

▸ Anistreplase is made from streptokinase and Lys-plasminogen
▸ When activated, the complex converts plasminogen to plasmin

Adverse effects in *Italics* are most common; those in **Bold** are life-threatening

A

▶ Plasmin lyses formed thrombi, which results in reperfusion of coronary arteries

Effects on hemodynamic parameters
▶ Unchanged or decreased BP

Contraindications/cautions
▶ **Contraindications:** anistreplase or streptokinase allergy, active internal bleeding, CVA, intracranial or intraspinal surgery or trauma within 2 mo, intracranial neoplasm, arteriovenous malformation, aneurysm, bleeding diathesis, severe/uncontrolled HTN
▶ **Cautions:** cerebrovascular disease, GI or GU bleeding within 10 d, recent (within 10 d) major surgery (CABG, obstetrical delivery, organ biopsy, or puncture of a noncompressible vessel), SBP ≥ 180 mmHg, DBP ≥ 110 mmHg, left heart thrombus, subacute bacterial endocarditis, acute pericarditis, hemostatic defects including those secondary to severe hepatic or renal disease, age > 75 y, diabetic hemorrhagic retinopathy or other hemorrhagic ophthalmic conditions, septic thrombophlebitis, oral anticoagulant therapy

Available form
▶ *IV injection:* 30 U/vial

IV facts
Preparation
▶ Slowly add 5 mL Sterile Water for Injection by directing stream of fluid against side of vial.
▶ Gently roll vial, mixing dry powder and fluid. **Do not shake.** Minimize foaming.
▶ Solution will be a colorless to pale yellow transparent solution. Inspect for particulate matter and discoloration.
▶ Withdraw entire contents of vial.
▶ Do not further dilute solution or add to any infusion fluids.
▶ Discard drug if not administered with 30 min of reconstitution.

Dosage
▶ Administer only by IV injection as soon as possible after onset of symptoms.
▶ Administer 30 U IV over 2–5 min into an IV line or vein.

Compatibility
Do not administer anistreplase with any other drugs.

Adverse effects in *Italics* are most common; those in **Bold** are life-threatening

Pharmacokinetics

Route	Onset	Peak	Duration
IV	Immediate	45 min	4–6 h; systemic hyperfibrinolytic state may persist for 2 d

Metabolism: Plasma; $T_{1/2}$: 70–120 min

Adverse effects
▸ *CNS:* **Intracranial hemorrhage,** agitation, dizziness, paresthesia, tremor, vertigo
▸ *CV:* **Dysrhythmia, hypotension, cardiac rupture, cholesterol embolism,** chest pain, emboli, vasculitis
▸ *Resp:* Dyspnea, lung edema, hemoptysis
▸ *GI:* **GI bleeding, retroperitoneal bleeding,** nausea, vomiting
▸ *GU:* **GU tract bleeding,** mild proteinuria
▸ *Allergic:* **Anaphylaxis,** urticaria, itching, flushing, rash
▸ *Hematologic: Bleeding,* **hemorrhage,** thrombocytopenia, anemia
▸ *Musc/Skel:* Arthralgia, myopathy, symptomatic weakness, fatigue, rhabdomyolysis
▸ *Misc:* Fever, epistaxis, vasculitis, ankle edema

Clinically important drug–drug interactions
▸ Increased hemorrhage with vitamin K antagonists, heparin, oral anticoagulants, drugs that alter platelet function (aspirin, dipyridamole, abciximab, tirofiban, eptifibatide, ticlopidine, clopidogrel)

⊙ NURSING CONSIDERATIONS

Assessment
▸ *History:* Anistreplase or streptokinase allergy, active internal bleeding, CVA within 2 mo, intracranial or intraspinal surgery or neoplasm, arteriovenous malformation, aneurysm, recent major surgery, obstetrical delivery, organ biopsy, puncture of noncompressible blood vessel, recent serious GI bleed, recent serious trauma, recent CPR, hemostatic defects, cerebrovascular disease, SBE, severe uncontrolled HTN, liver disease, age

Adverse effects in *Italics* are most common; those in **Bold** are life-threatening

(A)

▶ *Physical:* P, BP, R, T, ECG, I & O, neurologic checks, skin assessment, presence of bleeding, peripheral perfusion, liver evaluation, chest pain assessment, coagulation studies, CBC, type and crossmatch, CPK, CPK-MB, cardiac troponin, myoglobin, urine, stool, and emesis guaiac

Implementation

▶ Monitor for bleeding or hemorrhage.
▶ Carefully assess recent puncture sites and sites of lines/tubes (catheter insertion sites, cutdown sites, needle puncture sites, recent surgical incisions).
▶ Initiate bleeding precautions. Avoid nonessential handling of the patient.
▶ Avoid IM injections before, during, and for 24 h after therapy. Do not attempt central venous access or arterial puncture unless absolutely necessary. If arterial puncture is necessary, use an upper extremity vessel that is accessible to manual pressure.
▶ Apply pressure to arterial and venous puncture sites for least 30 min or until hemostasis is achieved.
▶ Apply pressure or pressure dressings to control superficial bleeding.
▶ If possible, draw blood for laboratory analysis from an existing saline lock.
▶ Take BP with manual BP cuff or ensure that NIBP cuff does not inflate excessively above patient's SBP.
▶ Shave patient with an electric razor.
▶ Monitor coagulation studies.
▶ Guaiac urine, feces, and emesis.
▶ Assess for chest pain (type, character, location, intensity, radiation) and monitor ECG before, during, and after therapy. Assess for ST segment changes.
▶ Monitor BP, P, R, and neurologic status continuously.
▶ Have resuscitative equipment/medications readily available in case of anaphylaxis, dysrhythmias, respiratory failure, or hemorrhage.
▶ Initiate other interventions as standard for patients with AMI.
▶ Because of increased likelihood of resistance due to antistreptokinase antibody, drug may not be effective if administered between 5 d and 6 mo of prior anistreplase or streptokinase administration or with streptococcal infections.

⬤ **atenolol** *(a ten' o lole)* Apo-Atenol (CAN), Gen-Atenolol (CAN), Novo-Atenol (CAN), Tenolin (CAN), Tenormin

Pregnancy Category C

Adverse effects in *Italics* are most common; those in **Bold** are life-threatening

Drug classes
Beta-adrenergic blocker (β_1 selective)
Antihypertensive

Indications
▸ Treatment of angina due to coronary atherosclerosis
▸ Treatment of hypertension with or without other antihypertensive agents
▸ Treatment of hemodynamically stable patients with acute myocardial infarction (AMI)
▸ Unlabeled uses: SVT, PVCs, migraine prophylaxis, alcohol withdrawal syndrome, rebleeding of esophageal varices, anxiety

Therapeutic actions
▸ Acts on β_1 (myocardial) receptors to decrease influence of sympathetic nervous system on the heart, excitability of the heart, myocardial contractility, cardiac workload, oxygen consumption, BP, and release of renin
▸ Inhibits β_2 receptors at higher doses

Effects on hemodynamic parameters
▸ Decreased BP
▸ Decreased CO
▸ Decreased HR

Contraindications/cautions
▸ **Contraindications:** beta-blocker allergy, sinus bradycardia, second- or third-degree heart block, cardiogenic shock, CHF unless secondary to a tachydysrhythmia treatable with beta-blockers
▸ **Cautions:** peripheral or mesenteric vascular disease, chronic bronchitis, emphysema, bronchospastic disease, diabetes, hepatic or renal dysfunction, thyrotoxicosis, muscle weakness

Available forms
▸ *Injection:* 5 mg/10 mL
▸ *Tablets:* 25, 50, 100 mg

IV facts
Preparation
▸ May be diluted in D5W/0.9%NS; D5W; or 0.9%NS.

Dosage
▸ Initiate drug as soon as possible after diagnosis.
▸ *AMI:* 5 mg IV over 5 min followed by 5 mg IV 10 min later.
▸ See next page for conversion to oral dosing.

Adverse effects in *Italics* are most common; those in **Bold** are life-threatening

A

Compatibility
Atenolol may be given through the same IV line as meperidine, meropenem, morphine.

Oral dosage
▶ *HTN:* 50 mg/d PO; after 1–2 wk, may increase dose to 100 mg.
▶ *Angina pectoris:* 50 mg/d PO. If optimal response not achieved in 1 wk, increase to 100 mg/d PO; up to 200 mg/d may be needed.
▶ *AMI:* If patient tolerates the IV 10-mg dose, give a 50-mg tablet PO 10 min after last IV dose, followed by a 50-mg PO dose 12 h later. Thereafter, give 100 mg/d PO or 50 mg PO bid for at least 7 d.
▶ *Hemodialysis:* 50 mg PO after each dialysis session; severe hypotension can occur.
▶ *Geriatric or renal impaired:* Reduce dose because atenolol is excreted through kidneys. The following dosages are recommended:

Creatinine Clearance (mL/min/1.73m²)	Half-life (h)	Maximum Dosage
15–35	16–27	50 mg/d
< 15	> 27	25 mg/d

TREATMENT OF OVERDOSE/ANTIDOTE
Discontinue drug or decrease dosage. Initiate general supportive and resuscitative measures. Initiate gastric lavage or induce emesis to remove drug after oral ingestion. Place patient in supine position with legs elevated. Treat symptomatic bradycardia with atropine, epinephrine, isoproterenol, or a pacemaker; cardiac failure with a digitalis glycoside, diuretic, or aminophylline; hypotension with vasopressors, such as dopamine, dobutamine, norepinephrine; hypoglycemia with IV glucose; PVCs with lidocaine; seizures with diazepam. Give glucagon (5–10 mg IV over 30 s, followed by infusion of 5 mg/h) for severe beta-blocker overdose. Atenolol can be removed by dialysis.

Pharmacokinetics

Route	Onset	Peak	Duration
IV	Immediate	5 min	24 h
Oral	Varies	2–4 h	24 h

$T_{1/2}$: 6–7 h
Excretion: Urine, feces

Adverse effects in *Italics* are most common; those in **Bold** are life-threatening

Adverse effects

- **CNS:** *Fatigue,* dizziness, vertigo, lightheadedness, depression, lethargy, drowsiness, dreaming, headache, psychoses
- **CV: Bradycardia, pulmonary edema, CHF,** *AV block,* postural hypotension, peripheral vasoconstriction
- **Resp: Bronchospasm,** dyspnea, crackles, wheezes
- **GI:** Diarrhea, nausea, ischemic colitis, renal and mesenteric arterial thrombosis, elevated liver enzymes
- **Derm:** Rash, psoriasis
- **Allergic: Bronchospasm, laryngospasm,** rash, fever, sore throat, respiratory distress
- **Misc:** Raynaud's phenomenon, lupus syndrome, hyperglycemia or hypoglycemia, development of antinuclear antibodies, dry eyes, impotence

Clinically important drug–drug interactions

- Increased effects with calcium channel blockers, quinidine, digitalis, oral contraceptives
- Increased postural hypotension with prazosin
- Decreased effects with nonsteroidal anti-inflammatory drugs
- Reduced clearance of lidocaine
- Life-threatening HTN when clonidine is discontinued for patients on beta-blocker therapy or when both drugs are discontinued simultaneously
- Hypertension followed by severe bradycardia with epinephrine
- May potentiate, counteract, or have no effect on nondepolarizing muscle relaxants

● NURSING CONSIDERATIONS

Assessment

- *History:* Beta-blocker allergy, cardiogenic shock, CHF unless secondary to a tachydysrhythmia treatable with beta-blockers, peripheral or mesenteric vascular disease, chronic bronchitis, emphysema, bronchospastic diseases, diabetes, hepatic or renal dysfunction, thyrotoxicosis, muscle weakness, angina
- *Physical:* P, BP, R, ECG, I & O, SpO_2, weight, neurologic checks, reflexes, heart sounds auscultation, chest pain assessment, orthostatic BP, edema, skin condition, adventitious lung sounds, JVD, abdominal assessment, bowel sounds, serum electrolytes, UA, serum glucose, CBC; liver, thyroid, and renal function tests

Implementation

- Exercise extreme caution when calculating and preparing IV doses; atenolol is a very potent drug; small dosage errors can cause serious adverse effects.
- Carefully monitor P, BP, R, and ECG during IV administration.

Adverse effects in *Italics* are most common; those in **Bold** are life-threatening

▶ Have emergency equipment (defibrillator, drugs, intubation equipment, oxygen) on standby in case bronchospasm or adverse reaction occurs.

▶ Assess for early evidence of heart failure as evidenced by increased weight, neck vein distention, oliguria, peripheral edema, crackles over lung fields, dyspnea, decreased SpO_2, cough, decreased activity tolerance, increased respiratory distress when lying flat, S_3 heart sound, tachycardia, hepatomegaly, and confusion.

▶ Patients with history of severe anaphylactic reactions may be more reactive on reexposure to the allergen and may be unresponsive to usual doses of epinephrine.

▶ Do not discontinue drug abruptly after chronic therapy. (Hypersensitivity to catecholamines may have developed, causing exacerbation of angina, MI, and ventricular dysrhythmias.) Taper drug gradually over 2 wk with monitoring.

▶ Consult with physician about withdrawing drug if patient is to undergo surgery (withdrawal is controversial).

▶ Diluted solution is stable for 48 h.

▶ May give with or without food.

⬤ atracurium besylate (*a tra cure' ee um*) Tracrium
Pregnancy Category C

Drug class
Nondepolarizing neuromuscular blocking agent

Indications
▶ Is an adjunct to general anesthesia to facilitate intubation
▶ Provides skeletal muscle relaxation during surgery or mechanical ventilation

Therapeutic actions
▶ Prevents neuromuscular transmission and produces paralysis by blocking effect of acetylcholine at the myoneural junction

Effects on hemodynamic parameters
▶ Decreased BP

Contraindications/cautions
▶ **Contraindications:** atracurium besylate or benzyl alcohol (if used from multidose vials) allergy
▶ **Cautions:** neuromuscular disease, myasthenia gravis, Eaton-Lambert syndrome, cardiovascular disease, malignant hyperthermia, electrolyte imbalance, respiratory depression, pulmonary disease, carcinomatosis, asthma, history of anaphylaxis

Adverse effects in *Italics* are most common; those in **Bold** are life-threatening

Available form
▸ *IV injection:* 10 mg/mL

IV facts
Preparation
▸ For a continuous infusion, dilute 20–50 mg in 100 mL D5W/0.9%NS; D5W; or 0.9%NS to achieve a concentration of 200–500 mcg/mL.

Dosage and titration
▸ *Initial bolus dose:* 400–500 mcg/kg IV.
▸ *Maintenance dose for ICU patients:* Usual dose is 11–13 mcg/kg/min by continous IV infusion.
▸ Titrate infusion by 1–2 mcg/kg/min to maintain desired neuromuscular blockade. Dose range is 4.5–29.5 mcg/kg/min.

Titration Guide

atracurium besylate									
50 mg in 100 mL									
	Body Weight								
lb	88	99	110	121	132	143	154	165	176
kg	40	45	50	55	60	65	70	75	80
Dose ordered in mcg/kg/min	**Amounts to Infuse in mL/h**								
4.5	22	24	27	30	32	35	38	41	43
5	24	27	30	33	36	39	42	45	48
6	29	32	36	40	43	47	50	54	58
7	34	38	42	46	50	55	59	63	67
8	38	43	48	53	58	62	67	72	77
9	43	49	54	59	65	70	76	81	86
10	48	54	60	66	72	78	84	90	96
11	53	59	66	73	79	86	92	99	106
12	58	65	72	79	86	94	101	108	115
13	62	70	78	86	94	101	109	117	125
14	67	76	84	92	101	109	118	126	134
16	77	86	96	106	115	125	134	144	154
18	86	97	108	119	130	140	151	162	173
20	96	108	120	132	144	156	168	180	192
22	106	119	132	145	158	172	185	198	211
24	115	130	144	158	173	187	202	216	230
26	125	140	156	172	187	203	218	234	250
28	134	151	168	185	202	218	235	252	269
29.5	142	159	177	195	212	230	248	266	283

Adverse effects in *Italics* are most common; those in **Bold** are life-threatening

					Body Weight					
lb	187	198	209	220	231	242	253	264	275	286
kg	85	90	95	100	105	110	115	120	125	130
Dose ordered in mcg/kg/min					Amounts to Infuse in mL/h					
4.5	46	49	51	54	57	59	62	65	68	70
5	51	54	57	60	63	66	69	72	75	78
6	61	65	68	72	76	79	83	86	90	94
7	71	76	80	84	88	92	97	101	105	109
8	82	86	91	96	101	106	110	115	120	125
9	92	97	103	108	113	119	124	130	135	140
10	102	108	114	120	126	132	138	144	150	156
11	112	119	125	132	139	145	152	158	165	172
12	122	130	137	144	151	158	166	173	180	187
13	133	140	148	156	164	172	179	187	195	203
14	143	151	160	168	176	185	193	202	210	218
16	163	173	182	192	202	211	221	230	240	250
18	184	194	205	216	227	238	248	259	270	281
20	204	216	228	240	252	264	276	288	300	312
22	224	238	251	264	277	290	304	317	330	343
24	245	259	274	288	302	317	331	346	360	374
26	265	281	296	312	328	343	359	374	390	406
28	286	302	319	336	353	370	386	403	420	437
29.5	301	319	336	354	372	389	407	425	443	460

Compatibility

Atracurium besylate may be given through the same IV line as cefazolin, cefuroxime, cimetidine, dobutamine, dopamine, epinephrine, esmolol, etomidate, fentanyl, gentamicin, heparin, hydrocortisone, isoproterenol, lorazepam, LR solution, midazolam, morphine, nitroglycerin, ranitidine, sodium nitroprusside, trimethoprim-sulfamethoxazole, vancomycin.

Incompatibility

Do not administer through the same IV line as diazepam, propofol, thiopental.

> **TREATMENT OF OVERDOSE/ANTIDOTE**
> Discontinue drug or decrease dosage. Decrease infusion rate or temporarily discontinue infusion until patient is stabilized. Continue to maintain a patent airway and provide mechanical ventilation. Pyridostigmine bromide, neostigmine, or edrophonium in conjunction with atropine or glycopyrrolate may reverse skeletal muscle relaxation.

Adverse effects in *Italics* are most common; those in **Bold** are life-threatening

Pharmacokinetics

Route	Onset	Peak	Duration
IV	2–2.5 min	3–5 min	60–70 min

Metabolism: Plasma; $T_{1/2}$: 20 min

Adverse effects

- *CV:* Hypotension, vasodilatation, tachycardia, bradycardia
- *Resp: **Apnea,*** bronchospasm, laryngospasm
- *Derm:* Rash, urticaria, reaction at injection site
- *Allergic:* **Anaphylactic reactions** (bronchospasm, flushing, redness, hypotension, tachycardia)
- *Musc/Skel:* Inadequate block, prolonged block

Clinically important drug–drug interactions

- Intensified neuromuscular blockage with diuretics, general anesthetics, antibiotics (aminoglycosides, polypeptides), lithium, verapamil, trimethaphan, procainamide, quinidine, magnesium sulfate
- Synergistic or antagonist effect when given concurrently with other muscle relaxants
- Resistance to or reversal of drug's neuromuscular blocking action with phenytoin, theophylline
- Reversed neuromuscular blockade with acetylcholinesterase inhibitors (neostigmine, edrophonium, pyridostigmine)
- Prolonged weakness with corticosteroids

⊙ NURSING CONSIDERATIONS

Assessment

- *History:* Atracurium besylate or benzyl alcohol allergy, neuromuscular disease, myasthenia gravis, Eaton-Lambert syndrome, cardiovascular disease, malignant hyperthermia, respiratory depression, pulmonary disease, carcinomatosis, asthma, anaphylaxis
- *Physical:* T, P, BP, R, ECG, I & O, IV site, weight, neurologic checks, skin assessment, level of sedation, respiratory status, method of mechanical ventilation, adventitious lung sounds, muscle strength, presence of pain, peripheral nerve stimulator response, serum electrolytes, acid–base balance

Implementation

- Exercise extreme caution when calculating and preparing doses; atracurium besylate is a very potent drug; small dosage errors can cause serious adverse effects.
- Always administer an infusion using an IV infusion pump.
- Do not administer unless equipment for intubation, artifical respiration, oxygen therapy, and reversal agents is read-

Adverse effects in *Italics* are most common; those in **Bold** are life-threatening

ily available. Atracurium besylate should be administered by people who are skilled in management of critically ill patients, cardiovascular resuscitation, and airway management.
⬩ Use the smallest dose possible to achieve desired patient response.
⬩ Monitor patient's response to therapy with a peripheral nerve stimulator.
⬩ Monitor BP, R, and ECG closely during infusion to monitor effectiveness of therapy.
⬩ Atracurium besylate does not affect consciousness, pain threshold, or cerebration. Administer adequate sedatives and analgesics before giving atracurium besylate.
⬩ Atracurium besylate produces paralysis. Provide oral and skin care. Administer artifical tears to protect corneas. May need to tape eyes closed. Position patient appropriately.
⬩ Use infusion within 24 h of mixing.

◉ atropine sulfate *(a' troe peen)*
Pregnancy Category C

Drug classes
Anticholinergic
Antimuscarinic
Parasympatholytic
Antiparkinsonism drug
Antidote

Indications
⬩ Antidote (with external cardiac massage) for cardiovascular collapse from the injudicious use of a cholinergic drug, pilocarpine, physostigmine, or isoflurophate
⬩ Treatment of severe bradycardia and syncope due to a hyperactive carotid sinus reflex
⬩ Relief of AV heart block when increased vagal tone is a major factor in the conduction defect as in some cases due to digitalis toxicity
⬩ Treatment of closed head injuries that cause acetylcholine to be released or to be present in cerebrospinal fluid, which in turn causes abnormal EEG patterns, stupor, and abnormal neurologic signs
⬩ Antisialogogue for preanesthetic medication to prevent or reduce respiratory tract secretions
⬩ Management of peptic ulcer
⬩ Treatment of anticholinesterase poisoning from organophosphorus insecticides; antidote for mushroom poisoning due to muscarine

Adverse effects in *Italics* are most common; those in **Bold** are life-threatening

- Treatment of parkinsonism; relieves tremor and rigidity
- Relief of pylorospasm, hypertonicity of small intestine and hypermotility of colon
- Relief of biliary and ureteral colic and bronchial spasm
- Diminishment of the tone of detrusor muscle of urinary bladder in treatment of urinary tract disorders
- Control of the crying and laughing episodes in patients with brain lesions

Therapeutic actions
- Inhibits muscarinic actions of acetylcholine at postganglionic parasympathetic neuroeffector sites, including smooth muscle, secretory glands, and CNS sites
- Small doses inhibit salivary and bronchial secretions and sweating
- Moderate doses dilate pupils, inhibit accommodation, and increase HR
- Larger doses decrease motility of GI and urinary tracts
- Very large doses inhibit gastric acid secretion

Effects on hemodynamic parameters
- Increased HR (moderate doses)

Contraindications/cautions
- **Contraindications:** atropine or anticholinergic drug allergy, narrow-angle glaucoma, adhesions between iris and lens, tachycardia, myocardial ischemia, unstable cardiovascular status in acute hemorrhage, asthma, myasthenia gravis, achalasia, pyloroduodenal stenosis, pyloric obstruction, paralytic ileus, intestinal atony of elderly or debilitated patients, severe ulcerative colitis, toxic megacolon, hepatic disease
- **Cautions:** elderly or debilitated patients, febrile patients, type II AV block, new third-degree heart block, renal disease, prostatic hypertrophy, prostatism, coronary artery disease, CHF, dysrhythmias, hypertension, chronic lung disease, hyperthyroidism, autonomic neuropathy, Down syndrome, spastic paralysis, brain damage

Available forms
- *Injection:* 0.05, 0.1, 0.3, 0.4, 0.5, 0.8, 1 mg/mL
- *Tablets:* 0.4 mg

IV/IM/SC/endotracheal facts
Preparation
- Give undiluted or dilute in 10 mL Sterile Water for Injection.

Adverse effects in *Italics* are most common; those in **Bold** are life-threatening

A

Dosage
- *Bradycardia and heart block in advanced cardiac life support:* 0.5–1 mg IVP. Repeat in 3–5 min up to total of 0.04 mg/kg.
- *Ventricular asystole in advanced cardiac life support:* 1 mg IVP. Repeat in 3–5 min up to total of 0.04 mg/kg.
- *Cardiac arrest (endotracheal administration):* Give 1–2 mg diluted in 10 mL of sterile water or normal saline.
- *Systemic administration:* 0.4–0.6 mg IV, IM, or SC.
- *Surgery:* 0.5 mg (0.4–0.6 mg) IV, IM, or SC prior to induction of anesthesia.
- *Reversal of muscarinic blockade of anticholinesterases:* 0.6–1.2 mg IV for each 0.5–2.5 mg of neostigmine methylsulfate or 10–20 mg of pyridostigmine bromide.
- *Poisoning:* For poisoning due to cholinesterase inhibitor insecticides, give at least 2–3 mg parenterally and repeat until signs of atropine intoxication appear. For "rapid" type of mushroom poisoning, give in doses sufficient to control parasympathetic signs before coma and CV collapse supervene.

Compatibility
Atropine may be given through the same IV line as amrinone, etomidate, famotidine, heparin, hydrocortisone, meropenem, nafcillin, potassium choride, sufentanil, vitamin B complex with C.

Incompatibility
Do not administer through the same IV line as sodium bicarbonate, norepinephrine, metaraminol, thiopental.

> ### TREATMENT OF OVERDOSE/ANTIDOTE
> Discontinue drug or decrease dosage. Initiate general supportive and resuscitative measures. May administer neostigmine methylsulfate 0.25–2.5 mg IV and repeat as needed. Physostigmine 0.2–0.4 mg by slow IV injection (may repeat as needed up to 6 mg) has been used to reverse anticholinergic effects. Treat fever with physical cooling measures.

Pharmacokinetics
Route	Onset	Peak	Duration
IV	Immediate	2–4 min	4–6 h
IM	10–15 min	30 min	4 h
SC	Varies	1–2 h	4 h

Metabolism: Hepatic; $T_{1/2}$: 2.5 h
Excretion: Urine

Adverse effects in *Italics* are most common; those in **Bold** are life-threatening

Adverse effects

▸ *CNS: Blurred vision, mydriasis, cycloplegia, photophobia,* increased intraocular pressure, headache, flushing, nervousness, weakness, dizziness, insomnia, mental confusion or excitement (after even small doses in the elderly)
▸ *CV: Palpitations, bradycardia (low doses), tachycardia (high doses)*
▸ *GI: Dry mouth, altered taste perception, nausea,* vomiting, dysphagia, heartburn, constipation, bloated feeling, paralytic ileus, gastroesophageal reflux
▸ *GU: Urinary hesitancy and retention,* impotence
▸ *Allergic:* **Anaphylaxis**
▸ *Misc:* Nasal congestion, decreased sweating

Clinically important drug–drug interactions

▸ Increased anticholinergic effects with other anticholinergics, TCAs, certain antihistamines, certain antiparkinsonian drugs, MAO inhibitors
▸ Decreased effectiveness of phenothiazines but increased incidence of paralytic ileus
▸ Decreased antipsychotic effectiveness of haloperidol with atropine

● NURSING CONSIDERATIONS

Assessment

▸ *History:* Atropine or anticholinergic drug allergy, narrow-angle glaucoma, adhesions between iris and lens, tachycardia, myocardial ischemia, unstable cardiovascular status in acute hemorrhage, asthma, myasthenia gravis, achalasia, pyloroduodenal stenosis, pyloric obstruction, paralytic ileus, intestinal atony of elderly or debilitated patients, severe ulcerative colitis, toxic megacolon, hepatic disease, renal disease, prostatic hypertrophy, prostatism, coronary artery disease, CHF, dysrhythmias, hypertension, chronic lung disease, hyperthyroidism, autonomic neuropathy, Down syndrome, spastic paralysis, brain damage, previous drug ingestion
▸ *Physical:* T, P, BP, R, ECG, I & O, IV site, weight, neurologic checks, reflexes, ophthalmologic exam, adventitious lung sounds, bowel sounds, prostate palpation, liver and renal function tests

Implementation

▸ Carefully monitor patient's HR, BP, and ECG during the course of therapy.
▸ Have emergency equipment (defibrillator, drugs, oxygen, intubation equipment) on standby in case anaphylaxis or adverse reaction occurs.

Adverse effects in *Italics* are most common; those in **Bold** are life-threatening

▶ Assess for urinary retention; insert Foley catheter as needed.
▶ Ensure adequate hydration; prevent high fever by providing environmental control.
▶ Drug affects pupil size; pupil size not a reliable diagnostic sign.

B

⬤ **bretylium tosylate** *(bre til' ee um)* Bretylol, Bretylate (CAN)

Pregnancy Category C

Drug classes
Antidysrhythmic
Adrenergic neuronal blocker

Indications
▶ Prophylaxis and therapy of ventricular fibrillation
▶ Treatment of life-threatening ventricular dysrhythmias (ventricular tachycardia and fibrillation) that are resistant to first-line antidysrhythmics (lidocaine)
▶ Unlabeled use: second-line agent for advanced cardiac life support during CPR

Therapeutic actions
▶ Type II antidysrhythmic: prolongs repolarization, prolongs refractory period, increases ventricular fibrillation threshold, increases automaticity

Effects on hemodynamic parameters
▶ Mildly increased arterial BP followed by a modest decrease in arterial BP

Contraindications/cautions
▶ **Contraindications:** bretylium is used in life-threatening conditions, benefits usually outweigh any possible risks of therapy
▶ **Cautions:** hypotension, renal disease, severe aortic stenosis, severe pulmonary HTN; use for digitalized patients only if etiology of dysrhythmia does not appear to be digitalis toxicity and other antidysrhythmic drugs are not effective

Available forms
▶ *IV injection:* 50 mg/mL
▶ *Premixed IV infusion:* 500 mg (2 mg/mL) and 1000 mg (4 mg/mL) in 250 mL D5W

Adverse effects in *Italics* are most common; those in **Bold** are life-threatening

IV/IM facts
Preparation
▸ If a premixed IV infusion is not available, add 1–2 g bretylium to 250–500 mL of Calcium Chloride (54.4 mEq/L) in D5W; D5W/LR; D5W/0.45%NS; D5W/0.9%NS; D5W with 40 mEq potassium/L; D5W; LR; Mannitol 20%; 0.9%NS; Sodium Bicarbonate 5%; or Sodium Lactate (1/6 Molar) Injection. For fluid restricted patients, add 400 mg bretylium to 50 mL (8 mg/mL) of a compatible IV fluid.
▸ For IM use, give undiluted.

Dosage and titration
▸ *Immediate life-threatening dysrhythmias:* **Initial dose:** 5 mg/kg undiluted by rapid IV injection. If dysrhythmia persists, increase dosage to 10 mg/kg and repeat as necessary. **Maintenance dose:** 1–2 mg/min IV or 5–10 mg/kg over > 8 min q6h.
▸ *Other ventricular dysrhythmias:* **Initial dose:** 5–10 mg/kg IV over > 8 min. Give subsequent doses at 1- to 2-h intervals if dysrhythmia persists. **Maintenance dose:** Give the same dosage q6h or continuous infusion of 1–2 mg/min.
▸ *IM dosage:* **Initial dose:** 5–10 mg/kg IM. Give subsequent doses at 1- to 2-h intervals if dysrhythmia persists. **Maintenance dose:** Give the same dosage q6–8h. Do not give > 5 mL in any one site. Do not inject into or near a major nerve. Rotate injection sites. Repeated injection into the same site may cause atrophy and necrosis of muscle tissue, fibrosis, vascular degeneration, and inflammatory changes.

Titration Guide

bretylium tosylate	
2 g in 250 mL	
mg/min	mL/h
1	8
2	15

Therapeutic serum level
▸ 0.5–1.5 mcg/mL

Compatibility
Bretylium tosylate may be given through the same IV line as amiodarone, amrinone, diltiazem, dobutamine, famotidine, isoproterenol, ranitidine.

Incompatibility
Do not administer through the same IV line as propofol or warfarin.

Adverse effects in *Italics* are most common; those in **Bold** are life-threatening

TREATMENT OF OVERDOSE/ANTIDOTE
Decrease infusion rate or temporarily discontinue infusion until patient is stabilized. Treat initial hypertension with nitroprusside or another short-acting IV antihypertensive agent. Do not use long-acting drugs that may potentiate hypotensive effects of bretylium. Treat hypotension with fluid therapy, dopamine, and norepinephrine.

Pharmacokinetics

Route	Onset	Peak	Duration
IV (V-fibrillation)	5 min		24 h
IV (V-tach, PVCs)	20 min–2 h		24 h
IM	Varies	6–9 h	

$T_{1/2}$: 6.9–8.1 h
Excretion: Urine

Adverse effects

◗ *CNS:* Vertigo, dizziness, lightheadedness, syncope
◗ *CV: Hypotension, postural hypotension,* transient hypertension, dysrhythmias, CHF, angina, substernal pressure
◗ *GI: Nausea, vomiting* (with rapid IV administration)

Clinically important drug–drug interactions

◗ Increased digitalis toxicity
◗ Increased pressor effects of dopamine, norepinephrine, catecholamines

◉ NURSING CONSIDERATIONS

Assessment

◗ *History:* Hypotension, renal disease, severe aortic stenosis, severe pulmonary HTN, use of digitalis glycosides
◗ *Physical:* T, P, BP, R, ECG, I & O, IV site, weight, chest pain assessment, neurologic checks, skin assessment, peripheral pulses, orthostatic BP, adventitious lung sounds

Implementation

◗ Exercise extreme caution when calculating and preparing doses; bretylium is a very potent drug; small dosage errors can cause serious adverse effects.
◗ Always administer infusion using an IV pump.
◗ Drug is for short-term use only.
◗ Keep patient supine during therapy and monitor for postural hypotension.
◗ Change patient to oral antidysrhythmic therapy as soon as possible.

Adverse effects in *Italics* are most common; those in **Bold** are life-threatening

▸ Increase dosage interval for patients with renal failure.
▸ Protect patient's airway if emesis occurs.

● bumetanide (byoo met' a nide) Bumex, Burinex (CAN)
Pregnancy Category C

Drug class
Loop diuretic

Indications
▸ Edema associated with CHF, cirrhosis, renal disease (including nephrotic syndrome)
▸ Acute pulmonary edema (IV)
▸ Unlabeled use: treatment of adult nocturia

Therapeutic actions
▸ Inhibits the reabsorption of sodium and chloride from the ascending limb of the loop of Henle
▸ Increases potassium excretion
▸ Decreases uric acid excretion and increases serum uric acid
▸ Affects phosphate reabsorption in proximal tubule, leading to phosphaturia

Contraindications/cautions
▸ **Contraindications:** bumetanide or sulfonamide allergy, electrolyte depletion, anuria, severe renal failure, hepatic coma
▸ **Cautions:** SLE, gout, diabetes mellitus, hypercholesteremia, sulfonamide sensitivity

Available forms
▸ *Injection:* 0.25 mg/mL
▸ *Tablets:* 0.5, 1, 2 mg

IV/IM facts
Preparation
▸ May be given undiluted or diluted in D5W; LR; or 0.9%NS.

Dosage
▸ Use only for patients with impaired GI absorption or who cannot take oral form. Begin oral therapy as soon as possible.
▸ 0.5–1 mg IV over 1–2 min or IM. If response insufficient, give a second or third dose at 2- to 3-h intervals. Do not exceed 10 mg/d.
▸ *Renal function impairment:* Continuous infusion of 12 mg IV over 12 h may be more effective and less toxic than intermittent bolus therapy.

Adverse effects in *Italics* are most common; those in **Bold** are life-threatening

B

Compatibility
Bumetanide may be given through the same IV line as allopurinol, amifostine, aztreonam, cefepime, cladribine, diltiazem, filgrastim, granisetron, lorazepam, melphalan, meperidine, morphine, piperacillin-tazobactam, propofol, teniposide, thiotepa, vinorelbine.

Incompatibility
Do not administer through the same IV line as midazolam.

Oral dosage
▶ 0.5–2 mg/d PO as a single dose. If diuretic response not adequate, give a second or third dose at 4- to 5-h intervals, up to 10 mg/d. Intermittent dosage schedule: give on alternate days or for 3–4 d with rest periods of 1–2 d between; safest and most effective for ongoing control of edema.

> **TREATMENT OF OVERDOSE/ANTIDOTE**
> Discontinue drug or decrease dosage. Initiate general supportive and resuscitative measures. Replace fluid and electrolyte losses. Carefully monitor urine and electrolyte output and serum electrolyte levels.

Pharmacokinetics
Route	Onset	Peak	Duration
IV	Minutes	15–30 min	0.5–1 h
Oral	30–60 min	60–120 min	4–6 h

Metabolism: Liver, $T_{1/2}$: 60–90 min (prolonged in renal disease)
Excretion: Urine

Adverse effects
▶ *CNS: Headache, encephalopathy, dizziness,* vertigo, paresthesias, fatigue, weakness, asterixis, drowsiness, fatigue, blurred vision, tinnitus, irreversible hearing loss
▶ *CV:* **Circulatory collapse,** *hypotension,* ECG changes, dehydration, cardiac arrhythmias, thrombophlebitis, chest pain
▶ *GI: Nausea,* anorexia, vomiting, diarrhea, abdominal pain, gastric irritation and pain, dry mouth, acute pancreatitis, jaundice
▶ *GU:* **Renal failure,** polyuria, nocturia, glycosuria, increased BUN and creatinine
▶ *Hematologic:* **Thrombocytopenia,** leukopenia, anemia
▶ *Derm:* Pain, phlebitis at injection site
▶ *Fluid/electrolytes: Hypochloremia, hypokalemia, hyponatremia, hypomagnesemia, hypocalcemia*
▶ *Misc: Muscle cramps,* metabolic alkalosis, hyperventilation,

Adverse effects in *Italics* are most common; those in **Bold** are life-threatening

arthritic pain, fatigue, hives, photosensitivity, rash, pruritus, sweating, nipple tenderness, premature ejaculation, difficulty maintaining erection, hyperglycemia, azotemia

Clinically important drug–drug interactions

▸ Decreased diuresis and natriuresis with NSAIDs
▸ Increased cardiac glycoside toxicity (secondary to hypokalemia)
▸ Increased ototoxicity if taken with aminoglycoside antibiotics, cisplatin
▸ Increased lithium toxicity
▸ Reduced natriuresis and hyperreninemia with probenecid
▸ Decreased urine and sodium excretion with indomethacin
▸ Enhanced effects of antihypertensives
▸ Increased profound diuresis and serious electrolyte abnormalities with thiazide diuretics

◉ NURSING CONSIDERATIONS

Assessment

▸ *History:* Bumetanide allergy, electrolyte depletion, anuria, severe renal failure, hepatic coma, SLE, gout, diabetes mellitus, hypercholesteremia
▸ *Physical:* P, R, BP, ECG, I & O, weight, neurologic checks, skin assessment, skin turgor, mucous membranes, edema, hearing, peripheral perfusion, orthostatic BP, respiratory effort, adventitious lung sounds, liver evaluation, bowel sounds, CBC, serum electrolytes (including calcium), serum glucose, liver and renal function tests, uric acid, UA, urine electrolytes

Implementation

▸ Closely monitor serum electrolytes, liver function, and CBC.
▸ Give with food or milk to prevent GI upset.
▸ Give single dose early in day so increased urination will not disturb sleep.
▸ Minimize postural hypotension by helping the patient change positions slowly.
▸ Evaluate for hypokalemia as evidenced by muscle weakness, fatigue, paralytic ileus, ECG changes, anorexia, nausea, vomiting, abdominal distention, dizziness, polyuria.
▸ Carefully assess fluid balance. Too frequent administration may lead to profound water loss, electrolyte depletion, dehydration, reduced blood volume, or circulatory collapse with possible vascular thrombosis and embolism.
▸ Provide diet rich in potassium or give supplemental potassium.
▸ Use diluted solution within 24 h.

Adverse effects in *Italics* are most common; those in **Bold** are life-threatening

C

● calcium chloride *(kal' see um klor' ride)*

Pregnancy Category C

Drug class
Electrolyte

Indications
▶ Treatment in cardiac resuscitation, particularly after open heart surgery, when epinephrine fails to improve weak or ineffective myocardial contractions
▶ To reverse severe hyperkalemia as evidenced on ECG, pending correction of increased potassium in the extracellular fluid
▶ Treatment of hypocalcemia associated with tetany due to parathyroid deficiency, vitamin D deficiency, or alkalosis
▶ Prevention of hypocalcemia during exchange transfusions
▶ Adjunctive therapy in treatment of insect bites or stings, such as black widow spider bites, to relieve muscle cramping
▶ Treatment of sensitivity reactions characterized by urticaria
▶ Treatment of acute symptoms of lead colic, rickets, or osteomalacia

Therapeutic actions
▶ Is an essential element needed for functional integrity of nervous and muscular systems, cardiac contractility, and coagulation
▶ Is an enzyme cofactor and affects the secretory activity of endocrine and exocrine glands
▶ Increases cardiac contractility in hypocalcemia
▶ Decreases cardiac effects of hyperkalemia
▶ Decreases adverse neuromuscular effects of hypermagnesemia

Effects on hemodynamic parameters
▶ Increased or decreased SVR
▶ Increased BP
▶ Increased CO

Contraindications/cautions
▶ **Contraindications:** calcium allergy, renal calculi, hypercalcemia, ventricular fibrillation, digitalized patients
▶ **Caution:** hypocalcemia of renal insufficiency

Available form
▶ *Injection:* 10%–13.6 mEq/g; 27.3% calcium

Adverse effects in *Italics* are most common; those in **Bold** are life-threatening

IV/intraventricular facts
Preparation
▸ Warm solution to body temperature in nonemergencies.
▸ May be undiluted or diluted in D5W/LR; D5W/0.25%NS; D5W/0.45%NS; D5W/0.9%NS; D5W; D10W; or 0.9%NS.
▸ Calcium chloride is for IV or intraventricular use only.

Dosage
▸ Do not inject at a rate exceeding 0.5–1 mL/min.
▸ *Cardiac resuscitation:* 7–14 mEq IV.
▸ *Intraventricular dose:* 3–11 mEq injected into the ventricular cavity. Do not inject into the myocardium.
▸ *Hypocalcemic disorders:* 7–14 mEq IV q1–3d depending on patient's response. Repeated injections may be necessary.
▸ *Hyperkalemic ECG disturbances of cardiac function:* Adjust dosage by constant monitoring of ECG changes during administration.
▸ *Magnesium toxicity:* 7 mEq IV promptly. Observe patient for signs of recovery before giving additional doses.
▸ *Hypocalcemic tetany:* 4.5–16 mEq IV. Repeat until positive response occurs.

Normal calcium level
▸ 8.5–10.5 mg/dL

Compatibility
Calcium chloride may be given through the same IV line as amrinone, dobutamine, epinephrine, esmolol, morphine, paclitaxel.

Incompatibility
Do not administer through the same IV line as phosphates, propofol, sodium bicarbonate, soluble carbonates, sulfates, tartrates.

> **TREATMENT OF OVERDOSE/ANTIDOTE**
> Discontinue drug or decrease dosage. Initiate general supportive and resuscitative measures. Infuse sodium chloride and administer a potent natriuretic agent, such as furosemide.

Pharmacokinetics

Route	Onset	Peak	Duration
IV	Immediate	3–5 min	30–120 min

Excretion: Feces, urine

Adverse effects
▸ *CNS:* Tingling
▸ *CV:* **Cardiac arrest, dysrhythmias,** *bradycardia,* syncope, peripheral vasodilation, decreased BP

Adverse effects in *Italics* are most common; those in **Bold** are life-threatening

- **GI:** *Constipation;* metallic, calcium, or chalky taste
- **Misc:** *Phlebitis at IV site,* extravasation with necrosis, pain at IV site, sense of oppression or "heat waves"

Clinically important drug–drug interactions
- Increased hypercalcemia related to bone release of calcium and decreased calcium excretion with thiazide diuretics
- Decreased mean peak plasma levels and bioavailability of atenolol
- Increased dysrhythmias and digitalis toxicity with digitalis glycoside
- Reversed clinical effects and toxicities with verapamil
- Patients with renal failure who receive sodium polystyrene sulfonate and calcium may experience metabolic alkalosis and reduced potassium binding capacity

⬤ NURSING CONSIDERATIONS

Assessment
- *History:* Calcium allergy, renal calculi, ventricular fibrillation, digitalis use, renal insufficiency
- *Physical:* T, P, BP, R, ECG, I & O, IV site, neurologic checks, reflexes, adventitious lung sounds, renal function tests, serum electrolytes, digitalis level, UA

Implementation
- Carefully monitor patient's HR, BP, ECG, and serum electrolytes during the course of therapy.
- Carefully monitor patient's IV site. Avoid infiltration because it may cause tissue necrosis and sloughing. Use a small needle in a large vein. Use a central line if possible.
- ECG: hypocalcemia may be evidenced by a long QT interval; T wave may become flattened or inverted; hypercalcemia may be evidenced by a short QT interval; QRS may be prolonged.
- Keep patient supine 30–60 min after IV injection.
- Assess for hypocalcemia as evidenced by Chvostek's or Trousseau's signs, muscle twitching, laryngospasm, or paresthesias.
- Assess for toxicity as evidenced by markedly elevated plasma calcium level, weakness, lethargy, intractable nausea, vomiting, or coma.
- Do not use interchangeably with calcium gluconate.

⬤ **calcium gluconate** *(kal' see um gloo' koh nate)*
Pregnancy Category C

Drug class
Electrolyte

Indications

▶ Treatment of hypocalcemia associated with tetany due to parathyroid deficiency, vitamin D deficiency, or alkalosis
▶ Prevention of hypocalcemia during exchange transfusions
▶ Adjunctive therapy in treatment of insect bites or stings, such as black widow spider bites, to relieve muscle cramping
▶ Treatment of sensitivity reactions characterized by urticaria
▶ Treatment of acute symptoms of lead colic, rickets, or osteomalacia
▶ To decrease in capillary permeability in allergic conditions, nonthrombocytopenic purpura, and exudative dermatoses, such as dermatitis herpetiformis
▶ Treatment of cardiac toxicity associated with hyperkalemia if patient is not receiving digitalis therapy

Therapeutic actions

▶ Is an essential element needed for functional integrity of nervous and muscular systems, cardiac contractility, and coagulation
▶ Is an enzyme cofactor; affects the secretory activity of endocrine and exocrine glands
▶ Increases cardiac contractility in hypocalcemia
▶ Decreases cardiac effects of hyperkalemia
▶ Decreases adverse neuromuscular effects of hypermagnesemia

Effects on hemodynamic parameters

▶ Increased or decreased SVR
▶ Increased BP
▶ Increased CO

Contraindications

▶ **Contraindications:** calcium allergy, renal calculi, hypercalcemia, ventricular fibrillation, digitalized patients

Available forms

▶ *Injection:* 10%–4.65 mEq/g; 9.3% calcium
▶ *Tablets:* 500, 650, 975 mg; 1 g; 9.3% calcium

IV facts
Preparation

▶ Warm solution to body temperature in nonemergencies.
▶ May be undiluted or diluted in D5W/LR; D5W/0.18%NS; D5W/0.45%NS; D5W/0.9%NS; D5W; D10W; D20W; LR; 0.9%NS; 3%NS; Polysal M with Dextrose 5%; or Sodium Lactate (1/6 Molar) Injection.

Dosage

▶ Do not give by direct IV injection faster than 0.5–2 mL/min. When giving by intermittent or continuous infusion, do not

Adverse effects in *Italics* are most common; those in **Bold** are life-threatening

exceed 200 mg/min. An infusion is preferred over direct IV injection.

- 2.3–9.3 mEq as required. Daily dose range is 4.65–70 mEq IV.
- *Emergency treatment for hypocalcemia:* 7–14 mEq IV.
- *Hyperkalemia with secondary cardiac toxicity:* 2.25–14 mEq IV while monitoring the ECG. If needed, repeat doses after 1 to 2 min.
- *Magnesium toxicity:* 4.5–9 mEq IV. Adjust subsequent doses to patient response.
- *Hypocalcemic tetany:* 4.5–16 mEq IV. Repeat until positive response occurs.
- *Exchange transfusion:* 1.35 mEq IV concurrent with each 100 mL of citrated blood.

Normal calcium level
- 8.5–10.5 mg/dL

Compatibility
Calcium gluconate may be given through the same IV line as allopurinol, aztreonam, cefepime, ciprofloxacin, dobutamine, enalaprilat, epinephrine, famotidine, filgrastim, heparin with hydrocortisone, labetalol, melphalan, netilmicin, piperacillin-tazobactam, potassium chloride, sargramostim, tacrolimus, teniposide, tolazoline, vinorelbine.

Incompatibility
Do not administer through the same IV line as cefamandole, cefazolin, cephalothin, cephradine, citrates, fluconazole, indomethacin sodium trihydrate, sodium bicarbonate, soluble carbonates, phosphates, sulfates.

Oral dosage
- 500–2000 mg PO bid–qid.

TREATMENT OF OVERDOSE/ANTIDOTE
Discontinue drug or decrease dosage. Initiate general supportive and resuscitative measures. Infuse sodium chloride, and administer a potent natriuretic agent, such as furosemide.

Pharmacokinetics

Route	Onset	Peak	Duration
IV	Immediate	Immediate	30–120 min

Excretion: Feces, urine

Adverse effects
- *CNS:* Tingling

Adverse effects in *Italics* are most common; those in **Bold** are life-threatening

▸ *CV:* **Cardiac arrest, dysrhythmias,** *bradycardia,* syncope, peripheral vasodilation, decreased BP
▸ *GI: Constipation;* metallic, calcium, or chalky taste
▸ *Misc: Phlebitis at IV site,* extravasation with necrosis, pain at IV site, sense of oppression or "heat waves"

Clinically important drug–drug interactions
▸ Hypercalcemia related to bone release of calcium and decreased calcium excretion with thiazide diuretics
▸ Decreased mean peak plasma levels and bioavailability of atenolol
▸ Dysrhythmias and digitalis toxicity with digitalis glycosides
▸ Reversed clinical effects and toxicities of verapamil
▸ Patients with renal failure who receive sodium polystyrene sulfonate and calcium may experience metabolic alkalosis and reduced potassium-binding capacity

● NURSING CONSIDERATIONS

Assessment
▸ *History:* Calcium allergy, renal calculi, digitalis use
▸ *Physical:* T, P, BP, R, ECG, I & O, IV site, neurologic checks, reflexes, adventitious lung sounds, renal function tests, serum electrolytes, digitalis level, UA

Implementation
▸ Carefully monitor patient's HR, BP, ECG, and serum electrolytes during the course of therapy.
▸ Carefully monitor patient's IV site. Avoid infiltration because it may cause necrosis and sloughing. Use a small needle in a large vein. Use a central line if possible.
▸ ECG: hypocalcemia may be evidenced by a long QT interval; T wave may become flattened or inverted; hypercalcemia may be evidenced by a short QT interval; QRS may be prolonged.
▸ Keep patient supine for 30–60 min after IV injection.
▸ Assess for hypocalcemia as evidenced by Chvostek's or Trousseau's signs, muscle twitching, laryngospasm, or paresthesias.
▸ Assess for toxicity as evidenced by markedly elevated plasma calcium level, weakness, lethargy, intractable nausea, vomiting, or coma.
▸ Calcium gluconate is preferred over calcium chloride because it is less irritating.
▸ Do not use interchangeably with calcium chloride.

Adverse effects in *Italics* are most common; those in **Bold** are life-threatening

◉ captopril *(kap' toe pril)* Apo-Capto (CAN), Capoten, Gen-Captopril (CAN), Novo-Captopril (CAN), Nu-Capto (CAN)

**Pregnancy Category C (first trimester)
and D (second and third trimesters)**

Drug classes
Angiotensin-converting enzyme (ACE) inhibitor
Antihypertensive

Indications
▸ Treatment of hypertension alone or with thiazide diuretics
▸ Treatment of heart failure in patients unresponsive to diuretic and digitalis therapy; used with diuretics and digitalis
▸ Treatment of left ventricular dysfunction after myocardial infarction (MI)
▸ Treatment of diabetic nephropathy
▸ Unlabeled uses: treatment of hypertensive crisis, rheumatoid arthritis, hypertension related to scleroderma renal crisis, idiopathic edema, Batter's syndrome, Raynaud's syndrome; diagnosis of anatomic renal artery stenosis, renovascular hypertension, primary aldosteronism

Therapeutic actions
▸ Suppresses renin-angiotensin-aldosterone system; blocks ACE from converting angiotensin I to angiotensin II, a powerful vasoconstrictor; leads to decreased blood pressure, decreased aldosterone secretion, a small increase in serum potassium levels, and sodium and fluid loss
▸ Increased prostaglandin synthesis also may be involved in the antihypertensive action

Effects on hemodynamic parameters
▸ Decreased BP
▸ Decreased SVR/PVR
▸ Decreased PCWP
▸ Increased CO

> **Contraindications/cautions**
> ▸ **Contraindications:** captopril allergy, angioedema related to previous treatment with an ACE inhibitor
> ▸ **Cautions:** neutropenia, agranulocytosis, salt/volume depletion, impaired renal function

Available forms
▸ *Tablets:* 12.5, 25, 50, 100 mg

Adverse effects in *Italics* are most common; those in **Bold** are life-threatening

Oral dosage

▸ *Accelerated or malignant hypertension:* Discontinue other antihypertensive therapy. Give captopril 25 mg PO bid or tid. Under close supervision, increase dose q24h until desired response is achieved.

▸ *Hypertension:* 25 mg PO bid or tid. If satisfactory response is not noted within 1–2 wk, increase to 50 mg PO bid or tid. If blood pressure is not controlled, add a thiazide diuretic and increase captopril dosage at 1- to 2-wk intervals until highest usual antihypertensive dose is reached. Usual dose is 25–150 mg bid or tid. Do not exceed 450 mg/d.

▸ *CHF:* 6.25–12.5 mg PO tid for patients with normal or low blood pressure who are on diuretics or who are hyponatremic or hypovolemic. Titrate dose to achieve intended effects. Usual dose is 50–100 mg PO tid. Do not exceed 450 mg/d. Use in conjunction with diuretic and digitalis therapy.

▸ *Left ventricular dysfunction after MI:* Start as early as 3 d after MI. Give 6.25 mg PO, then 12.5 mg PO tid. Increase to 25 mg PO tid over next several days to target dose of 50 mg tid.

▸ *Diabetic nephropathy:* 25 mg PO tid. May use in conjunction with diuretics, beta-blockers, vasodilators, other antihypertensives.

▸ *Patients with renal impairment:* Excretion is reduced in renal failure, so patients may respond to smaller, less frequent doses. Reduce initial dosage; titrate dosage over 1- to 2-wk interval to smallest effective dose. Use a loop diuretic if diuretic therapy is needed.

> **TREATMENT OF OVERDOSE/ANTIDOTE**
> Discontinue drug or decrease dosage. Initiate general supportive and resuscitative measures. Initiate IV infusion of normal saline to treat hypotension. Treat anaphylaxis or angioedema with epinephrine and maintain a patent airway. May be removed by hemodialysis.

Pharmacokinetics

Route	Onset	Peak	Duration
Oral	15–30 min	30–90 min	6–12 h

$T_{1/2}$: <2 h
Excretion: Urine

Adverse effects

▸ *CNS:* **CVA,** *insomnia, sleep disturbances, paresthesias, headache, dizziness, fatigue, malaise,* somnolence, ataxia, confusion, depression, nervousness

---

Adverse effects in *Italics* are most common; those in **Bold** are life-threatening

▶ **CV: AMI, cardiac arrest,** *palpitations, tachycardia,* dysrhythmias, chest pain, CHF, orthostatic hypotension, hypotension, Raynaud's syndrome, cerebrovascular insufficiency, syncope
▶ **Resp:** *Cough, dyspnea,* asthma, bronchospasm, rhinitis, eosinophilic pneumonitis
▶ **GI:** *Dysgeusia, gastric irritation, aphthous ulcers, peptic ulcer,* glossitis, taste loss, weight loss, jaundice, cholestasis, vomiting, nausea, diarrhea, anorexia, constipation, dry mouth pancreatitis
▶ **GU:** *Proteinuria,* oliguria, nephrotic syndrome, polyuria, urinary frequency, worsening renal failure, azotemia, increased BUN and creatinine, impotence
▶ **Derm: Stevens-Johnson syndrome,** *rash, pruritus,* pallor, alopecia, flushing
▶ **Hematologic: Neutropenia, agranulocytosis**
▶ **Allergic: Anaphylaxis, angioedema**
▶ **Misc:** Gynecomastia, asthenia, blurred vision, fever, myalgia, arthralgia, vasculitis, positive ANA titer

Clinically important drug–drug interactions
▶ Decreased bioavailability of captopril when used within 2 h of antacids
▶ Decreased hypotensive effects when used with indomethacin
▶ Increased effects with phenothiazines
▶ Increased blood levels and decreased total clearance when used with probenecid
▶ Increased hypersensitivity reactions when given with allopurinol
▶ Increased digoxin and lithium toxicity
▶ Increased hyperkalemia with potassium, potassium-sparing diuretics
▶ Increased severe hypotension when patient is on diuretic therapy, salt-restricted diet, or dialysis
▶ Enhanced by vasodilator drugs, such as nitroglycerin or nitrates; if possible, discontinue these drugs before starting captopril

● NURSING CONSIDERATIONS
Assessment
▶ *History:* Captopril or other ACE inhibitor allergy, neutropenia, agranulocytosis, salt/volume depletion, impaired renal function
▶ *Physical:* P, BP, R, ECG, I & O, weight, neurologic checks, vision assessment, cardiac auscultation, edema, skin assessment, adventitious lung sounds, orthostatic BP, bowel sounds, serum electrolytes, liver and renal function tests, UA, CBC

Adverse effects in *Italics* are most common; those in **Bold** are life-threatening

Implementation
- Monitor patient closely for hypotension secondary to reduced fluid volume (excessive perspiration and dehydration, vomiting, diarrhea); excessive hypotension may occur.
- Administer 1 h before meals.
- Change patient's position slowly to avoid postural hypotension.
- Have emergency equipment (defibrillator, drugs, oxygen, intubation equipment) on standby in case anaphylaxis or adverse reaction occurs.
- Alert surgeon and mark patient's chart with notice that captopril is being taken; the angiotensin II formation subsequent to compensatory renin release during surgery will be blocked; hypotension may be reversed with volume expansion.

⬤ cefazolin sodium *(sef a' zoe lin)* Ancef, Kefzol, Zolicef

Pregnancy Category B

Drug classes
Antibiotic: cephalosporin (first generation)

Indications
- Respiratory tract infections caused by *Streptococcus pneumoniae, Staphylococcus aureus,* group A β-hemolytic streptococci, *Klebsiella* species, *Haemophilus influenzae*
- Dermatologic infections caused by *S. aureus,* group A β-hemolytic streptococci, other strains of streptococci
- GU infections caused by *Escherichia coli, Proteus mirabilis, Klebsiella* species, sensitive strains of enterobacter, and enterococci
- Biliary tract infections caused by *E. coli,* streptococci, *P. mirabilis, Klebsiella* species, *S. aureus*
- Septicemia caused by *S. pneumoniae, S. aureus, E. coli, P. mirabilis, Klebsiella* species
- Bone and joint infections caused by *S. aureus*
- Genital infections caused by *E. coli, P. mirabilis, Klebsiella* species, sensitive strains of enterococci
- Endocarditis caused by *S. aureus,* group A β-hemolytic streptococci
- Preoperative or postoperative prophylaxis

Therapeutic actions
- Bactericidal: inhibits synthesis of bacterial cell wall, causing cell death

Adverse effects in *Italics* are most common; those in **Bold** are life-threatening

Contraindications/cautions
▶ **Contraindications:** allergy to cephalosporins
▶ **Cautions:** allergy to penicillin, impaired renal function

Available forms
▶ *Powder for injection:* 250, 500 mg; 1, 5, 10, 20 g
▶ *Premixed frozen injection:* 500 mg, 1 g

IV/IM facts
Preparation
▶ *Premixed IV injection:* Obtain bag and thaw at room temperature. Do not force thaw by immersion in water or by microwave irradiation. Do not refreeze.
▶ *ADD-Vantage vials:* Reconstitute only with D5W or 0.9%NS. Activate the ADD-Vantage vial by pulling the inner cap from the drug vial. Allow drug and diluent to mix.
▶ *Other vials:* Reconstitute using Bacteriostatic Water for Injection, Sodium Chloride for Injection, or Sterile Water for Injection as follows:

Vial Size	Diluent to Add	Available Volume	Concentration
250 mg	2 mL	2 mL	125 mg/mL
500 mg	2 mL	2.2 mL	225 mg/mL
1 g	2.5 mL	3 mL	330 mg/mL

Shake well until dissolved.
▶ *Direct IV administration:* Further dilute reconstituted drug with at least 10 mL Sterile Water for Injection. **Intermittent IV infusion:** Further dilute the drug in 50 to 100 mL of D5W/LR; D5W/0.2%NS; D5W/0.45%NS; D5W/0.9%NS; D5W; D10W; Invert Sugar 5% or 10% in Sterile Water for Injection; *Ionosol B* with 5% Dextrose; LR; 0.9%NS; *Normosol- M* in D5W; *Plasma-Lyte* with 5% Dextrose; or Ringer's Injection.
▶ *IM:* Reconstitute as above and give without further dilution.

Dosage
▶ Give IV by direct injection over 3–5 min or by intermittent infusion.
▶ Give IM into a large muscle mass.
▶ *Mild infections caused by susceptible gram-positive cocci:* 250–500 mg IV or IM q8h.
▶ *Moderate-to-severe infections:* 500–1000 mg IV or IM q6–8h.
▶ *Pneumococcal pneumonia:* 500 mg IV or IM q12h.
▶ *Severe, life-threatening infections:* 1–1.5 g IV or IM q6h.
▶ *Acute uncomplicated urinary tract infections:* 1 g IV or IM q12h.

Adverse effects in *Italics* are most common; those in **Bold** are life-threatening

- *Preoperative prophylaxis:* 1 g IV or IM 0.5 to 1 before surgery.
- *Postoperative prophylaxis:* 0.5–1 g IV or IM q6–8h for 24 h after surgery. May continue for 3–5 d after surgery.
- *Renal function impairment:* After loading dose appropriate for severity of the infection, refer to table below for maintenance dosages.

Creatinine Clearance (mL/min)	Mild to Moderate Infection	Severe Infection
≥ 55	250–500 mg q6–8h	500–1000 mg q6–8h
35–54	250–500 mg q ≥ 8h	500–1000 mg q ≥ 8h
11–34	125–250 mg q12h	250–500 mg q12h
≤ 10	125–250 mg q18–24h	250–500 mg q18–24h

Compatibility
Cefazolin may be given through the same IV line as acyclovir, allopurinol, amifostine, atracurium, aztreonam, calcium gluconate, cyclophosphamide, diltiazem, enalaprilat, esmolol, famotidine, filgrastim, fluconazole, fludarabine, foscarnet, gallium, granisetron, heparin, insulin (regular), labetalol, lidocaine, magnesium sulfate, melphalan, meperidine, midazolam, morphine, multivitamins, ondansetron, pancuronium, perphenazine, propofol, sargramostim, tacrolimus, teniposide, theophylline, thiotepa, vecuronium, vitamin B complex with C.

Incompatibility
Do not administer through the same IV line as aminoglycosides, idarubicin, pentamidine, vinorelbine.

TREATMENT OF OVERDOSE/ANTIDOTE
Discontinue drug or decrease dosage. Initiate general supportive and resuscitative measures. Treat anaphylaxis with epinephrine, oxygen, IV steroids, and airway management. If seizures occur, administer anticonvulsants. Consider hemodialysis for an overwhelming overdosage.

Pharmacokinetics

Route	Onset
IV	Immediate
IM	Rapid

$T_{1/2}$: 90–120 min
Excretion: Urine

Adverse effects
- *CNS:* **Seizures,** hemiparesis, extreme confusion

Adverse effects in *Italics* are most common; those in **Bold** are life-threatening

- **GI:** **Pseudomembranous colitis, liver toxicity,** *diarrhea,* nausea, vomiting, anorexia, transient hepatitis, abdominal pain, oral candidiasis; transient increase in ALT, AST, and alkaline phosphatase
- **GU:** Transient increase in BUN
- **Allergic:** **Anaphylaxis, Stevens-Johnson syndrome,** eosinophilia, itching, drug fever, rash
- **Hematologic:** **Neutropenia, leukopenia, thrombocytopenia, thrombocythemia**
- **Misc:** *Superinfections,* pain or phlebitis at injection site, genital and anal pruritus, serum sickness

Clinically important drug–drug interactions
- Increased and prolonged drug levels related to decreased renal excretion with probenecid
- Increased nephrotoxicity with aminoglycosides
- Increased bleeding with oral anticoagulants
- Disulfiram-like reaction possible if alcohol is taken within 72 h of cefazolin administration

⬤ NURSING CONSIDERATIONS

Assessment
- *History:* Allergy to cephalosporins or penicillin, impaired renal function
- *Physical:* T, P, R, BP, I & O, IV or IM site, neurologic checks, skin assessment, respiratory status, abdominal assessment, bowel sounds, culture and sensitivity tests of infected area, renal and liver function tests, UA, CBC

Implementation
- Obtain specimens for culture and sensitivity of infected area before beginning therapy. May begin drug before results are available.
- Have emergency equipment (defibrillator, drugs, oxygen, intubation equipment) on standby in case anaphylactic reaction occurs.
- Assess for evidence of anaphylaxis; if suspected, discontinue drug immediately and notify provider.
- Monitor renal, hepatic, and hematopoietic function.
- Initiate seizure precautions for patients receiving high doses.
- Monitor for occurrence of superinfections; treat as appropriate.
- Discontinue drug at any sign of colitis; initiate appropriate supportive treatment.
- Solution may appear pale yellow to yellow without a change in potency. Solution is stable for 24 h at room temperature or

Adverse effects in *Italics* are most common; those in **Bold** are life-threatening

4 d if refrigerated; redissolve by warming to room temperature and agitating slightly.

● **cefepime hydrochloride** *(sef' ah pime)*
Maxipime

Pregnancy Category B

Drug classes
Antibiotic: cephalosporin (third generation)

Indications
▶ Uncomplicated and complicated urinary tract infections caused by *Escherichia coli, Klebsiella pneumoniae, Proteus mirabilis*
▶ Uncomplicated skin and skin structure infections caused by *Staphylococcus aureus, Streptococcus pyogenes*
▶ Moderate to severe pneumonia caused by *Streptococcus pneumoniae, Pseudomonas aeruginosa, K. pneumoniae, Enterobacter* species
▶ Empiric therapy for febrile neutropenic patients
▶ Complicated intra-abdominal infections caused by *E. coli,* viridans group streptococci, *P. aeruginosa, K. pneumoniae, Enterobacter* species, *Bacteroides fragilis;* use in combination with metronidazole

Therapeutic actions
▶ Bactericidal: inhibits synthesis of bacterial cell wall, causing cell death

Contraindications/cautions
▶ **Contraindications:** allergy to cephalosporins
▶ **Cautions:** allergy to penicillin, impaired renal function, gastrointestinal disease (especially colitis)

Available forms
▶ *Powder for injection:* 500 mg; 1, 2 g

IV/IM facts
Preparation
▶ *ADD-Vantage vials:* Reconstitute only with 50 to 100 mL D5W or 0.9%NS. Activate the ADD-Vantage vial by pulling the inner cap from the drug vial. Allow drug and diluent to mix.
▶ *Other vials/bottles for IV use:* Reconstitute other vials/bottles with D5W/LR; D5W/0.9%NS; D5W; D10W; *Normosol-R* or *Normosol-M* in D5W; 0.9%NS; or Sodium Lactate (1/6 Molar) Injection as follows:

C

Package Size	Diluent to Add (mL)	Available Volume (mL)	Concentration (mg/mL)
500-mg vial	5	5.6	100
1-g vial	10	11.3	100
2-g vial	10	12.5	160
1-g bottle	50	50	20
2-g bottle	50	50	40

◗ *IV:* Further dilute the drug in 50 to 100 mL of one of the above compatible IV solutions.
◗ *IM:* Reconstitute (500-mg vial with 1.3 mL or 1-g vial with 2.4 mL) with D5W; Lidocaine Hydrochloride 0.5% or 1%; 0.9%NS; Sterile Bacteriostatic Water for Injection with Parabens or Benzyl Alcohol; or Sterile Water for Injection. Give without further dilution.

Dosage
◗ Give IV infusion over 30 min.
◗ Give IM into a large muscle mass.
◗ *Mild to moderate uncomplicated or complicated UTI:* 0.5–1 g IV or IM q12h for 7–10 d.
◗ *Severe uncomplicated or complicated UTI:* 2 g IV q12h for 10 d.
◗ *Moderate to severe pneumonia:* 1–2 g IV q12h for 10 d.
◗ *Moderate to severe uncomplicated skin and skin structure infections:* 2 g IV q12h for 10 d.
◗ *Empiric therapy for febrile neutropenic patients:* 2 g IV q8h for 7 d or until neutropenia is resolved.
◗ *Complicated intra-abdominal infections:* 2 g IV q12h for 7–10 d.
◗ *Hemodialysis patients:* At completion of each dialysis session, give a repeat dose that is equivalent to the initial dose.
◗ *Renal function impairment:* After loading dose of 1–2 g IV, refer to table below for maintenance dosages.

Creatinine Clearance (mL/min)	Mild Infection	Moderate Infection	Severe Infection
> 60	500 mg q12h	1 g q12h	2 g q12h
30–60	500 mg q24h	1 g q24h	2 g q24h
11–29	500 mg q24h	500 mg q24h	1 g q24h
< 11	250 mg q24h	250 mg q24h	500 mg q24h

Compatibility
Cefepime may be given through the same IV line as ampicillin-sulbactam, aztreonam, bleomycin, bumetanide, buprenorphine, butorphanol, calcium gluconate, carboplatin, carmustine, cyclophosphamide, cytarabine, dactinomycin, dexamethasone, fluconazole, fludarabine, fluorouracil, furosemide, granisetron,

Adverse effects in *Italics* are most common; those in **Bold** are life-threatening

hydrocortisone, hydromorphone, imipenem-cilastatin, leuco-vorin, lorazepam, melphalan, mesna, methotrexate, methylpred-nisolone, metronidazole, paclitaxel, piperacillin-tazobactam, ran-itidine, sargramostim, sodium bicarbonate, thiotepa, ticarcillin-clavulanate, trimethoprim-sulfamethoxazole, zidovudine.

Incompatibility
Do not administer through the same IV line as acyclovir, am-photericin B, chlordiazepoxide, chlorpromazine, cimetidine, ciprofloxacin, cisplatin, dacarbazine, daunorubicin, diazepam, diphenhydramine, dobutamine, dopamine, doxorubicin, drop-eridol, enalaprilat, etoposide, famotidine, filgrastim, floxuridine, gallium, ganciclovir, haloperidol, hydroxyzine, idarubicin, ifos-famide, magnesium sulfate, mannitol, mechlorethamine, meperi-dine, metoclopramide, mitomycin, mitoxantrone, morphine, nal-buphine, ofloxacin, ondansetron, plicamycin, prochlorperazine, promethazine, streptozocin, vancomycin, vinblastine, vincristine.

> **TREATMENT OF OVERDOSE/ANTIDOTE**
> Discontinue drug or decrease dosage. Initiate general sup-portive and resuscitative measures. If renal insufficiency oc-curs, hemodialysis is recommended to remove the drug from the body.

Pharmacokinetics

Route	Onset	Peak
IV	Immediate	5 min
IM	30 min	1.5 h

$T_{1/2}$: 102–138 min
Excretion: Urine

Adverse effects
▸ *CNS:* **Seizures,** headache
▸ *GI:* **Pseudomembranous colitis, liver toxicity,** *diarrhea,* nausea, vomiting, oral candidiasis
▸ *GU:* **Acute renal failure**
▸ *Allergic:* **Anaphylaxis, angioedema,** *rash,* pruritus
▸ *Hematologic:* **Bone marrow depression**
▸ *Misc:* *Superinfections,* pain or phlebitis at injection site, en-cephalopathy (in renally impaired patients treated with un-adjusted doses), positive direct Coombs' test

Clinically important drug–drug interactions
▸ Increased and prolonged drug levels related to decreased re-nal excretion with probenecid

Adverse effects in *Italics* are most common; those in **Bold** are life-threatening

▸ Nephrotoxicity and ototoxicity with aminoglycosides
▸ Nephrotoxicity with loop diuretics

◯ NURSING CONSIDERATIONS

Assessment
▸ *History:* Allergy to cephalosporins or penicillin, impaired renal function, gastrointestinal disease
▸ *Physical:* T, P, R, BP, I & O, IV or IM site, neurologic checks, skin assessment, respiratory status, abdominal assessment, bowel sounds, culture and sensitivity tests of infected area, renal and liver function tests, UA, CBC

Implementation
▸ Obtain specimens for culture and sensitivity of infected area before beginning therapy. May begin drug before results are available.
▸ Have emergency equipment (defibrillator, drugs, oxygen, intubation equipment) on standby in case anaphylactic reaction occurs.
▸ Assess for evidence of anaphylaxis; if suspected, discontinue drug immediately and notify provider.
▸ Monitor renal, hepatic, and hematopoietic function.
▸ Monitor for occurrence of superinfections; treat as appropriate.
▸ Have vitamin K available in case of hypoprothrombinemia.
▸ Discontinue drug at any sign of colitis; initiate appropriate supportive treatment.
▸ Store dry powder at between 2° and 25°C in a dry area. After reconstitution, drug is stable for 24 h at room temperature and for 7 d when refrigerated.

◯ **cefoxitin sodium** *(se fox' i tin)* Mefoxin
Pregnancy Category B

Drug classes
Antibiotic: cephalosporin (second generation)

Indications
▸ Lower respiratory tract infections caused by *Streptococcus pneumoniae, Staphylococcus aureus,* streptococci, *Escherichia coli, Klebsiella* species, *Haemophilus influenzae, Bacteroides* species
▸ Dermatologic infections caused by *S. aureus, Staphylococcus epidermidis,* streptococci, *E. coli, Proteus mirabilis, Klebsiella* species, *Bacteroides* species, *Clostridium* species, *Peptococcus* species, *Peptostreptococcus* species
▸ UTIs caused by *E. coli, P. mirabilis, Klebsiella* species, *Morganella morganii, Proteus rettgeri, Proteus vulgaris, Providen-*

Adverse effects in *Italics* are most common; those in **Bold** are life-threatening

cia species; uncomplicated gonorrhea caused by *Neisseria gonorrhoeae*
▸ Intra-abdominal infections caused by *E. coli, Klebsiella* species, *Bacteroides* species, *Clostridium* species
▸ Gynecologic infections caused by *E. coli, N. gonorrhoeae, Bacteroides* species, *Clostridium* species, *Peptococcus* species, *Peptostreptococcus* species, group B streptococci
▸ Septicemia caused by *S. pneumoniae, S. aureus, E. coli, Klebsiella* species, *Bacteroides* species
▸ Bone and joint infections caused by *S. aureus*
▸ Preoperative or postoperative prophylaxis

Therapeutic actions
▸ Bactericidal: inhibits synthesis of bacterial cell wall, causing cell death

Contraindication/cautions
▸ **Contraindication:** allergy to cephalosporins
▸ **Cautions:** allergy to penicillin, impaired renal function, gastrointestinal disease (especially colitis)

Available forms
▸ *Powder for injection:* 1, 2 g
▸ *Premixed frozen injection:* 1, 2 g in 5% Dextrose in Water

IV/IM facts
Preparation
▸ **Premixed IV injection:** Obtain bag and thaw at room temperature. Do not force thaw by immersion in water or by microwave irradiation. Do not refreeze.
▸ **Vials/bottles for IM or IV use:** Reconstitute using Sterile Water for Injection as follows:

Package Size	Diluent to Add (mL)	Available Volume (mL)	Concentration (mg/mL)
1-g vial (IM)	2	2.5	400
2-g vial (IM)	4	5	400
1-g vial (IV)	10	10.5	95
2-g vial (IV)	10 or 20	11.1 or 21	180 or 95
1-g bottle (IV)	50 or 100	50 or 100	20 or 10
2-g bottle (IV)	50 or 100	50 or 100	40 or 20

▸ **IV: Direct administration:** May give as reconstituted. **Intermittent infusion:** Further dilute the drug in 50 to 100 mL of D5W/LR; D5W/0.2%NS; D5W/0.45%NS; D5W/0.9%NS; D5W; D10W; Invert Sugar 5% or 10% in Sterile Water for Injection or 0.9%NS; *Ionosol B* with 5% Dextrose; LR; Mannitol 10% in Wa-

ter; 0.9%NS; *Normosol-M* in D5W; Ringer's Injection; Sodium Bicarbonate 5%; or Sodium Lactate (1/6 Molar) Injection.
▶ *IM:* Reconstitute as above and give without further dilution.

Dosage

▶ Dosage and route of administration are based on the organism, severity of the infection, and the patient's condition. Dose range is 1–2 g IV or IM q6–8h.
▶ Give IV by direct injection over 3–5 min or by intermittent infusion over 15–30 min.
▶ Give IM into a large muscle mass.
▶ *Uncomplicated infections:* 1 g IV q6–8h.
▶ *Moderately severe or severe infections:* 1 g IV q4h or 2 g IV q6– 8h.
▶ *Infections commonly requiring higher dosages:* 2 g IV q4h or 3 g IV q6h.
▶ *Uncomplicated gonorrhea:* 2 g IM with probenecid 1 g PO.
▶ *Surgical prophylactic use:* 2 g IV 30 to 60 min before surgery followed by 2 g q6h for ≤ 24 h.
▶ *Transurethral prostatectomy:* 1 g IV prior to surgery and then 1 g q8h for ≤ 5 d.
▶ *Hemodialysis patients:* Give a 1- to 2-g loading dose IV after each hemodialysis. Give maintenance dose as indicated on the table below.
▶ *Renal function impairment:* After loading dose of 1–2 g IV, refer to the table below for maintenance dosages.

Creatinine Clearance (mL/min)	Maintenance Dosage
30–50	1–2 g q8–12h
10–29	1–2 g q12–24h
5–9	0.5–1 g q12–24h
< 5	0.5–1 g q24–48h

Compatibility

Cefoxitin may be given through the same IV line as acyclovir, amifostine, aztreonam, cyclophosphamide, diltiazem, famotidine, fluconazole, foscarnet, granisetron, hydromorphone, magnesium sulfate, meperidine, morphine, ondansetron, perphenazine, propofol, teniposide, thiotepa.

Incompatibility

Do not administer through the same IV line as aminoglycosides, filgrastim, hetastarch, pentamidine.

Adverse effects in *Italics* are most common; those in **Bold** are life-threatening

TREATMENT OF OVERDOSE/ANTIDOTE
Discontinue drug or decrease dosage. Initiate general supportive and resuscitative measures. Treat anaphylaxis with epinephrine, oxygen, IV steroids, and airway management. If seizures occur, administer anticonvulsants. Consider hemodialysis for an overwhelming overdosage.

Pharmacokinetics

Route	Onset
IV	Immediate
IM	Rapid

$T_{1/2}$: 40–60 min
Excretion: Urine

Adverse effects
- *CNS:* Exacerbation of myasthenia gravis
- *GI:* **Pseudomembranous colitis, liver toxicity,** diarrhea, nausea, vomiting, abdominal pain, oral candidiasis, transient hepatitis; transient increase in ALT, AST, LDH, and alkaline phosphatase
- *GU:* **Acute renal failure,** elevated BUN and creatinine
- *Allergic:* **Anaphylaxis, toxic epidermal necrolysis, exfoliative dermatitis, angioedema,** itching, drug fever, rash
- *Hematologic:* **Neutropenia, leukopenia, thrombocytopenia, thrombocythemia, eosinophilia,** anemia, bone marrow depression, positive direct Coombs' test
- *Misc:* *Superinfections;* pain or phlebitis at injection site, serum sickness

Clinically important drug–drug interactions
- Increased and prolonged drug levels related to decreased renal excretion with probenecid
- Nephrotoxicity with aminoglycosides

◉NURSING CONSIDERATIONS

Assessment
- *History:* Allergy to cephalosporins or penicillin, impaired renal function, gastrointestinal disease, colitis
- *Physical:* T, P, R, BP, I & O, IV or IM site, neurologic checks, skin assessment, respiratory status, abdominal assessment, bowel sounds, culture and sensitivity tests of infected area, renal and liver function tests, UA, CBC

Implementation
- Obtain specimens for culture and sensitivity of infected area before beginning therapy. May begin drug before results are available.

Adverse effects in *Italics* are most common; those in **Bold** are life-threatening

C

- Have emergency equipment (defibrillator, drugs, oxygen, intubation equipment) on standby in case anaphylactic reaction occurs.
- Assess for evidence of anaphylaxis; if suspected, discontinue drug immediately and notify provider.
- Monitor renal, hepatic, and hematopoietic function.
- Monitor for occurrence of superinfections; treat as appropriate.
- Discontinue drug at any sign of colitis; initiate appropriate supportive treatment.
- Store dry powder at < 30°C in a dry area. Powder and reconstituted solution darken with storage, but this does not affect potency. Reconstituted drug is stable for 24 h at room temperature and for 48 h when refrigerated.

⬤ ceftriaxone sodium *(sef try ax' one)* Rocephin
Pregnancy Category B

Drug classes
Antibiotic: cephalosporin (third generation)

Indications
- Lower respiratory tract infections caused by *Streptococcus pneumoniae, Staphylococcus aureus, Klebsiella pneumoniae, Haemophilus influenzae, Escherichia coli, Proteus mirabilis, Enterobacter aerogenes, Serratia marcescens, Haemophilus parainfluenzae*
- UTIs caused by *E. coli, K. pneumoniae, Proteus vulgaris, P. mirabilis, Morganella morganii*
- Gonorrhea caused by *Neisseria gonorrhoeae*
- Intra-abdominal infections caused by *E. coli, K. pneumoniae, Bacteroides fragilis, Clostridium* species, *Peptostreptococcus* species
- Pelvic inflammatory disease caused by *N. gonorrhoeae*
- Skin and skin structure infections caused by *S. aureus, Enterobacter cloacae, P. mirabilis, Staphylococcus epidermidis, Pseudomonas aeruginosa, E. coli, Klebsiella oxytoca, K. pneumoniae, M. morganii, Peptostreptococcus* species, *S. marcescens, Acinetobacter calcoaceticus, B. fragilis, Streptococcus pyogenes, Viridans* group streptococci
- Septicemia caused by *E. coli, S. pneumoniae, H. influenzae, S. aureus, K. pneumoniae*
- Bone and joint infections caused by *S. aureus, P. mirabilis, S. pneumoniae, E. coli, K. pneumoniae, Enterobacter* species
- Meningitis caused by *H. influenzae, S. pneumoniae, N. meningitidis*
- Prophylaxis for patients undergoing coronary artery bypass

Adverse effects in *Italics* are most common; those in **Bold** are life-threatening

surgery or surgical procedures classified as contaminated or potentially contaminated
▸ Unlabeled use: treatment of Lyme disease

Therapeutic actions
▸ Bactericidal: inhibits synthesis of bacterial cell wall, causing cell death

Contraindications/cautions
▸ **Contraindications:** allergy to cephalosporins
▸ **Cautions:** allergy to penicillin, impaired hepatic or renal function, gastrointestinal disease (especially colitis), impaired vitamin K synthesis, low vitamin K stores (chronic hepatic disease, malnutrition)

Available forms
▸ *Powder for injection:* 250, 500 mg; 1, 2, 10 g
▸ *Premixed frozen injection:* 1, 2 g

IV/IM facts
Preparation
▸ *Premixed IV injection:* Obtain bag and thaw at room temperature. Do not force thaw by immersion in water or by microwave irradiation. Do not refreeze.
▸ *ADD-Vantage vials:* Activate the ADD-Vantage vial by pulling the inner cap from the drug vial. Allow drug and diluent to mix.
▸ *Vials/bottles for IM or IV use:* Reconstitute using Bacteriostatic Water with 0.9% Benzyl Alcohol; D5W; 0.9%NS; or Sterile Water for Injection as follows:

Package Size	Diluent to Add (mL)	Resulting Concentration (mg/mL)
250 mg (IV)	2.4	100
250 mg (IM)	0.9	250
500 mg (IV)	4.8	100
500 mg (IM)	1.8	250
1 g (IV)	9.6	100
1 g (IM)	3.6	250
2 g (IV)	19.2	100
2 g (IM)	7.2	250
1 g (IVPB)	10	
2 g (IVPB)	20	

▸ *IV:* **Intermittent infusion:** Further dilute the drug in 50 to 100 mL of D5W/0.45%NS; D5W/0.9%NS; D5W; D10W; 0.9%NS; or Sterile Water for Injection.
▸ *IM:* Reconstitute as above and give without further dilution.

Adverse effects in *Italics* are most common; those in **Bold** are life-threatening

Dosage
◗ Give IV by intermittent infusion over 30 minutes.
◗ Give IM into a large muscle mass.
◗ Usual dose is 1–2 g/d IM or IV or in equally divided doses bid. Do not exceed 4 g/d.
◗ *Surgical prophylaxis:* Single 1-g dose IV 0.5–2 h before surgery.
◗ *Meningitis/endocarditis:* 1–2 g IV q12h for 10–14 d (meningitis) or for ≥ 4 wk (endocarditis).
◗ *Lyme disease:* 2 g/d IV for 14–28 d.
◗ *Uncomplicated gonococcal infection:* 125 mg IM as a single dose.
◗ *Disseminated gonococcal infection:* 1 g IV or IM q24h.
◗ *Renal or hepatic function impairment:* No dosage adjustment needed except do not exceed 2 g/d if patient has both renal and hepatic dysfunction.

Compatibility
Ceftriaxone may be administered through the same IV line as acyclovir, allopurinol, amifostine, aztreonam, diltiazem, fludarabine, foscarnet, gallium, granisetron, heparin, melphalan, meperidine, methotrexate, morphine, paclitaxel, propofol, sargramostim, sodium bicarbonate, tacrolimus, teniposide, theophylline, thiotepa, zidovudine.

Incompatibility
Do not administer through the same IV line as aminoglycosides, amsacrine, filgrastim, fluconazole, labetalol, pentamidine, vancomycin, vinorelbine.

> ### TREATMENT OF OVERDOSE/ANTIDOTE
> Discontinue drug or decrease dosage. Initiate general supportive and resuscitative measures. Treat anaphylaxis with epinephrine, oxygen, IV steroids, and airway management. If seizure occurs, administer anticonvulsants.

Pharmacokinetics

Route	Onset
IV	Immediate
IM	Rapid

Metabolism: Liver, intestine; $T_{1/2}$: 5.8–8.7 h
Excretion: Urine, bile, feces

Adverse effects
◗ *CNS:* Headache, dizziness
◗ *GI:* **Pseudomembranous colitis,** *diarrhea, elevated AST and ALT,* nausea, vomiting, dysgeusia, elevated alkaline

Adverse effects in *Italics* are most common; those in **Bold** are life-threatening

phosphatase and bilirubin, sonographic abnormalities of the gallbladder
▸ *GU:* **Nephrotoxicity,** elevated BUN and creatinine, casts in urine
▸ *Derm: Pain, induration, and tenderness at injection site;* diaphoresis, flushing; phlebitis at IV site
▸ *Allergic:* **Anaphylaxis,** rash, pruritus, fever, chills
▸ *Hematologic: Eosinophilia, thrombocytosis, leukopenia,* **thrombocytopenia, neutropenia,** hemolytic anemia, anemia, lymphopenia, prolonged PT
▸ *Misc: Superinfections,* serum sickness

Clinically important drug–drug interactions
▸ Increased and prolonged drug levels related to decreased renal excretion with probenecid
▸ Increased nephrotoxicity with aminoglycosides

●NURSING CONSIDERATIONS

Assessment
▸ *History:* Allergy to cephalosporins or penicillin, impaired hepatic or renal function, gastrointestinal disease, colitis, impaired vitamin K synthesis, low vitamin K stores, chronic hepatic disease, malnutrition
▸ *Physical:* T, P, R, BP, I & O, IV or IM site, neurologic checks, skin assessment, respiratory status, abdominal assessment, bowel sounds, culture and sensitivity tests of infected area, renal and liver function tests, UA, CBC, PT

Implementation
▸ Obtain specimens for culture and sensitivity of infected area before beginning therapy. May begin drug before results are available.
▸ Have emergency equipment (defibrillator, drugs, oxygen, intubation equipment) on standby in case anaphylactic reaction occurs.
▸ Assess for evidence of anaphylaxis; if suspected, discontinue drug immediately and notify provider.
▸ Monitor renal, hepatic, and hematopoietic function.
▸ Vitamin K 10 mg weekly may be needed if the PT is prolonged.
▸ Monitor ceftriaxone blood levels in patients with severe renal impairment and in patients with both renal and hepatic impairment.
▸ Monitor for occurrence of superinfections; treat as appropriate.
▸ Discontinue drug at any sign of colitis; initiate appropriate supportive treatment.
▸ The solution's color ranges from light yellow to amber, depending on the length of storage, concentration, and diluent used.

Adverse effects in *Italics* are most common; those in **Bold** are life-threatening

▶ Stability of reconstituted and diluted solution depends on diluent, concentration, and type of container (eg, glass, PVC). Check manufacturer's insert for specific details.
▶ Protect from light during storage.

⬤ charcoal, activated *(char' kole)* Actidose-Aqua, Actidose with Sorbitol, CharcoAid, Charcodote (CAN), Liqui-Char

Drug class
Antidote

Indications
▶ Emergency treatment in poisoning by most drugs and chemicals

Therapeutic actions
▶ Inhibits GI absorption of toxic substances—adsorbs toxic substances in the GI tract by forming an effective barrier between any remaining particulate material and the GI mucosa
▶ Maximum amount of toxin absorbed is 100–1000 mg/g charcoal

Contraindications/cautions
▶ **Contraindications:** unconsciousness, semiconsciousness; ineffective for poisoning or overdose of mineral acids and alkalies
▶ **Cautions:** not necessarily contraindicated but not effective in ethanol, methanol, and iron salts poisonings

Available Forms
▶ *Powder:* 15, 30, 40, 120, 240 g and UD 30 g
▶ *Suspension:* 12.5, 15, 25, 30, 50 g
▶ *Granules:* 15 g in 120 mL

Oral dosage
▶ For maximum effect, administer activated charcoal within 30 min after poison ingestion.
▶ Induce emesis (unless contraindicated) before giving activated charcoal.
▶ Give drug only to conscious patients.
▶ Prepare suspension of powder in 6–8 oz of water; taste may be gritty and disagreeable. Add sorbitol to improve taste.
▶ 25–100 g PO, NG, or OG or 1 g/kg PO, NG, or OG or

Adverse effects in *Italics* are most common; those in **Bold** are life-threatening

approximately 10 times the amount of poison ingested as an oral suspension (4–8 oz water).

▸ *Gastric dialysis:* 20–40 g q6h for 1–2 d for severe poisonings.

Pharmacokinetics
Not absorbed systemically. Excreted in the feces.

Adverse effects
▸ *GI: Vomiting* (related to rapid ingestion of high doses), *constipation, diarrhea,* black stools; loose stools, vomiting, dehydration (if given with sorbitol)

Clinically important drug–drug interactions
▸ Do not administer concurrently with syrup of ipecac because adsorption and inactivation of either drug may be decreased.
▸ Effectiveness of other medications may be decreased because of their adsorption by activated charcoal.

● NURSING CONSIDERATIONS
Assessment
▸ *History:* Type of poisoning or overdose, unconsciousness, semiconsciousness
▸ *Physical:* BP, P, R, neurologic checks, respiratory effort, stools, bowel sounds

Implementation
▸ Have emergency equipment (defibrillator, drugs, oxygen, intubation equipment) nearby.
▸ Maintain patent airway. Aspiration of charcoal has produced airway obstruction and death.
▸ Repeat dose if emesis occurs soon after dose.
▸ Do not mix charcoal with milk, ice cream, or sherbet because its adsorptive capacity will decrease.
▸ Patient's stools will be black.
▸ Store in closed containers; activated charcoal adsorbs gases from the air and will lose its effectiveness with prolonged exposure to air.

● cimetidine (*sye met' i deen*) Apo-Cimetidine (CAN), Gen-Cimetidine (CAN), Novo-Cimetine (CAN), Nu-Cimet (CAN), Tagamet, Tagamet HB

Pregnancy Category B

Drug class
Histamine H_2 antagonist

Adverse effects in *Italics* are most common; those in **Bold** are life-threatening

Indications
▶ Short-term treatment and maintenance therapy of active duodenal ulcer
▶ Short-term treatment of benign gastric ulcer
▶ Treatment of pathological hypersecretory conditions (Zollinger-Ellison syndrome, systemic mastocytosis, multiple endocrine adenomas)
▶ Prophylaxis of acute upper GI bleeding in critically ill patients
▶ Treatment of erosive gastroesophageal reflux disease (GERD)
▶ Relief of symptoms of heartburn, acid indigestion, sour stomach (OTC use)
▶ Unlabeled uses: treatment of peptic ulcer; prevention of aspiration pneumonitis; prophylaxis of stress ulcers; prevention of gastric NSAID damage; treatment of hyperparathyroidism and secondary hyperparathyroidism in chronic hemodialysis patients; potentially useful for tinea capitis, herpes virus infection, hirsute women; treatment of chronic idiopathic urticaria; may be useful in anaphylaxis, pruritus, urticaria, and contact dermatitis; protection against hepatotoxicity with acetaminophen overdose; treatment of dyspepsia; to improve survival in colorectal cancer

Therapeutic actions
▶ Reversibly and competitively blocks histamine at the H_2 receptors, especially those in the gastric parietal cells
▶ Inhibits secretions caused by histamine, muscarinic agonists, and gastrin
▶ Inhibits fasting and nocturnal secretions and secretions caused by food, insulin, caffeine, pentagastrin, and betazole
▶ Reduces volume and hydrogen ion concentration of gastric juice
▶ Inhibits the cytochrome P450 oxidase system that affects other drugs

Contraindications/cautions
▶ **Contraindications:** cimetidine allergy
▶ **Cautions:** impaired renal or hepatic function, age > 50 years

Available forms
▶ *Injection:* 150 mg/mL, 300 mg/2 mL
▶ *Premixed injection:* 300 mg in 50 mL 0.9%NS
▶ *Tablets:* 100, 200, 300, 400, 800 mg
▶ *Liquid:* 300 mg/5 mL

Adverse effects in *Italics* are most common; those in **Bold** are life-threatening

IV/IM facts
Preparation
▸ *Direct IV injection:* Dilute in D5W/LR; D5W/0.45%NS; D5W/0.9%NS; D10W/0.9%NS; D5W; D10W; Invert Sugar 5% or 10% in Water; LR; Mannitol 10% in Water; 0.9%NS; *Normosol* M in Dextrose 5%; *Normosol* R; Ringer's injection; Sodium Bicarbonate 5%; or Sterile Water for Injection to a total volume of 20 mL.
▸ *Intermittent IV infusion:* Use premixed solution or dilute 300 mg in at least 50 mL of a compatible IV solution (see above).
▸ *Continuous IV infusion:* Dilute 900 mg in 100–1000 mL of a compatible IV fluid (see above).
▸ *IM:* Give undiluted.

Dosage
▸ *Direct injection:* Inject IV over ≥ 2 min.
▸ *Intermittent IV infusion:* 300 mg in 50 mL IV over 15–20 min.
▸ *Continuous IV infusion:* 37.5 mg/h IV. May precede with a 150-mg loading dose administered by IV infusion.
▸ *Prevention of upper GI bleeding:* 50 mg/h by continuous IV infusion. If creatinine clearance < 30 mL/min, give half the recommended dose. Do not use beyond 7 d.
▸ *Pathological hypersecretory conditions/intractable ulcers/patients unable to take oral medications:* 300 mg IV or IM q6–8h. Do not exceed 2400 mg/d.

Compatibility
Cimetidine may be given through the same IV line as acyclovir, amifostine, aminophylline, amrinone, atracurium, aztreonam, cisplatin, cladribine, cyclophosphamide, cytarabine, diltiazem, doxorubicin, enalaprilat, esmolol, filgrastim, fluconazole, fludarabine, foscarnet, gallium, granisetron, haloperidol, heparin, hetastarch, idarubicin, labetalol, melphalan, meropenem, methotrexate, midazolam, ondansetron, paclitaxel, pancuronium, piperacillin-tazobactam, propofol, sargramostim, tacrolimus, teniposide, theophylline, thiotepa, tolazoline, vecuronium, vinorelbine, zidovudine.

Incompatibility
Do not administer through the same IV line as allopurinol, amsacrine, cefepime, indomethacin, warfarin.

Oral dosage
▸ *Active duodenal ulcer:* 800 mg PO at hs, 300 mg PO qid at meals and hs, or 400 mg PO bid. Continue for 4–6 wk.
▸ *Maintenance therapy for duodenal ulcer:* 400 mg PO at hs.
▸ *Active benign gastric ulcer:* 800 mg PO at hs or 300 mg PO qid at meals and hs.

Adverse effects in *Italics* are most common; those in **Bold** are life-threatening

- *GERD:* 1600 mg PO daily in divided doses (800 mg bid or 400 mg qid) for 12 wk.
- *Pathological hypersecretory syndrome:* 300 mg PO qid at meals and hs. Individualize doses; **do not exceed 2400 mg/d.**
- *Heartburn, acid indigestion:* 200 mg PO with water as symptoms occur. Do not exceed 400 mg/24 h.
- *Geriatric or impaired renal function:* Accumulation may occur. Use lowest effective dose. 300 mg PO q12h is recommended. May increase q8h if patient tolerates drug.

TREATMENT OF OVERDOSE/ANTIDOTE
Discontinue drug or decrease dosage. Initiate general supportive and resuscitative measures. Remove unabsorbed drug from GI tract. Physostigmine may arouse obtunded patients with cimetidine-induced CNS toxicity.

Pharmacokinetics

Route	Onset	Peak
IV/IM	Rapid	30 min
Oral	Varies	45–90 min

Metabolism: Hepatic; $T_{1/2}$: 2 h
Excretion: Urine

Adverse effects

- ***CNS:*** *Dizziness, somnolence, headache, confusion, hallucinations,* peripheral neuropathy, symptoms of brain stem dysfunction (dysarthria, ataxia, diplopia)
- ***CV:*** **Dysrhythmias,** hypotension (IV use)
- ***Resp:*** **Bronchospasm**
- ***GI:*** *Diarrhea,* increased serum transaminases
- ***Allergic:*** **Anaphylaxis,** fever, rash, vasculitis
- ***Hematologic:*** **Agranulocytosis, granulocytopenia, thrombocytopenia,** autoimmune hemolytic/aplastic anemia
- ***Misc:*** *Impotence* (reversible), gynecomastia, pain at IM injection site, gouty arthritis, increased plasma creatinine

Clinically important drug–drug interactions

- Decreased white blood cell counts with antimetabolites, alkylating agents, other drugs known to cause neutropenia
- Increased serum levels and toxicity of alcohol, beta-adrenergic blocking agents, carbamazepine, chloroquine, certain benzodiazepines (alprazolam, chlordiazepoxide, diazepam, flurazepam, triazolam), lidocaine, metronidazole, nifedipine, pentoxifylline, phenytoin, procainamide, quinidine, theophylline, tricyclic antidepressants, warfarin-type anticoagulants
- Decreased efficacy with cigarette smoking

Adverse effects in *Italics* are most common; those in **Bold** are life-threatening

▸ Decreased serum digoxin, fluconazole concentrations
▸ Increase effects of flecainide, succinylcholine
▸ Increased toxic effects of narcotic analgesics
▸ Decreased effects of tocainide

● NURSING CONSIDERATIONS

Assessment
▸ *History:* Cimetidine allergy, impaired renal or hepatic function, age, smoking history
▸ *Physical:* P, BP, R, ECG, I & O, neurologic checks, skin assessment, adventitious lung sounds, respiratory effort, liver evaluation, abdominal exam, presence of pain, gastric pH, CBC, liver and renal function tests, emesis and stool guaiac

Implementation
▸ Monitor ECG and BP closely during IV administration.
▸ Give drug with meals and at hs.
▸ Administer IM dose undiluted deep into large muscle group.
▸ Symptomatic improvement does not rule out gastric cancer, which did occur in preclinical studies.
▸ Do not administer simultaneously with antacids.

● ciprofloxacin hydrochloride
(si proe flox' a sin) Cipro, Cipro I.V.

Pregnancy Category C

Drug classes
Antibacterial: fluoroquinolone

Indications
▸ Lower respiratory infections caused by *Escherichia coli, Klebsiella pneumoniae, Enterobacter cloacae, Proteus mirabilis, Pseudomonas aeruginosa, Haemophilus influenzae, Haemophilus parainfluenzae, Streptococcus pneumoniae, Moraxella catarrhalis*
▸ Skin and skin structure infections caused by *E. coli, K. pneumoniae, E. cloacae, P. mirabilis, Proteus vulgaris, Providencia stuartii, Morganella morganii, Citrobacter freundii, Streptococcus pyogenes, P. aeruginosa, S. aureus, Staphylococcus epidermidis*
▸ Bone/joint infections caused by *E. cloacae, Serratia marcescens, P. aeruginosa*
▸ Acute sinusitis caused by *H. influenzae, S. pneumoniae, M. catarrhalis*
▸ Urinary tract infections (UTIs) caused by *E. coli, K. pneumoniae, E. cloacae, S. marcescens, P. mirabilis, Providencia rettgeri, M. morganii, Citrobacter diversus, C. freundii, P. aeruginosa, S. epidermidis, Enterococcus faecalis*

◗ Used with metronidazole for complicated intra-abdominal infections caused by *E. coli, P. aeruginosa, P. mirabilis, K. pneumoniae, B. fragilis*
◗ Infectious diarrhea caused by *E. coli, Campylobacter jejuni, Shigella flexneri, Shigella sonnei*
◗ Typhoid fever caused by *Salmonella typhi*
◗ Sexually transmitted diseases caused by *Neisseria gonorrhoeae*
◗ Treatment of chronic bacterial prostatitis caused by *E. coli, P. mirabilis*

Therapeutic actions

◗ Bactericidal: interferes with the enzyme DNA gyrase, which is needed for synthesis of bacterial DNA

Contraindications/cautions

◗ **Contraindications:** allergy to ciprofloxacin or other quinolone antimicrobials
◗ **Cautions:** renal dysfunction; CNS disorders, such as seizures, severe cerebral arteriosclerosis, or epilepsy; use of theophylline; dehydration

Available forms

◗ *Injection:* 200, 400 mg
◗ *Premixed injection:* 200, 400 mg
◗ *Tablets:* 100, 250, 500, 750 mg
◗ *Suspension, oral:* 5 g/100 mL, 10 g/100mL

IV facts

Preparation

◗ If a premixed bag is not available, dilute vials with D5W or 0.9%NS. Further dilute drug in D5W/0.225%NS; D5W/0.45%NS; D5W; D10W; Fructose 10% in Water; LR; 0.9%NS; or Ringer's Injection to a final concentration of 1–2 mg/mL.

Dosage

◗ Give each IV dose over 60 min. During infusion through a Y-site, temporarily discontinue the administration of the primary solution.
◗ *Mild/moderate UTI:* 200 mg IV q12h.
◗ *Severe/complicated UTI:* 400 mg IV q12h.
◗ *Complicated intra-abdominal infection:* 400 mg IV q12h.
◗ *Nosocomial pneumonia:* 400 mg IV q8h.
◗ *Mild/moderate lower respiratory tract, bone or joint, or skin or skin structure infection:* 400 mg IV q12h.
◗ *Severe/complicated lower respiratory tract, bone or joint, or skin or skin structure infection:* 400 mg IV q8h.
◗ *Impaired renal function:* If creatinine clearance is > 30 mL/min, give usual dosage. If creatinine clearance is 5–29 mL/min, give 200–400 mg IV q18–24h.

Adverse effects in *Italics* are most common; those in **Bold** are life-threatening

Compatibility

Ciprofloxacin may be given through the same IV line as amifostine, amino acids, aztreonam, calcium gluconate, ceftazidime, digoxin, diltiazem, diphenhydramine, dobutamine, dopamine, gallium, gentamicin, granisetron, hydroxyzine, lidocaine, lorazepam, metoclopramide, midazolam, midodrine, piperacillin, potassium acetate, potassium chloride, potassium phosphates, promethazine, propofol, ranitidine, tacrolimus, teniposide, thiotepa, tobramycin, verapamil.

Incompatibility

Do not administer through the same IV line as aminophylline, ampicillin-sulbactam, cefepime, dexamethasone, furosemide, heparin, hydrocortisone, methylprednisolone, mezlocillin, phenytoin, sodium phosphates, warfarin.

Oral dosage

▸ *Mild/moderate UTI:* 250 mg PO q12h.
▸ *Severe/complicated UTI:* 500 mg PO q12h.
▸ *Complicated intra-abdominal infection:* 500 mg PO q12h.
▸ *Mild/moderate lower respiratory tract, bone or joint, or skin or skin structure infection:* 500 mg PO q12h.
▸ *Severe/complicated lower respiratory tract, bone or joint, or skin or skin structure infection:* 750 mg PO q8h.
▸ *Typhoid fever:* 500 mg PO q12h.
▸ *Infectious diarrhea:* 500 mg PO q12h.
▸ *Acute sinusitis:* 500 mg PO q12h.
▸ *Urethral/cervical gonococcal infections:* 250 mg PO as a single dose.
▸ *Impaired renal function:* If creatinine clearance is > 50 mL/min, give usual dosage; if 30–50 mL/min, give 250 to 500 mg PO q12h; if 5–29, give 250 to 500 mg PO q24h. For patients receiving hemodialysis or peritoneal dialysis, give 250–500 mg PO q24h after dialysis.

TREATMENT OF OVERDOSE/ANTIDOTE

Discontinue drug or decrease dosage. Initiate general supportive and resuscitative measures. Empty the stomach by inducing vomiting or by gastric lavage. Maintain adequate hydration.

Pharmacokinetics

Route	Onset	Peak
IV	Rapid	End of infusion
Oral	Varies	1–2 h

Metabolism: Hepatic; $T_{1/2}$: 5–6 h (IV); 4 h (PO)
Excretion: Urine, feces, bile

Adverse effects in *Italics* are most common; those in **Bold** are life-threatening

C

Adverse effects
▶ *CNS:* **Seizures,** *headache, CNS disturbance, restlessness,* paranoia, dysphasia, ataxia, dizziness, insomnia, fatigue, somnolence, depression, blurred vision, dizziness, lightheadedness, weakness, irritability
▶ *GI:* **Pseudomembranous colitis, pancreatitis, GI bleeding,** *nausea, diarrhea,* vomiting, dry mouth, abdominal pain, bad taste
▶ *GU:* **Renal failure,** crystalluria, renal calculi, hematuria, frequent urination
▶ *Derm:* *IV site reaction,* dermatitis, purpura, pruritus, urticaria, cutaneous candidiasis, increased perspiration
▶ *Allergic:* **Anaphylaxis, angioedema**
▶ *Hematologic:* *Eosinophilia; elevated BUN, AST, ALT, LDH, bilirubin,* serum creatinine, PT and alkaline phosphatase; decreased WBC, neutrophil count, Hct, and Hgb
▶ *Misc:* Fever, rash, elevated glucose and triglycerides, Achilles and other tendon rupture

Clinically important drug–drug interactions
▶ Decreased therapeutic effect with iron salts, sucralfate
▶ Decreased absorption with antacids, didanosine, iron salts, sucralfate, zinc salts
▶ Increased effects with azlocillin
▶ Decreased renal clearance and increased serum concentrations with probenecid
▶ Decreased total body clearance of caffeine
▶ Increased nephrotoxic effects of cyclosporine
▶ Reduced serum levels of phenytoin
▶ Increased severe and fatal hypoglycemia with sulfonylurea glyburide
▶ Enhanced effects of warfarin and increased risk of bleeding
▶ Increased serum levels and potentially fatal toxic effects of theophyllines if taken concurrently with ciprofloxacin

⬤ NURSING CONSIDERATIONS

Assessment
▶ *History:* Allergy to ciprofloxacin or other quinolone antimicrobials, renal dysfunction; CNS disorders, such as seizures, severe cerebral arteriosclerosis, and epilepsy; use of theophylline, dehydration
▶ *Physical:* T, P, R, BP, I & O, IV or IM site, neurologic checks, skin assessment, adventitious lung sounds, hydration status, bowel sounds, abdominal assessment, bowel sounds, culture and sensitivity tests of infected area, renal and liver function tests, UA, CBC, PT, serum glucose

Adverse effects in *Italics* are most common; those in **Bold** are life-threatening

Implementation

▸ Obtain specimens for culture and sensitivity of infected area before beginning therapy. May begin drug before results are available.

▸ Have emergency equipment (defibrillator, drugs, oxygen, intubation equipment) on standby in case anaphylactic reaction occurs.

▸ Assess for evidence of anaphylaxis; if suspected, discontinue drug immediately and notify provider.

▸ Monitor renal, hepatic, and hematopoietic function.

▸ Monitor for occurrence of superinfections; treat as appropriate.

▸ Discontinue drug at any sign of colitis; initiate appropriate supportive treatment.

▸ Give oral drug 1 h before or 2 h after meals with a glass of water. Dairy products reduce the drug's absorption; avoid concurrent use.

▸ Ensure that patient is well hydrated. Avoid alkalinity of the urine.

▸ Do not give antacids within 4 h before or 2 h after dosing.

▸ Diluted drug appears clear or colorless to slightly yellow.

▸ Diluted drug is stable up to 14 d refrigerated or at room temperature.

⬤ **cisapride** *(sis' a pride)* Prepulsid (CAN), Propulsid
Pregnancy Category C

Drug class
GI stimulant

Indication
▸ Symptomatic treatment of nocturnal heartburn due to gastroesophageal reflux disease in patients not responding adequately to lifestyle modifications, antacids, and gastric-reducing agents

Therapeutic actions
▸ Enhances the release of acetylcholine in the myenteric plexus, thus improving GI motility and peristalsis

Contraindications/cautions
▸ **Contraindications:** cisapride allergy, prolonged QT interval, torsades de pointes, long QT syndrome, sinus node dysfunction, second- or third-degree heart block, renal failure, ventricular dysrhythmias, ischemic heart disease,

(contraindications continued on next page)

Adverse effects in *Italics* are most common; those in **Bold** are life-threatening

C

CHF, uncorrected hypokalemia or hypomagnesemia, potential for rapid reduction in potassium levels, respiratory failure, concomitant medications known to prolong QT interval and increase risk of dysrhythmias (see drug interactions below), patients in whom an increase in GI motility could be harmful (GI hemorrhage, mechanical obstruction, perforation); concomitant administration of oral ketoconazole, itraconazole, oral or IV fluconazole, oral or IV erythromycin, clarithromycin, troleandomycin, nefazodone, indinavir, or ritonavir
▸ **Caution:** elderly patients

Available forms
▸ *Tablets:* 10, 20 mg
▸ *Suspension:* 1 mg/mL

Oral Dosage
▸ Use minimum effective dose. Begin with 10 mg PO qid at least 15 min before meals and at hs. Some patients will require 20 mg qid to achieve intended results. Discontinue if nocturnal heartburn is not relieved.
▸ *Hepatic insufficiency:* Give half the normal daily dose.

TREATMENT OF OVERDOSE/ANTIDOTE
Discontinue drug or decrease dosage. Initiate general supportive and resuscitative measures. Treatment should include gastric lavage or activated charcoal.

Pharmacokinetics

Route	Onset	Peak
Oral	30–60 min	1–1.5 h

Metabolism: Hepatic; $T_{1/2}$: 6–12 h
Excretion: Urine, feces

Adverse effects
▸ *CNS:* **Seizures,** *headache,* insomnia, anxiety, nervousness, somnolence, confusion, depression, hallucinations, tremor, migraine, extrapyramidal effects
▸ *CV:* **Life-threatening cardiac dysrhythmias** (ventricular tachycardia, ventricular fibrillation, torsades de pointes) and prolonged QT interval when used in combination drug regimens; palpitations, tachycardia
▸ *Resp: Rhinitis, sinusitis, upper respiratory infections,* coughing
▸ *GI: Abdominal pain, diarrhea, constipation, nausea,*

Adverse effects in *Italics* are most common; those in **Bold** are life-threatening

flatulence, bloating, dyspepsia, elevated liver enzymes, hepatitis, dry mouth
▸ *GU:* Urinary tract infection, micturition frequency, incontinence
▸ *Derm:* Rash, pruritus
▸ *Allergic:* **Bronchospasm, angioedema,** urticaria
▸ *Hematologic:* **Thrombocytopenia, leukopenia, aplastic anemia, pancytopenia**
▸ *Misc:* Pain, fever, viral infection, arthralgia, abnormal vision, vaginitis, gynecomastia, female breast enlargement

Clinically important drug–drug interactions
▸ Decreased effects with anticholinergics
▸ Serious ventricular arrhythmias with class IA/III antidysrhythmics, antidepressants, antipsychotics, astemizole, azole antifungals, bepridil, clarithromycin, erythromycin, troleandomycin, protease inhibitors, sparfloxacin, terodiline
▸ Increased peak plasma level with cimetidine; increased absorption of cimetidine and ranitidine with cisapride
▸ Increased coagulation times with oral anticoagulants
▸ Enhanced sedative effects of benzodiazepines and alcohol
▸ Increased gastric emptying, and absorption of other drugs possibly affected

⬤ NURSING CONSIDERATIONS
Assessment
▸ *History:* Cisapride allergy, prolonged QT interval, torsades de pointes, long QT syndrome, sinus node dysfunction, second- or third-degree heart block, renal failure, ventricular dysrhythmias, ischemic heart disease, CHF, uncorrected hypokalemia or hypomagnesemia, potential for rapid reduction in potassium levels, respiratory failure, concomitant medications, GI hemorrhage, mechanical obstruction, perforation, age
▸ *Physical:* P, R, BP, I & O, ECG, QTc, neurologic checks, adventitious lung sounds, abdominal exam, presence of heartburn, serum electrolytes, liver and renal function tests, CBC

Implementation
▸ Monitor for dysrhythmias.
▸ Monitor QT interval and QTc.
▸ Monitor drug levels of other drugs that may be affected by accelerated gastric emptying.

⬤ **cisatracurium besylate** *(sis ah trah* **cure'** *ee um)*
    Nimbex
Pregnancy Category B

Adverse effects in *Italics* are most common; those in **Bold** are life-threatening

C

Drug class
Nondepolarizing neuromuscular blocking agent

Indications
◗ Is an adjunct to general anesthesia to facilitate intubation
◗ Provides skeletal muscle relaxation during surgery or mechanical ventilation

Therapeutic actions
◗ Prevents neuromuscular transmission and produces paralysis by binding competitively to cholinergic receptors on the motor end-plate to antagonize action of acetylcholine

Contraindications/cautions
◗ **Contraindications:** hypersensitivity to cisatracurium or bis-benzylisoquinolinium agents; some forms contain benzyl alcohol
◗ **Cautions:** renal or hepatic function impairment, elderly patients, myasthenia gravis, carcinomatosis, burns, hemiparesis or paraparesis, acid–base or serum electrolyte abnormalities

Available forms
◗ *IV injection:* 2, 10 mg/mL

IV facts
Preparation
◗ May give bolus undiluted.
◗ For a continuous infusion, dilute the drug in D5W/0.9%NS; D5W; or 0.9%NS to achieve a concentration of 0.1 mg/mL (using the 2 mg/mL solution, add 10 mg to 95 mL; using 10 mg/mL solution, add 10 mg to 99 mL) or 0.4 mg/mL (using the 2 mg/mL solution, add 40 mg to 80 mL; using 10 mg/mL solution, add 40 mg to 96 mL).

Dosage and titration
◗ Initial adult dose: For intubation: 0.15–0.2 mg/kg IV over 5–10 s as components of a propofol/nitrous oxide/oxygen induction-intubation technique. Should produce good or excellent conditions for intubation in 1.5–2 min.
◗ *Infusion in the ICU:* 3 mcg/kg/min IV (range 0.5–10.2 mcg/kg/min).
◗ *Elderly/renal function impairment:* Slower time to onset; extend interval between administration and the intubation attempt to achieve adequate intubation conditions.

Adverse effects in *Italics* are most common; those in **Bold** are life-threatening

Titration Guide

cisatracurium besylate									
Using 10 mg/mL solution, 40 mg in 96 mL									

	Body Weight									
lb	88	99	110	121	132	143	154	165	176	187
kg	40	45	50	55	60	65	70	75	80	85
Dose ordered in mcg/kg/min	Amounts to Infuse in mL/h									
0.5	3	3	4	4	5	5	5	6	6	6
1	6	7	8	8	9	10	11	11	12	13
2	12	14	15	17	18	20	21	23	24	26
3	18	20	23	25	27	29	32	34	36	38
4	24	27	30	33	36	39	42	45	48	51
5	30	34	38	41	45	49	53	56	60	64
6	36	41	45	50	54	59	63	68	72	77
7	42	47	53	58	63	68	74	79	84	89
8	48	54	60	66	72	78	84	90	96	102
9	54	61	68	74	81	88	95	101	108	115
10	60	68	75	83	90	98	105	113	120	128

	Body Weight									
lb	198	209	220	231	242	253	264	275	286
kg	90	95	100	105	110	115	120	125	130
Dose ordered in mcg/kg/min	Amounts to Infuse in mL/h								
0.5	7	7	8	8	8	9	9	9	10
1	14	14	15	16	17	17	18	19	20
2	27	29	30	32	33	35	36	38	39
3	41	43	45	47	50	52	54	56	59
4	54	57	60	63	66	69	72	75	78
5	68	71	75	79	83	86	90	94	98
6	81	86	90	95	99	104	108	113	117
7	95	100	105	110	116	121	126	131	137
8	108	114	120	126	132	138	144	150	156
9	122	128	135	142	149	155	162	169	176
10	135	143	150	158	165	173	180	188	195

Compatibility
Cisatracurium may be given through the same IV line as sufentanil, alfentanil, fentanyl, midazolam, droperidol.

Adverse effects in *Italics* are most common; those in **Bold** are life-threatening

Incompatibility

Do not administer through the same IV line as ketorolac or propofol.

> **TREATMENT OF OVERDOSE/ANTIDOTE**
> Discontinue drug or decrease dosage. Initiate general supportive and resuscitative measures. Continue to maintain a patent airway and provide mechanical ventilation. Do not give antagonists (such as neostigmine and edrophonium) when complete neuromuscular block is evident or suspected. Use a peripheral nerve stimulator to evaluate recovery and antagonism of neuromuscular block.

Pharmacokinetics

Route	Onset	Peak	Duration
IV	Immediate	2 min	64–121 min

Metabolism: Liver; $T_{1/2}$: 22–29 min; metabolite 3.1–3.3 h
Excretion: Hofmann elimination, urine, feces

Adverse effects

▶ *CV:* Bradycardia, hypotension
▶ *Resp: Apnea,* **bronchospasm**
▶ *Misc:* Flushing, rash

Clinically important drug–drug interactions

▶ Increased resistance to neuromuscular blocking action with phenytoin, carbamazepine
▶ Faster onset of maximum block with prior administration of succinylcholine
▶ Prolonged duration of action with isoflurane or enflurane given with nitrous oxide/oxygen
▶ Enhanced neuromuscular blockade with aminoglycosides, tetracyclines, bacitracin, polymyxins, lincomycin, clindamycin, colistin, sodium colistimethate, magnesium salts, lithium, local anesthetics, procainamide, quinidine

● NURSING CONSIDERATIONS

Assessment

▶ *History:* Hypersensitivity to cisatracurium, bis-benzylisoquinolinium agents, or benzyl alcohol; renal or hepatic function impairment, age, myasthenia gravis, carcinomatosis, burns, hemiparesis or paraparesis, acid–base or serum electrolyte abnormalities

Adverse effects in *Italics* are most common; those in **Bold** are life-threatening

▸ *Physical:* T, P, BP, R, ECG, I & O, IV site, weight, orientation, mental status, level of sedation, respiratory status, method of mechanical ventilation, adventitious lung sounds, presence of pain, muscle strength, peripheral nerve stimulator response, serum electrolytes, acid–base balance, renal and liver function studies

Implementation

▸ Exercise extreme caution when calculating and preparing doses; cisatracurium is a very potent drug; small dosage errors can cause serious adverse effects.
▸ Always administer an infusion through an IV infusion pump.
▸ Do not administer unless equipment for intubation, artifical respiration, oxygen therapy, and reversal agents is readily available. Cisatracurium should be administered by people who are skilled in management of critically ill patients, cardiovascular resuscitation, and airway management.
▸ Use the smallest effective dose to achieve desired patient response.
▸ Monitor patient's response to therapy with a peripheral nerve stimulator.
▸ Monitor BP, R, and ECG closely during infusion to monitor effectiveness of therapy.
▸ Cisatracurium does not affect consciousness, pain threshold, or cerebration. Administer adequate sedatives and analgesics before giving cisatracurium.
▸ Cisatracurium produces paralysis. Provide oral and skin care. Administer artifical tears to protect corneas. May need to tape eyes closed. Position patient appropriately.
▸ Protect vials from light and refrigerate.
▸ Diluted drug is good for 24 h when refrigerated.

● **clonidine hydrochloride** *(kloe' ni deen)*

Antihypertensives: Apo-Clonidine (CAN), Catapres, Catapres-TTS (transdermal preparation), Nu-Clonidine (CAN)

Pregnancy Category C

Drug classes
Antihypertensive
Centrally acting sympatholytic

Indications
▸ Hypertension (step 2 drug in stepped-care approach)
▸ Unlabeled uses: alcohol withdrawal, atrial fibrillation, attention deficit hyperactivity disorder, cyclosporine-associated

---

Adverse effects in *Italics* are most common; those in **Bold** are life-threatening

nephrotoxicity, diabetic diarrhea, hypertensive "urgencies" (diastolic blood pressure > 120 mmHg), mania, menopausal flushing, methadone/opiate detoxification, postherpetic neuralgia, psychosis in schizophrenic patients, reduction of allergen-induced inflammatory reactions in patients with extrinsic asthma, restless leg syndrome, smoking cessation facilitation, ulcerative colitis

Therapeutic actions
- Inhibits sympathetic cardioaccelerator and vasoconstrictor centers
- Stimulates peripheral alpha-adrenergic receptors, resulting in reduced sympathetic outflow from CNS, decreased peripheral resistance, renal vascular resistance, HR, and BP

Effects on hemodynamic parameters
- Decreased BP
- Decreased HR
- Decreased SVR

Contraindications/cautions
- **Contraindications:** allergy to clonidine or any adhesive layer components of transdermal system
- **Cautions:** severe coronary insufficiency, conduction disturbances, recent MI, cerebrovascular disease, chronic renal failure

Available forms
- *Tablets:* 0.1, 0.2, 0.3 mg
- *Transdermal:* 0.1, 0.2, 0.3 mg/24 h

Oral/transdermal dosage
- *Initial dose:* 0.1 mg PO bid. Elderly patients may benefit from a lower dose.
- *Maintenance dose:* Continue increments of 0.1 mg/d made at weekly intervals until desired response achieved. Common range is 0.2–0.6 mg/d given in divided doses. Maximum dose is 2.4 mg/d. Minimize sedation by giving majority of daily dose at hs.
- *Transdermal system:* Start with 0.1-mg system. Apply system to hairless area of intact skin of upper arm or torso once every 7 d. Change skin site for each application. If system loosens while wearing, apply adhesive overlay directly over system to ensure adhesion. If desired BP reduction is not achieved in 1–2 wk, add another 0.1-mg system or use a larger system. Dosage > two 0.3-mg systems usually does not improve efficacy. Antihypertensive effect may not commence until

Adverse effects in *Italics* are most common; those in **Bold** are life-threatening

2–3 d after application. When substituting transdermal systems, a gradual reduction of prior dosage is advised. Previous antihypertensive medication may have to be continued, particularly with severe hypertension.

▸ *Renal function impairment:* Adjust dosage according to degree of renal impairment; carefully monitor patient.

TREATMENT OF OVERDOSE/ANTIDOTE

Discontinue drug or decrease dosage. Initiate general supportive and resuscitative measures. Establish respiration, initiate gastric lavage, and administer activated charcoal. Magnesium sulfate will increase the rate of transport through the GI tract. Treat bradycardia with atropine; hypotension with dopamine and IV fluids; rebound hypertension with IV furosemide, diazoxide, or alpha-blocking agents, such as phentolamine. Tolazoline in IV doses of 10 mg at 30-min intervals may reverse clonidine's effects if other efforts fail. Naloxone may be a useful adjunct to treat clonidine-induced respiratory depression, hypotension, or coma.

Pharmacokinetics

Route	Onset	Peak	Duration
Oral	30–60 min	3–5 h	24 h
Transdermal	Slow	2–3 d	7 d

Metabolism: Hepatic; $T_{1/2}$: 12–16 h (tablets)
Excretion: Urine

Adverse effects
Tablets

▸ **CNS:** *Drowsiness, sedation, dizziness,* headache, dreams, nightmares, insomnia, hallucinations, delirium, nervousness, agitation, restlessness, anxiety, depression, blurred vision
▸ **CV:** CHF, syncope, chest pain, orthostatic symptoms, palpitations, tachycardia, bradycardia, Raynaud's phenomenon, sinus node arrest, Wenckebach's phenomenon, ventricular trigeminy, conduction disturbances, dysrhythmias, sinus bradycardia
▸ **GI:** *Dry mouth, constipation,* abdominal pain, anorexia, malaise, nausea, vomiting, mild transient abnormalities in liver function tests, hepatitis, parotitis
▸ **GU:** *Impotence, decreased libido,* Peyronie's disease, dysuria, nocturia, frequency, urinary tract infection, renal failure
▸ **Musc/Skel:** Weakness, fatigue, muscle or joint pain, cramps of lower limbs

Adverse effects in *Italics* are most common; those in **Bold** are life-threatening

- **Derm:** Rash, pruritus, angioneurotic edema, hives, urticaria, alopecia
- **Metabolic:** Weight gain, transient elevation of blood glucose or serum creatine phosphokinase, gynecomastia
- **Misc:** Increased sensitivity to alcohol, dry nasal mucosa, pallor, fever, weakly positive Coombs' test, burning and dryness of eyes

Transdermal system
- **CNS: Cerebrovascular accident,** *drowsiness,* fatigue, headache, lethargy, sedation, insomnia, nervousness, dizziness, irritability
- **CV:** Chest pain, increases in BP
- **GI:** *Dry mouth,* constipation, nausea, change in taste, dry throat
- **GU:** Impotence, sexual dysfunction
- **Derm:** Transient localized skin reactions, pruritus, erythema, allergic contact sensitization and contact dermatitis, localized vesiculation, hyperpigmentation, rash, urticaria, angioedema of face and tongue

Clinically important drug–drug interactions
- Potentiated CNS-depressive effects of alcohol, barbiturates, or other sedating drugs
- Reduced antihypertensive effects with TCAs, prazosin
- Bradycardia and AV block with use with drugs that affect sinus node function or AV nodal conduction (digitalis, calcium channel-blockers, beta-blockers)
- Reduced effectiveness of levodopa

● NURSING CONSIDERATIONS

Assessment
- *History:* Allergy to clonidine or any adhesive layer components of transdermal system, severe coronary insufficiency, conduction disturbances, recent MI, cerebrovascular disease, chronic renal failure
- *Physical:* P, BP, R, ECG, I & O, weight, neurologic checks, muscle strength, reflexes, vision, ophthalmologic exam, cardiac auscultation, edema, skin assessment, adventitious lung sounds, palpation of salivary glands, bowel sounds, voiding patterns, breast exam, serum electrolytes, liver and renal function tests

Implementation
- Do not discontinue abruptly but reduce dose gradually over 2–4 d to avoid rebound hypertension, tachycardia, flushing, nausea, vomiting, dysrhythmias. Hypertensive encephalopathy,

Adverse effects in *Italics* are most common; those in **Bold** are life-threatening

cerebrovascular accident, and death have occurred after abrupt cessation of clonidine.

▸ Reevaluate therapy if clonidine tolerance occurs; giving a concomitant diuretic increases the antihypertensive efficacy of clonidine.

▸ If patient experiences isolated, mild, localized skin irritation before completing 7 d of transdermal use, system may be removed and replaced with a new system at a fresh site.

▸ Remove transdermal clonidine systems before attempting defibrillation or cardioversion because of potential for altered electrical conductivity that may increase risk of arcing.

▸ Perform periodic eye examinations because retinal degeneration has been noted in animal studies.

▸ Continue clonidine to within 4 h of surgery and resume as soon as possible after surgery.

⬤ **clopidogrel** *(cloe pid' oh grel)* Plavix

Pregnancy Category B

Drug classes
Adenosine diphosphate (ADP) receptor antagonist
Antiplatelet agent

Indications
▸ Reduction of atherosclerotic events (AMI, CVA, vascular death) in patients with documented atherosclerosis
▸ Particularly useful after coronary angioplasty or under conditions in which acute vessel closure due to intimal edema or thrombosis is a significant risk
▸ Alternative to aspirin for patients with aspirin sensitivity, intolerance, or when aspirin produces poor response

Therapeutic actions
▸ Inhibits binding of ADP to its platelet receptor
▸ Blocks fibrinogen binding to the GP IIb/IIIa receptor
▸ Irreversibly inhibits platelet aggregation

Contraindications/cautions
▸ **Contraindications:** clopidogrel allergy, active pathological bleeding
▸ **Cautions:** bleeding disorders, recent trauma or surgery, liver function impairment

Available form
▸ Tablets: 75 mg

Adverse effects in *Italics* are most common; those in **Bold** are life-threatening

Oral dosage
▸ Some physicians may order 300–375 mg PO before coronary artery stent placement.
▸ 75 mg/d PO with or without food.

TREATMENT OF OVERDOSE/ANTIDOTE
Discontinue drug or decrease dosage. Initiate general resuscitative and supportive measures. A platelet transfusion may be appropriate if quick reversal of drug's effects is required.

Pharmacokinetics
Route	Onset	Peak	Duration
Oral	Rapid	1 h	3–4 h

Metabolism: Hepatic; $T_{1/2}$: 8 h; once drug achieves steady state inhibition after 3–7 d of therapy, it inhibits 40% to 60% of platelet aggregation; after stopping clopidogrel therapy, platelet aggregation and bleeding times return to baseline in about 3–7 d
Excretion: Urine, feces

Adverse effects
▸ *CNS: Headache, dizziness,* weakness, fatigue, depression
▸ *CV: Chest pain,* edema, hypertension
▸ *Resp: Upper respiratory tract infection,* dyspnea, rhinitis, bronchitis, coughing
▸ *GI:* **GI bleeding,** *abdominal pain, dyspepsia,* diarrhea, nausea, ulcers, anorexia, elevated liver transaminases
▸ *Hematologic:* **Neutropenia, agranulocytosis, thrombotic thrombocytopenic purpura, bleeding diatheses,** epistaxis
▸ *Musc/Skel: Arthralgia, back pain*
▸ *Dermatologic: Skin rash,* pruritus
▸ *Misc:* Hypercholesterolemia, urinary tract infection, pain, influenza-like symptoms

Clinically important drug–drug interactions
▸ Occult GI blood loss with NSAIDs
▸ Prolonged bleeding time, but no conclusive data exist about its effect on warfarin
▸ Interference with metabolism of phenytoin, tamoxifen, tolbutamide, warfarin, torsemide, fluvastatin, many NSAIDs, but no conclusive data are available; use with caution

● NURSING CONSIDERATIONS

Assessment
▸ *History:* Clopidogrel allergy, active pathological bleeding, bleeding disorders, recent trauma or surgery, liver function impairment

Adverse effects in *Italics* are most common; those in **Bold** are life-threatening

▸ *Physical:* T, P, R, BP, ECG, I & O, neurologic checks, skin assessment, orthostatic BP, peripheral perfusion, bowel sounds, liver evaluation, pain assessment, adventitious lung sounds, presence of bleeding, CBC, coagulation studies, liver function tests, serum cholesterol; urine, stool, and emesis guaiac

Implementation
▸ Monitor CBC before use and frequently while initiating therapy; if neutropenia or TTP is suspected (fever, weakness, difficulty speaking, seizures, yellowing of skin or eyes, dark or bloody urine, pallor, or petechiae), discontinue drug immediately.
▸ Monitor patient for any sign of excessive bleeding (eg, bruises, dark urine and stools), and monitor bleeding times.
▸ Provide increased precautions against bleeding during invasive procedures; bleeding will be prolonged.
▸ Check stools, urine, and emesis for occult blood.
▸ Monitor the patient's WBC, Hgb, Hct, APTT, and platelet values; notify provider of abnormal values. Be prepared to transfuse platelets if platelet count is < 50,000 cells/mcL.
▸ Mark patient's chart indicating that patient is receiving clopidogrel to alert medical personnel of increased risk of bleeding in cases of surgery or diagnostic procedures.
▸ Provide small, frequent meals if GI upset occurs (not as common as with aspirin).
▸ Provide comfort measures and arrange for analgesics if headache occurs.

⬤ **co-trimoxazole** *(trimethoprim and sulfamethoxazole)* (koe try *mox'* oh zole), Bactrim, Bactrim DS, Bactrim IV, Cotrim, Cotrim D.S., Septra, Septra I.V., Sulfatrim, TMP-SMZ

Pregnancy Category C

Drug class
Anti-infective

Indications
▸ Urinary tract infections (UTIs) due to susceptible strains of *Escherichia coli, Klebsiella* and *Enterobacter* species, *Morganella morganii, Proteus mirabilis,* and *Proteus vulgaris* (oral and parenteral)
▸ *Shigellosis* enteritis caused by susceptible strains of *Shigellosis flexneri* and *Shigellosis sonnei* (oral and parenteral)
▸ *Pneumocystis carinii* pneumonia (oral and parenteral)
▸ Prophylaxis of *P. carinii* pneumonia (oral)
▸ Acute exacerbations of chronic bronchitis due to susceptible strains of *Haemophilus influenzae* and *Streptococcus pneumoniae* (oral)

Adverse effects in *Italics* are most common; those in **Bold** are life-threatening

- Travelers' diarrhea due to susceptible strains of enterotoxigenic *E. coli* (oral)
- Unlabeled uses: treatment of cholera and salmonella-type infections and nocardiosis; prophylaxis of neutropenic patients with *P. carinii* infections or leukemia to reduce the incidence of gram-negative rod bacteremia; prophylaxis of bacterial infection after renal transplantation; treatment of acute and chronic prostatitis

Therapeutic actions

- Bacteriocidal: blocks two consecutive steps in the bacterial biosynthesis of essential nucleic acids and proteins (sulfamethoxazole [SMZ] inhibits bacterial synthesis of dihydrofolic acid by competing with para-aminobenzoic acid; trimethoprim [TMP] blocks the production of tetrahydrofolic acid by inhibiting the enzyme dihydrofolate reductase)

Contraindications/cautions
- **Contraindications:** hypersensitivity to TMP or sulfonamides, megaloblastic anemia due to folate deficiency, streptococcal pharyngitis
- **Cautions:** severe allergy or bronchial asthma, G-6-PD deficiency, impaired renal or hepatic function, *P. carinii pneumonitis* in patients with AIDS, bone marrow depression, possible folate deficiency (elderly patients, chronic alcoholics, anticonvulsant therapy, malabsorption syndrome, malnutrition)

Available forms

- *Injection:* 80 mg TMP and 400 mg SMZ per 5 mL, 80 mg/mL SMZ, 16 mg/mL TMP per 5 mL
- *Tablets:* 80 mg TMP and 400 mg SMZ
- *Tablets, double strength:* 160 mg TMP and 800 mg SMZ
- *Oral suspension:* 40 mg TMP and 200 mg SMZ per 5 mL

IV facts
Preparation
- Add contents of each 5-mL ampule to 125 mL of D5W. Do not refrigerate; use within 6 h. If 5 mL was diluted in 100 mL D5W, use within 4 h. If fluid restriction needed, add each 5-mL ampule to 75 mL of D5W and use within 2 h.

Dosage
- Give each IV dose over 60–90 min. If administered by an infusion device, thoroughly flush all lines to remove any residual drug.
- *Severe UTI and shigellosis:* 8–10 mg/kg/d (based on TMP) IV in 2–4 divided doses q6–12h for up to 14 d for UTI or 5 d for shigellosis.

Adverse effects in *Italics* are most common; those in **Bold** are life-threatening

▸ *P. carinii pneumonia:* 15–20 mg/kg/d (based on TMP) IV in 3–4 divided doses q6–8h for up to 14 d.

Compatibility

Co-trimoxazole may be given through the same IV line as: acyclovir, aldesleukin, allopurinol, amifostine, atracurium, aztreonam, cefepime, cyclophosphamide, diltiazem, enalaprilat, esmolol, filgrastim, fludarabine, gallium, granisetron, hydromorphone, labetalol, lorazepam, magnesium sulfate, melphalan, meperidine, morphine, pancuronium, perphenazine, piperacillin-tazobactam, sargramostim, tacrolimus, teniposide, thiotepa, vecuronium, zidovudine.

Incompatibility

Do not administer through the same IV line as fluconazole, midazolam, vinorelbine.

Oral dosage

▸ *Urinary tract and shigellosis:* 160 mg TMP/800 mg SMZ PO q12h for 10–14 d for UTI or 5 d for shigellosis.
▸ *Travelers' diarrhea:* 160 mg TMP/800 mg SMZ PO q12h for 5 d.
▸ *Acute exacerbations of chronic bronchitis:* 160 mg TMP/800 SMZ PO q12h for 14 d.
▸ *Treatment of P. carinii pneumonia:* 15–20 mg/kg TMP/100 mg/kg SMZ PO per day in divided doses q6h for 14–21 d.
▸ *Prophylaxis of P. carinii pneumonia:* 160 mg TMP/800 mg SMZ PO q24h.
▸ *Impaired renal function:* If creatinine clearance is > 30 mL/min, give usual dosage; if 15–30 mL/min, give half the usual regimen; if < 15 mL/min, drug not recommended.

TREATMENT OF OVERDOSE/ANTIDOTE

Discontinue drug or decrease dosage. Initiate general supportive and resuscitative measures. Empty the stomach by inducing vomiting or by gastric lavage. If urine output is low and renal function is normal, force oral fluids and administer IV fluids. Acidifying urine will increase renal elimination of TMP. Hemodialysis is moderately effective in eliminating TMP and SMZ.

Pharmacokinetics

Route	Onset	Peak
IV	Immediate	1–1.5 h
Oral	Rapid	1–4 h

Metabolism: Hepatic; $T_{1/2}$: IV: 11.3 h TMP, 12.8 h SMZ; Oral: 8–11 h TMP, 10–12 h SMZ
Excretion: Urine

Adverse effects in *Italics* are most common; those in **Bold** are life-threatening

C

Adverse effects
- *CNS:* **Convulsions,** headache, depression, ataxia, hallucinations, tinnitus, vertigo, insomnia, apathy, fatigue, weakness, nervousness, peripheral neuritis, aseptic meningitis
- *GI:* **Hepatitis (including cholestatic jaundice and hepatic necrosis), pseudomembranous colitis, pancreatitis,** *nausea, vomiting, anorexia,* emesis, glossitis, stomatitis, abdominal pain, elevated serum transaminases and bilirubin
- *GU:* **Renal failure, toxic nephrosis with oliguria and anuria,** interstitial nephritis, elevated BUN and creatinine, crystalluria
- *Derm:* *Allergic skin reactions (rash, urticaria),* local pain and irritation with IV administration
- *Allergic:* **Anaphylaxis, Stevens-Johnson syndrome, toxic epidermal necrolysis, angioedema,** drug fever, allergic myocarditis, pruritus, rash, erythema multiforme
- *Hematologic:* **Agranulocytosis; aplastic, hemolytic, or megaloblastic anemia; thrombocytopenia, leukopenia, neutropenia, eosinophilia**
- *Misc:* Hyperkalemia, hyponatremia, serum sickness-like syndrome, arthralgia, myalgia, sore throat, pulmonary infiltrates, shortness of breath

Clinically important drug–drug interactions
- Prolonged PT with warfarin
- Decreased effects of cyclosporine; increased risk of nephrotoxicity
- Increased serum levels of either drug when given with dapsone
- Increased thrombocytopenia in elderly patients who take diuretics
- Decreased clearance and prolonged half-life of phenytoin
- Increased methotrexate concentrations and increased risk of bone marrow depression
- Increased hypoglycemia associated with use of sulfonylureas
- Reduced renal clearance and increased serum levels of zidovudine

● NURSING CONSIDERATIONS

Assessment
- *History:* Hypersensitivity to TMP or sulfonamides, megaloblastic anemia due to folate deficiency, streptococcal pharyngitis, severe allergy or bronchial asthma, G-6-PD deficiency, impaired renal or hepatic function, *P. carinii pneumonitis,* AIDS, bone marrow depression, folate deficiency,

Adverse effects in *Italics* are most common; those in **Bold** are life-threatening

age, chronic alcoholism, anticonvulsant therapy, malabsorption syndrome, malnutrition

▸ *Physical:* T, P, R, BP, I & O, IV site, neurologic checks, skin assessment, adventitious lung sounds, hydration status, abdominal assessment, bowel sounds, culture and sensitivity tests of infected area, renal and liver function tests, UA, CBC, PT

Implementation

▸ Obtain specimens for culture and sensitivity of infected area before beginning therapy. May begin drug before results are available.
▸ Have emergency equipment (defibrillator, drugs, oxygen, intubation equipment) on standby in case anaphylactic reaction occurs.
▸ Assess for evidence of anaphylaxis; if suspected, discontinue drug immediately and notify provider.
▸ Monitor renal, hepatic, and hematopoietic function.
▸ Monitor for occurrence of superinfections; treat as appropriate.
▸ Discontinue drug at any sign of colitis; initiate appropriate supportive treatment.
▸ Give oral drug with a full glass of water.
▸ Ensure that patient is well hydrated.
▸ After entering a multidose vial, use the remaining contents within 48 h.

⬤ **cyclosporine** *(sye' kloe spor een)* cyclosporin A
Neoral, Sandimmune, SangCya

Pregnancy Category C

Drug class
Immunosuppressant

Indications

▸ Prophylaxis for organ rejection in kidney, liver, and heart allogeneic transplants; Sandimmune is given in conjunction with adrenal corticosteroids; Neoral has been used in combination with azathioprine and corticosteroids
▸ Treatment of chronic rejection in patients previously treated with other immunosuppressive agents (Sandimmune)
▸ Treatment of severe active rheumatoid arthritis when the disease has not adequately responded to methotrexate (Neoral)
▸ Treatment of nonimmunocompromised patients with severe, plaque psoriasis who failed to respond to at least one systemic therapy or for whom other systemic therapies are contraindicated or cannot be tolerated

Adverse effects in *Italics* are most common; those in **Bold** are life-threatening

C

- Unlabeled uses: limited but successful use in pancreas, bone marrow, and heart/lung transplants; alopecia areata, aplastic anemia, atopic dermatitis, Behçet's disease, biliary cirrhosis, corneal transplantation, Crohn's disease, ulcerative colitis, dermatomyositis, diabetes mellitus, lupus nephritis, multiple sclerosis, myasthenia gravis, nephrotic syndrome, pemphigus and pemphigoid, polymyositis, psoriatic arthritis, pulmonary sarcoidosis, pyoderma gangrenosum, uveitis

Therapeutic actions
- Exact mechanism of immunosuppressant unknown; specifically and reversibly inhibits immunocompetent lymphocytes in the G_0 or G_1 phase of the cell cycle; inhibits T-helper and T-suppressor cells, lymphokine production, and release of interleukin-2 or T-cell growth factor

Contraindications/cautions
- **Contraindications:** cyclosporine allergy, allergy to polyoxyethylated castor oil (injection only); psoriasis or rheumatoid arthritis with abnormal renal function, uncontrolled hypertension (HTN), or malignancy (Neoral); concomitant use with PUVA or UVB in psoriasis patients (Neoral)
- **Cautions:** impaired renal or liver function, malabsorption, HTN, hyperkalemia, convulsive disorders

Available forms
- *IV solution:* 50 mg/mL
- *Capsules:* 25, 50, 100 mg
- *Oral solution:* 100 mg/mL

IV facts
Preparation
- Immediately before use, dilute 50 mg in 20–100 mL of D5W or 0.9%NS. Use nonleaching IV tubing.

Dosage
- 5–6 mg/kg IV infused over 2–6 h beginning 4–12 h before transplantation. Continue postoperatively as a single daily dose until patient tolerates oral therapy.

Therapeutic serum levels
- 24-h trough values: 250–800 ng/mL (whole blood), 50–300 ng/mL (plasma)

Compatibility
Cyclosporine may be given through the same IV line as cefmetazole, propofol, sargramostim.

Adverse effects in *Italics* are most common; those in **Bold** are life-threatening

Oral dosage

▸ *Allogenic transplants, Sandimmune:* 15 mg/kg PO 4–12 h before transplantation. Continue postoperatively for 1–2 wk. Then taper by 5%/wk to a maintenance level of 5–10 mg/kg/d.

▸ *Allogenic transplants, Neoral:* Initial dose varies depending on transplanted organ and use of other drugs. In newly transplanted patients, initial dose is the same as the initial oral dose of Sandimmune. Divide total daily dose into 2 equal daily doses. Adjust dosage to achieve desired cyclosporine levels.

> **TREATMENT OF OVERDOSE/ANTIDOTE**
> Discontinue drug or decrease dosage. Initiate general supportive and resuscitative measures. Induce emesis if ≤ 2 h after oral ingestion. Drug is not cleared well by charcoal hemoperfusion.

Pharmacokinetics

Route	Onset	Peak
IV	Rapid	3.5 h
Oral	Varies	1.5–2 h

Metabolism: Hepatic; $T_{1/2}$: 5–18 h Neoral; 10–27 h Sandimmune
Excretion: Bile, feces, urine

Adverse effects

▸ *CNS:* **Convulsions,** *tremor,* confusion, headache, paresthesias
▸ *CV:* *Hypertension,* chest pain
▸ *GI:* **Hepatotoxicity,** *gum hyperplasia, nausea, vomiting, diarrhea,* anorexia, gastritis, peptic ulcer, hiccups
▸ *GU:* **Nephrotoxicity,** *renal dysfunction,* glomerular capillary thrombosis, hyperuricemia
▸ *Allergic:* **Anaphylaxis**
▸ *Hematologic:* Leukopenia, lymphoma
▸ *Misc:* *Hirsutism,* acne, lymphomas, infections, hyperkalemia, hypomagnesemia, brittle finger nails

Clinically important drug–drug interactions

▸ Increased nephrotoxicity with other nephrotoxic agents (erythromycin)
▸ Increased digoxin, etoposide toxicity
▸ Severe myopathy or rhabdomyolysis with lovastatin
▸ Increased toxicity if taken with amiodarone, androgens, colchicine, corticosteroids, diltiazem, imipenem-cilastatin, metoclopramide, nicardipine
▸ Increased plasma concentration of cyclosporine with ketoconazole, fluconazole

Adverse effects in *Italics* are most common; those in **Bold** are life-threatening

▶ Increased renal failure with foscarnet
▶ Decreased therapeutic effect with hydantoins, probucol, rifampin, rifabutin, sulfonamides, terbinafine

● NURSING CONSIDERATIONS

Assessment
▶ *History:* Cyclosporine or polyoxyethylated castor oil allergy, psoriasis, rheumatoid arthritis, HTN, malignancy, use of PUVA or UVB, impaired renal or liver function, malabsorption, hyperkalemia, convulsive disorders
▶ *Physical:* T, P, R, BP, I & O, weight, neurologic checks, skin assessment, peripheral perfusion, liver evaluation, bowel sounds, gum evaluation, renal and liver function tests, CBC, UA, serum electrolytes, cyclosporine drug levels

Implementation
▶ Monitor renal and liver function tests prior to and during therapy; marked decreases in function may require dosage adjustment or discontinuation.
▶ Continuously monitor patients receiving IV cyclosporine for at least the first 30 min after starting the infusion. Have emergency equipment (defibrillator, drugs, oxygen, intubation equipment) on standby in case anaphylaxis or adverse reaction occurs.
▶ Monitor for evidence of infection related to immunosuppression.
▶ Sandimmune may be given with adrenal corticosteroids but not with other immunosuppressants.
▶ Routinely monitor serum drug levels and adjust dosage as indicated.
▶ Monitor for CNS toxicity as evidenced by headache, flushing, confusion, seizures, ataxia, mania, depression, encephalopathy, sleep problems, and blurred vision.
▶ Monitor BP; heart transplant patients may require concomitant antihypertensive therapy.
▶ Neoral and Sandimmune are not bioequivalent; do not use interchangeably.
▶ Give drug on a consistent schedule with regard to time of day and meal schedule.
▶ Using a glass container, mix oral solution with milk, chocolate milk, or orange juice at room temperature. Do not mix with grapefruit juice. Stir well, and administer at once. Do not allow mixture to stand before drinking. Rinse glass with more diluent to ensure that the total dose is taken.
▶ Do not refrigerate oral solution; store at room temperature; use within 2 mo after opening.
▶ Protect IV solution from light.

Adverse effects in *Italics* are most common; those in **Bold** are life-threatening

D

● **dalteparin** *(dahl' tep ah rin)* Fragmin

Pregnancy Category B

Drug classes
Antithrombotic agent
Low–molecular-weight (LMW) heparin

Indications
▸ Treatment of unstable angina and non-Q-wave myocardial infarction for the prevention of ischemic complications in patients on concurrent aspirin therapy
▸ Prevention of deep vein thrombosis, which may lead to pulmonary embolism, following abdominal or hip replacement surgery
▸ Unlabeled uses: systemic anticoagulation in venous and arterial thromboembolic complications

Therapeutic actions
▸ LMW heparin drug with an average weight about half the molecular weight of standard heparin
▸ Blocks Factors Xa and thrombin in the clotting cascade by antithrombin III, thus preventing thrombus formation

Contraindications/cautions
▸ **Contraindications:** hypersensitivity to dalteparin, heparin, pork products; severe thrombocytopenia; uncontrolled bleeding
▸ **Cautions:** hypertensive or diabetic retinopathy, impaired renal or liver function, heparin-induced thrombocytopenia, platelet defects, bacterial endocarditis, uncontrolled hypertension (HTN); recent brain, spinal, or ophthalmological surgery; history of gastrointestinal or intracranial bleeding, bleeding diathesis, other patients at risk for bleeding; congenital or acquired bleeding disorders, active ulceration, angiodysplastic GI disease, hemorrhagic stroke, patients receiving other platelet inhibitors

Available forms
▸ *Injection:* 16 mg/0.2 mL; 32 mg/0.2 mL; 64 mg/0.2 mL

SC facts

Dosage
▸ *Systemic anticoagulation:* 200 IU/kg SC qd or 100 IU/kg SC bid.

Adverse effects in *Italics* are most common; those in **Bold** are life-threatening

- *Unstable angina/non-Q-wave MI:* 120 IU/kg, but not more than 10,000 IU SQ q/2h with concurrent aspirin therapy (unless contraindicated) until the patient is stabilized.
- *Patients undergoing abdominal surgery at risk for thromboembolic complications:* 2500 IU/d SC starting 1–2 h before surgery and repeated qd for 5–10 d postoperatively.
- *Patients undergoing hip replacement surgery at risk for thromboembolic complications:* 2500 IU SC ≤ 2 h before surgery. Give second dose of 2500 IU SC the evening of the day of surgery (≥ 6 h after first dose). Then give 5000 IU SC qd for 5–10 d. Or give 5000 IU SC starting the evening before surgery, followed by 5000 IU/d SC starting the evening of the day of surgery. Continue 5–10 d.
- *High-risk patients:* 5000 IU SC the evening before surgery and repeat qd for 5–10 d postoperatively. For patients with malignancy, give the first 5000-IU dose as 2500 IU SC 1–2 h before surgery with an additional 2500-IU dose 12 h later; then give 5000 IU/d for 5–10 d.

TREATMENT OF OVERDOSE/ANTIDOTE

Discontinue drug or decrease dosage. Initiate general supportive and resuscitative measures. Drug's effect may be stopped by protamine sulfate (1%) 1 mg (IV over 10 minutes) for every 100 anti-Xa IU of dalteparin. If the APTT remains prolonged 2–4 h after first infusion, may repeat protamine sulfate at half the first dose. Be aware that protamine sulfate may cause hypotension or anaphylactic reactions.

Pharmacokinetics

Route	Onset	Peak
SC	Rapid	4 h

$T_{1/2}$: 3–5 h
Excretion: Urine

Adverse effects

- *Allergic:* **Anaphylaxis,** chills, fever, urticaria, asthma, rash
- *Hematologic:* **Hemorrhage; thrombocytopenia;** *bruising;* elevated AST, ALT; hyperkalemia, wound hematoma, injection site hematoma
- *Misc:* Fever, pain, local irritation, hematoma, erythema, skin necrosis at site of injection

Clinically important drug–drug interactions

- Increased bleeding tendencies with oral anticoagulants, salicylates, NSAIDs, antiplatelet drugs

Adverse effects in *Italics* are most common; those in **Bold** are life-threatening

◉ NURSING CONSIDERATIONS

Assessment

‣ *History:* Hypersensitivity to dalteparin, heparin, pork products; severe thrombocytopenia, uncontrolled bleeding, hypertensive or diabetic retinopathy, impaired renal or liver function, heparin-induced thrombocytopenia, platelet defects, bacterial endocarditis, uncontrolled HTN; recent brain, spinal, or ophthalmological surgery; history of gastrointestinal or intracranial bleeding, bleeding diathesis, risk for bleeding, congenital or acquired bleeding disorders, active ulceration, angiodysplastic GI disease, hemor-rhagic stroke, use of other platelet inhibitors

‣ *Physical:* T, P, BP, R, ECG, weight, peripheral perfusion, skin assessment, presence of bleeding, surgical incision assessment, injection site assessment, character of output from indwelling drains, CBC, coagulation studies, kidney and liver function tests; urine, stool, emesis guaiac

Implementation

‣ Give deep subcutaneous injections; *do not* give dalteparin by IM injection. Patient should be lying down; inject into a U-shaped area around navel, the upper outer side of thigh, or upper outer quadrangle of buttock; vary injection site daily. Introduce the whole length of the needle into a skin fold held between the thumb and forefinger; hold skin fold throughout the injection.

‣ Apply pressure to all injection sites after needle is withdrawn, but do not massage site; inspect injection sites for signs of hematoma.

‣ Do not mix with other injections or infusions.

‣ Alert all health care providers that patient is on dalteparin.

‣ If thromboembolic episode should occur despite therapy, discontinue and initiate appropriate therapy.

‣ Have emergency equipment (defibrillator, drugs, oxygen, intubation equipment) on standby in case of anaphylaxis.

‣ Provide safety measures (electric razor, soft toothbrush) to prevent injury and minimize risk for bleeding.

‣ Assess patient for signs of bleeding.

‣ Routinely monitor CBC, UA, and stool guaiac during treatment. No monitoring of blood clotting times is needed because drug only slightly affects PT and APTT.

‣ LMW heparins cannot be used interchangeably with other LMW heparins or unfractionated heparin.

‣ Have protamine sulfate (dalteparin antidote) on standby in case of overdose.

‣ Store at room temperature.

Adverse effects in *Italics* are most common; those in **Bold** are life-threatening

● **dantrolene sodium** *(dan' troe leen)* Dantrium, Dantrium Intravenous

Pregnancy Category C

Drug class
Skeletal muscle relaxant, direct acting

Indications
▸ Management of fulminant hypermetabolism of skeletal muscle characteristic of malignant hyperthermia; preoperatively or postoperatively to prevent or attenuate malignant hyperthermia in patients susceptible to malignant hyperthermia (IV)
▸ Preoperatively to prevent or attenuate malignant hyperthermia in patients susceptible to malignant hyperthermia; following malignant hyperthermia crisis to prevent recurrence of malignant hyperthermia (oral)
▸ Control of clinical spasticity resulting from upper motor neuron disorders, such as spinal cord injury, stroke, cerebral palsy, or multiple sclerosis; chronic use justified if drug significantly reduces painful or disabling spasticity, reduces intensity or degree of nursing care, or rids patient of annoying spasticity (oral)
▸ Unlabeled uses: heat stroke, neuroleptic malignant syndrome, exercise-induced muscle pain

Therapeutic actions
▸ Prevents acute catabolic processes common to malignant hypermetabolic crisis
▸ Reverses hypermetabolic process of malignant hyperthermia
▸ Produces muscle relaxation by dissociating excitation-contraction coupling in skeletal muscle, probably by interfering with release of calcium from the sarcoplasmic reticulum

Contraindications/cautions
▸ **Contraindications:** dantrolene allergy, active hepatic disease (hepatitis, cirrhosis), treatment of skeletal muscle spasm resulting from rheumatic disorders; when spasticity is needed to sustain upright posture, balance in locomotion, or to obtain or maintain increased function
▸ **Cautions:** impaired pulmonary function, severely impaired cardiac function due to myocardial disease, history of liver disease or dysfunction, females and patients > 35 y (increased risk of potentially fatal hepatocellular disease)

Available forms
▸ *Powder for injection:* 20 mg/vial
▸ *Capsules:* 25, 50, 100 mg

Adverse effects in *Italics* are most common; those in **Bold** are life-threatening

IV facts
Preparation
▸ Add 60 mL Sterile Water for Injection (without a bacteriostatic agent) to each vial; shake until solution is clear.
▸ Do not transfer to glass bottles; may precipitate.
▸ Protect solution from light and use within 6 h.

Dosage
▸ *Preoperative prophylaxis of malignant hyperthermia:* 2.5 mg/kg IV over 1 h infused 1 h before anesthesia.
▸ *Treatment of malignant hyperthermia:* 1 mg/kg by continuous rapid IV push and continuing until symptoms subside or dose of 10 mg/kg is given. If physiologic and metabolic abnormalities reappear, repeat regimen.
▸ *Postcrisis follow-up:* Use oral drug (see below) unless not practical. Start with 1 mg/kg IV or more as clinical situation dictates.

Incompatibility
Dantrolene is incompatible with acidic solutions; D5W; 0.9%NS.

Oral dosage
▸ *Preoperative prophylaxis of malignant hyperthermia:* 4–8 mg/kg/d PO in 3–4 divided doses for 1–2 d before surgery with last dose 3–4 h before surgery. Adjust within recommended dosage range to avoid drowsiness, skeletal muscle weakness, or excessive GI irritation.
▸ *Postcrisis follow-up:* 4–8 mg/kg/d PO in 4 divided doses for 1–3 d to prevent recurrence.
▸ *Chronic spasticity:* Establish therapeutic goal before starting therapy. Increase dosage until the maximum performance compatible with the dysfunction is reached. Begin with 25 mg/d PO; increase to 25 mg PO bid–qid; then by increment of 25 mg up to 100 mg bid–qid if needed. Most patients will respond to 400 mg/d or less. Maintain each dosage level 4–7 d to evaluate response. Discontinue drug after 45 d if benefits are not evident.

TREATMENT OF OVERDOSE/ANTIDOTE
Discontinue drug or decrease dosage. Initiate general supportive and resuscitative measures. Begin gastric lavage. Administer large quantities of IV fluids to prevent crystalluria.

Adverse effects in *Italics* are most common; those in **Bold** are life-threatening

Pharmacokinetics

Route	Onset
IV	Rapid
PO	Slow

Metabolism: Hepatic; $T_{1/2}$: 4–8 h (IV); 9 h (oral)
Excretion: Urine

Adverse effects

Oral

- *CNS:* **Seizures,** *drowsiness, dizziness, weakness, malaise, fatigue,* speech disturbance, headache, lightheadedness, visual disturbance, diplopia, insomnia, mental depression, mental confusion, increased nervousness
- *CV:* Tachycardia, erratic blood pressure, phlebitis, pleural effusion with pericarditis
- *GI:* **Hepatitis,** *diarrhea,* constipation, GI bleeding, anorexia, dysphagia, gastric irritation, abdominal cramps
- *GU:* Increased urinary frequency, hematuria, crystalluria, difficult erection, urinary incontinence, nocturia, dysuria, urinary retention
- *Derm:* Abnormal hair growth, acne-like rash, pruritus, urticaria, eczematoid eruption, sweating
- *Hematologic:* **Aplastic anemia, leukopenia, lymphocytic lymphoma**
- *Musc/Skel:* Myalgia, backache
- *Misc:* Chills, fever, feeling of suffocation, excessive tearing

Parenteral

- None of the serious reactions reported with long-term oral dantrolene use has been associated with short-term IV therapy.
- **Death, pulmonary edema,** thrombophlebitis, urticaria, erythema

Clinically important drug–drug interactions

- Decreased plasma protein binding with clofibrate and warfarin
- Increased hyperkalemia and myocardial depression or collapse with verapamil

⬤ NURSING CONSIDERATIONS

Assessment

- *History:* Dantrolene allergy; active hepatic disease; treatment of skeletal muscle spasm resulting from rheumatic disorders; need for spasticity to sustain upright posture, balance in locomotion, or obtain or maintain increased function; impaired pulmonary function; severely impaired cardiac function due to myocardial disease; liver disease or dysfunction; gender; age

Adverse effects in *Italics* are most common; those in **Bold** are life-threatening

‣ *Physical:* T, P, BP, R, ECG, I & O, IV site, weight, neurologic checks, muscle strength assessment, presence of muscle spasticity, skin assessment, activity tolerance, adventitious lung sounds, bowel sounds, UA, liver function tests, serum electrolytes

Implementation

‣ IV use is not a substitute for other treatment for malignant hyperthermia. Discontinue suspected triggering agents, increase oxygen delivery, manage metabolic acidosis, institute cooling if needed, monitor urine output, and monitor electrolyte balance.
‣ Monitor IV sites and ensure that extravasation does not occur; drug is very alkaline and irritates tissues.
‣ Use lowest possible dose to achieve desired effects.
‣ Perform liver function tests during therapy; discontinue therapy if results are abnormal.
‣ Discontinue therapy if symptoms of hepatitis, such as jaundice, appear. Restart drug only if absolutely necessary and when patient is hospitalized.
‣ Withdraw drug for 2–4 d to confirm therapeutic benefits; exacerbated spasticity may confirm clinical impression and justify use of this potentially dangerous drug.
‣ Drug caused cancer in animals; risk to humans is not known. Weigh this risk against potential benefits of drug therapy.

● deferoxamine mesylate *(de fer ox' a meen)*
Desferal

Pregnancy Category C

Drug classes
Antidote
Chelating agent

Indications
‣ Adjunct therapy for acute iron intoxication
‣ Treatment of chronic iron overload
‣ Unlabeled uses: management of aluminum accumulation in bone in renal failure and aluminum-induced dialysis encephalopathy; treatment in some cancers and Alzheimer's disease

Therapeutic actions
‣ Chelates unbound iron and forms ferrioxamine, which is excreted by the kidneys

Contraindications
‣ **Contraindications:** deferoxamine allergy, severe renal disease, anuria, primary hemochromatosis

Adverse effects in *Italics* are most common; those in **Bold** are life-threatening

Available form
◗ *Powder for injection:* 500 mg/vial

IV/IM/SC facts
Preparation
◗ Add 2 mL Sterile Water for Injection to each vial. For IV use, add drug to D5W; LR; or 0.9%NS. Protect from light.

Dosage
◗ May give slow IV infusion, IM, or by continuous SC mini-infusion. IM is the preferred route if patient is not in shock.
◗ *Acute iron intoxication:* 1 g IV by slow infusion ($\leq$ 15mg/kg/h) or IM. Then 500 mg IV or IM q4h for 2 doses. Subsequently, give 0.5 g q4–12h based on clinical response. Do not exceed 6 g/d. As soon as possible, switch from IV to IM administration.
◗ *Chronic iron overload:* Individualize dosage. 0.5–1 g/d IM. Give 2 g IV with, but separate from, each unit of blood. Do not exceed IV infusion rate of 15 mg/kg/h. Or 1–2 g/d (20–40 mg/kg/d) SC over 8–12 h.

Compatibility
Information not available. Do not mix or administer with other drugs.

> **TREATMENT OF OVERDOSE/ANTIDOTE**
> Discontinue drug or decrease dosage. Initiate general supportive and resuscitative measures. There is no specific antidote. Deferoxamine is dialyzable.

Pharmacokinetics

Route	Onset
IV, IM	Rapid

Metabolism: Plasma enzymes; $T_{1/2}$: 1 h
Excretion: Urine, feces through bile

Adverse effects
◗ *CV:* **Shock** and hypotension with rapid IV use; tachycardia
◗ *GI:* Abdominal discomfort, diarrhea
◗ *Derm:* Irritation, pain, erythema, wheal formation, swelling, pruritus, and induration at SC injection site
◗ *Allergic:* **Anaphylaxis**
◗ *Acute iron intoxication:* Red urine; generalized erythema with rapid IV use
◗ *Misc:* Dysuria, leg cramps, fever, ocular and auditory disturbances (blurred vision, cataracts, visual loss, tinnitus, hearing loss; impaired peripheral, color, and night vision)

Adverse effects in *Italics* are most common; those in **Bold** are life-threatening

⦿NURSING CONSIDERATIONS

Assessment
▸ *History:* Deferoxamine allergy, severe renal disease, anuria, primary hemochromatosis
▸ *Physical:* P, BP, R, I & O, IV site, neurologic checks, skin assessment, respiratory effort, adventitious lung sounds, edema, abdominal exam, vision and hearing exam, CBC, kidney and liver function tests, UA, serum iron levels

Implementation
▸ Always administer IV and SC infusions using an IV infusion pump.
▸ Monitor I & O. Iron chelate is excreted by kidneys; urine may turn red.
▸ Rapid IV infusion may cause flushing of skin, urticaria, hypotension, and shock.
▸ Monitor infusion and injection sites for redness, inflammation, pain, pruritus, swelling.
▸ Have emergency equipment (defibrillator, drugs, oxygen, intubation equipment) on standby in case anaphylaxis or adverse reaction occurs.
▸ For acute iron intoxication, deferoxamine is an adjunct to other standard treatments, such as induction of emesis with syrup of ipecac; gastric lavage; maintenance of airway; control of shock with IV fluids, blood, oxygen, and vasopressors; and correction of acidosis.
▸ Monitor for visual or auditory disturbances.
▸ Do not store reconstituted solutions for more than 1 wk.

⦿ desmopressin acetate
(1-deamino-8-D-arginine vasopressin) *(des moe press' in)*
DDAVP, Octostim (CAN), Stimate

Pregnancy Category B

Drug class
Hormone

Indications
▸ DDAVP:
  ▸ Treatment of neurogenic diabetes insipidus (parenteral, oral, intranasal)
  ▸ Maintenance of hemostasis in patients with hemophilia A or von Willebrand's disease with Factor VIII levels > 5% (parenteral, intranasal)
  ▸ Treatment of primary nocturnal enuresis (intranasal)

Adverse effects in *Italics* are most common; those in **Bold** are life-threatening

- Stimate:
  - Maintenance of hemostasis in patients with hemophilia A or von Willebrand's disease with Factor VIII levels > 5%
- Unlabeled use: Treatment of chronic autonomic failure

Therapeutic actions
- Is a synthetic analog of human antidiuretic hormone
- Promotes reabsorption of water in the renal tubule to decrease urine output and maintain fluid volume
- In large doses, increases levels of clotting Factor VIII to control bleeding

Contraindications/cautions
- **Contraindications:** allergy to desmopressin acetate or its components, hemophilia A with Factor VIII levels ≤ 5%, hemophilia B, patients with Factor VIII antibodies, type I or type IIB von Willebrand's disease; impaired level of consciousness (intranasal)
- **Cautions:** coronary artery insufficiency, hypertensive cardiovascular disease, water intoxication, electrolyte imbalance, patients at risk for thrombosis

Available forms
- *Injection:* 4 mcg/mL
- *Tablets:* 0.1, 0.2 mg
- *Nasal solution:* 0.1 mg/mL, DDAVP; 1.5 mg/mL, Stimate

IV/SC facts
Preparation
- May be given undiluted or diluted in 50 mL of sterile physiologic saline.

Dosage
- *Diabetes insipidus:* 2–4 mcg/d IV or SC in 2 divided doses; titrate for an adequate diurnal rhythm of water turnover.
- *Hemophilia A or von Willebrand's disease:* 0.3 mcg/kg diluted in sterile physiologic saline IV over 15–30 min. Determine need for repeated administration based on patient response and laboratory values.

Compatibility
Do not mix or give with other drugs.

Oral/intranasal dosage
- *Diabetes insipidus:* 0.05 mg PO bid (range 0.1–1.2 mg divided 2–3 times a day); 0.1–0.4 mL/d intranasally as a single dose or divided into 2–3 doses. Adjust according to water turnover pattern.

Adverse effects in *Italics* are most common; those in **Bold** are life-threatening

▸ *Hemophilia A or von Willebrand's disease:* Administer 1 spray per nostril by nasal insufflation to provide total dose of 300 mcg. Determine need for repeated administration based on patient response and laboratory values.
▸ *Primary nocturnal enuresis:* 0.2 mL (20 mcg) intranasally at HS; dose range is 10–40 mcg. Give half the dose per nostril. Adjust according to patient's response.

TREATMENT OF OVERDOSE/ANTIDOTE
Discontinue drug or decrease dosage. Initiate general supportive and resuscitative measures.

Pharmacokinetics

Route	Onset	Peak	Duration
IV/SC	30 min	1.5–2 h	
Oral	1 h	0.9–1.5 h	7 h
Nasal	15–60 min	1.5 h	5–21 h

$T_{1/2}$: Fast phase, 7.8 min; slow phase, 75.5 min

Adverse effects
▸ *CNS:* Transient headache
▸ *CV:* Chest pain, edema, palpitations, tachycardia, blood pressure changes
▸ *Resp:* Nasal congestion, upper respiratory infection, cough, nostril pain, nosebleed
▸ *GI:* Mild abdominal pain, nausea, vomiting
▸ *GU:* Vulval pain, fluid retention, water intoxication, hyponatremia
▸ *Derm: Local erythema, swelling, burning pain at injection site,* skin rash, facial flushing
▸ *Allergic:* **Anaphylaxis**
▸ *Misc:* Eye edema, conjunctivitis, epistaxis, lacrimation disorder, sore throat

Clinically important drug–drug interactions
▸ Large doses enhance other pressor agents
▸ Increased effects may occur with carbamazepine, chlorpropamide

⬤ NURSING CONSIDERATIONS
Assessment
▸ *History:* Allergy to desmopressin acetate or its components, type IIB von Willebrand's disease, coronary artery insufficiency, hypertensive cardiovascular disease, water intoxication, risk for thrombosis

Adverse effects in *Italics* are most common; those in **Bold** are life-threatening

▸ *Physical:* P, BP, R, ECG, I & O, IV site, weight, neurologic checks, vision assessment, cardiac auscultation, edema, adventitious lung sounds, nasal mucous membranes, bowel sounds, electrolyte levels, UA, plasma and urine osmolality, Factor VIII coagulant activity, Factor VIII antigen and ristocetin cofactor, skin bleeding time, PTT

Implementation
▸ Carefully monitor P, BP, and ECG during IV administration.
▸ Carefully monitor electrolyte levels during therapy.
▸ Have emergency equipment (defibrillator, drugs, oxygen, intubation equipment) on standby in case anaphylaxis occurs.
▸ Prime the Stimate spray pump prior to its first use. To prime pump, press down four times. Discard bottle after 25 doses.
▸ Administer intranasally by drawing solution into the rhinyle or flexible calibrated plastic tube supplied with preparation. Insert one end of tube into nostril; blow on the other end to deposit solution deep into nasal cavity. May also use nasal spray pump.
▸ Monitor condition of nasal passages during long-term therapy; inappropriate administration can lead to nasal ulcerations.
▸ Individualize dosage to establish a diurnal pattern of water turnover; estimate response by adequate duration of sleep and adequate, not excessive, water turnover. Also monitor lab reports to determine effectiveness of therapy.
▸ Refrigerate nasal solution.
▸ Do not expose desmopressin to light or heat.

● dexamethasone sodium phosphate
(dex a meth' a sone) Dalalone, Decadron Phosphate, Decaject, Dexasone, Dexone, Hexadrol Phosphate, Solurex

Pregnancy Category C

Drug classes
Corticosteroid
Glucocorticoid, long-acting
Hormone

Indications
▸ Management of a wide variety of endocrine, rheumatic, collagen, dermatologic, allergic, gastrointestinal, respiratory, hematologic, neoplastic, edematous disorders
▸ Management of cerebral edema associated with primary or metastatic brain tumor, craniotomy, or head injury
▸ Adjunct therapy for unresponsive shock
▸ Management of acute allergic disorders

Adverse effects in *Italics* are most common; those in **Bold** are life-threatening

Therapeutic actions

▸ Is a glucocorticoid with more rapid onset and shorter duration of action when compared to less soluble preparations
▸ Suppresses inflammation and normal immune response
▸ Causes profound and varied metabolic effects
▸ Has minimal sodium-retaining properties

Contraindications/cautions

▸ **Contraindications:** hypersensitivity to dexamethasone or sulfites; systemic infections, especially tuberculosis, fungal infections, amebiasis, vaccinia and varicella, and antibiotic-resistant infections
▸ **Cautions:** renal or hepatic disease, amebiasis, cerebral malaria, hypothyroidism, ulcerative colitis with impending perforation, diverticulitis, active or latent peptic ulcer, inflammatory bowel disease, fresh intestinal anastomoses, psychotic tendencies, hypertension, thromboembolic disorders, osteoporosis, convulsive disorders, ocular herpes simplex, myasthenia gravis, Cushing's syndrome, metastatic carcinoma, antibiotic-resistant infections, diabetes mellitus, recent acute myocardial infarction (AMI), elderly patients

Available forms

▸ *Injection:* 4, 10, 20, 24 mg/mL

IV/IM facts
Preparation

▸ May be given undiluted or diluted in D5W or 0.9%NS.

Dosage

▸ Dosage requirements vary and must be individualized on the basis of the disease and the response of the patient. Use smallest effective dose.
▸ *Systemic administration:* 0.5–9 mg/d IV over 1 min.
▸ *Cerebral edema:* 10 mg IV over 1 min followed by 4–6 mg IM q6h until maximum response noted, usually within 12–24 h. Reduce dosage after 2–4 d and gradually discontinue over 5–7 d. Then continue oral drug if needed.
▸ *Unresponsive shock:* Range of 1–6 mg/kg to 40 mg as single IV injection over 1 min. Follow with repeated IV injections q2–6h while shock persists.

Compatibility

Dexamethasone may given through the same IV line as acyclovir, allopurinol, amifostine, amikacin, amsacrine, aztreonam, cefepime, cisplatin, cladribine, cyclophosphamide, cytarabine, doxorubicin, famotidine, filgrastim, fluconazole, fludarabine, foscarnet, granisetron, heparin, lorazepam, mel-

---

Adverse effects in *Italics* are most common; those in **Bold** are life-threatening

phalan, meperidine, meropenem, morphine, ondansetron, paclitaxel, piperacillin-tazobactam, potassium chloride, sargramostim, sodium bicarbonate, sufentanil, tacrolimus, teniposide, theophylline, thiotepa, vinorelbine, vitamin B complex with C, zidovudine.

Incompatibility
Do not administer through the same IV line as ciprofloxacin, idarubicin, midazolam.

> **TREATMENT OF OVERDOSE/ANTIDOTE**
> Discontinue drug or decrease dosage. Initiate general supportive and resuscitative measures.

Pharmacokinetics

Route	Onset	Duration
IV	Rapid	2–3 d

Metabolism: Hepatic; $T_{1/2}$: 110–210 min
Excretion: Urine

Adverse effects

- *CNS:* **Convulsions,** *depression, mood swings,* increased intracranial pressure, vertigo, headache, psychic disturbances
- *CV:* **Myocardial rupture after recent AMI, fat embolism,** *hypertension,* thrombophlebitis, dysrhythmias secondary to electrolyte imbalances
- *GI:* Peptic ulcer, bowel perforation, pancreatitis, abdominal distention, ulcerative esophagitis, nausea, hiccups, increased appetite
- *Derm:* *Impaired wound healing, petechiae, ecchymoses, increased sweating, thin and fragile skin, acne,* burning or tingling after IV injection, allergic dermatitis, urticaria, angioneurotic edema
- *Allergic:* **Anaphylaxis**
- *Fluid/Electrolytes:* Sodium and fluid retention, CHF, hypokalemia, hypokalemic alkalosis, metabolic alkalosis, hypocalcemia
- *Musc/Skel:* *Muscle weakness,* steroid myopathy, muscle mass loss, osteoporosis, vertebral compression fractures, pathologic fractures, tendon rupture
- *Endocrine:* *Secondary adrenocortical and pituitary unresponsiveness,* decreased carbohydrate tolerance, diabetes mellitus, cushingoid state, menstrual irregularities, negative nitrogen balance
- *EENT:* Cataracts, increased intraocular pressure, glaucoma

Adverse effects in *Italics* are most common; those in **Bold** are life-threatening

▸ **Misc:** *Increased susceptibility to infection, masking of signs of infection*

Clinically important drug–drug interactions

▸ Decreased effects of anticholinesterases with corticotropin; profound muscular depression possible
▸ Decreased blood levels and lessened effects with phenytoin, phenobarbital, ephedrine, rifampin
▸ Decreased serum levels of salicylates
▸ Altered response to coumarin anticoagulants, such as warfarin
▸ Increased hypokalemia when given with potassium-depleting diuretics
▸ Increased requirements for insulin, sulfonylurea drugs
▸ Increased digitalis toxicity related to hypokalemia

● NURSING CONSIDERATIONS

Assessment

▸ *History:* Hypersensitivity to dexamethasone or sulfites; systemic infections, especially tuberculosis, fungal infections, amebiasis, vaccinia and varicella, and antibiotic-resistant infections; renal or hepatic disease; amebiasis; cerebral malaria; hypothyroidism; ulcerative colitis with impending perforation; diverticulitis; active or latent peptic ulcer; inflammatory bowel disease; fresh intestinal anastomoses; psychotic tendencies; hypertension; thromboembolic disorders; osteoporosis; convulsive disorders; ocular herpes simplex; Cushing's syndrome; metastatic carcinoma; diabetes mellitus; recent AMI; age
▸ *Physical:* T, P, R, BP, I & O, weight, neurologic checks, peripheral perfusion, skin assessment, ophthalmologic exam, evidence of infection, respiratory effort, adventitious lung sounds, abdominal assessment, upper GI x-ray (history or symptoms of peptic ulcer), muscle strength, serum electrolytes, renal and liver function tests, adrenal function tests, CBC, serum glucose

Implementation

▸ Evaluate for hypokalemia as evidenced by muscle weakness, fatigue, paralytic ileus, ECG changes (flat or inverted T wave, U wave, ST segment depression, atrial and ventricular dysrhythmias), anorexia, nausea, vomiting, abdominal distention, dizziness, or polyuria.
▸ Assess for hypocalcemia as evidenced by Chvostek's or Trousseau's signs, muscle twitching, laryngospasm, paresthesias, or ECG changes (prolonged QT interval, prolonged ST segment).
▸ Have emergency equipment (defibrillator, drugs, oxygen, intubation equipment) on standby in case anaphylaxis or adverse reaction occurs.

D

- Give daily doses before 9:00 AM to mimic normal peak corticosteroid blood levels.
- Increase dosage when patient is subject to stress.
- Taper doses when discontinuing high-dose or long-term therapy. Symptoms of adrenal insufficiency from too rapid withdrawal include nausea, fatigue, anorexia, dyspnea, hypotension, hypoglycemia, myalgia, fever, malaise, arthralgia, dizziness, desquamation of skin, and fainting.
- Do not give live virus vaccines with immunosuppressive doses of corticosteroids.

⦿ dextran, high molecular weight

(dex' tran) Dextran 70, Dextran 75, Gendex 75, Gentran 70, Macrodex

Pregnancy Category C

Drug class
Plasma expander

Indications
- Treatment of shock or impending shock due to surgery or trauma, hemorrhage, or burns; to be used only in emergency situations when blood or blood products are not available

Therapeutic actions
- Is a synthetic polysaccharide used to approximate the colloidal properties of albumin
- Improves BP, pulse rate, respiratory exchange, and renal function in patients with hypovolemia or hypotensive shock
- Expands plasma volume slightly in excess of volume infused

Effects on hemodynamic parameters
- Increased BP
- Decreased HR
- Increased CVP
- Increased CO
- Decreased SVR

Contraindications/cautions
- **Contraindications:** dextran allergy; marked hemostatic defects or cardiac decompensation; renal disease with severe oliguria or anuria; severe CHF, pulmonary edema, or bleeding disorders; when use of sodium chloride could be clinically detrimental

(contraindications continued on next page)

Adverse effects in *Italics* are most common; those in **Bold** are life-threatening

> **Cautions:** impaired renal clearance, thrombocytopenia, pathological abdominal conditions or bowel surgery, patients receiving corticosteroids or corticotropin

Available forms
▸ *Injection:* 6% dextran 75 in D5W; 6% dextran 70 in D5W; 6% dextran 75 in 0.9%NS; 6% dextran 70 in 0.9%NS

IV facts
Preparation
▸ No further preparation is needed. Ensure that the solution is clear.

Dosage
▸ Administer by IV infusion only. 500–1000 mL at a rate of 20–40 mL/min IV in an emergency. Do not exceed 20 mL/kg during the first 24 h.

> **TREATMENT OF OVERDOSE/ANTIDOTE**
> Discontinue drug or decrease dosage. Initiate general supportive and resuscitative measures.

Pharmacokinetics

Route	Onset	Duration
IV	Minutes	12 h

Metabolism: Enzymatically degraded; $T_{1/2}$: 24 h
Excretion: Urine, feces

Adverse effects
▸ *CV:* Hypotension, CHF, hypervolemia, edema
▸ *Resp:* **Pulmonary edema**
▸ *GI:* Nausea, vomiting
▸ *Derm:* Infection at injection site, extravasation, venous thrombosis or phlebitis at injection site
▸ *Allergic:* **Anaphylaxis,** urticaria, nasal congestion, wheezing, chest tightness, dyspnea, mild hypotension
▸ *Hematologic:* Prolonged bleeding time, bleeding, decreased coagulation
▸ *Misc:* Fever, joint pain, hypernatremia

● NURSING CONSIDERATIONS

Assessment
▸ *History:* Dextran allergy; marked hemostatic defects or cardiac decompensation; renal disease; severe CHF, pulmonary edema, or bleeding disorders; when use of sodium chloride

Adverse effects in *Italics* are most common; those in **Bold** are life-threatening

could be clinically detrimental; impaired renal clearance; thrombocytopenia; pathological abdominal conditions or bowel surgery; use of corticosteroids or corticotropin
▶ *Physical:* T, P, BP, R, I & O, SpO$_2$, CVP, weight, skin assessment, peripheral perfusion, respiratory effort, adventitious lung sounds, edema, JVD, hydration status, presence of bleeding, liver and renal function tests, CBC, UA, coagulation studies, serum electrolytes, serum osmolarity

Implementation
▶ Closely monitor VS, I & O, and CVP.
▶ Dextran is not a substitute for whole blood or plasma proteins.
▶ Immediately discontinue if evidence of an allergic reaction occurs.
▶ Assess for evidence of fluid overload or electrolyte imbalance.
▶ Discontinue drug if urine output does not increase after 500 mL given.
▶ May interfere with blood typing and crossmatching if samples are taken after a dextran infusion. If blood is drawn after the infusion, the saline-agglutination and indirect antiglobulin methods may be used for type and crossmatching.
▶ Dextran may cause blood to coagulate in the tubing. Flush the tubing well with 0.9%NS before transfusing blood.

⬤ dextran, low molecular weight
(dex' tran) Dextran 40, Gentran 40, 10% LMD, Rheomacrodex

Pregnancy Category C

Drug class
Plasma expander

Indications
▶ Treatment of shock or impending shock due to surgery or trauma, hemorrhage, or burns; to be used only in emergency situations when blood or blood products are not available
▶ Priming fluid in pump oxygenators during extracorporeal circulation
▶ Prophylaxis against DVT and PE in patients undergoing procedures known to be associated with a high incidence of thromboembolic complications

Therapeutic actions
▶ Is a synthetic polysaccharide used to approximate the colloidal properties of albumin
▶ Enhances blood flow, especially in the microcirculation, by increasing blood volume, venous return, and cardiac output; decreasing blood viscosity and peripheral vascular resistance;

Adverse effects in *Italics* are most common; those in **Bold** are life-threatening

and reducing aggregation of erythrocytes and other cellular elements of blood by coating them and maintaining their electronegative charges

▸ Is more advantageous than blood and other priming fluids when used as priming solution for extracorporeal circulation; advantages include decreased destruction of erythrocytes and platelets, reduced intravascular hemagglutination, and maintained electronegativity of erythrocytes and platelets

▸ When used as prophylaxis against thrombosis and thromboembolism, it inhibits mechanisms essential to thrombus formation, such as vascular stasis and platelet adhesiveness, and alters the structure and lysability of fibrin clots

Effects on hemodynamic parameters
▸ Increased BP
▸ Decreased HR
▸ Increased CVP
▸ Increased CO
▸ Decreased SVR

Contraindications/cautions
▸ **Contraindications:** dextran allergy, marked hemostatic defects or cardiac decompensation, renal disease with severe oliguria or anuria, when use of sodium chloride could be clinically detrimental
▸ **Cautions:** impaired renal function, thrombocytopenia; severe CHF, pulmonary edema, or bleeding disorders; active hemorrhage when increased microcirculatory flow could result in additional blood loss; diabetes if dextran solution contains dextrose

Available forms
▸ *Injection:* 10% dextran 40 in D5W; 10% dextran 40 in 0.9%NS

IV facts
Preparation
▸ No further preparation is needed. Ensure that the solution is clear.

Dosage
▸ Administer by IV infusion only.
▸ *Adjunctive therapy in shock:* Infuse the first 10 mL/kg rapidly IV; then give the remaining dose more slowly. Do not exceed 20 mL/kg during the first 24 h. After the first 24 h, do not exceed total daily dose of 10 mL/kg. Do not continue > 5 d.
▸ *Hemodiluent in extracorporeal circulation:* Generally, 10–20 mL/kg is added to the perfusion circuit. Do not exceed 20 mL/kg.

Adverse effects in *Italics* are most common; those in **Bold** are life-threatening

▶ *Prophylactic therapy of venous thrombosis and thromboembolism:* Individualize based on the patient's risk. 500–1000 mL (approximately 10 mL/kg) IV on the day of surgery. Continue 500 mL/d IV for an additional 2–3 d. Thereafter, may give 500 mL every second or third day for up to 2 wk.

Compatibility
Dextran may be given through the same IV line as enalaprilat or famotidine.

TREATMENT OF OVERDOSE/ANTIDOTE
Discontinue drug or decrease dosage. Initiate general supportive and resuscitative measures.

Pharmacokinetics

Route	Onset	Duration
IV	Minutes	12 h

Metabolism: Enzymatically degraded; $T_{1/2}$: 3 h
Excretion: Urine, feces

Adverse effects
▶ *CV:* Hypotension, CHF, hypervolemia, edema
▶ *Resp:* **Pulmonary edema**
▶ *GU:* **Renal failure**
▶ *Derm:* Infection at injection site, extravasation, venous thrombosis or phlebitis at injection site
▶ *Allergic:* **Anaphylaxis, bronchospasm,** mild cutaneous eruptions, urticaria, hypotension, nausea, vomiting, headache, dyspnea, fever, tightness of the chest, wheezing
▶ *Hematologic:* Prolonged bleeding time, decreased coagulation, bleeding
▶ *Misc:* Fever, hypernatremia

● NURSING CONSIDERATIONS

Assessment
▶ *History:* Dextran allergy; marked hemostatic defects or cardiac decompensation; renal disease; when use of sodium chloride could be clinically detrimental; impaired renal function, thrombocytopenia; severe CHF, pulmonary edema, or bleeding disorders; active hemorrhage; diabetes
▶ *Physical:* T, P, BP, R, I & O, SpO$_2$, CVP, weight, skin assessment, peripheral perfusion, respiratory effort, adventitious lung sounds, edema, JVD, hydration status, presence of bleeding, liver and renal function tests, CBC, UA, coagulation studies, serum electrolytes, serum osmolarity

Adverse effects in *Italics* are most common; those in **Bold** are life-threatening

Implementation
▸ Closely monitor VS, I & O, and CVP.
▸ Dextran is not a substitute for whole blood or plasma proteins.
▸ Immediately discontinue if evidence of an allergic reaction occurs.
▸ Assess for evidence of fluid overload or electrolyte imbalance.
▸ Discontinue drug if urine output does not increase after 500 mL given.
▸ May interfere with blood typing and crossmatching if samples are taken after a dextran infusion.
▸ Dextran may cause blood to coagulate in the tubing. Flush the tubing well with 0.9%NS before transfusing blood.

⬤ **dextrose** d-Glucose *(dex' trose)* Glucose
Pregnancy Category C

Drug classes
Carbohydrate
Caloric agent

Indications
▸ 2.5%, 5%, 10%: used for peripheral infusion to provide calories whenever fluid and caloric replacement are required
▸ 50%: treatment of insulin hypoglycemia (hyperinsulinemia or insulin shock) to restore blood glucose levels
▸ 10%, 20%, 30%, 40%, 50%, 60%, 70% (hypertonic): used for infusion after admixture with other solutions, such as amino acids
▸ Unlabeled uses: hypertonic 25%–50% solutions used as an irritant to produce adhesive pleuritis and to reduce cerebrospinal pressure and cerebral edema caused by delirium tremens or acute alcohol injection

Therapeutic actions
▸ Undergoes oxidation to carbon dioxide and water
▸ Provides calories and hydration, may decrease body protein and nitrogen losses, promotes glycogen deposition, and decreases or prevents ketosis if sufficient doses are given
▸ Provides 3.4 calories/g of d-glucose monohydrate

Contraindications/cautions
▸ **Contraindications:** diabetic coma with high blood sugar, corn or corn product allergy, concentrated solution with intracranial or intraspinal hemorrhage, delirium tremens in dehydrated patients, severe hydration anuria, hepatic coma, or glucose-galactose malabsorption syndrome

(contraindications continued on next page)

Adverse effects in *Italics* are most common; those in **Bold** are life-threatening

D

◗ **Cautions:** overhydration, congested states, pulmonary edema, diabetes mellitus, carbohydrate intolerance, chronic uremia

Available forms
◗ *Dextrose in water for injection:* 2.5%, 5%, 10%, 20%, 25%, 30%, 40%, 50%, 60%, 70%

IV facts
Preparation
◗ May be given undiluted through a central venous catheter. When treating hypoglycemia in emergency situations, may give up to 50% slowly into a large peripheral vein.

Dosage
◗ Determine blood glucose levels before injecting; in emergencies, administer glucose without waiting for test results.
◗ Concentration and dose depend on patient's age, weight, and clinical condition. Add electrolytes as needed to maintain fluid and electrolyte status.
◗ The maximum rate at which dextrose can be infused without producing glycosuria is 0.5 g/kg/h. 95% is retained when infused at 0.8 g/kg/h.
◗ *Insulin-induced hypoglycemia:* 10–25 g IV. May need to repeat in severe cases.
◗ *Severe cases of hypoglycemia:* Larger or repeated single doses up to 10–12 mL of 25% dextrose may be required. May need to infuse 10% dextrose continuously to stabilize blood glucose levels.

Normal fasting glucose level
◗ 65–115 mg/dL

Incompatibility
Do not administer through the same IV line as blood.

TREATMENT OF OVERDOSE/ANTIDOTE
Discontinue drug or decrease dosage. Initiate general supportive and resuscitative measures.

Pharmacokinetics
Route	Onset	Peak	Duration
IV	Rapid	Rapid	Brief

Metabolism: Oxidized to carbon dioxide and water
Excretion: If renal threshold is exceeded, the kidneys excrete dextrose

Adverse effects in *Italics* are most common; those in **Bold** are life-threatening

Adverse effects

▸ **CNS:** Mental confusion, unconsciousness
▸ **CV: Pulmonary edema,** fluid overload, hypovolemia, dehydration
▸ **Endocrine:**   Hyperglycemia, hyperosmolar syndrome, glycosuria, rebound hypoglycemia
▸ **Misc:** Fever, infection at injection site, tissue necrosis, venous thrombosis or phlebitis extending from injection site, extravasation, vitamin B complex deficiency, hypokalemia

Clinically important drug–drug interaction

▸ Give cautiously to patients receiving corticosteroids, corticotropin

⬤ NURSING CONSIDERATIONS

Assessment

▸ *History:* Diabetic coma with high blood sugar, corn or corn product allergy, intracranial or intraspinal hemorrhage, delirium tremens in dehydrated patients, severe hydration anuria, hepatic coma, glucose-galactose malabsorption syndrome, overhydration, congested states, pulmonary edema, diabetes mellitus, carbohydrate intolerance, chronic uremia
▸ *Physical:* T, P, BP, R, I & O, IV site, weight, neurologic checks, skin assessment, respiratory effort, adventitious lung sounds, edema, nutritional status, ABG, serum electrolytes, serum and urine glucose

Implementation

▸ Administer hypertonic dextrose solutions through a central line except in emergency situations.
▸ If concentrated dextrose is abruptly withdrawn, give 5%–10% dextrose to avoid rebound hypoglycemia.
▸ Do not administer concentrated solutions SC or IM.
▸ Monitor serum glucose frequently during therapy.
▸ Monitor for evidence of hyperglycemia and hypoglycemia.
▸ Monitor for evidence of hypervolemia and hypovolemia.
▸ Thiamine-deficient patients may experience a sudden onset or worsening of Wernicke's encephalopathy after administering glucose; administer thiamine before or along with dextrose-containing fluids.

⬤ **diazepam** *(dye az' e pam)* Apo-Diazepam (CAN), Diastat, Diazemuls (CAN), Diazepam Intensol, Valium

Pregnancy Category D

C-IV controlled substance

Adverse effects in *Italics* are most common; those in **Bold** are life-threatening

D

Drug classes
Sedative/hypnotic (benzodiazepine)
Antianxiety agent
Anticonvulsant
Skeletal muscle relaxant, centrally acting

Indications
▶ Management of anxiety disorders or for short-term relief of symptoms of anxiety
▶ Antiepileptic: adjunct in status epilepticus and severe recurrent convulsive seizures (parenteral); adjunct in convulsive disorders (oral); to control bouts of increased seizure activity for selected, refractory patients with epilepsy on stable regimens of antiepileptic agents (rectal)
▶ Preoperative: relief of anxiety and tension and to lessen recall in patients prior to surgical procedures, cardioversion, and endoscopic procedures (parenteral)
▶ Acute alcohol withdrawal; may be useful in symptomatic relief of acute agitation, tremor, delirium tremens, and hallucinosis
▶ Muscle relaxant: adjunct for relief of reflex skeletal muscle spasm due to local pathology (inflammation of muscles or joints) or secondary to trauma; spasticity caused by upper motor neuron disorders (cerebral palsy and paraplegia); athetosis, stiff-man syndrome
▶ Treatment of tetanus (parenteral)
▶ Unlabeled use: treatment of panic attack
▶ Orphan drug use: Management of selected, refractory patients with epilepsy on stabile regimens of antiepileptic drugs who require intermittent use of diazepam to control bouts of increased seizure activity (rectal viscous solution)

Therapeutic actions
▶ Exact mechanism of action not understood
▶ Potentiates GABA, an inhibitory neurotransmitter, to produce CNS depression
▶ May act in spinal cord and at supraspinal sites to produce muscle relaxation
▶ Anticonvulsant properties of diazepam due to enhanced presynaptic inhibition

Effects on hemodynamic parameters
▶ May decrease RR
▶ May decrease BP

Adverse effects in *Italics* are most common; those in **Bold** are life-threatening

Contraindications/cautions
▸ **Contraindications:** benzodiazepine or diazepam allergy, acute narrow-angle glaucoma, shock, coma, acute alcoholic intoxication
▸ **Cautions:** elderly or debilitated patients, impaired liver or kidney function, limited pulmonary reserve

Available forms
▸ *Injection:* 5 mg/mL
▸ *Tablets:* 2, 5, 10 mg
▸ *Oral solution:* 5 mg/5 mL, 5 mg/mL, 1 mg/mL
▸ *Rectal gel:* 10, 15, 20 mg

IV/IM facts
Preparation
▸ Diazepam has been diluted in infusion solutions, but this is not recommended.

Dosage
▸ Usual dose is 2–20 mg IV or IM. Larger doses may be required for some patients. Give each 5 mg over 1 min using a large vein. If injected into IV tubing, inject as close to vein as possible.
▸ *Anxiety:* 2–10 mg IV or IM; repeat in 3–4 h if needed.
▸ *Status epilepticus:* 5–10 mg, preferably by slow IV. May repeat q5–10 min up to total dose of 30 mg. If needed, repeat therapy in 2–4 h; other drugs are preferable for long-term control.
▸ *Cardioversion:* 5–15 mg IV 5–10 min before procedure.
▸ *Preoperative:* 10 mg IM.
▸ *Alcohol withdrawal:* 10 mg IV or IM initially, then 5–10 mg in 3–4 h if needed.
▸ *Endoscopic procedures:* 10 mg IV or less is usually adequate, but may give up to 20 mg IV just before procedure or 5–10 mg IM 30 min prior to procedure. Reduce or omit dosage of narcotics.
▸ *Muscle spasm:* 5–10 mg IV or IM initially, then 5–10 mg in 3–4 h if needed.
▸ *Elderly or debilitated:* 2–5 mg IV or IM initially. Gradually increase dose as needed and tolerated.

Compatibility
Diazepam may be given through the same IV site as cefmetazole, dobutamine, nafcillin, quinidine, sufentanil.

Incompatibility
Do not administer through the IV line as atracurium, cefepime, diltiazem, fluconazole, foscarnet, heparin, hydromorphone,

---

Adverse effects in *Italics* are most common; those in **Bold** are life-threatening

meropenem, pancuronium, potassium chloride, propofol, vecuronium, vitamin B complex with C.

Oral/rectal dosage
▶ *Anxiety disorders, skeletal muscle spasm, convulsive disorders:* 2–10 mg PO bid–qid.
▶ *Alcohol withdrawal:* 10 mg PO tid–qid first 24 h; reduce to 5 mg PO tid–qid as needed.
▶ *Elderly or debilitated:* 2–2.5 mg PO qd–bid. Increase gradually as needed and tolerated.
▶ *Rectal:* 0.2 mg/kg PR. Calculate recommended dosage by rounding up to next available unit dose. May give second dose 4–12 h after first dose. Do not treat more than five episodes per month or more than one episode q5d.

TREATMENT OF OVERDOSE/ANTIDOTE
Discontinue drug or decrease dosage. Initiate general supportive and resuscitative measures. Administer IV fluids. Treat hypotension with norepinephrine or metaraminol. Dialysis is of limited value. Flumazenil may completely or partially reverse the sedative effects. Before initiating flumazenil, secure airway, provide ventilation, and ensure adequate IV access. Initiate immediate gastric lavage for oral diazepam overdose.

Pharmacokinetics

Route	Onset	Peak	Duration
IV	1–5 min	30 min	15–60 min
IM	15–30 min	30–45 min	3 h
Oral	30–60 min	1–2 h	3 h

Metabolism: Hepatic; $T_{1/2}$: 20–80 h
Excretion: Urine

Adverse effects
▶ *CNS: Transient, mild drowsiness initially; sedation, depression, lethargy, apathy, fatigue, lightheadedness, disorientation, restlessness, confusion, mild paradoxical excitatory reactions* during first 2 wk of treatment; crying, delirium, headache, slurred speech, dysarthria, stupor, rigidity, tremor, vertigo, euphoria, nervousness, difficulty concentrating, vivid dreams, psychomotor retardation, extrapyramidal symptoms, visual and auditory disturbances, diplopia, nystagmus, depressed hearing, nasal congestion
▶ *CV: **Bradycardia,** CV collapse, hypotension*

Adverse effects in *Italics* are most common; those in **Bold** are life-threatening

- **GI:** *Constipation, diarrhea,* dry mouth, changes in salivation, nausea, anorexia, vomiting, difficulty swallowing, hepatic dysfunction, jaundice; elevated LDH, alkaline phosphatase, ALT, and AST
- **GU:** *Incontinence, urinary retention, changes in libido,* menstrual irregularities
- **Derm:** Phlebitis and thrombosis at IV site, urticaria, skin rash, dermatitis
- **Dependence:** *Drug dependence with withdrawal syndrome* when drug is discontinued
- **Misc:** Hiccups, fever, diaphoresis, muscular disturbances; pain, burning, and redness after IM injection

Clinically important drug–drug interactions

- Increased CNS depression, hypotension, or muscular weakness when used with narcotics, barbiturates, MAO inhibitors, alcohol
- Delayed clearance with cimetidine, oral contraceptives, disulfiram, fluoxetine, isoniazid, ketoconazole, metoprolol, propoxyphene, propranolol, valproic acid
- Increased digoxin serum concentrations
- Reduced GI absorption with ranitidine
- Decreased effects with rifampin, theophyllines

● NURSING CONSIDERATIONS

Assessment

- *History:* Diazepam or benzodiazepine allergy, acute narrow-angle glaucoma, shock, coma, acute alcoholic intoxication, pregnancy, age, debilitation, impaired liver or kidney function, limited pulmonary reserve
- *Physical:* P, BP, R, I & O, IV site, weight, neurologic checks, anxiety, tremors, agitation, hallucinations, level of sedation, muscle strength, muscle spasm, skin assessment, ophthalmologic exam, edema, adventitious lung sounds, liver and renal function tests, UA, CBC

Implementation

- Do not administer intra-arterially; may produce arteriospasm or gangrene.
- Change from IV to oral therapy ASAP.
- Do not use small veins (dorsum of hand or wrist) for IV injection. Assess IV site frequently.
- Reduce dose of narcotic analgesics with IV diazepam; eliminate use or reduce dose by at least one third.
- Carefully monitor P, BP, and R during IV administration.
- Maintain bed rest for 3 h for patients receiving parenteral benzodiazepines. Initiate fall precautions.

Adverse effects in *Italics* are most common; those in **Bold** are life-threatening

- Monitor EEG in patients treated for status epilepticus; seizures may recur after initial control, presumably because of short duration of drug effect.
- Monitor liver and kidney function, CBC during long-term therapy.
- Taper dosage gradually after long-term therapy, especially for epileptic patients.
- Follow federal, state, and institutional policies for dispensing controlled substances.

⬤ **diazoxide** *(di az ok' sid)* Hyperstat, Proglycem

Pregnancy Category C

Drug classes
Antihypertensive
Thiazide diuretic
Glucose-elevating agent (oral)

Indications
- Parenteral: emergency reduction of blood pressure; treatment of nonmalignant and malignant hypertension
- Oral: management of hypoglycemia due to hyperinsulinism; inoperable islet cell adenoma or carcinoma; extrapancreatic malignancy

Therapeutic actions
- Reduces blood pressure by relaxing smooth muscle in peripheral arterioles
- Increases blood glucose by inhibiting pancreatic insulin release and by an extrapancreatic effect
- Decreases sodium and water excretion

Effects on hemodynamic parameters
- Increased HR (parenteral and oral)
- Decreased BP (parenteral)
- Increased CO (parenteral)
- Decreased SVR (parenteral)

Contraindications/cautions
- **Contraindications:** diazoxide, thiazide, or other sulfonamide derivative allergy; treatment of compensatory hypertension, such as that associated with aortic coarctation or arteriovenous shunt; dissecting aortic aneurysm, functional hypoglycemia
- **Cautions:** CHF, edema, pheochromocytoma, impaired cerebral or cardiac circulation, renal function impairment

Adverse effects in *Italics* are most common; those in **Bold** are life-threatening

Available forms
▸ *Injection:* 15 mg/mL
▸ *Capsules:* 50 mg
▸ *Oral elixir:* 50 mg/mL

IV/IM facts
Preparation
▸ Administer undiluted.

Dosage
▸ Give 1–3 mg/kg (maximum of 150 mg) IV within 30 s. May repeat dose at 5- to 15-min intervals until desired decrease in blood pressure is achieved. Repeat doses q4–24h until oral antihypertensive medication is instituted. Treatment is seldom needed for longer than 4–5 d; do not use for > 10 d.

Incompatibility
Do not administer through the same IV line as hydralazine or propranolol.

Oral dosage
▸ Starting dose is 3 mg/kg/d PO in three equal doses q8h. Usual daily dose is 3–8 mg/kg/d in 2–3 equal doses q8–12h. Patients with refractory hyperglycemia may require higher doses. Reduce dose in renal disease.

> **TREATMENT OF OVERDOSE/ANTIDOTE**
> Discontinue drug or decrease dosage. Initiate general supportive and resuscitative measures. Hypotension can usually be controlled with the Trendelenburg maneuver. Dopamine or norepinephrine may be used to treat hypotension. Treat excessive hyperglycemia with insulin; restore fluid and electrolytes. Diazoxide may be removed by hemodialysis.

Pharmacokinetics

Route	Onset	Peak	Duration
IV	Within 1 min	2–5 min	3–12 h
Oral	1 h	8 h	

Metabolism: Hepatic; $T_{1/2}$: 21–45 h
Excretion: Urine

Adverse effects
▸ *CNS:* Cerebral ischemia, cerebral infarction, sweating, flushing, sensation of warmth, headache, dizziness, lightheadedness, lethargy, euphoria, weakness, tinnitus, apprehension, anxiety, malaise

Adverse effects in *Italics* are most common; those in **Bold** are life-threatening

▶ *CV:* **Acute myocardial infarction, sodium and water retention with repeated doses,** *hypotension, palpitations, tachycardia,* CHF, myocardial ischemia, dysrhythmias, ECG changes, hypertension, chest discomfort, nonanginal chest tightness

▶ *Resp:* Dyspnea, choking sensation, cough

▶ *GI: Nausea, vomiting,* diarrhea, abdominal discomfort, anorexia, alterations in taste, parotid swelling, dry mouth, ileus, constipation, elevated liver enzymes, pancreatitis

▶ *GU: Glycosuria, increased serum uric acid,* renal toxicity, decreased creatinine clearance and urinary output, reversible nephrotic syndrome

▶ *Derm:* Warmth or pain along injected vein, cellulitis without sloughing or phlebitis at injection site of extravasation, skin rash

▶ *Allergic:* Hypersensitivity reactions

▶ *Endocrine:* **Diabetic ketoacidosis, hyperosmolar nonketotic coma,** hyperglycemia

▶ *Hematologic:* Thrombocytopenia with or without purpura; neutropenia, eosinophilia, decreased hemoglobin/hematocrit, excessive bleeding, decreased IgG

▶ *Misc: Hirsutism,* fever, lymphadenopathy, gout

Clinically important drug–drug interactions

▶ Loss of seizure control with concurrent administration of diazoxide with ethotoin, fosphenytoin, mephenytoin, or phenytoin

▶ Enhanced hyperglycemic, antihypertensive, and hyperuricemic effects with thiazides or other diuretics

▶ Enhanced by other antihypertensives

▶ Potentiates coumarin and its derivatives

▶ Hyperglycemia with sulfonylurea drugs

▶ Do not administer Hyperstat within 6 h of hydralazine, reserpine, alphaprodine, methyldopa, beta-blockers, prazosin, minoxidil, nitrites, and other papaverine-like compounds

● NURSING CONSIDERATIONS

Assessment

▶ *History:* Diazoxide, thiazide, or other sulfonamide-derivative allergy; compensatory hypertension, such as that associated with aortic coarctation or arteriovenous shunt; dissecting aortic aneurysm; functional hypoglycemia; CHF; edema; pheochromocytoma; impaired cerebral or cardiac circulation; renal function impairment

▶ *Physical:* P, BP, R, ECG, I & O, IV site, weight, neurologic checks, reflexes, vision, cardiac auscultation, edema, orthostatic BP, adventitious lung sounds, JVD, bowel sounds, skin condition, status of nasal mucous membranes, voiding pat-

Adverse effects in *Italics* are most common; those in **Bold** are life-threatening

tern, lymph node palpation, urine glucose and ketones, renal and hepatic function tests, UA; serum electrolytes, glucose, and uric acid levels; CBC

Implementation

▸ Exercise extreme caution when calculating and preparing doses. Diazoxide is a very potent drug; small dosage errors can cause serious adverse effects.
▸ Carefully monitor P, BP, R, and ECG during IV administration.
▸ Have insulin and tolbutamide nearby in case hyperglycemic reaction occurs.
▸ Have dopamine and norepinephrine nearby in case of severe hypotensive reaction.
▸ Monitor serum glucose, BUN, electrolytes, creatinine, and renal and liver function tests frequently.
▸ Assess for evidence of fluid retention and CHF.

Parenteral diazoxide

▸ Monitor BP closely during administration until stable and then q30–60 min.
▸ Administer injection/infusion with patient in a supine position. Keep patient in supine position for at least 1 h after diazoxide injection is given.
▸ Change patient's position slowly to avoid postural hypotension.
▸ Protect parenteral drug from light, heat, and freezing.
▸ Give Hyperstat only by IV injection, taking care to avoid extravasation. If SC leakage occurs, treat with warm compress and rest.

Oral diazoxide

▸ Administer drug on a regular schedule.
▸ Reassure patient that hirsutism will resolve when drug is discontinued.
▸ Protect oral elixir from light.

⬤ digoxin (di jox' in) Lanoxin, Lanoxicap
Pregnancy Category A

Drug classes
Cardiac glycoside
Inotropic agent
Antidysrhythmic

Indications
▸ CHF
▸ Atrial fibrillation

Adverse effects in *Italics* are most common; those in **Bold** are life-threatening

▸ Atrial flutter
▸ Paroxysmal atrial tachycardia

Therapeutic actions

▸ Alters sodium potassium-ATPase system, resulting in intracellular K^+ loss and gain of Na^+ and Ca^{2+}
▸ Increases force and velocity of myocardial systolic contraction
▸ Slows HR
▸ Decreases conduction velocity through the AV node
▸ Inhibits sodium potassium-activated ATPase
▸ In higher doses, increases sympathetic outflow from the CNS to cardiac and peripheral sympathetic nerves

Effects on hemodynamic parameters

▸ Decreased HR
▸ Increased CO
▸ Decreased or unchanged CVP
▸ Decreased or unchanged PCWP
▸ Increased or unchanged SVR

Contraindications/cautions

▸ **Contraindications:** digitalis allergy, ventricular fibrillation, ventricular tachycardia, heart block, sick sinus syndrome, treatment of obesity, atrial dysrhythmias associated with hypermetabolic states, sinus tachycardia without heart failure
▸ **Cautions:** elderly, renal insufficiency, acute myocardial infarction (AMI), severe pulmonary disease, idiopathic hypertrophic subaortic stenosis, Wolff-Parkinson-White syndrome, constrictive pericarditis, hypothyroidism, hypokalemia, hypercalcemia, hypomagnesemia, suspected digitalis toxicity

Available forms

▸ *Injection:* 0.1, 0.25 mg/mL
▸ *Tablets:* 0.125, 0.25, 0.5 mg
▸ *Capsules:* 0.05, 0.1, 0.2 mg
▸ *Oral elixir:* 0.05 mg/mL

IV facts

Preparation

▸ Give undiluted or diluted in fourfold or greater volume of D5W; LR; 0.9%NS; or Sterile Water for Injection.

Dosage

▸ Administer IV only when need for rapid digitalization is urgent or when drug cannot be taken orally.
▸ Dose selection is based on patient's disease that requires

treatment, weight, renal function, age, concomitant disease states, other drugs that may affect digoxin, and response to previous doses of digoxin.

▸ Peak digoxin stores of 8–12 mcg/kg generally provide therapeutic effects with minimum risk for toxicity; however, stores of 10–15 mcg/kg may be required for patients with atrial fibrillation or atrial flutter. A typical 70-kg patient requires 600–1000 mcg (0.6–1.0 mg) digoxin to achieve 8–15 mcg/kg peak body stores.

▸ *Loading dose:* 400–600 mcg (0.4–0.6 mg) IV with additional doses of 100–300 mcg (0.1–0.3 mg) q4–8h. Give each dose over 5 min.

▸ *Maintenance dose:* 125–500 mcg/d (0.125–0.5 mg) IV.

Therapeutic serum level
▸ 0.5–2.0 ng/mL

Compatibility
Digoxin may be given through the same IV line as amrinone, cefmetazole, ciprofloxacin, diltiazem, famotidine, heparin, meperidine, meropenem, midazolam, milrinone, morphine, potassium chloride, propofol, tacrolimus, vitamin B complex with C.

Incompatibility
Manufacturer recommends that digoxin not be admixed with other drugs. Do not administer through the same IV line as fluconazole or foscarnet.

Oral dosage
▸ *Loading dose:* 500–700 mcg (0.5–0.7 mg) PO with additional doses of 125–375 mcg (0.125–0.375 mg) PO q6–8h.

▸ *Maintenance dose:* 125–500 mcg/d (0.125–0.5 mg) PO.

TREATMENT OF OVERDOSE/ANTIDOTE
Discontinue drug or decrease dosage. Initiate general supportive and resuscitative measures. Correct factors that may contribute to toxicity, such as hypoxia, acid–base disturbances, and aggravating agents, such as catecholamines. Administer potassium salts if patient is hypokalemic. Atropine or a temporary pacemaker may be helpful for advanced heart block. Treat dysrhythmias with lidocaine, propranolol, or procainamide. Administer digoxin immune fab to neutralize digoxin. With massive digitalis ingestion, administer large doses of activated charcoal to prevent absorption and bind digoxin in the gut during enteroenteric recirculation. Emesis or gastric lavage may be indicated, especially if ingestion occurred within past 30 min.

Adverse effects in *Italics* are most common; those in **Bold** are life-threatening

D

Pharmacokinetics

Route	Onset	Peak	Duration
IV	5–30 min	1–4 h	4–5 d
Oral	30–120 min	2–6 h	6–8 d

Metabolism: Some hepatic; $T_{1/2}$: 34–44 h
Excretion: Urine

Adverse effects

▸ *CNS: Headache, weakness,* drowsiness, visual disturbances, psychosis
▸ *CV:* **Dysrhythmias**
▸ *GI: GI upset,* anorexia, vomiting, diarrhea
▸ *Derm:* Skin rash
▸ *Misc:* Gynecomastia

Clinically important drug–drug interactions

▸ Serious dysrhythmias with rapid calcium administration
▸ Rise in serum digoxin concentration with quinidine, verapamil, amiodarone, propafenone, indomethacin, itraconazole, alprazolam
▸ Increased digoxin absorption with erythromycin, tetracycline, clarithromycin, propantheline, diphenoxylate
▸ Digoxin toxicity with potassium-depleting corticosteroids, diuretics
▸ Low serum concentrations with antacids, kaolin-pectin, sulfasalazine, neomycin, cholestyramine, certain anticancer drugs
▸ Increased dose requirements with thyroid administration
▸ Increased dysrhythmias with sympathomimetics, succinylcholine
▸ Complete heart block with beta-adrenergic blockers, calcium channel-blockers
▸ Caution needed when combining digoxin with any drug that may cause deteriorated renal function

◉ NURSING CONSIDERATIONS

Assessment

▸ *History:* Allergy to digitalis preparations, sick sinus syndrome, obesity, atrial dysrhythmias associated with hypermetabolic states, sinus tachycardia without heart failure, age, renal insufficiency, AMI, severe pulmonary disease, idiopathic hypertrophic subaortic stenosis, Wolff-Parkinson-White syndrome, constrictive pericarditis, hypothyroidism, suspected digitalis toxicity
▸ *Physical:* P, BP, R, ECG, I & O, IV site, weight; neurologic checks, vision, cardiac auscultation, peripheral pulses,

Adverse effects in *Italics* are most common; those in **Bold** are life-threatening

peripheral perfusion, edema, adventitious lung sounds, abdominal percussion, bowel sounds, serum digoxin level, electrolyte levels, liver and renal function tests, UA

Implementation
- Monitor apical pulse for 1 min before administering. Withhold dose if HR < 50–60 or as ordered by prescriber. Assess changes from baseline rhythm or rate.
- Carefully monitor P, BP, R, and ECG during IV administration.
- Digitalis effect may be seen on ECG as prolonged PR interval, scooped ST depression, and relatively short QT interval.
- Carefully monitor electrolyte levels during therapy.
- Avoid giving with meals; this will delay absorption.
- Have emergency equipment (defibrillator, drugs, oxygen, intubation equipment) on standby in case toxicity occurs.
- Monitor serum digoxin levels.
- Decrease dose in renal failure.
- Digoxin toxicity is often first manifested by anorexia, nausea, vomiting, headache, fatigue, depression, confusion, and hallucination. Vision problems are less common. Suspect digoxin toxicity for patients with dysrhythmias or a change in rhythm.

⬤ digoxin immune fab (ovine) *(di jox' in)*
digoxin-specific antibody fragments, Digibind

Pregnancy Category C

Drug class
Antidote

Indications
- Life-threatening digoxin or digitoxin intoxication (dysrhythmias, serum potassium levels of > 5 mEq/L, digoxin level > 10 ng/mL)

Therapeutic actions
- Binds digoxin molecules making them unavailable for binding at their site of action
- Fab fragment-digoxin complex accumulates in blood and is excreted by kidneys

Contraindications/cautions
- **Contraindications:** none known
- **Cautions:** poor cardiac function, electrolyte abnormalities, renal impairment; consider skin testing for patients at high risk for hypersensitivity or with sheep allergy

Available form
- *Powder for injection:* 38 mg/vial

Adverse effects in *Italics* are most common; those in **Bold** are life-threatening

IV facts
Preparation
▶ Dissolve contents of each vial with 4 mL of Sterile Water for Injection. Mix gently to give a clear, colorless, isosmotic solution with a protein concentration of 9.5 mg/mL.
▶ May be further diluted with sterile isotonic saline.

Dosage
▶ Determine dosage based on serum digoxin level or estimated digoxin ingested. If no estimate is available and serum digoxin cannot be obtained, use 800 mg (20 vials), which should treat most life-threatening ingestions.
▶ *Estimated fab fragment dose based on amount of digoxin ingested:*

Est. Number of 0.25-mg Caps Ingested	Dose of Fab Fragments (mg)	Number of Vials
25	380	10
50	760	20
75	1140	30
100	1520	40
150	2280	60
200	3040	80

▶ *Estimated fab fragment dose based on serum digoxin concentration:*

	Serum Digoxin Concentration						
	(ng/mL)						
	1	2	4	8	12	16	20
Wt (kg)	**Adult (Dose in Vials)**						
40	0.5	1	2	3	5	7	8
60	0.5	1	3	5	7	10	12
70	1	2	3	6	9	11	14
80	1	2	3	7	10	13	16
100	1	2	4	8	12	16	20

▶ Equations also are available for calculating exact dosage from serum digoxin or digitoxin concentrations.
▶ Administer dose IV over 30 min through a 0.22-mcm filter.
▶ If cardiac arrest is imminent, administer as a bolus injection.

Compatibility
Do not mix digoxin immune fab with any other drugs or give through the same IV line as other drugs.

Adverse effects in *Italics* are most common; those in **Bold** are life-threatening

TREATMENT OF OVERDOSE/ANTIDOTE
Discontinue drug or decrease dosage. Initiate general supportive and resuscitative measures. Treat anaphylaxis using aminophylline, oxygen, volume expansion, diphenhydramine, corticosteroids, and airway management.

Pharmacokinetics

Route	Onset	Peak	Duration
IV	30 min (variable)	Unknown	4–6 h

$T_{1/2}$: 15–20 h
Excretion: Urine

Adverse effects
▸ *CV:* Reemergence of heart failure or rapid ventricular response in patients with atrial fibrillation
▸ *Derm:* Skin rash
▸ *Allergic:* **Anaphylaxis**
▸ *Misc:* Hypokalemia

Clinically important drug–drug interactions
▸ Reversed effects with digitalis glycosides
▸ Aggravated digitalis toxic dysrhythmias with catecholamines

◉ NURSING CONSIDERATIONS

Assessment
▸ *History:* Allergy to sheep products, poor cardiac function, electrolyte abnormalities, renal impairment
▸ *Physical:* P, BP, R, ECG, I & O, IV site, cardiac auscultation, peripheral perfusion, adventitious lung sounds, serum electrolytes, renal function tests, serum digoxin level

Implementation
▸ If possible before administering digoxin immune fab, obtain serum digoxin levels because drug interferes with digoxin measurement.
▸ Carefully monitor T, P, BP, R, ECG, and K^+ levels during administration.
▸ Severe digitalis intoxication will shift serum K^+ concentrations from inside to outside the cell, which may result in life-threatening hyperkalemia. However, this elevation may lead to increased renal excretion of K^+. Therefore, patients may have hyperkalemia with a total body deficit of K^+. When drug reverses digoxin's effect, K^+ shifts back inside the cell, which may result in sudden hypokalemia.
▸ Maintain life-support equipment and emergency drugs on standby.

Adverse effects in *Italics* are most common; those in **Bold** are life-threatening

- Serum digoxin levels will be very high and will be unreliable until drug is eliminated from the body.
- Do not redigitalize patient until digoxin immune fab has been eliminated from the body—several days to a week or longer in cases of renal insufficiency.
- Assess for recurrent heart failure and dysrhythmias.
- If suicide is suspected, consider toxicity from other drugs.
- Skin testing may be done for patients considered at high risk for allergies.
  - Dilute 0.1 mL of reconstituted drug in 9.9 mL sterile isotonic saline.
  - Inject 0.1 mL of the 1:100 dilution intradermally and observe for a urticarial wheal surrounded by a zone of erythema.
  - Read test at 20 min.
  - If test causes a systemic reaction, apply a tourniquet above the site and treat for anaphylaxis. If further treatment with digoxin immune fab is absolutely essential, pretreat patient with corticosteroids and diphenhydramine.

⬤ diltiazem hydrochloride *(dil tye' a zem)*
Alti-Diltiazem (CAN), Apo-Diltiaz (CAN), Cardizem, Cardizem CD, Cardizem SR, Dilacor XR, Gen-Diltiazem (CAN), Novo-Diltazem (CAN), Nu-Diltiaz (CAN), Tiamate, Tiazac

Pregnancy Category C

Drug classes
Calcium channel-blocker
Antianginal agent
Antihypertensive

Indications
- Angina pectoris due to coronary artery spasm (Prinzmetal's variant angina)
- Effort-associated angina; chronic stable angina not controlled by beta-adrenergic blockers, nitrates
- Essential hypertension (sustained release)
- Treatment of hypertension (sustained release, Tiamate)
- Prophylaxis of paroxysmal supraventricular tachycardia (parenteral)
- Atrial fibrillation and atrial flutter (parenteral)

Therapeutic actions
- Inhibits movement of calcium ions across the membranes of myocardial and smooth muscle cells
- Depresses mechanical contraction of myocardial and smooth muscle
- Depresses automaticity of pacemaker cells

Adverse effects in *Italics* are most common; those in **Bold** are life-threatening

- Depresses SA and AV conduction velocity and thus ventricular rate in atrial fibrillation and atrial flutter
- Dilates coronary arteries and arterioles and peripheral arterioles
- Decreases myocardial energy consumption
- Increases myocardial oxygen delivery in patients with Prinzmetal's angina

Effects on hemodynamic parameters
- Decreased or unchanged HR
- Increased or decreased CO
- Decreased SVR
- Decreased BP

Contraindications/cautions
- **Contraindications:** diltiazem allergy, sick sinus syndrome, second- or third-degree heart block (unless functioning pacemaker is present), hypotension, acute myocardial infarction (AMI), pulmonary congestion, ventricular tachycardia, cardiogenic shock, patients with atrial fibrillation or atrial flutter associated with an accessory bypass tract (Wolff-Parkinson-White syndrome, short PR syndrome); IV diltiazem is contraindicated within a few hours of IV beta-blocker administration
- **Cautions:** CHF, concomitant use of beta-blockers or digitalis, impaired hepatic or renal function

Available forms
- *Injection:* 5 mg/mL
- *Tablets:* 30, 60, 90, 120 mg
- *Extended-release tablets:* 120, 180, 240 mg
- *Extended-release capsules:* 360 mg
- *SR capsules:* 60, 90, 120, 180, 240, 300 mg

IV facts
Preparation
- May give bolus dose undiluted.
- Add 125–250 mg (25–50 mL) to 100–250 mL of D5W/0.45%NS; D5W; or 0.9%NS.
- A commonly used concentration is 1 mg/mL (125 mg added to 100 mL).

Dosage and titration
- *Bolus dose:* 0.25 mg/kg IV over 2 min. After 15 min, may give a second bolus dose of 0.35 mg/kg IV over 2 min. Additional IV boluses may be given on an individual basis.
- *Infusion:* 5–10 mg/h IV. Increase infusion rate by 5 mg/h up to 15 mg/h as needed to reduce HR. Avoid infusing drug for > 24 h.

Titration Guide

diltiazem hydrochloride					
125 mg in 125 mL					
(result of adding 125 mg to 100 mL)					

mg/h	1	2	3	4	5	6
mL/h	1	2	3	4	5	6

mg/h	7	8	9	10	11	12
mL/h	7	8	9	10	11	12

mg/h	13	14	15
mL/h	13	14	15

Compatibility

Diltiazem may be given through the same IV line as albumin, amikacin, amphotericin B, aztreonam, bretylium, bumetanide, cefazolin, cefotaxime, cefotetan, cefoxitin, ceftazidime, ceftriaxone, cefuroxime, cimetidine, ciprofloxacin, clindamycin, digoxin, dobutamine, dopamine, doxycycline, epinephrine, erythromycin, esmolol, fentanyl, fluconazole, gentamicin, hetastarch, hydromorphone, imipenem-cilastatin, labetalol, lidocaine, lorazepam, meperidine, metoclopramide, metronidazole, midazolam, milrinone, morphine, multivitamins, nicardipine, nitroglycerin, nitroprusside sodium, norepinephrine, oxacillin, penicillin G potassium, pentamidine, piperacillin, potassium chloride, potassium phosphates, ranitidine, theophylline, ticarcillin, ticarcillin-clavulanate, tobramycin, trimethoprim-sulfamethoxazole, vancomycin, vecuronium.

Incompatibility

Do not administer through the same IV line as diazepam, furosemide, phenytoin, rifampin, thiopental.

Oral dosage

▶ *Tablets:* Start with 30 mg PO qid before meals and hs; gradually increase dosage at 1- to 2-d intervals to 180–360 mg PO in 3 to 4 divided doses.
▶ *Sustained/extended release:* Adjust dosage when maximum antihypertensive effect is achieved (around 14 d). Cardizem SR: Initially 60–120 mg PO bid; optimum range is 240–360 mg/d. Cardizem CD: Initially 180–240 mg PO qd for hypertension (usual range 240–360 mg qd) and 120–180 mg PO qd (up for 480 mg qd) for angina. Dilacor XR: Initially, 180–240 mg PO

qd (up to 540 mg qd) for hypertension and 120 mg PO qd (up to 480 mg qd) for angina.

TREATMENT OF OVERDOSE/ANTIDOTE
Discontinue infusion or decrease dosage. Initiate general supportive and resuscitative measures. IV calcium, atropine, beta-adrenergic agonists, isoproterenol, and pacing may reverse the hemodynamic effects of diltiazem. Monitor cardiac and respiratory function. Initiate gastric lavage, and administer emetics to patients with recent oral overdose.

Pharmacokinetics

Route	Onset	Peak	Duration
IV	Within 3 min	2–7 min	1–3 h after bolus dose; 0.5–10 h after stopping infusion
Oral	30–60 min	2–3 h	
SR	30–60 min	6–11 h	

Metabolism: Hepatic; $T_{1/2}$: 3½–6 h; 5–7 h (SR); 3.4 h (IV)
Excretion: Urine

Adverse effects

▸ *CNS: Dizziness, lightheadedness, headache, asthenia,* fatigue, somnolence
▸ *CV:* **Asystole,** *peripheral edema, bradycardia, AV block,* hypotension, dysrhythmias, bundle branch block, angina
▸ *GI: Nausea,* hepatic injury, constipation, abdominal discomfort
▸ *Misc: Flushing,* rash, micturition disorder, gait abnormality, eye irritation, burning at injection site, amblyopia

Clinically important drug–drug interactions

▸ Increased serum levels and toxicity of cyclosporine
▸ Increased bioavailability with cimetidine, ranitidine
▸ Increased carbamazepine serum levels or toxicity
▸ Severe hypotension or increased fluid volume requirements with fentanyl
▸ Enhanced effects of theophyllines
▸ Reduced lithium levels
▸ Additive antihypertensive effect when used with other antihypertensive agents
▸ Bradycardia and heart block with digitalis, beta-blockers

● NURSING CONSIDERATIONS

Assessment

▸ *History:* Diltiazem allergy, sick sinus syndrome, presence of functioning pacemaker, hypotension, AMI, pulmonary con-

Adverse effects in *Italics* are most common; those in **Bold** are life-threatening

gestion, cardiogenic shock, atrial fibrillation or atrial flutter associated with an accessory bypass tract, recent IV beta-blocker administration, CHF, concomitant use of beta-blockers or digitalis, impaired hepatic or renal function
▶ *Physical:* P, BP, R, ECG, I & O, weight, neurologic checks, skin assessment, peripheral perfusion, edema, adventitious lung sounds, abdominal assessment, liver and renal function tests, UA

Implementation
▶ Exercise extreme caution when calculating and preparing IV doses. Diltiazem is a very potent drug; small dosage errors can cause serious adverse effects. Avoid inadvertent bolus of drug.
▶ Always administer IV diltiazem through an IV infusion pump.
▶ Administer Dilacor XR in the morning on an empty stomach.
▶ Swallow SR, CD, and XR forms whole. Do not open capsules, chew, or crush.
▶ Monitor patient carefully (BP, cardiac rhythm, I & O) while drug is being titrated to therapeutic dose.
▶ Monitor BP carefully if patient is on concurrent doses of nitrates.
▶ Monitor cardiac rhythm regularly during stabilization of dosage and periodically during long-term therapy.
▶ Oral antiarrhythmic therapy is often started within 3 h of the IV bolus dose.
▶ Have patient make gradual position changes to minimize postural hypotension.
▶ Keep solution and vials refrigerated until use.
▶ Once diluted, solution is stable for 24 h.

dimercaprol *(dye mer kap' role)* BAL in Oil

Pregnancy Category C

Drug classes
Antidote
Chelating agent

Indications
▶ Treatment of arsenic, gold, and mercury poisoning
▶ Treatment of acute lead poisoning when used with calcium edetate disodium
▶ Treatment of acute mercury poisoning if therapy begun within 1 to 2 h

Therapeutic actions
▶ Forms complexes with arsenic, gold, and mercury by chelation, which increases urinary and fecal elimination of these metals

Adverse effects in *Italics* are most common; those in **Bold** are life-threatening

Contraindications/cautions
- **Contraindications:** dimercaprol allergy; hepatic or renal insufficiency, except postarsenical jaundice; iron, cadmium, or selenium poisoning
- **Cautions:** acute renal insufficiency that develops during therapy, G-6-PD deficiency

Available form
- *Injection:* 100 mg/mL

IM facts
Dosage
- Give by deep IM injection only.
- Begin therapy as early as possible, along with other supportive measures.
- *Mild arsenic or gold poisoning:* 2.5 mg/kg IM qid for 2 d, then bid on the third day, and qd thereafter for 10 days.
- *Severe arsenic or gold poisoning:* 3 mg/kg IM q4h for 2 d, then qid on the third day, and bid thereafter for 10 days.
- *Mercury poisoning:* 5 mg/kg IM initially, then 2.5 mg/kg qd or bid for 10 d.
- *Acute lead encephalopathy:* 4 mg/kg IM and then at 4-h intervals in combination with calcium edetate disodium. For less severe poisoning, may reduce dose to 3 mg/kg IM after first dose. Continue treatment for 2 to 7 d.

TREATMENT OF OVERDOSE/ANTIDOTE
Discontinue drug or decrease dosage. Initiate general supportive and resuscitative measures.

Pharmacokinetics

Route	Onset	Peak	Duration
IM	Rapid	30–60 min	3–4 h

Metabolism: Hepatic; $T_{1/2}$: short
Excretion: Urine, feces

Adverse effects
- ***CNS:*** *Headache,* tingling of hands, anxiety, weakness, unrest
- ***CV:*** *Rise in BP, tachycardia*
- ***GI:*** *Nausea, vomiting;* burning sensation of lips, mouth, throat; feeling of constriction or pain in throat, chest, hands; abdominal pain
- ***Misc:*** **Nephrotoxicity,** conjunctivitis, lacrimation, blepharal spasm, rhinorrhea, salivation, burning sensation of penis,

---

Adverse effects in *Italics* are most common; those in **Bold** are life-threatening

sweating of forehead and hands, local pain at injection site, painful sterile abscesses

Clinically important drug–drug interaction
▶ Increased toxicity with iron

◉ NURSING CONSIDERATIONS

Assessment
▶ *History:* Dimercaprol allergy, hepatic or renal insufficiency, postarsenical jaundice, type of poisoning, G-6-PD deficiency
▶ *Physical:* P, BP, R, I & O, weight, neurologic checks, reflexes, skin assessment, edema, peripheral sensation, abdominal exam, CBC, liver and kidney function tests, UA, serum levels of heavy metals

Implementation
▶ Carefully monitor P, BP, and R; increased BP and P may occur.
▶ Monitor I & O to detect any alteration in urine function.
▶ Alkalinize urine to increase excretion of chelated complex.
▶ Patient may experience loss of sensation in extremities; assess extremities for injuries.

◉ **diphenhydramine hydrochloride**
(*dye fen hye' dra meen*) AllerMax Caplets, Banophen Caplets, Benadryl, Benadryl Dye-Free Allergy Liqui Gels, Benadryl Allergy Kapseals, Benadryl Allergy Ultratabs, Diphen AF, Diphenhist Captabs, Diphen Cough, Dormin, Genahist, Hyrexin-50, Miles Nervine, Nighttime Sleep Aid, Nytol, Scot-Tussin Allergy DM, Siladryl, Sleep-eze 3, Sleepwell 2-nite, Sominex, Tusstat

Pregnancy Category B

Drug classes
Antihistamine
Sedative
Antiparkinsonism agent

Indications
▶ Hypersensitivity reactions (type I): adjunctive therapy for anaphylactic reactions; relief of symptoms associated with perennial and seasonal allergic rhinitis; vasomotor rhinitis; allergic conjunctivitis; mild, uncomplicated urticaria and angioedema; amelioration of allergic reactions to blood or plasma; dermatographism
▶ Nighttime sleep aid (oral only)
▶ Treatment of vertigo; prevention of motion sickness (oral only)

Adverse effects in *Italics* are most common; those in **Bold** are life-threatening

- For control of cough due to colds or allergy
- Parkinsonism (including drug-induced parkinsonism and extrapyramidal reactions) in elderly who are intolerant of more potent agents, for milder forms of the disorder in other age groups, and in combination with centrally acting anticholinergic drugs

Therapeutic actions

- Competitively blocks the effects of histamine at H_1 receptor sites
- Inhibits respiratory, vascular, and GI smooth muscle constriction; decreases capillary permeability, decreases histamine-activated exocrine secretions
- Exhibits strong atropine-like properties, which can potentiate the drying effect by suppressing exocrine glands
- Binds to central muscarinic receptors and produces antiemetic effects, decreasing nausea, vomiting, and motion sickness

Contraindications/cautions

- **Contraindications:** allergy to any antihistamines, patients receiving MAO inhibitors
- **Cautions:** elderly patients, predisposition to urinary retention, increased intraocular pressure, hyperthyroidism, CV disease, hypertension, narrow-angle glaucoma, stenosing peptic ulcer, symptomatic prostatic hypertrophy, asthma and other lower respiratory tract symptoms, bladder neck obstruction, pyloroduodenal obstruction

Available forms

- *Injection:* 50 mg/mL
- *Capsules:* 25, 50 mg
- *Tablets:* 25, 50 mg
- *Chewable tablets:* 12.5 mg
- *Liquid:* 6.25 mg/5 mL, 12.5 mg/5 mL
- *Solution:* 12.5 mg/5 mL
- *Elixir:* 12.5 mg/5 mL
- *Syrup:* 12.5 mg/5 mL

IV/IM facts
Preparation
- No additional preparation is needed.

Dosage
- *Hypersensitivity reactions/antiparkinsonism/motion sickness:* 10–50 mg IV or IM. Give each 25 mg over ≥ 1 min by direct injection or into tubing of running IV. If needed, may give up to 100 mg. Do not exceed 400 mg/d.
- *Elderly:* More likely to cause dizziness, sedation, syncope,

Adverse effects in *Italics* are most common; those in **Bold** are life-threatening

toxic confusional states, and hypotension in elderly patients; use with caution.

Compatibility
Diphenhydramine may be given through the same IV line as acyclovir, aldesleukin, amifostine, amsacrine, aztreonam, ciprofloxacin, cisplatin, cladribine, cyclophosphamide, cytarabine, doxorubicin, famotidine, filgrastim, fluconazole, fludarabine, gallium, granisetron, heparin, hydrocortisone, idarubicin, melphalan, meperidine, meropenem, methotrexate, ondansetron, paclitaxel, piperacillin-tazobactam, potassium chloride, propofol, sargramostim, sufentanil, tacrolimus, teniposide, thiotepa, vinorelbine, vitamin B complex with C.

Incompatibility
Do not administer through the same IV line as allopurinol, cefepime, cefmetazole, foscarnet.

Oral dosage
❯ *Hypersensitivity reactions/antiparkinsonism/motion sickness:* 25–50 mg PO q4–8h.
❯ *Nighttime sleep aid:* 50 mg PO at hs.
❯ *Treatment vertigo:* 25–50 mg PO tid–qid.
❯ *Antitussive:* 25 mg PO q4h using only syrup. Do not exceed 100 mg/d.

TREATMENT OF OVERDOSE/ANTIDOTE
Discontinue drug or decrease dosage. Initiate general supportive and resuscitative measures. Induce emesis in conscious patients. Perform gastric lavage in unconscious patients. Administer activated charcoal. Correct acidosis and electrolyte imbalances. Avoid stimulants, analeptics, and epinephrine. Treat hypotension with vasopressors, dysrhythmias with propranolol, and convulsions with IV diazepam. IV physostigmine may reverse central anticholinergic effects.

Pharmacokinetics
Route	Onset	Peak	Duration
IV	Rapid	1–4 h	4–8 h
IM	20–30 min	1–4 h	4–8 h
Oral	15–30 min	1–4 h	4–7 h

Metabolism: Hepatic; $T_{1/2}$: 2.5–7 h
Excretion: Urine

Adverse effects in *Italics* are most common; those in **Bold** are life-threatening

Adverse effects
- *CNS:* **Convulsions,** *drowsiness, sedation, dizziness, disturbed coordination,* fatigue, confusion, restlessness, excitation, nervousness, tremor, headache, blurred vision, diplopia, acute labyrinthitis, paresthesia
- *CV:* Hypotension, palpitations, bradycardia, tachycardia, extrasystoles
- *Resp:* *Thickening of bronchial secretions,* chest or throat tightness, wheezing, nasal stuffiness, dry mouth, dry nose, dry throat, sore throat
- *GI:* *Epigastric distress,* anorexia, increased appetite and weight gain, nausea, vomiting, diarrhea, constipation
- *GU:* Urinary frequency, dysuria, urinary retention, early menses, decreased libido, impotence
- *Allergic:* **Anaphylaxis,** urticaria, rash
- *Hematologic:* **Hemolytic anemia, thrombocytopenia, agranulocytosis**
- *Misc:* Excessive perspiration, chills

Clinically important drug–drug interactions
- Increased and prolonged anticholinergic effects with MAO inhibitors
- Enhanced effects with alcohol, other CNS depressants, hypnotics, sedatives, tranquilizers

● NURSING CONSIDERATIONS

Assessment
- *History:* Allergy to any antihistamines, current use of MAO inhibitors, age, predisposition to urinary retention, increased intraocular pressure, hyperthyroidism, CV disease, hypertension, narrow-angle glaucoma, stenosing peptic ulcer, symptomatic prostatic hypertrophy, asthma and other lower respiratory tract symptoms, bladder neck obstruction, pyloroduodenal obstruction
- *Physical:* P, R, BP, neurologic checks, skin assessment, presence of vertigo or insomnia, vision exam, parkinsonism or extrapyramidal symptoms, presence of anaphylactic or allergic reaction, adventitious lung sounds, bowel sounds, hydration status, nausea or vomiting, prostate palpation, CBC

Implementation
- Give IV forms when patient is lying down.
- Have emergency equipment (defibrillator, drugs, oxygen, intubation equipment) on standby in case anaphylaxis or adverse reaction occurs.
- Avoid SC administration.

Adverse effects in *Italics* are most common; those in **Bold** are life-threatening

D

▸ May give with or without food; administer with food if GI upset occurs.
▸ Do not crush capsules or coated tablets; may crush scored tablets.
▸ Administer syrup form if patient is unable to take tablets.
▸ Monitor patient response; adjust dosage to lowest effective dose.
▸ Initiate fall precautions; assist patient if he or she is out of bed.

⬤ disopyramide phosphate
*(dye soe **peer' a mide**)* Norpace, Norpace CR, Rythmodan (CAN)

Pregnancy Category C

Drug class
Antidysrhythmic

Indications
▸ Treatment of life-threatening ventricular dysrhythmias
▸ Unlabeled use: treatment of paroxysmal supraventricular tachycardia

Therapeutic actions
▸ Type Ia antidysrhythmic: decreases rate of diastolic depolarization
▸ Decreases automaticity
▸ Decreases the rate of rise of the action potential
▸ Prolongs the refractory period of cardiac muscle cells
▸ Decreases the disparity in refractoriness between infarcted and adjacent normally perfused myocardium
▸ Does not affect alpha- or beta-adrenergic receptors
▸ Shortens sinus node recovery time; lengthens atrial and ventricular refractoriness
▸ Has anticholinergic effects

Contraindications/cautions
▸ **Contraindications:** disopyramide allergy, cardiogenic shock, second- or third-degree block (unless functioning pacemaker is present), congenital QT prolongation, sick sinus syndrome, asymptomatic premature ventricular contractions, uncompensated or marginally compensated CHF or hypotension (unless secondary to the dysrhythmia)
▸ **Cautions:** myocarditis, cardiomyopathy, Wolff-Parkinson-White syndrome, bundle branch block, diabetes, impaired renal or hepatic function, hyperkalemia, hypokalemia, urinary retention, glaucoma, myasthenia gravis

Adverse effects in *Italics* are most common; those in **Bold** are life-threatening

Available forms
- *Capsules:* 100, 150 mg
- *Extended-release capsules:* 100, 150 mg

Oral dosage
- Evaluate patient carefully and monitor cardiac response closely to determine the correct dosage for each patient.
- *Usual dosage:* 400–800 mg/d PO. For patients < 50 kg, give 400 mg/d. Divide total daily dose giving immediate-release forms q6h or extended-release forms q12h.
- *Initial loading dose for rapid control of ventricular dysrhythmias:* 300 mg (200 mg for patients < 50 kg) PO (immediate release).
- *Maintenance dose:* 150 mg PO q6h. If no response or no evidence of toxicity within 6 h of loading dose, give 200 mg PO q6h. If no response within 48 h, discontinue drug or carefully monitor subsequent doses of 250 or 300 mg PO q6h.
- *Severe refractory ventricular tachycardia:* Up to 400 mg PO q6h.
- *Cardiomyopathy:* Do not give a loading dose. Limit initial dosage to 100 mg q6–8h.
- *Hepatic or moderate renal (creatinine clearance > 40 mL/min) insufficiency:* 100 mg PO q6h (immediate-release forms) or 200 mg q12h (extended-release forms).
- *Severe renal insufficiency:* May give or omit loading dose of 150 mg PO. Then give 100 mg (immediate-release form) at intervals shown below.

Creatinine Clearance (mL/min)	Interval
30–40	q8h
15–30	q12h
< 15	q24h

- *Transfer to disopyramide from other antidysrhythmics:* Use regular maintenance dosing without a loading dose 6–12 h after last dose of quinidine or 3–6 h after last dose of procainamide.
- *Conversion from immediate- to controlled-release forms:* Start controlled release 6 h after last dose of immediate form.

Therapeutic serum level
- 2–8 mcg/mL

> **TREATMENT OF OVERDOSE/ANTIDOTE**
> Discontinue drug or decrease dosage. Initiate general supportive and resuscitative measures. Prompt vigorous treatment is needed even in the absence of symptoms. Initiate
> *(treatment continued on next page)*

emesis, gastric lavage, or a cathartic followed by activated charcoal. Useful treatments may include isoproterenol, dopamine, cardiac glycosides, diuretics, intra-aortic balloon counterpulsation, mechanical ventilation, hemodialysis, or charcoal hemoperfusion. Implement pacing for progressive AV block. Neostigmine can reverse the drug's anticholinergic effects.

Pharmacokinetics

Route	Onset	Peak	Duration
Oral	30–60 min	2 h	1.5–8.5 h

Metabolism: Hepatic; $T_{1/2}$: 4–10 h
Excretion: Urine

Adverse effects

▸ *CNS: Dizziness, fatigue, headache, blurred vision, dry nose/eyes/throat,* nervousness, depression, insomnia
▸ *CV:* **Dysrhythmias,** CHF, hypotension, cardiac conduction disturbances, edema, shortness of breath, syncope, chest pain, elevated cholesterol/triglycerides
▸ *GI: Nausea, bloating, dry mouth, constipation, pain, gas,* anorexia, diarrhea, vomiting, elevated liver enzymes, reversible cholestatic jaundice
▸ *GU: Urinary hesitancy and retention,* impotence, elevated BUN and creatinine
▸ *Derm:* Rash, itching
▸ *Allergic:* **Anaphylaxis**
▸ *Musc/Skel: Muscle weakness, malaise, aches pains*
▸ *Misc:* Hypoglycemia, fever, respiratory difficulty, lupus erythematosus symptoms

Clinically important drug–drug interactions

▸ Decreased disopyramide plasma levels and enhanced anticholinergic effects with hydantoins, rifampin
▸ QRS complex or QT prolongation with other antidysrhythmics
▸ Increased disopyramide plasma levels, dysrhythmias, and QTc interval with erythromycin
▸ Increased disopyramide serum levels or decreased quinidine levels when used with quinidine

● NURSING CONSIDERATIONS

Assessment

▸ *History:* Disopyramide allergy, cardiogenic shock, functioning pacemaker, congenital QT prolongation, sick sinus

Adverse effects in *Italics* are most common; those in **Bold** are life-threatening

syndrome, CHF, hypotension, myocarditis, cardiomyopathy, Wolff-Parkinson-White syndrome, diabetes, impaired renal or hepatic function, hyperkalemia, hypokalemia, urinary retention, glaucoma, myasthenia gravis

▸ *Physical:* P, R, BP, ECG, I & O, weight, neurologic checks, intraocular pressure, edema, respiratory effort, cardiac auscultation, JVD, orthostatic BP, adventitious lung sounds, abdominal assessment, skin assessment, liver evaluation, UA, renal and liver function tests, blood glucose, serum electrolytes, disopyramide level

Implementation

▸ Closely monitor patients for dysrhythmias because drug may be prodysrhythmic.

▸ Check to see that patients with atrial flutter or fibrillation have been digitalized before starting procainamide.

▸ ECG changes associated with disopyramide therapy include prolonged PR interval, QRS duration, QT interval, and JT interval.

▸ Monitor for evidence of toxicity as evidenced by widened QRS complex and QT interval, worsened CHF, hypotension, varying conduction disturbances, bradycardia, or asystole.

▸ Have emergency equipment (defibrillator, drugs, oxygen, intubation equipment) on standby in case an allergic or adverse reaction occurs.

▸ Minimize postural hypotension by helping the patient change positions slowly.

▸ Differentiate the extended-release form from the regular.

▸ Do not break or crush sustained-release tablets.

● dobutamine hydrochloride

(doe' byoo ta meen) Dobutrex

Pregnancy Category C

Drug classes
Vasopressor
Beta-1 selective adrenergic stimulant
Inotropic agent

Indications
▸ For inotropic support in short-term treatment of adults with cardiac decompensation due to depressed contractility, resulting from either organic heart disease or cardiac surgical procedures

---

Adverse effects in *Italics* are most common; those in **Bold** are life-threatening

Therapeutic actions
▶ Direct-acting inotropic agent stimulates beta receptors in the heart, increasing the force of myocardial contraction while producing mild chronotropic, hypertensive, arrhythmogenic, and vasodilative effects
▶ Increases CO in patients with depressed cardiac function

Effects on hemodynamic parameters
▶ Increased CO
▶ Increased SV
▶ Decreased SVR
▶ Increased CVP
▶ Decreased PCWP
▶ Increased or unchanged HR

Contraindications/cautions
▶ **Contraindications:** dobutamine or bisulfite allergy, idiopathic hypertrophic subaortic stenosis
▶ **Cautions:** preexisting ventricular ectopy, acute myocardial infarction (AMI), hypovolemia, hypertension, atrial fibrillation; marked mechanical obstruction, as in severe valvular aortic stenosis

Available forms
▶ *IV injection:* 12.5 mg/mL
▶ *Premixed IV infusion:* 0.5, 1, 2, and 4 mg/mL

IV facts
Preparation
▶ If a premixed IV infusion is not available, add 250 mg dobutamine to at least 50 mL (preferably 250–500 mL) of D5W/LR; D5W/0.45%NS; D5W/0.9%NS; D5W; D10W; Isolyte M with 5% Dextrose; LR; Osmitrol 20% in Water for Injection; Normosol-M in D5W; 0.45%NS; 0.9%NS; or Sodium Lactate (1/6 Molar) Injection.
▶ Commonly used concentrations are 1000 mcg/mL (250 mg in 250 mL) or 2000 mcg/mL (500 mg in 250 mL). The 2000 mcg/mL concentration is preferred for patients with volume overload. Do not exceed 5000 mcg/mL concentration.

Dosage and titration
▶ Usual dosage is 2.5–15 mcg/kg/min IV. Start infusion at 2.5 mcg/kg/min and increase by 2.5 mcg/kg/min until desired CO achieved. Titrate infusion based on patient's hemodynamic status. Rarely, infusion rates up to 40 mcg/kg/min have been used.
▶ When discontinuing the infusion, gradually decrease the dose.

Adverse effects in *Italics* are most common; those in **Bold** are life-threatening

Titration Guide

dobutamine hydrochloride									
500 mg in 250 mL									
Body Weight									
lb	88	99	110	121	132	143	154	165	176	187
kg	40	45	50	55	60	65	70	75	80	85

Dose ordered in mcg/kg/min	Amounts to Infuse in mL/h									
2.5	3	3	4	4	5	5	5	6	6	6
5	6	7	8	8	9	10	11	11	12	13
7.5	9	10	11	12	14	15	16	17	18	19
10	12	14	15	17	18	20	21	23	24	26
12.5	15	17	19	21	23	24	26	28	30	32
15	18	20	23	25	27	29	32	34	36	38
17.5	21	24	26	29	32	34	37	39	42	45
20	24	27	30	33	36	39	42	45	48	51
25	30	34	38	41	45	49	53	56	60	64
30	36	41	45	50	54	59	63	68	72	77
35	42	47	53	58	63	68	74	79	84	89
40	48	54	60	66	72	78	84	90	96	102

Body Weight									
lb	198	209	220	231	242	253	264	275	286
kg	90	95	100	105	110	115	120	125	130

Dose ordered in mcg/kg/min	Amounts to Infuse in mL/h								
2.5	7	7	8	8	8	9	9	9	10
5	14	14	15	16	17	17	18	19	20
7.5	20	21	23	24	25	26	27	28	29
10	27	29	30	32	33	35	36	38	39
12.5	34	36	38	39	41	43	45	47	49
15	41	43	45	47	50	52	54	56	59
17.5	47	50	53	55	58	60	63	66	68
20	54	57	60	63	66	69	72	75	78
25	68	71	75	79	83	86	90	94	98
30	81	86	90	95	99	104	108	113	117
35	95	100	105	110	116	121	126	131	137
40	108	114	120	126	132	138	144	150	156

Compatibility

Dobutamine may be given through the same IV line as amifostine, amiodarone, amrinone, atracurium, aztreonam, bretylium, calcium chloride, calcium gluconate, ciprofloxacin, cladribine, diazepam, diltiazem, dopamine, enalaprilat, epinephrine, famotidine, fentanyl, fluconazole, granisetron, haloperidol, hydromorphone, insulin (regular), labetalol, lidocaine, lorazepam, magnesium sulfate, meperidine, milrinone, nicardipine, nitroglycerin, nitroprusside sodium, norepinephrine, pancuronium, potassium chloride, propofol, ranitidine, streptokinase, tacrolimus, theophylline, thiotepa, tobramycin, tolazoline, vecuronium, verapamil, zidovudine.

Incompatibility

Do not administer through the same IV line as acyclovir, alteplase, aminophylline, cefepime, cefmetazole, foscarnet, indomethacin, phytonadione, piperacillin-tazobactam, thiopental, warfarin.

TREATMENT OF OVERDOSE/ANTIDOTE

Discontinue drug or decrease dosage. Initiate general supportive and resuscitative measures. Initiate resuscitative measures as indicated. Treat severe ventricular dysrhythmias with propranolol or lidocaine.

Pharmacokinetics

Route	Onset	Peak	Duration
IV	1–2 min	10 min	5–10 min

Metabolism: Hepatic; $T_{1/2}$: 2 min
Excretion: Urine

Adverse effects

▶ *CNS: Headache*
▶ *CV: Elevated HR, elevated SBP, increased PVCs,* hypotension, angina, palpitations, shortness of breath
▶ *GI: Nausea*
▶ *Derm:* Phlebitis at infusion site

Clinically important drug–drug interactions

▶ May be ineffective in patients who recently received a beta-blocker
▶ Higher CO and lower PCWP with nitroprusside than when either drug is used alone
▶ Increased dysrhythmias with bretylium
▶ Increased severe hypertension with guanethidine, oxytocic drugs
▶ Increased vasopressor effect with TCAs

Adverse effects in *Italics* are most common; those in **Bold** are life-threatening

◉ NURSING CONSIDERATIONS

Assessment

▸ *History:* Dobutamine or bisulfite allergy; idiopathic hypertrophic subaortic stenosis; preexisting ventricular ectopy; AMI, hypovolemia, hypertension, marked mechanical obstruction as in severe valvular aortic stenosis

▸ *Physical:* T, P, BP, R, CO, PCWP, SVR, CVP, ECG, I & O, IV site, weight, pulse pressure, skin assessment, adventitious lung sounds, heart murmur, hydration status, serum electrolytes

Implementation

▸ Exercise extreme caution when calculating and preparing doses. Dobutamine is a very potent drug; small dosage errors can cause serious adverse effects. Always dilute drug before use; avoid inadvertent bolus of drug.

▸ Always administer through an IV infusion pump.

▸ Administer into large veins of antecubital fossa rather than hand or ankle veins. Use a central line whenever possible.

▸ Correct hypovolemia before administering dobutamine.

▸ Digitalize patients who have atrial fibrillation with a rapid ventricular rate before giving dobutamine; dobutamine facilitates AV conduction.

▸ Monitor ECG, CO, PCWP, BP, and urine output closely during infusion. Adjust dose and rate accordingly.

▸ Monitor infusion site closely for evidence of infiltration or phlebitis.

▸ Once diluted, solution is stable for 24 h.

▸ Do not freeze.

▸ Drug solution may turn pink; however, this does not change its effectiveness.

◉ dopamine hydrochloride *(doe' pa meen)*

Intropin

Pregnancy Category C

Drug classes

Vasopressor
Alpha-adrenergic stimulant
Beta-1 selective adrenergic stimulant
Dopaminergic receptor activator

Indications

▸ To correct hemodynamic imbalances present in shock due to myocardial infarction, trauma, endotoxic septicemia, open heart surgery, renal failure, and chronic cardiac decompensation in CHF

Adverse effects in *Italics* are most common; those in **Bold** are life-threatening

D

Therapeutic actions
▶ Acts directly and by release of norepinephrine from sympathetic nerve terminals
▶ Dopaminergic receptors mediate dilation of vessels in the renal and splanchnic beds to increase renal perfusion and function
▶ Beta-1 receptors mediate a positive inotropic effect (increased myocardial contractility, heart rate, cardiac output, automaticity, and AV conduction)
▶ At doses greater than 10 mcg/kg/min, alpha receptors mediate vasoconstriction and override dopamine's dopaminergic effects

Effects on hemodynamic parameters
▶ < 3 mcg/kg/min: unchanged or increased CO, unchanged or increased HR, decreased SVR, increased renal perfusion, increased urine output
▶ 3–10 mcg/kg/min: increased CO, increased HR, increased SVR, increased BP
▶ > 10 mcg/kg/min: increased CO, increased HR, markedly increased SVR, increased PVR, increased BP, decreased renal perfusion and urine output

Contraindications/cautions
▶ **Contraindications:** dopamine allergy, pheochromocytoma, tachydysrhythmias, ventricular fibrillation, **hypovolemia (dopamine is not a substitute for blood, plasma, fluids, or electrolytes, which should be restored promptly when a loss occurs)**
▶ **Cautions:** atherosclerosis, arterial embolism, sulfite sensitivity, Raynaud's disease, cold injury, frostbite, diabetic endarteritis, Buerger's disease

Available forms
▶ *IV injection:* 40, 80, 160 mg/mL
▶ *Premixed IV infusion:* 0.8 mg/mL (250 or 500 mL); 1.6 mg/mL (250 or 500 mL); 3.2 mg/mL (250 mL)

IV facts
Preparation
▶ Either dilute dopamine before using or use a premixed solution.
▶ Add 200–800 mg dopamine to 250–500 mL of D5W/LR; D5W/0.45%NS; D5W/0.9%NS; D5W; D10W/0.18%NS; D10W; LR; Mannitol 20% in Water; 0.9%NS; Sodium Bicarbonate 5%; or Sodium Lactate (1/6 Molar) Injection.

Adverse effects in *Italics* are most common; those in **Bold** are life-threatening

▸ Commonly used concentrations are 1600 mcg/mL (400 mg in 250 mL) or 3200 mcg/mL (800 mg in 250 mL). The 3200 mcg/mL concentration is preferred for patients with volume overload.

Dosage and titration

▸ *Patients likely to respond to modest increments of cardiac contractility and renal perfusion:* Start IV infusion at 2–5 mcg/kg/min. Titrate infusion to patient response.
▸ *Patients who are seriously ill:* Start IV infusion at 5 mcg/kg/min. Increase rate by 5–10 mcg/kg/min increments up to 20–50 mcg/kg/min. Most patients require less than 20 mcg/kg/min.
▸ When discontinuing the infusion, gradually decrease the dose because sudden cessation may lead to hypotension.

Titration Guide

dopamine hydrochloride									
400 mg in 250 mL									
Body Weight									
lb	88	99	110	121	132	143	154	165	176	187
kg	40	45	50	55	60	65	70	75	80	85

Dose ordered in mcg/kg/min	Amounts to Infuse in mL/h									
1	2	2	2	2	2	2	3	3	3	3
2	3	3	4	4	5	5	5	6	6	6
3	5	5	6	6	7	7	8	8	9	10
4	6	7	8	8	9	10	11	11	12	13
5	8	8	9	10	11	12	13	14	15	16
6	9	10	11	12	14	15	16	17	18	19
8	12	14	15	17	18	20	21	23	24	26
10	15	17	19	21	23	24	26	28	30	32
12	18	20	23	25	27	29	32	34	36	38
14	21	24	26	29	32	34	37	39	42	45
16	24	27	30	33	36	39	42	45	48	51
18	27	30	34	37	41	44	47	51	54	57
20	30	34	38	41	45	49	53	56	60	64
25	38	42	47	52	56	61	66	70	75	80
30	45	51	56	62	68	73	79	84	90	96
35	53	59	66	72	79	85	92	98	105	112
40	60	68	75	83	90	98	105	113	120	128
45	68	76	84	93	101	110	118	127	135	143
50	75	84	94	103	113	122	131	141	150	159

Adverse effects in *Italics* are most common; those in **Bold** are life-threatening

					Body Weight				
lb	198	209	220	231	242	253	264	275	286
kg	90	95	100	105	110	115	120	125	130
Dose ordered in mcg/kg/min				Amounts to Infuse in mL/h					
1	3	4	4	4	4	4	5	5	5
2	7	7	8	8	8	9	9	9	10
3	10	11	11	12	12	13	14	14	15
4	14	14	15	16	17	17	18	19	20
5	17	18	19	20	21	22	23	23	24
6	20	21	23	24	25	26	27	28	29
8	27	29	30	32	33	35	36	38	39
10	34	36	38	39	41	43	45	47	49
12	41	43	45	47	50	52	54	56	59
14	47	50	53	55	58	60	63	66	68
16	54	57	60	63	66	69	72	75	78
18	61	64	68	71	74	78	81	84	88
20	68	71	75	79	83	86	90	94	98
25	84	89	94	98	103	108	113	117	122
30	101	107	113	118	124	129	135	141	146
35	118	125	131	138	144	151	158	164	171
40	135	143	150	158	165	173	180	188	195
45	152	160	169	177	186	194	203	211	219
50	169	178	188	197	206	216	225	234	244

Compatibility

Dopamine may be given through the same IV line as aldesleukin, amifostine, amiodarone, amrinone, atracurium, aztreonam, cefmetazole, ciprofloxacin, cladribine, diltiazem, dobutamine, enalaprilat, epinephrine, esmolol, famotidine, fentanyl, fluconazole, foscarnet, granisetron, haloperidol, heparin, hydrocortisone, hydromorphone, labetalol, lidocaine, lorazepam, meperidine, methylprednisolone, metronidazole, midazolam, milrinone, morphine, nicardipine, nitroglycerin, nitroprusside sodium, norepinephrine, ondansetron, pancuronium, piperacillin-tazobactam, potassium chloride, propofol, ranitidine, sargramostim, streptokinase, tacrolimus, theophylline, thiotepa, tolazoline, vecuronium, verapamil, vitamin B complex with C, warfarin, zidovudine.

Incompatibility

Do not administer through the same IV line as acyclovir, alteplase, cefepime, indomethacin, insulin (regular), thiopental.

Adverse effects in *Italics* are most common; those in **Bold** are life-threatening

TREATMENT OF OVERDOSE/ANTIDOTE
Discontinue drug or decrease dosage. Initiate general supportive and resuscitiative measures. Consider giving phentolamine. See below for treatment of drug infiltration.

Pharmacokinetics

Route	Onset	Peak	Duration
IV	5 min	10 min	<10 min

Metabolism: Hepatic; $T_{1/2}$: 2 min
Excretion: Urine

Adverse effects
▸ *CV: Ectopic beats, tachycardia, angina, palpitations, hypotension, vasoconstriction, dyspnea,* bradycardia, **hypertension,** widened QRS
▸ *GI: Nausea, vomiting*
▸ *Derm:* Tissue necrosis at infusion site, gangrene with prolonged use
▸ *Misc:* Headache, piloerection, azotemia

Clinically important drug–drug interactions
▸ Severe hypertension with MAO inhibitors
▸ Decreased effect with tricyclic antidepressants
▸ Decreased antihypertensive effects of guanethidine
▸ Seizures, severe hypotension, bradycardia when infused with phenytoin
▸ Increased hypertension with alseroxylon, deserpidine, furazolidone, methyldopa

◉ NURSING CONSIDERATIONS

Assessment
▸ *History:* Dopamine allergy, pheochromocytoma, **hypovolemia,** atherosclerosis, arterial embolism, sulfite sensitivity, Raynaud's disease, cold injury, frostbite, diabetic endarteritis, Buerger's disease
▸ *Physical:* T, P, BP, R, CO, PCWP, CVP, ECG, I & O, IV site, weight, pulse pressure, skin assessment, peripheral pulses and perfusion, adventitious lung sounds, hydration status, acid–base status, serum electrolytes, Hct, renal function tests, ABG

Implementation
▸ Exercise extreme caution when calculating and preparing doses. Dopamine is a very potent drug; small dosage errors

Adverse effects in *Italics* are most common; those in **Bold** are life-threatening

can cause serious adverse effects. Always dilute drug before use; avoid inadvertent bolus of drug.

> Always administer through an IV infusion pump.
> Closely monitor HR, BP, and ECG. Continuous arterial pressure monitoring is preferred.
> Administer into large veins of antecubital fossa rather than hand or ankle veins. Use a central line whenever possible.
> Correct hypovolemia before administering drug.
> Correct acid–base imbalances because acidosis lessens the response to vasopressors.
> Monitor infusion site closely for evidence of infiltration or phlebitis. If extravasation occurs, prevent sloughing and necrosis by using a fine hypodermic needle to infiltrate area with 5–10 mg phentolamine in 10–15 mL 0.9%NS.
> Use the smallest dose possible to achieve intended effects.
> Reduce initial dosage by 1/10 in patients who have been on MAO inhibitors.
> Once diluted, solution is stable for 24 h.
> During storage, protect drug solutions from light.
> Drug solution should be clear and colorless.

● droperidol (droe pear' ih dall) Inapsine
Pregnancy Category C

Drug classes
Tranquilizer
Antiemetic

Indications
> To produce tranquilization and reduce nausea and vomiting in surgical and diagnostic procedures
> Current use with a narcotic analgesic to produce tranquility and decrease anxiety and pain
> Premedication, induction, and adjunct in maintenance of general and regional anesthesia
> Unlabeled use: antiemetic in cancer chemotherapy

Therapeutic actions
> Produces marked tranquilization, sedation, and antiemetic effects
> Produces mild alpha-adrenergic blockade, peripheral vascular dilatation
> Reduces pressor effect of epinephrine

Effects on hemodynamic parameters
> Decreased BP
> Decreased SVR
> Decreased PCWP (especially if abnormally high)

Adverse effects in *Italics* are most common; those in **Bold** are life-threatening

Contraindications/cautions
▸ **Contraindication:** droperidol allergy
▸ **Cautions:** renal or hepatic function impairment; elderly, poor risk, or debilitated patients; pheochromocytoma; risk for dysrhythmias

Available form
▸ *Injection:* 2.5 mg/mL

IV/IM facts
Preparation
▸ Withdraw appropriate dose into syringe. May be given undiluted or added to 250 mL D5W or LR.

Dosage
▸ *Antiemetic:* 1–4 mg IV q3–6h.
▸ *Premedication:* 2.5–10 mg IM 30–60 min preoperatively.
▸ *Use without general anesthesia in diagnostic procedures:* 2.5–10 mg IM 30–60 min before procedure. May give additional 1.25–2.5 mg IV.

Compatibility
Droperidol may be given through the same IV line as amifostine, aztreonam, bleomycin, cisplatin, cladribine, cyclophosphamide, cytarabine, doxorubicin, famotidine, filgrastim, fluconazole, fludarabine, granisetron, hydrocortisone, idarubicin, melphalan, meperidine, metoclopramide, mitomycin, ondansetron, paclitaxel, potassium chloride, propofol, sargramostim, teniposide, thiotepa, vinblastine, vincristine, vinorelbine, vitamin B complex with C.

Incompatibility
Do not administer through the same IV line as allopurinol, cefepime, cefmetazole, fluorouracil, foscarnet, furosemide, leucovorin, nafcillin, piperacillin-tazobactam.

TREATMENT OF OVERDOSE/ANTIDOTE
Discontinue drug or decrease dosage. Initiate general supportive and resuscitative measures. Treat hypotension with IV fluids, and elevate patient's legs. If hypotension continues, treat with pressors other than epinephrine.

Adverse effects in *Italics* are most common; those in **Bold** are life-threatening

Pharmacokinetics

Route	Onset	Peak	Duration
IV/IM	3–10 min	30 min	2–4 h (altered consciousness may persist 12 h)

Metabolism: Hepatic; $T_{1/2}$: 2.2 h
Excretion: Urine, feces

Adverse effects

▶ *CNS: Postoperative drowsiness,* dizziness, postoperative hallucinations, transient mental depression, restlessness, hyperactivity, anxiety, extrapyramidal symptoms (dystonia, akathisia, oculogyric crisis)
▶ *CV: Hypotension, tachycardia,* hypertension
▶ **Resp: Respiratory depression, apnea, respiratory arrest, laryngospasm, bronchospasm,** muscular rigidity
▶ *Misc:* Shivering

Clinically important drug–drug interactions

▶ Enhanced by other CNS depressant drugs (barbiturates, tranquilizers, opioids, general anesthetics); decrease droperidol dosage
▶ Paradoxically decreased blood pressure with epinephrine

● NURSING CONSIDERATIONS

Assessment

▶ *History:* Droperidol allergy, renal or hepatic function impairment, age, debilitation, pheochromocytoma, risk for dysrhythmias
▶ *Physical:* T, P, BP, R, ECG, I & O, neurologic checks, orthostatic BP, cardiac auscultation, skin assessment, adventitious lung sounds, abdominal assessment, presence of nausea or vomiting, renal and hepatic function tests

Implementation

▶ Use for anesthesia only if trained to give anesthetic agents.
▶ Carefully monitor P, BP, R, and ECG during IV administration.
▶ Have emergency equipment (defibrillator, drugs, oxygen, intubation equipment) on standby in case adverse reaction occurs.
▶ Monitor patient closely for extrapyramidal symptoms.
▶ Minimize postural hypotension by helping the patient slowly change positions.
▶ Protect drug from light.

Adverse effects in *Italics* are most common; those in **Bold** are life-threatening

E

⬤ **enalapril maleate** *(e nal' a pril)* Vasotec

⬤ **enalaprilat** Vasotec I.V.

Pregnancy Category C (first trimester) and D (second and third trimesters)

Drug classes
ACE inhibitor
Antihypertensive

Indications
▸ Treatment of hypertension alone or in combination with other antihypertensive drugs, especially thiazide diuretics
▸ Treatment of congestive heart failure
▸ Treatment of asymptomatic left ventricular dysfunction

Therapeutic actions
▸ Suppresses renin-angiotensin-aldosterone system; blocks ACE from converting angiotensin I to angiotensin II, a powerful vasoconstrictor; leads to decreased blood pressure, decreased aldosterone secretion, a small increase in serum potassium levels, and sodium and fluid loss
▸ Increased prostaglandin synthesis also may be involved in the antihypertensive action

Effects on hemodynamic parameters
▸ Decreased BP
▸ Decreased PCWP
▸ Decreased SVR/PVR
▸ May decrease CVP

Contraindications/cautions
▸ **Contraindications:** enalapril allergy, angioedema related to previous treatment with an ACE inhibitor
▸ **Cautions:** impaired renal function, salt/volume depletion, heart failure, high-dose diuretic therapy, recent intensive diuresis, renal dialysis, diabetes

Available forms
▸ *Injection:* 1.25 mg/mL
▸ *Tablets:* 2.5, 5, 10, 20 mg

IV facts
Preparation
▸ Give undiluted or diluted with up to 50 mL D5W/LR; D5W/0.9%NS; D5W; Isolyte E; or 0.9%NS.

Adverse effects in *Italics* are most common; those in **Bold** are life-threatening

E

Dosage and titration
⏵ *Hypertension; converting to IV therapy from oral therapy:* 1.25 mg IV over 5 min q6h. A response is usually seen within 15 min, but peak effects may not occur for 4 h. Do not exceed 20 mg/d.
⏵ *Patients taking diuretics:* 0.625 mg IV over 5 min. If adequate response is not seen after 1 h, repeat the 0.625-mg dose. Give additional doses of 1.25 mg q6h.
⏵ *Patients with renal impairment:* If creatinine clearance > 30 mL/min, give 1.25 mg IV over 5 min q6h. If creatinine clearance ≤ 30 mL/min, give initial dose of 0.625 mg. May repeat this dose after 1 h if clinical response is not adequate. Additional doses of 1.25 mg may be given at 6-h intervals.

Compatibility
IV enalaprilat may be given through the same IV line as allopurinol, amifostine, amikacin, aminophylline, ampicillin, ampicillin-sulbactam, aztreonam, butorphanol, calcium gluconate, cefazolin, cefoperazone, ceftazidime, ceftizoxime, chloramphenicol, cimetidine, cladribine, clindamycin, dextran 40, dobutamine, dopamine, erythromycin, esmolol, famotidine, fentanyl, filgrastim, ganciclovir, gentamicin, granisetron, heparin, hetastarch, hydrocortisone, labetalol, lidocaine, magnesium sulfate, melphalan, meropenem, methylprednisolone, metronidazole, morphine, nafcillin, nicardipine, nitroglycerin, nitroprusside sodium, penicillin G potassium, phenobarbital, piperacillin, piperacillin-tazobactam, potassium chloride, potassium phosphates, propofol, ranitidine, sodium acetate, teniposide, thiotepa, tobramycin, trimethoprim-sulfamethoxazole, vancomycin, vinorelbine.

Incompatibility
Do not administer through the same IV line as amphotericin B, cefepime, phenytoin.

Oral dosage
⏵ *Hypertension for patients not taking diuretics:* 5 mg/d PO. Adjust dosage based on patient response. Usual range is 10–40 mg/d as a single dose or in 2 divided doses.
⏵ *Hypertension for patients taking diuretics:* If possible, discontinue diuretic for 2–3 d. If not possible to discontinue, give initial dose of 2.5 mg PO and monitor for excessive hypotension.
⏵ *Hypertension, converting to oral therapy from IV therapy:* 5 mg/d PO with subsequent doses based on patient response.
⏵ *Patients with hypertension and renal impairment:* If creatinine clearance is between 30 and 80 mL/min, start with 5 mg PO qd. If creatinine clearance ≤ 30 mL/min, start with 2.5 mg/d PO. For dialysis patients, start with 2.5 mg on dialysis days. Titrate dosage up to 40 mg/d.
⏵ *Heart failure:* 2.5 mg/d or bid PO in conjunction with diuret-

Adverse effects in *Italics* are most common; those in **Bold** are life-threatening

ics and digitalis. Maintenance dose is 2.5–20 mg/d given in 2 divided doses. Maximum daily dose is 40 mg in divided doses.

▸ *Asymptomatic left ventricular dysfunction:* 2.5 mg PO bid; target maintenance dose is 20 mg/d in 2 divided doses.

▸ *Patients with heart failure and renal impairment or hyponatremia:* Start at 2.5 mg/d PO. Titrate as tolerated to a maximum daily dose of 40 mg in divided doses.

TREATMENT OF OVERDOSE/ANTIDOTE

Discontinue drug or decrease dosage. Initiate general supportive and resuscitative measures. Treat hypotension with supportive measures including an IV 0.9%NS infusion. Treat angioedema with antihistamines and SC epinephrine, and maintain a patent airway. Drug may be removed by dialysis.

Pharmacokinetics

Route	Onset	Peak	Duration
IV	Within 15 min	1–4 h	6 h
Oral	Within 60 min	3–4 h	24 h

$T_{1/2}$: 11 h
Excretion: Urine

Adverse effects

▸ *CNS:* **CVA,** *headache,* fatigue, dizziness, nervousness, confusion, blurred vision

▸ *CV:* **AMI, cardiac arrest, pulmonary embolism,** *hypotension,* chest pain, dysrhythmias, palpitations, pulmonary edema, postural hypotension

▸ *Resp:* **Bronchospasm,** *cough,* bronchitis, dyspnea, pneumonia, rhinorrhea, sore throat, hoarseness, upper respiratory infection, pulmonary infiltrates

▸ *GI:* **Hepatic failure,** *nausea, diarrhea,* constipation, ileus, hepatitis

▸ *GU:* **Renal failure,** oliguria, flank pain, gynecomastia, impotence

▸ *Derm:* **Stevens-Johnson syndrome, toxic epidermal necrolysis,** exfoliative dermatitis, flushing, rash, urticaria, pruritus, diaphoresis

▸ *Allergic:* **Anaphylaxis,** angioedema

▸ *Hematologic:* **Neutropenia, thrombocytopenia,** bone marrow depression

▸ *Musc/Skel:* Muscle cramps, arthralgia, myalgia

▸ *Misc:* Fever, blurred vision, positive ANA

Clinically important drug–drug interactions

▸ Increased hypotension with diuretics

Adverse effects in *Italics* are most common; those in **Bold** are life-threatening

▪ Attenuated potassium loss caused by thiazide-type diuretics
▪ Increased hyperkalemia with potassium-sparing diuretics, potassium supplements, potassium-containing salts
▪ Increased lithium toxicity
▪ Decreased hypotensive effect with indomethacin

● NURSING CONSIDERATIONS

Assessment

▪ *History:* Enalapril allergy, impaired renal function, angioedema related to previous treatment with an ACE inhibitor, salt/volume depletion, heart failure, high-dose diuretic therapy, diabetes, renal dialysis
▪ *Physical:* T, P, BP, R, SVR, PCWP, CVP, I & O, weight, neurologic checks, skin assessment, peripheral sensation, peripheral perfusion, orthostatic BP, edema, JVD, mucous membranes, bowel sounds, liver evaluation, UA, renal and liver function tests, CBC, serum glucose

Implementation

▪ Exercise extreme caution when calculating and preparing IV doses.
▪ Monitor patient closely; peak effect may take 4 h. Do not administer second dose until checking BP.
▪ Monitor patients on diuretic therapy for excessive hypotension following the first few doses of enalapril.
▪ Have emergency equipment (defibrillator, drugs, oxygen, intubation equipment) on standby in case anaphylaxis or adverse reaction occurs.
▪ Monitor patient closely in any situation that may lead to a fall in BP secondary to reduced fluid volume (excessive perspiration, dehydration, vomiting, diarrhea) because excessive hypotension may occur.
▪ Monitor for postural hypotension, especially in hypovolemic patients. Help patients change positions slowly to minimize risk of postural hypotension.
▪ African American hypertensive patients have a smaller average response to enalaprilat therapy than non-African American patients.
▪ Alert surgeon and mark patient's chart with notice that enalapril is being taken; the angiotensin II formation subsequent to compensatory renin release during surgery will be blocked. Correct this hypotension with volume expansion.
▪ After being diluted, drug remains stable for up to 24 h at room temperature.

● enoxaparin *(en ocks' a pear in)* Lovenox
Pregnancy Category B

Drug classes
Antithrombotic agent
Low-molecular-weight (LMW) heparin

Indications
▸ Used in conjunction with aspirin to prevent ischemic complications of USA and non–Q-wave MI
▸ Prevention of deep vein thrombosis, which may lead to pulmonary embolism following abdominal surgery or hip or knee replacement
▸ Used in conjunction with warfarin sodium for treatment of acute DVT with and without pulmonary embolism
▸ Unlabeled uses: systemic anticoagulation in venous and arterial thromboembolic complications; secondary prophylaxis for recurrent thromboembolic events

Therapeutic actions
▸ LMW heparin drug whose average weight is about 62% less than unfractionated standard heparin
▸ Blocks Factors Xa and thrombin (IIa) in the clotting cascade by antithrombin III and thus prevents thrombus formation
▸ Compared to other LMW heparins, enoxaparin has a low molecular weight and a high anti-Xa to anti-IIa activity ratio, nearly three times that of standard unfractionated heparin

Contraindications/cautions
▸ **Contraindications:** hypersensitivity to enoxaparin, heparin, or pork products; severe thrombocytopenia; uncontrolled bleeding
▸ **Cautions:** risk for bleeding, impaired renal or hepatic function, bacterial endocarditis, HTN; recent brain, spinal, or ophthalmological surgery; hemorrhagic stroke, history of gastrointestinal or intracranial bleeding, bleeding disorders, less severe thrombocytopenia, heparin-induced thrombocytopenia, diabetic retinopathy, elderly patients

Available forms
▸ *Injection:* 30 mg/0.3 mL; 40 mg/0.4 mL; 60 mg/0.6 mL; 80 mg/0.8 mL; 100 mg/1 mL

SC facts
Dosage
▸ *USA/NQWMI:* 1 mg/kg SC q12h with aspirin for at least 2 d or until patient is stable (usually 2–8 d).

Adverse effects in *Italics* are most common; those in **Bold** are life-threatening

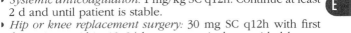
- *Systemic anticoagulation:* 1 mg/kg SC q12h. Continue at least 2 d and until patient is stable.
- *Hip or knee replacement surgery:* 30 mg SC q12h with first dose given within 12–24 h postoperatively provided hemostasis is established. Continue until risk of DVT has diminished or up to 14 d.
- *Abdominal surgery:* 40 mg SC qd with initial dose 2 h prior to surgery. Continue postoperatively up to 12 d.
- *DVT/PE:* 1 mg/kg SC q12h or 1.5 mg/kg SC qd.

TREATMENT OF OVERDOSE/ANTIDOTE
Discontinue drug or decrease dosage. Initiate general supportive and resuscitative measures. Drug's effect may be stopped by 1 mg protamine sulfate (1%) for q 1 mg of enoxaparin. Give protamine IV over 10 min. If the APTT remains prolonged 2–4 h after first infusion, may repeat protamine sulfate at half the first dose. Be aware that protamine sulfate may cause hypotension or anaphylaxis.

Pharmacokinetics

Route	Onset	Peak
SC	Rapid	3–5 h

$T_{1/2}$: 4.5 h
Excretion: Urine

Adverse effects
- *GI:* Nausea
- *Derm:* Pain, local irritation, hematoma, erythema, skin necrosis at site of injection
- *Allergic:* Chills, fever, urticaria, asthma, rash
- *Hematologic:* **Hemorrhage, thrombocytopenia, hypochromic anemia,** *bleeding, bruising,* hematoma at injection site; elevated AST, ALT levels
- *Misc:* Fever, neuraxial hematoma, confusion, peripheral edema

Clinically important drug–drug interactions
- Increased bleeding tendencies with oral anticoagulants, salicylates, NSAIDs, antiplatelet drugs

⬤ NURSING CONSIDERATIONS

Assessment
- *History:* Hypersensitivity to enoxaparin, heparin, or pork products; severe thrombocytopenia, uncontrolled bleeding, risk for bleeding, impaired renal or hepatic function, bacterial endocarditis, HTN; recent brain, spinal, or ophthalmological

Adverse effects in *Italics* are most common; those in **Bold** are life-threatening

surgery; hemorrhagic stroke, history of gastrointestinal or intracranial bleeding, bleeding disorders, heparin-induced thrombocytopenia, diabetic retinopathy, age

▸ *Physical:* T, P, R, BP, ECG, weight, skin assessment, peripheral perfusion, presence of bleeding, surgical incision assessment, injection site assessment, character of output from indwelling drains, Homan's sign, CPK, CPK-MB, cardiac troponin, myoglobin, APTT, CBC, renal function tests; urine, stool, and emesis guaiac

Implementation

▸ Give by deep SC injection; *do not* give by IM injection.
▸ Administer by deep SC injection while patient is lying down. Alternate between the left and right anterolateral and left and right posterolateral abdominal wall. Introduce whole length of needle into a skin fold held between the thumb and forefinger; hold skin fold throughout injection.
▸ Apply pressure to all injection sites after needle is withdrawn but do not massage site; inspect injection sites for signs of hematoma.
▸ Do not mix with other injections.
▸ Provide safety measures (electric razor, soft toothbrush) to prevent injury and minimize risk for bleeding.
▸ Assess patient for signs of bleeding.
▸ Routinely monitor CBC, UA, and stool guaiac during treatment. No monitoring of blood clotting times is needed as drug only slightly affects PT and APTT.
▸ LMW heparins cannot be used interchangeably with other LMW heparins or unfractionated heparin.
▸ Alert all health care providers that patient is on enoxaparin.
▸ Discontinue drug and initiate appropriate therapy if thromboembolic episode occurs despite enoxaparin therapy.
▸ Have protamine sulfate (enoxaparin antidote) on standby in case of overdose.
▸ Store at room temperature; fluid should be clear and colorless to pale yellow.

◉ **epinephrine** *(ep i nef' rin)* Sus-Phrine Ana-Guard

◉ **epinephrine hydrochloride**

Adrenalin Chloride, AsthmaNefrin, Epipen, microNefrin, Nephron, S-2

Pregnancy Category C

Drug classes
Sympathomimetic drug
Alpha-adrenergic agonist

Adverse effects in *Italics* are most common; those in **Bold** are life-threatening

β$_1$- and β$_2$-adrenergic agonist
Cardiac stimulant
Vasopressor
Bronchodilator

Indications

◗ Intravenous: Resuscitation in acute ventricular standstill; treatment and prophylaxis of cardiac arrest and attacks of transitory AV heart block with syncopal seizures (Adams-Stokes syndrome); treatment of syncope due to complete heart block or carotid sinus hypersensitivity; treatment of acute hypersensitivity (anaphylactoid) reactions; symptomatic relief of serum sickness, urticaria, angioneurotic edema; acute asthmatic attacks to relieve bronchospasm not controlled by inhalation or SC injection; resuscitation in cardiac arrest after anesthetic accidents; additive to local anesthetic solutions for injection to prolong their duration of action and limit systemic absorption
◗ Injection: Relief of respiratory distress of anaphylaxis, bronchial asthma, chronic bronchitis, emphysema, or other obstructive pulmonary diseases
◗ Nebulization: Temporary relief from acute paroxysms (shortness of breath, tightness of chest, wheezing) of bronchial asthma or postintubation; microNefrin: chronic obstructive pulmonary disease, chronic bronchitis, bronchiolitis, bronchial asthma, and other peripheral airway diseases

Therapeutic actions

◗ Naturally occurring neurotransmitter, the effects of which are mediated by alpha or beta receptors in target organs
◗ Beta-adrenergic drugs stimulate production of cAMP; cAMP inhibits release of mediators associated with hypersensitivity reactions and promotes relaxation by lowering intracellular calcium concentrations
◗ At usual doses, most prominent actions are on beta receptors of the heart and of vascular and other smooth muscle; β$_1$-adrenergic stimulation: increased myocardial contractility and conduction; β$_2$-adrenergic stimulation: bronchial dilation and vasodilation, enhancement of mucociliary clearance, inhibition of cholinergic neurotransmission
◗ At higher doses, alpha-adrenergic effects predominate (directly stimulates cardiac muscle, promotes nasal decongestion, increases ventricular muscle contraction, improves cerebral and coronary blood flow by preventing arterial collapse); produces peripheral circulatory vasoconstriction of arterioles in the skin, mucosa, and splanchnic areas
◗ Other adrenergic actions include contraction of GI and urinary sphincters, lipolysis, decreased GI tone, changes

in renin secretion, uterine relaxation, hepatic glycogenolysis/
gluconeogenesis, pancreatic beta cell secretion

Effects on hemodynamic parameters
▸ Increased or decreased SVR
▸ Increased systolic BP; decreased diastolic BP
▸ Increased HR
▸ Increased CO
▸ Increased PCWP
▸ Increased CVP
▸ Increased contractility

Contraindications/cautions
▸ **Contraindications:** allergy or hypersensitivity to epinephrine or components of preparation, narrow-angle glaucoma, nonanaphylactic shock, hypovolemia, organic brain damage, cerebral arteriosclerosis, tachydysrhythmias, cardiac dilation, coronary insufficiency, circulatory collapse or hypotension due to phenothiazines
▸ **Cautions:** elderly patients, cardiovascular disease, ischemic heart disease, hypertension, diabetes, hyperthyroidism, psychoneurotic individuals, bronchial asthma and emphysema with degenerative heart disease, thyrotoxicosis, Parkinson's disease, history of seizures, renal dysfunction

Available forms
▸ *Solution for injection:* 1:1000, 1:2000, 1:10,000, 1:100,000
▸ *Suspension for injection:* 1:200
▸ *Solution for inhalation:* 1:100, 1:1000, 1.125% base with racepinephrine

IV/IM/SC/endotracheal facts
Preparation
▸ To prepare a 1:10,000 solution, dilute 1 mL of a 1:1000 (1 mg/mL) solution in 9 mL of 0.9%NS for injection.
▸ For a continuous infusion, add 1 mg to 250 mL (4 mcg/mL) of D5W/LR; D5W; D10W; Dextrose-LR combinations; Dextrose-Ringer's combinations; Dextrose-Saline combinations; Fructose 10% in 0.9%NS or Water; Invert sugar 5% and 10% in 0.9%NS or Water; LR; 0.9%NS; Ringer's Injection; or Sodium lactate (1/6 Molar) Injection.

Dosage
▸ *Cardiac arrest (IV injection):* 1 mg (10 mL of 1:10,000 solution) IV q3–5min diluted to 10 mL with 0.9%NS. Consider intermediate dosing of 2 to 5 mg IV q3–5min; escalating doses of 1 mg–3 mg–5 mg IV 3 min apart, or high dosing of 0.1 mg/kg IV q3–5min.

Adverse effects in *Italics* are most common; those in **Bold** are life-threatening

- *Cardiac arrest (intracardial injection):* 0.1–1 mg (1–10 mL of 1:10,000 solution) intracardially (into left ventricle) q3–5min.
- *Cardiac arrest (endotracheal administration):* If IV access not available, perform five rapid insufflations, give 1 mg (diluted in 10 mL) directly into the tube, and follow with five quick insufflations.
- *Cardiac arrest/symptomatic bradycardia with profound hypotension (continuous infusion):* Add 30 mg epinephrine to 250 mL of D5W or 0.9%NS and run at 100 mL/h. Titrate to desired hemodynamic end point.
- *Shock/symptomatic bradycardia:* 2–10 mcg/min by continuous IV infusion.
- *Anaphylaxis:* 0.1–0.25 mg (1–2.5 mL of 1:10,000 solution) IV over 5–10 min. Repeat q5–15min as needed or begin an infusion of 1–4 mcg/min. May also give 0.1–1 mg (0.2–1 mL of 1:1000 solution) SC or IM; however, SC is preferred.
- *Respiratory distress:* 0.2–1 mg (0.2–1 mL of 1:1000 solution) SC or IM. Repeat q4h as needed.

Titration Guide

epinephrine hydrochloride				
1 mg in 250 mL				
mcg/min	1	2	3	4	5
mL/h	15	30	45	60	75

mcg/min	6	7	8	9	10
mL/h	90	105	120	135	150

Compatibility
Epinephrine may be given through the same IV line as amrinone, atracurium, calcium chloride, calcium gluconate, diltiazem, dobutamine, dopamine, famotidine, fentanyl, furosemide, heparin, hydrocortisone, hydromorphone, labetalol, lorazepam, midazolam, milrinone, morphine, nicardipine, nitroglycerin, norepinephrine, pancuronium, phytonadione, potassium chloride, propofol, vecuronium, vitamin B complex with C, warfarin.

Incompatibility
Do not administer through the same IV line as ampicillin or thiopental.

Nebulization dosage
- Add 0.5 mL of racemic epinephrine to 3 mL of diluent or 0.2–0.4 mL of microNefrin to 4.6–4.8 mL water. Administer for 15 min q3–4h.

Adverse effects in *Italics* are most common; those in **Bold** are life-threatening

TREATMENT OF OVERDOSE/ANTIDOTE

Discontinue drug or decrease dosage. Initiate general supportive and resuscitative measures. Rapidly acting vasodilators or alpha-blocking agents may counteract marked pressor effects and most toxic effects. Treat dysrhythmias with antidysrhythmics or beta-blockers. Treat overdose-induced pulmonary edema that interferes with respiration with an alpha-adrenergic blocker or intermittent positive pressure respiration. If patient is with prolonged hypotension, treat with another pressor, such as norepinephrine.

Pharmacokinetics

Route	Onset	Peak	Duration
IV	Immediate	20 min	20–30 min
SC	5–10 min	20 min	20–30 min
IM	5–10 min	20 min	20–30 min
Inhalation	3–5 min	20 min	1–3 h

Metabolism: Liver, nerve endings
Excretion: Urine

Adverse effects

- *CNS:* **Cerebral hemorrhage (from hypertension), subarachnoid hemorrhage,** *headache, dizziness, nervousness,* hemiplegia, anxiety, fear, restlessness, tremor, weakness, apprehensiveness, hallucinations, psychological disturbances, occlusion of central retinal artery
- *CV:* **Shock, aortic rupture, dysrhythmias,** hypertension, angina in patients with CAD, palpitations, tachycardia
- *Resp:* **Pulmonary edema,** respiratory difficulty
- *GI:* Nausea, vomiting
- *GU:* Constriction of renal blood vessels and oliguria with IV use, urinary retention and hesitancy
- *Derm:* Urticaria, wheal, and hemorrhage at injection site, necrosis with repeated injections at same site
- *Misc:* Flushing, hyperglycemia

Clinically important drug–drug interactions

- Antagonized vasoconstrictive and hypertensive effects with alpha-adrenergic blockers
- Excessive hypertension with propranolol, beta-blockers
- Enhanced pressor response with TCAs, furazolidone, methyldopa, MAO inhibitors, reserpine
- Hypotension with beta-adrenergic blockers
- Increased dysrhythmias with bretylium, cardiac glycosides, other sympathomimetic drugs

Adverse effects in *Italics* are most common; those in **Bold** are life-threatening

- Decreased vascular response with diuretics
- Decreased response to insulin, oral hypoglycemic drugs
- Reversed drug effects with ergot alkaloids, phenothiazines
- Severe hypertension with guanethidine, levothyroxine, antihistamines
- Decreased vasopressor effects with chlorpromazine, phenothiazines

◉ NURSING CONSIDERATIONS

Assessment
- *History:* Allergy or hypersensitivity to epinephrine or components of preparation, narrow-angle glaucoma, nonanaphylactic shock, hypovolemia, organic brain damage, cerebral arteriosclerosis, tachydysrhythmias, cardiac dilation, coronary insufficiency, circulatory collapse or hypotension due to phenothiazines, age, cardiovascular disease, ischemic heart disease, hypertension, diabetes, hyperthyroidism, psychoneurotic individuals, bronchial asthma and emphysema with degenerative heart disease, thyrotoxicosis, Parkinson's disease, seizures, renal dysfunction
- *Physical:* T, P, R, BP, CVP, SVR, PCWP, CO, SvO_2, SpO_2, ECG, I & O, IV site, weight, neurologic checks, skin assessment, intraocular pressure, respiratory effort, presence of retractions/accessory muscle use, adventitious lung sounds, peripheral pulses and perfusion, prostate palpation, UA, kidney function tests, serum and urine glucose, serum electrolytes, thyroid function tests, ABG

Implementation
- Use extreme caution when calculating and preparing doses. Epinephrine is a very potent drug; small errors in dosage can cause serious adverse effects.
- Always administer an infusion using an IV infusion pump.
- Assess vital signs and hemodynamic monitoring parameters frequently. Continuous arterial pressure monitoring is preferred.
- Administer into large veins of antecubital fossa rather than hand or ankle veins. Use a central line whenever possible.
- Monitor infusion site closely for evidence of infiltration or phlebitis. If extravasation occurs, prevent sloughing and necrosis by using a fine hypodermic needle to infiltrate area with 5–10 mg phentolamine in 10–15 mL 0.9% Sodium Chloride.
- Use the smallest effective dose.
- Correct hypovolemia before administering drug.
- Correct acid–base imbalances because acidosis lessens the response to vasopressors.

Adverse effects in *Italics* are most common; those in **Bold** are life-threatening

- Shake the suspension for injection well before withdrawing the dose. Suspension is for SC use only.
- Rotate SC injection sites to prevent necrosis; monitor injection sites frequently.
- Use minimal doses for minimal periods of time; "epinephrine-fastness" (a form of drug tolerance) can occur with prolonged use.
- Maintain a rapidly acting alpha-adrenergic blocker (phentolamine) or a vasodilator (a nitrite) on standby in case of excessive hypertensive reaction.
- Maintain an alpha-adrenergic blocker and equipment for intermittent positive pressure breathing or intubation on standby in case pulmonary edema occurs.
- Maintain antidysrhythmics and a beta-adrenergic blocker, such as propranolol, on standby in case cardiac dysrhythmias occur.
- Protect drug solutions from light, extreme heat, and freezing; do not use pink or brown solutions. Drug solutions should be clear and colorless.

⬤ epoetin alfa (e poe e' tin) erythropoietin, EPO
Epogen, Eprex (CAN), Procrit

Pregnancy Category C

Drug class
Recombinant human erythropoietin

Indications
- Treatment of anemia associated with chronic renal failure, including patients on dialysis and patients not on dialysis, to elevate or maintain the red blood cell level and to decrease the need for transfusions
- Treatment of anemia related to therapy with AZT in HIV-infected patients to elevate or maintain the red blood cell level and to decrease the need for transfusions
- Treatment of anemia related to chemotherapy in cancer patients to decrease the need for transfusions
- Treatment of anemic patients scheduled for elective, noncardiac, nonvascular surgery to reduce the need for allogeneic blood transfusions.
- Unlabeled use: pruritus associated with renal failure

Therapeutic actions
- A natural glycoprotein produced in the kidneys that stimu-

lates division and differentiation of erythroid progenitors in bone marrow

Contraindications/cautions
▶ **Contraindications:** uncontrolled hypertension; hypersensitivity to mammalian cell-derived products or to human albumin
▶ **Cautions:** hypertension, heart disease, CHF, porphyria

Available forms
▶ *Injection:* 2000; 3000; 4000; 10,000; 20,000 U/mL

IV/SC facts
Preparation
▶ Do not shake vial.
▶ For IV use, do not dilute drug; for SC use, may add bacteriostatic 0.9% Sodium Chloride Injection, USP, with benzyl alcohol 0.9% at a 1:1 ratio. The benzyl alcohol acts as a local anesthetic.
▶ The single-dose 1-mL vials contain no preservatives; use only once. When stored at 2° to 8°C, may use multidose vials for 21 d after initial entry.

Dosage
▶ *Chronic renal failure:* **Starting dose:** 50–100 U/kg IV or SC 3 times a week. Reduce dose if Hct approaches 36% or increases > 4 points in any 2-wk period. Increase dose if Hct does not increase by 5–6 points after 8 wk of therapy. **Maintenance dose:** Individualize based on Hct; range of 12.5–525 U/kg 3 times a wk for dialysis patients to 75–150 U/kg/wk for nondialysis patients. Target Hct range is 30%–36%.
▶ *Zidovudine-treated, HIV-infected patients:* Patients receiving zidovudine < 4200 mg/wk with serum erythropoietin levels ≤ 500 mU/mL: 100 U/kg IV or SC 3 times a wk for 8 wk. When desired response is achieved, titrate dose to maintain Hct with lowest possible dose.
▶ *Cancer patients on chemotherapy:* 150 U/kg SC 3 times a wk. After 8 wk, can be increased to 300 U/kg 3 times a wk.
▶ *Surgery:* Establish that Hgb is > 10 to ≤ 13 g/dL. 300 U/kg/d SC for 10 d before surgery, on the day of surgery, and for 4 d after surgery.

Compatibility
Do not give through an IV line containing other medications.

TREATMENT OF OVERDOSE/ANTIDOTE

Discontinue drug or decrease dosage. Initiate general supportive and resuscitative measures. If polycythemia is a concern, phlebotomy may be indicated to decrease hematocrit.

Pharmacokinetics

Route	Onset	Peak	Duration
SC	10 d	5–24 h serum levels; 2–6 wk for erythropoiesis	24 h (plasm erythropoietin levels)

$T_{1/2}$: 4–13 h
Excretion: Urine

Adverse effects

- **CNS: Seizures, CVA,** headache, fatigue
- **CV: MI,** *hypertension,* tachycardia, edema
- **Resp:** Shortness of breath
- **GI:** Nausea, vomiting, diarrhea
- **Misc:** Clotted vascular access, hyperkalemia, injection site stinging, flulike symptoms, rash

● NURSING CONSIDERATIONS

Assessment

- *History:* Uncontrolled hypertension; hypersensitivity to mammalian cell-derived products or to human albumin; hypertension, heart disease, CHF, porphyria
- *Physical:* P, R, BP, I & O, IV site, neurologic checks, skin assessment, respiratory effort, adventitious lung sounds, edema, renal function tests, CBC, iron levels, serum electrolytes

Implementation

- Confirm chronic, renal nature of anemia; not intended as a treatment for severe anemia or substitute for emergency transfusion.
- Monitor access lines for signs of clotting.
- Measure Hct reading before administration of each dose to determine dosage. If patient fails to respond within 8 wk of therapy, evaluate patient for other etiologies of the problem.
- Evaluate iron stores prior to and periodically during therapy. Supplemental iron may be ordered.
- Initiate seizure precautions.

● **eptifibatide** *(ep tiff ib' ah tide)* Integrilin
Pregnancy Category B

Adverse effects in *Italics* are most common; those in **Bold** are life-threatening

Drug class
Glycoprotein (GP) IIb/IIIa antagonist
Antiplatelet drug

Indications
▶ Treatment, in conjunction with heparin and aspirin, of acute coronary syndrome, including patients who are to be managed medically or those undergoing PCI

Therapeutic actions
▶ Reversibly inhibits platelet aggregation by preventing binding of fibrinogen, von Willebrand factor, and other adhesive ligands to GP IIb/IIIa

Contraindications/cautions
▶ **Contraindications:** eptifibatide allergy; recent (within 30 d) active internal bleeding, bleeding diathesis, or stroke; any hemorrhagic stroke; intracranial hemorrhage, neoplasm, arteriovenous malformation, or aneurysm; major surgery within previous 6 wk; severe uncontrolled HTN (SBP > 200 mmHg or DBP > 110 mmHg); use of another parenteral GP IIb/IIIa inhibitor; dependency on renal dialysis; platelet count < 100,000/mm³; serum creatinine ≥ 2.0 mg/dL (for 180 mcg/kg bolus and 2 mcg/kg/min infusion) or ≥ 4.0 mg/dL (for the 135 mcg/kg bolus and the 0.5 mcg/kg/min infusion)
▶ **Cautions:** elderly patients, concurrent anticoagulant therapy

Available forms
▶ *Injection:* 2 mg/mL
▶ *Premixed IV infusion:* 0.75 mg/mL

IV facts
Preparation
▶ Withdraw bolus dose from the 10-mL vial.
▶ Spike infusion vial with a vented infusion set using caution to center the spike within the circle of stopper top.

Dosage
▶ *Acute coronary syndrome:* **Bolus:** 180 mcg/kg IV over 1–2 min as soon as possible after diagnosis. **Maintenance infusion:** 2 mcg/kg/min IV until discharge, initiation of CABG surgery, or 72 h. Consider reducing dose to 0.5 mcg/kg/min at beginning of a PCI. Continue infusion for additional 20–24 h after PCI, allowing for up to 96 hours of therapy. Maximum bolus is 22.6 mg; maximum infusion rate is 15 mg/h.

Adverse effects in *Italics* are most common; those in **Bold** are life-threatening

▸ *PCI in patients not presenting with acute coronary syndrome:* **Bolus:** 135 mcg/kg IV over 1–2 min immediately before starting PCI. **Maintenance infusion:** 0.5 mcg/kg/min IV for 20–24 h.

Titration Guide

eptifibatide									
75 mg in 100 mL									
Body Weight									
lb	88	99	110	121	132	143	154	165	176	187
kg	40	45	50	55	60	65	70	75	80	85

Dose ordered in mcg/kg/min	Amounts to Infuse in mL/h									
0.5	2	2	2	2	2	3	3	3	3	3
2	6	7	8	9	10	10	11	12	13	14

Body Weight									
lb	198	209	220	231	242	253	264	275	286
kg	90	95	100	105	110	115	120	125	130

Dose ordered in mcg/kg/min	Amounts to Infuse in mL/h								
0.5	4	4	4	4	4	5	5	5	5
2	14	15	16	17	18	18	19	20	21

Compatibility
Eptifibatide may be given through the same IV line as alteplase, atropine, dobutamine, heparin, lidocaine, meperidine, metoprolol, midazolam, morphine, nitroglycerin, potassium chloride, verapamil.

Incompatibility
Do not administer through the same IV line as furosemide.

TREATMENT OF OVERDOSE/ANTIDOTE
Discontinue drug or decrease dosage. Initiate general and supportive measures. In vitro analysis has shown that dialysis may remove eptifibatide.

Adverse effects in *Italics* are most common; those in **Bold** are life-threatening

E

Pharmacokinetics

Route	Onset	Duration
IV	Immediate	4 h after infusion stopped

$T_{1/2}$: 2.5 h
Excretion: Urine

Adverse effects

- *CNS:* **Hemorrhagic stroke**
- *CV:* *Hypotension*
- *GI:* **GI bleeding**
- *GU:* **GU bleeding**
- *Allergic:* **Anaphylaxis**
- *Hematologic: Bleeding* **(retroperitoneal, venous and arterial access sites), thrombocytopenia**

Clinically important drug–drug interactions

- Increased bleeding with anticoagulant, thrombolytic, antithrombotic, aspirin, NSAIDs, other antiplatelet drugs

○ NURSING CONSIDERATIONS

Assessment

- *History:* Eptifibatide allergy, recent active internal bleeding, bleeding diathesis, stroke, intracranial hemorrhage, neoplasm, arteriovenous malformation, aneurysm, major surgery within previous 6 wk, severe uncontrolled HTN, use of another parenteral GP IIb/IIIa inhibitor, dependency on renal dialysis, age
- *Physical:* P, BP, R, ECG, I & O, IV site, weight, neurologic checks, skin assessment, arterial and venous access sites, chest pain assessment, peripheral perfusion, pain assessment, bowel sounds, presence of bleeding, CBC, CPK, CPK-MB, cardiac troponin, myoglobin, renal function tests, PT, PTT, ACT; urine, stool, and emesis guaiac

Implementation

- Administer infusion through an IV pump.
- Frequently assess potential bleeding sites, paying careful attention to arterial and venous puncture sites and femoral access site.
- While the arterial and/or venous sheath is in place, maintain patient on bed rest with head of the bed < 30 degrees. Keep affected extremity flat and straight.
- Adhere to strict anticoagulation guidelines per hospital protocol. Administer and adjust weight-adjusted heparin as ordered.

Adverse effects in *Italics* are most common; those in **Bold** are life-threatening

Discontinue heparin 2–4 h before sheath removal or according to hospital protocol.

▸ Remove sheaths when APTT is ≤ 45–50 s or the ACT is ≤ 175 to 180 s.

▸ Apply pressure to access site for at least 30 min after sheath removal.

▸ Following initial hemostasis, continue bed rest for 6–8 h or according to hospital policy. Apply a pressure dressing to site.

▸ If bleeding recurs, reapply manual or mechanical compression until hemostasis is achieved.

▸ Mark and measure the size of any hematoma, and monitor for evidence of enlargement.

▸ After achieving hemostasis, monitor the patient in hospital for at least 4 h.

▸ Assess for neurovascular compromise in affected leg. Palpate distal pulses and note extremity's color and warmth. Assess for pain, numbness, tingling of affected leg.

▸ Minimize arterial and venous punctures.

▸ If possible, draw blood from a saline lock.

▸ Do not insert intravenous access devices into noncompressible sites, such as the subclavian and jugular veins.

▸ Avoid intramuscular injections, urinary catheter insertion, and nasotracheal and nasogastric intubation whenever possible.

▸ Continue aspirin therapy.

▸ Discontinue antiplatelet drug infusions and determine a bleeding time before surgery if the patient requires CABG or other surgery.

▸ Check stools, urine, emesis for occult blood.

▸ Monitor the patient's WBC, Hgb, Hct, APTT, ACT, platelet, and creatinine values; notify provider of abnormal values. Be prepared to transfuse platelets if platelet count is < 50,000 cells/mcL.

▸ Have emergency equipment (defibrillator, drugs, oxygen, intubation equipment) on standby in case anaphylaxis or adverse reaction occurs.

▸ Monitor for evidence of adverse or allergic reactions to the drug. If a reaction is suspected, discontinue the drug and initiate resuscitative interventions.

▸ Medicate patient for back or groin pain.

▸ Use a manual blood pressure cuff or ensure that an automatic blood pressure cuff does not apply excessive pressure to the patient's arm.

▸ Shave patients using an electric razor.

▸ Protect drug from light until administration.

Adverse effects in *Italics* are most common; those in **Bold** are life-threatening

▸ Refrigerate vials.
▸ Discard any unused drug left in vial.

⬤ esmolol hydrochloride *(ess' moe lol)* Brevibloc
Pregnancy Category C

Drug class
Beta-adrenergic blocker (β_1 selective)

Indications
▸ Supraventricular tachycardia when rapid but short-term control of ventricular rate is desirable (atrial fibrillation, flutter, perioperative, postoperative, or emergent situations)
▸ Noncompensatory tachycardia when heart rate requires specific intervention

Therapeutic actions
▸ Blocks beta-adrenergic receptors in the heart and juxtaglomerular apparatus, reducing the influence of the sympathetic nervous system on these tissues
▸ Decreases excitability of heart
▸ Decreases release of renin
▸ At low doses, acts relatively selectively at the β_1-adrenergic receptors of the heart
▸ Inhibits β_2 receptors at higher doses

Effects on hemodynamic parameters
▸ Decreased CO
▸ Decreased BP
▸ Decreased HR
▸ Decreased myocardial oxygen consumption
▸ Decreased LVEDP
▸ Decreased PAP
▸ Increased PCWP at high doses

Contraindications/cautions
▸ **Contraindications:** sinus bradycardia, second- or third-degree heart block, cardiogenic shock, overt heart failure
▸ **Cautions:** hypotension, hypertension associated with hypothermia, bronchospastic disease, diabetes, impaired renal function; treatment of SVT when using vasoconstrictor drugs, such as dopamine, epinephrine, norepinephrine

Available forms
▸ *Injection:* 10 mg/mL, 250 mg/mL

Adverse effects in *Italics* are most common; those in **Bold** are life-threatening

IV facts
Preparation
▶ Draw up bolus dose with syringe from 100-mg vial that contains ready-to-use 10 mg/mL concentration.
▶ Add 2.5 g to 250 mL of D5W; D5W/KCl (40 mEq/L); D5W/LR; D5W/0.45%NS; D5W/0.9%NS; LR; 0.45%NS; 0.9%NS; or Sodium Bicarbonate 5%.
▶ Once diluted, solution is stable for 24 h.

Dosage and titration
▶ Administer loading dose of 500 mcg/kg/min IV over 1 min.
▶ Follow loading dose with infusion of 50 mcg/kg/min IV for 4 min.
▶ If desired effect not observed after 5 min, repeat the loading dose and increase the infusion rate to 100 mcg/kg/min.
▶ Continue titration procedure as above every 5 min—repeat loading dose and increase infusion rate by 50 mcg/kg/min. Infusion rates above 200 mcg/kg/min are not recommended.
▶ When near desired HR or BP, omit subsequent loading doses, titrate infusion up or down as indicated, and wait 5–10 min between titration intervals.
▶ Use caution if abrupt cessation of drug is indicated due to adverse reactions or site infiltration.

Titration Guide

esmolol hydrochloride									
Mix 2.5 g in 250 mL									
Body Weight									
lb	88	99	110	121	132	143	154	165	176	187
kg	40	45	50	55	60	65	70	75	80	85
Dose ordered in mcg/kg/min	Amounts to Infuse in mL/h								
25	6	7	8	8	9	10	11	11	12	13
50	12	14	15	17	18	20	21	23	24	26
75	18	20	23	25	27	29	32	34	36	38
100	24	27	30	33	36	39	42	45	48	51
125	30	34	38	41	45	49	53	56	60	64
150	36	41	45	50	54	59	63	68	72	77
175	42	47	53	58	63	68	74	79	84	89
200	48	54	60	66	72	78	84	90	96	102

	Body Weight								
lb	198	209	220	231	242	253	264	275	286
kg	90	95	100	105	110	115	120	125	130
Dose ordered in mcg/kg/min	Amounts to Infuse in mL/h								
25	14	14	15	16	17	17	18	19	20
50	27	29	30	32	33	35	36	38	39
75	41	43	45	47	50	52	54	56	59
100	54	57	60	63	66	69	72	75	78
125	68	71	75	79	83	86	90	94	98
150	81	86	90	95	99	104	108	113	117
175	95	100	105	110	116	121	126	131	137
200	108	114	120	126	132	138	144	150	156

Compatibility

Esmolol may be given through the same IV line as amikacin, aminophylline, amiodarone, ampicillin, atracurium, butorphanol, calcium chloride, cefazolin, cefmetazole, cefoperazone, ceftazidime, ceftizoxime, chloramphenicol, cimetidine, clindamycin, diltiazem, dopamine, enalaprilat, erythromycin, famotidine, fentanyl, gentamicin, heparin, hydrocortisone, insulin (regular), labetalol, magnesium sulfate, methyldopate, metronidazole, midazolam, morphine, nafcillin, nitroglycerin, nitroprusside sodium, norepinephrine, pancuronium, penicillin G potassium, phenytoin, piperacillin, polymyxin B, potassium chloride, potassium phosphates, propofol, ranitidine, sodium acetate, sodium bicarbonate, streptomycin, tacrolimus, trimethoprim-sulfamethoxazole, tobramycin, vancomycin, vecuronium.

Incompatibility

Do not administer through the same IV line as furosemide or warfarin.

TREATMENT OF OVERDOSE/ANTIDOTE

Discontinue infusion or decrease dosage. Initiate general supportive and resuscitative measures. Treat bradycardia with atropine; bronchospasm with an IV beta$_2$-stimulating drug and/or theophylline derivative; hypotension with fluids or pressors; cardiac failure with diuretics, a digitalis glycoside, dopamine, dobutamine, isoproterenol, or amrinone.

Adverse effects in *Italics* are most common; those in **Bold** are life-threatening

Pharmacokinetics

Route	Onset	Peak	Duration
IV	< 5 min	10–20 min	10–30 min

Metabolism: RBC esterases; $T_{1/2}$: 9 min
Excretion: Urine

Adverse effects

▸ **CNS:** **Seizures,** *lightheadedness, dizziness, headache, agitation, weakness, somnolence,* confusion
▸ **CV:** *Hypotension, peripheral ischemia,* bradycardia, pallor, chest pain, syncope, pulmonary edema, heart block
▸ **Resp:** **Bronchospasm,** wheezing, dyspnea, nasal congestion, crackles
▸ **GI:** *Nausea,* vomiting, dyspepsia, constipation, dry mouth, abdominal discomfort
▸ **Derm:** *Inflammation, induration,* edema, erythema, skin discoloration, burning, skin necrosis from extravasation at infusion site
▸ **Misc:** Speech disorder, midscapular pain, fever, rigors, abnormal vision, urinary retention, diaphoresis

Clinically important drug–drug interactions

▸ Increased therapeutic and toxic effects with verapamil
▸ Impaired antihypertensive effects with ibuprofen, indomethacin, piroxicam
▸ Hypotension or bradycardia with catecholamine-depleting drugs
▸ Increased digoxin levels
▸ Avoid concurrent use of dopamine, epinephrine, and norepinephrine; may block cardiac contractility when SVR is high
▸ Increased blood levels when given with IV morphine

◉ NURSING CONSIDERATIONS

Assessment

▸ *History:* Cardiogenic shock, overt heart failure, hypotension, hypertension, hypothermia, bronchospastic disease, diabetes, impaired renal function, use of vasoconstrictor drugs
▸ *Physical:* P, BP, R, I & O, ECG, IV site, weight, neurologic checks, adventitious lung sounds, abdominal assessment, serum electrolytes, serum glucose, renal function tests

Implementation

▸ Exercise extreme caution when calculating and preparing IV doses. Always dilute drug before use; avoid inadvertent bolus of drug.
▸ Always administer using an IV infusion pump.

Adverse effects in *Italics* are most common; those in **Bold** are life-threatening

- Administer into large veins. Avoid concentrations greater than 10 mg/mL. Use a central line whenever possible.
- Monitor the infusion site closely for evidence of infiltration or phlebitis.
- Continuously monitor blood pressure and ECG.
- Assist patient with changing positions to minimize postural hypotension.
- After HR is controlled and patient is stable, transition to oral antidysrhythmics, such as propranolol, digoxin, or verapamil. Reduce esmolol infusion rate by 50% 30 min after giving oral drug. Discontinue esmolol 1 h after the second dose of the oral drug.

⬤ **ethacrynic acid** *(eth a krin' ik)* Edecrin

⬤ **ethacrynic sodium** Edecrin Sodium
Pregnancy Category B

Drug class
Loop (high ceiling) diuretic

Indications
- Treatment of edema associated with CHF, cirrhosis, renal disease
- Adjunctive therapy for acute pulmonary edema (parenteral)
- Ascites due to malignancy, idiopathic edema, lymphedema
- Unlabeled use: treatment of glaucoma

Therapeutic actions
- Inhibits the reabsorption of sodium and chloride from the proximal and distal renal tubules and the loop of Henle, leading to a sodium-rich diuresis
- Is effective in many patients with significant degrees of renal insufficiency

Contraindications/cautions
- **Contraindications:** ethacrynic acid allergy, electrolyte imbalance, anuria, severe hepatic coma, increasing azotemia or oliguria
- **Cautions:** hypoproteinemia, hepatic impairment, metabolic alkalosis, HTN, SLE, gout, cardiovascular disease, diabetes, elderly and debilitated patients

Available forms
- *Powder for injection:* 50 mg/vial
- *Tablets:* 25, 50 mg

Adverse effects in *Italics* are most common; those in **Bold** are life-threatening

IV facts
Preparation
▶ Add 50 mL of D5W or 0.9%NS to vial. Do not use hazy or opalescent solutions.

Dosage
▶ *Usual dose:* 50 mg or 0.5 to 1 mg/kg IV. Do not exceed 100 mg. Give through the tubing of a running infusion or by direct IV injection over several minutes. May give IV infusion over 20–30 min. Usually, only one dose is needed. If a second dose is needed, give through a new injection site to avoid thrombophlebitis.

Compatibility
Ethacrynic acid may be given through the same IV line as heparin sodium with hydrocortisone, potassium chloride, vitamin B complex with C.

Incompatibility
Do not administer through the same IV line as solutions or drugs with a final pH < 5, whole blood or its derivatives.

Oral dosage
▶ *Initial therapy:* 50–200 mg PO daily to produce gradual weight loss of 2.2–4.4 kg/d. Adjust dose in 25- to 50-mg increments. Higher doses, up to 200 mg bid, may be required for severe, refractory edema.
▶ *Maintenance therapy:* Give intermittently using an alternate daily schedule or more prolonged periods of diuretic therapy interspersed with rest periods.
▶ *Concomitant diuretic therapy:* 25 mg PO initially. Change dose in 25-mg increments as needed.

TREATMENT OF OVERDOSE/ANTIDOTE
Discontinue drug or decrease dosage. Initiate general supportive and resuscitative measures. Induce emesis and perform gastric lavage for oral overdose. Correct dehydration, electrolyte imbalance, hepatic coma, and hypotension.

Pharmacokinetics

Route	Onset	Peak	Duration
IV	Within 5 min	15–30 min	2 h
Oral	Within 30 min	2 h	6–8 h

Metabolism: Hepatic; $T_{1/2}$: 1 h
Excretion: Urine, bile

Adverse effects in *Italics* are most common; those in **Bold** are life-threatening

Adverse effects

▶ **CNS:** Headache, fatigue, apprehension, confusion, tinnitus, vertigo, deafness, blurred vision
▶ **CV:** *Hypotension, orthostatic hypotension,* volume depletion, dysrhythmias, thrombophlebitis
▶ **GI:** **Acute pancreatitis, GI bleed,** *nausea, anorexia, vomiting, dysphagia;* sudden, profuse watery diarrhea; jaundice, thirst
▶ **GU:** *Frequency,* hematuria
▶ **Derm:** Local irritation and pain with IV use, skin rash
▶ **Hematologic:** **Neutropenia, thrombocytopenia, agranulocytosis**
▶ **Metabolic:** Hypovolemia, hyperuricemia, metabolic alkalosis, hypokalemia, hyponatremia, hypochloremia, hypocalcemia, hyperglycemia, increased serum creatinine
▶ **Misc:** Fever, muscle cramps

Clinically important drug–drug interactions

▶ Increased cardiac glycoside (digitalis) toxicity (secondary to hypokalemia)
▶ Increased ototoxicity with aminoglycoside and some cephalosporin antibiotics
▶ Enhanced anticoagulant effects of warfarin
▶ Reduced diuretic, natriuretic, and antihypertensive effects with nonsteroidal anti-inflammatory agents
▶ Profound diuresis and electrolyte abnormalities with thiazide diuretics
▶ Increased lithium toxicity

◉ NURSING CONSIDERATIONS

Assessment

▶ *History:* Ethacrynic acid allergy, electrolyte imbalance, anuria, severe hepatic coma, increasing azotemia or oliguria, hypoproteinemia, hepatic impairment, metabolic alkalosis, HTN, SLE, gout, cardiovascular disease, diabetes, age, debilitation
▶ *Physical:* T, P, R, BP, ECG, I & O, IV site, weight, neurologic checks, eighth cranial nerve function, skin assessment, hearing, orthostatic BP, hydration status, skin turgor, adventitious lung sounds, peripheral edema, liver evaluation, abdominal assessment, presence of ascites, bowel sounds, CBC, serum electrolytes (including calcium, magnesium), serum glucose, liver and renal function tests, uric acid level, UA, ABG

Implementation

▶ Give IV infusion using an IV pump.
▶ Minimize postural hypotension by helping the patient change positions slowly.

Adverse effects in *Italics* are most common; those in **Bold** are life-threatening

- Rapid and aggressive diuresis may result in hemoconcentration and lead to thromboembolism.
- Administer oral doses with food or milk to prevent GI upset.
- Administer early in the day so that increased urination does not disturb sleep.
- Measure and record daily weights to monitor fluid changes.
- Monitor serum electrolytes, hydration, liver function.
- Provide potassium-rich diet or supplemental potassium.
- Discard unused IV solution after 24 h.

F

● Factor IX concentrates *(fac' tor nine)*

● Factor IX complex (human)

● coagulation Factor IX (human)
AlphaNine SD, Benefix, Hemonyne, Immunine VH (CAN), Konyne 80, Mononine, Profilnine SD, Proplex T

Pregnancy Category C

Drug class
Antihemophilic agent

Indications
- Treatment of Factor IX deficiency (hemophilia B, Christmas disease) to prevent or control bleeding
- Treatment of bleeding episodes in patients with hemophilia A who have inhibitors to Factor VIII (Proplex T, Konyne 80 only)
- Reversal of coumarin anticoagulant-induced hemorrhage when prompt reversal is required (Konyne 80)
- Prevention or control of bleeding episodes in patients with Factor VII deficiency (Proplex T only)

Therapeutic actions
- Raises plasma level of Factor IX to prevent or minimize hazards of hemorrhage
- Activated Factor IX, in combination with activated Factor VIII, activates Factor X; results in conversion of prothrombin to thrombin and formation of a fibrin clot
- Increases blood levels of Factors II, VII, IX, X
- Human Factor IX complex consists of plasma fractions involved in the intrinsic pathway of blood coagulation; causes an increase in blood levels of clotting Factors II, VII, IX, and X

Adverse effects in *Italics* are most common; those in **Bold** are life-threatening

F

Contraindications/cautions
▸ **Contraindications:** mouse protein (mononine) allergy, Factor VII deficiencies (except as listed above for Proplex T, Konye 80), heparin allergy (for products containing heparin), liver disease with evidence of intravascular coagulation or fibrinolysis
▸ **Cautions:** liver disease, postoperative patients

Available forms
▸ *Injection:* varies with brand, see label

IV facts
Preparation
▸ Warm product to room temperature before reconstituting.
▸ Prepare using diluent and needles supplied with product.
▸ Factor IX complex: Reconstitute *only* with Sterile Water for Injection. Warm unopened diluent and concentrate to room temperature. Insert transfer-needle cartridge into diluent bottle's stopper. Invert diluent bottle and penetrate rubber seal on concentrate bottle. Hold diluent bottle to direct diluent against wall of concentrate bottle; vacuum will draw diluent into concentrate bottle. Swirl continuously until dissolved. Withdraw dose using supplied filter needle; replace filter needle with injection needle. Use within 3 h of reconstitution. Do not refrigerate after reconstitution.
▸ Coagulation Factor IX: Insert one end of double-end needle into diluent vial. Invert diluent vial and insert other end of needle into drug vial. Direct diluent over entire surface of drug cake. Rotate vial to ensure complete wetting of cake. Remove diluent vial to release the vacuum; then remove double-end needle from the drug vial. Gently swirl vial until powder is dissolved. Use within 3 h of reconstitution. Use plastic disposable syringes to administer drug. Attach the supplied vented filter to a syringe; *do not inject air into the drug vial.* Insert vented filter spike into vial. Invert vial, and position filter spike so that orifice is at inside edge of stopper. Withdraw solution into syringe. Discard filter spike.

Dosage
▸ Dosage depends on severity of deficiency and severity of bleeding; follow treatment carefully with Factor IX level assays. To calculate dosage, use the following formulae: **Recombinant Factor IX:** 1.2 IU/kg × body weight (kg) × desired increase (% of normal). **Human-derived Factor IX:**

1 IU/kg × body weight (kg) × desired increase (% of normal). Administer qd to bid (once every 2–3 d may suffice to maintain lower effective levels) IV.

▸ Generally, one unit of human-derived Factor IX activity/kg will increase circulating Factor IX by 1% of normal; one IU of recombinant Factor IX/kg of body weight will increase circulatory Factor IX by 0.8 IU/dL.

▸ Rate of administration varies with product. Infuse slowly IV; 100–200 IU/min IV or 2–3 mL/min IV is suggested. If headache, flushing, or pulse or BP changes occur, stop infusion until symptoms subside; then resume at slower rate.

▸ *Preparation for and after surgery:* Maintain levels > 25% for at least 1 wk. Calculate each dose to raise levels to 40% to 60% of normal. Repeat dosage as needed.

▸ *Major trauma or surgery:* Amount needed to achieve 25%–50% of desired Factor IX or up to 75 U/kg. Repeat q18–30h as needed.

▸ *Minor spontaneous hemorrhage:* Amount needed to achieve 10% to 15% of desired Factor IX.

▸ *Maintenance dose:* Dose is usually 10–20 IU/kg/d IV. Individualize dose based on patient response.

▸ *Factor VII deficiency (Proplex T only):* Units required to raise blood level percentages: 0.5 U/kg × body weight (kg) × desired increase (% of normal). Repeat q4–6h as needed.

▸ *Reversal of coumarin effect:* 15 U/kg IV.

▸ *Treatment of bleeding episode for hemophilia A with inhibitors to Factor VIII:* 75 IU/kg IV. Give a second dose after 12 h if needed.

Compatibility

Do not admix or administer through the same IV line as other drugs.

TREATMENT OF OVERDOSE/ANTIDOTE
Decrease drug or discontinue dosage. Initiate general supportive and resuscitative measures.

Pharmacokinetics

Route	Onset	Duration
IV	Immediate	1–2 d

Metabolism: Plasma; $T_{1/2}$: 24–32 h

Adverse effects

▸ *CNS: Headache,* tingling, somnolence, lethargy
▸ *CV:* **AMI,** pulse and blood pressure changes

Adverse effects in *Italics* are most common; those in **Bold** are life-threatening

F

▶ *Resp:* **Pulmonary embolism, bronchospasm**
▶ *GI:* **Transmission of hepatitis,** *nausea,* vomiting
▶ *Derm:* Urticaria, hives, or stinging at injection site
▶ *Allergic:* **Anaphylaxis,** flushing, chills, fever
▶ *Hematologic: Thrombosis,* **DIC, transmission of HIV**

● NURSING CONSIDERATIONS

Assessment

▶ *History:* Mouse protein (mononine) allergy, Factor VII deficiencies, heparin allergy, liver disease with evidence of intravascular coagulation or fibrinolysis, liver disease, recent surgery
▶ *Physical:* T, P, BP, R, ECG, I & O, IV site, presence of bleeding, skin color, lesions, neurologic checks, peripheral perfusion, coagulation studies, clotting factor levels, liver function tests

Implementation

▶ Administer by IV route only.
▶ Have emergency equipment (defibrillator, drugs, oxygen, intubation equipment) on standby in case anaphylaxis or adverse reaction occurs.
▶ Generally a Factor IX level of 25%–50% is considered adequate for hemostasis, including major hemorrhages and surgery.
▶ Drug may transmit hepatitis or HIV; before administration, consider if this risk is justifiable.
▶ Monitor patient's clinical response and Factors IX, II, VII, and X levels regularly, and regulate dosage based on response.
▶ Monitor patient for any sign of thrombosis; use comfort and preventive measures when possible (exercise, support stockings, ambulation, positioning).

● **famotidine** *(fa moe' ti deen)* Pepcid, Pepcid AC, Pepcid AC Acid Controller, Pepcid RPD

Pregnancy Category B

Drug class

Histamine 2 (H_2) blocker

Indications

▶ Short-term treatment of active duodenal ulcer
▶ Maintenance therapy for duodenal ulcer patients at reduced dosage after healing of an active ulcer
▶ Short-term treatment of active benign gastric ulcer, GERD, and esophagitis due to GERD
▶ Treatment of pathological hypersecretory conditions (Zollinger-Ellison syndrome, multiple endocrine adenomas)

Adverse effects in *Italics* are most common; those in **Bold** are life-threatening

Therapeutic actions

‣ Competitively blocks action of histamine at the histamine receptors of the parietal cells of the stomach; inhibits basal gastric acid secretion and chemically induced gastric acid secretion

Contraindications/cautions

‣ **Contraindication:** famotidine allergy
‣ **Caution:** severe renal insufficiency

Available forms

‣ *Injection:* 10 mg/mL
‣ *Premixed IV infusion:* 20 mg/50 mL
‣ *Tablets:* 10, 20, 40 mg
‣ *Powder for oral suspension:* 40 mg/5 mL
‣ *Chewable tablets:* 10 mg
‣ *Orally disintegrating tablets:* 20, 40 mg

IV facts
Preparation

‣ *Direct IV injection:* Dilute 20 mg in D5W; D10W; LR; 0.9%NS; or Sterile Water for Injection to a total volume of 5–10 mL.
‣ *Intermittent IV infusion:* Use premixed solution or dilute 20 mg in 100 mL of a compatible IV solution (see above).

Dosage and titration

‣ *Pathological hypersecretory conditions, intractable ulcers, patients unable to take PO medications:* **Direct IV:** 20 mg IV over 2 min. **Intermittent infusion:** 20 mg IV over 15–30 min.
‣ *Patients with severe renal insufficiency:* Reduce dosage to 20 mg q hs or prolong dosing interval to 36–48 h as indicated by patient's clinical response.

Compatibility

Famotidine may be given through the same IV line as acyclovir, allopurinol, amifostine, aminophylline, amphotericin B, ampicillin, ampicillin-sulbactam, amrinone, amsacrine, atropine, aztreonam, bretylium, calcium gluconate, cefazolin, cefoperazone, cefotaxime, cefotetan, cefoxitin, ceftazidime, ceftizoxime, ceftriaxone, cefuroxime, cephalothin, cephapirin, chlorpromazine, cisplatin, cladribine, cyclophosphamide, cytarabine, dexamethasone, dextran 40, digoxin, diphenhydramine, dobutamine, dopamine, doxorubicin, droperidol, enalaprilat, epinephrine, erythromycin, esmolol, filgrastim, fluconazole, fludarabine, folic acid, furosemide, gentamicin, granisetron, haloperidol, heparin, hydrocortisone, hydromorphone, hydroxyzine, imipenem-cilastatin, insulin (regular), isoproterenol, labetalol, lidocaine, lorazepam, magnesium sulfate, melphalan, meperidine, methotrexate, methylprednisolone, metoclopramide, mezlocillin, midazolam, morphine, nafcillin, nitroglycerin, nitroprusside sodium, norepinephrine, ondansetron, oxacillin, paclitaxel, perphenazine, phenylephrine, phenytoin, phytonadione, piperacillin, potassium chloride, potassium phosphates, procainamide, propofol, sargramostim, sodium bicarbonate, teniposide, theophylline, thiamine, thiotepa, ticarcillin, ticarcillin-clavulanate, verapamil, vinorelbine.

Incompatibility
Do not administer through the same IV line as cefepime or piperacillin-tazobactam.

Oral dosage
▶ *Acute duodenal ulcer:* 40 mg PO q hs or 20 mg PO bid. Full dosage therapy generally is discontinued after 6–8 wk.
▶ *Maintenance therapy, duodenal ulcer:* 20 mg PO q hs.
▶ *Acute benign gastric ulcer:* 40 mg PO q hs.
▶ *GERD:* 20 mg PO bid for up to 6 wk.
▶ *Hypersecretory syndrome:* Initially, 20 mg PO q6h. Doses up to 160 mg PO q6h have been given.
▶ *Esophagitis:* 20–40 mg PO bid for up to 12 wk.
▶ *Patients with severe renal insufficiency:* Reduce dosage to 20 mg q hs or prolong dosing interval to 36–48 h as indicated by patient's clinical response.
▶ *Heartburn, acid indigestion, and sour stomach:* **Relief:** 10 mg PO with water. **Prevention:** 10 mg PO 1 h before eating a meal that is expected to cause symptoms. Can be used up to bid (up to 2 tablets in 24 h).

TREATMENT OF OVERDOSE/ANTIDOTE
Discontinue drug or decrease dosage. Initiate general supportive and resuscitative measures.

Pharmacokinetics

Route	Onset	Peak	Duration
IV	Within 30 min	0.5–3 h	10–12 h
Oral	Within 60 min	1–3 h	10–12 h

Metabolism: Hepatic; $T_{1/2}$: 2.5–3.5 h
Excretion: Urine

Adverse effects
▶ *CNS:* **Seizures,** *headache, dizziness,* malaise, somnolence, insomnia, confusion, hallucinations, depression, anxiety
▶ *CV:* Dysrhythmias, AV block, palpitations
▶ *Resp:* **Bronchospasm**
▶ *GI:* *Constipation, diarrhea,* anorexia, abdominal pain, jaundice, taste disorder, dry mouth, abnormal liver enzymes

Adverse effects in *Italics* are most common; those in **Bold** are life-threatening

- **Derm:** Dry skin, flushing, acne, pruritus, alopecia
- **Allergic:** **Anaphylaxis, angioedema,** rash, urticaria, conjunctival injection
- **Hematologic:** Thrombocytopenia, leukopenia
- **Musc/Skel:** Muscle cramps/pain, arthralgia
- **Misc:** Fever, decreased libido, tinnitus, fatigue

⬤ NURSING CONSIDERATIONS

Assessment
- *History:* Famotidine allergy, renal insufficiency
- *Physical:* T, P, R, BP, I & O, ECG, neurologic checks, skin assessment, adventitious lung sounds, liver evaluation, abdominal exam, pain assessment, liver and renal function tests, CBC, stool and emesis guaiac

Implementation
- May administer concurrent antacid therapy to relieve pain.
- Have emergency equipment (defibrillator, drugs, oxygen, intubation equipment) on standby in case anaphylaxis or adverse reaction occurs.
- Assess for abdominal pain and for blood in stool or emesis.
- If IV preparation is not used immediately, store diluted solutions in refrigerator and use within 48 h.

⬤ fat emulsion, intravenous
(fat ee mul' shun) Intralipid 10%, 20%; Liposyn II 10%, 20%; Liposyn III 10%, 20%

Pregnancy Category C

Drug class
Caloric agent

Indications
- Source of calories and essential fatty acids for patients requiring parenteral nutrition for extended periods
- Essential fatty acid deficiency

Therapeutic actions
- A preparation from soybean or safflower oil that provides neutral triglycerides, mostly unsaturated fatty acids; used as a source of energy, causing an increase in heat production, decrease in respiratory quotient, and increase in oxygen consumption

Contraindications/cautions
- **Contraindications:** allergy to eggs, disturbance of normal fat metabolism (hyperlipemia, lipoid nephrosis, acute pancreatitis)

(contraindications continued on next page)

Adverse effects in *Italics* are most common; those in **Bold** are life-threatening

> ▶ **Cautions:** severe liver damage, pulmonary disease, anemia, blood coagulation disorders, danger of fat embolism

Available forms
▶ *Injection:* 10% (50, 100, 200, 250, 500 mL), 20% (50, 100, 200, 250, 500 mL)

IV facts
Preparation
▶ Obtain a single dose container. Examine solution for "breaking or oiling out" of emulsion—seen as yellow streaking or accumulation of yellow droplets—or for formation of particulates; if present, discard solution.
▶ Do not use with filters.
▶ If given with amino acid-dextrose mixtures, keep lipid infusion line higher than amino acid-dextrose line. Lipid emulsion has a lower specific gravity, so it may be taken up into the amino acid-dextrose line.

Dosage
▶ Administer IV through peripheral vein or central venous catheter.
▶ *TPN:* **10%:** 1 mL/min IV for 15–30 min. If no adverse reactions occur, increase rate to 2 mL/min. Give only 500 mL the first day; increase dose the next day. Do not exceed 2.5 g/kg/d or 60% of total caloric intake. **20%:** 0.5 mL/min IV for 15–30 min. Infuse only 250 mL Liposyn II or 500 mL Intralipid the first day; increase dose the next day. Do not exceed 3 g/kg/d or 60% of total caloric intake.
▶ *Fatty acid deficiency:* Supply 8%–10% of caloric intake by IV fat emulsion.

Compatibility
Fat emulsion may be given through the same IV line as ampicillin, cefamandole, cefazolin, cefoxitin, cephapirin, clindamycin, digoxin, dopamine, erythromycin, furosemide, gentamicin, IL-2, isoproterenol, kanamycin, lidocaine, norepinephrine, oxacillin, penicillin G, potassium, ticarcillin, tobramycin.

Incompatibility
Do not administer through the same IV line as amikacin.

> **TREATMENT OF OVERDOSE/ANTIDOTE**
> Discontinue drug or decrease dosage. Initiate general supportive and resuscitative measures. Determine triglyceride concentrations or measure plasma light-scattering activity.

Adverse effects in *Italics* are most common; those in **Bold** are life-threatening

Pharmacokinetics

Route	Onset	Peak	Duration
IV	Unknown	Unknown	Unknown

Metabolism: Tissue

Adverse effects

‣ *CNS:* Headache, flushing, sleepiness, pressure over eyes, dizziness
‣ *CV:* Chest pain, fluid overload
‣ *Resp:* Dyspnea, cyanosis
‣ *GI:* Nausea, vomiting, hepatomegaly, jaundice due to cholestasis, splenomegaly, transient increases in liver function tests
‣ *Derm:* *Thrombophlebitis/irritation at infusion site*
‣ *Hematologic:* *Sepsis,* **thrombocytopenia, leukopenia,** hypercoagulability
‣ *Misc:* Fever, sweating, hyperlipidemia, overloading syndrome (focal seizures, fever, leukocytosis, splenomegaly, shock), brown pigmentation in reticuloendothelial system (IV fat pigment)

● NURSING CONSIDERATIONS

Assessment

‣ *History:* Allergy to eggs, fat metabolism disturbances, hyperlipemia, lipoid nephrosis, acute pancreatitis, severe liver damage, pulmonary disease, anemia, blood coagulation disorders, risk of fat embolism
‣ *Physical:* T, P, BP, R, I & O, ECG, IV site, weight, neurologic checks, adventitious lung sounds, fluid balance, nutritional status, liver function tests, serum electrolytes, coagulation studies, plasma lipid profile, CBC, serum albumin, serum transferrin, nitrogen balance

Implementation

‣ Always administer fat emulsion infusion using an IV pump.
‣ If patient develops symptoms of acute respiratory distress, pulmonary emboli, or interstitial pneumonitis, immediately stop the infusion and inspect it for precipitates. Institute appropriate interventions.
‣ Monitor carefully for fluid or fat overloading during infusion as evidenced by diluted serum electrolytes, overhydration, pulmonary edema, distended neck veins, metabolic acidosis, or impaired pulmonary diffusion capacity. If present, stop infusion. Reevaluate patient before restarting infusion at a lower rate.
‣ Monitor patient's serum lipid profile, weight, nitrogen balance, and response to therapy.

Adverse effects in *Italics* are most common; those in **Bold** are life-threatening

▶ Monitor for thrombosis or sepsis.
▶ Routinely monitor coagulation studies, liver function tests, lipid profile, and platelet count.
▶ Maximum infusion hang time for Intralipid is 12 h; other fat emulsions may hang for up to 24 h.
▶ Avoid freezing fat emulsions. Do not store or reuse partially used bottles.
▶ Do not resterilize solution for later use.

⬤ fenoldopam mesylate *(phen ole' doe pam)*
Corlopam

Pregnancy Category B

Drug classes
Antihypertensive

Indications
▶ Management of severe hypertensive emergencies when rapid, but quickly reversible, emergency reduction of blood pressure is indicated, including malignant hypertension with deteriorating end-organ function

Therapeutic actions
▶ An agonist for D_1-like dopamine receptors
▶ Binds to α_2-adrenoceptors

Effects on hemodynamic parameters
▶ Decreased BP
▶ Increased HR

> **Contraindications/cautions**
> ▶ **Contraindications:** fenoldopam allergy, hypotension
> ▶ **Cautions:** glaucoma, intraocular hypertension, hypokalemia, sulfite sensitivity

Available form
▶ *Injection:* 10 mg/mL

IV facts
Preparation
▶ Add 10 mg of drug to 250 mL D5W or 0.9%NS to achieve a final concentration of 40 mcg/mL.

Dosage and titration
▶ 0.01–0.3 mg/kg/min IV. Titrate by 0.05–0.1 mcg/kg/min increments no more frequently than q15min to achieve desired therapeutic effect. Drug has not been used > 48 h. Transition to oral antihypertensive therapy as soon as possible.

Adverse effects in *Italics* are most common; those in **Bold** are life-threatening

Titration Guide

fenoldopam mesylate										
10 mg in 250 mL										
Body Weight										
lb	88	99	110	121	132	143	154	165	176	187
kg	40	45	50	55	60	65	70	75	80	85
Dose ordered in mcg/kg/min	**Amounts to Infuse in mL/h**									
0.01	1	1	1	1	1	1	1	1	1	1
0.05	3	3	4	4	5	5	5	6	6	6
0.1	6	7	8	8	9	10	11	11	12	13
0.15	9	10	11	12	14	15	16	17	18	19
0.2	12	14	15	17	18	20	21	23	24	26
0.25	15	17	19	21	23	24	26	28	30	32
0.3	18	20	23	25	27	29	32	34	36	38

Body Weight										
lb	198	209	220	231	242	253	264	275	286	
kg	90	95	100	105	110	115	120	125	130	
Dose ordered in mcg/kg/min	**Amounts to Infuse in mL/h**									
0.01	1	1	2	2	2	2	2	2	2	
0.05	7	7	8	8	8	9	9	9	10	
0.1	14	14	15	16	17	17	18	19	20	
0.15	20	21	23	24	25	26	27	28	29	
0.2	27	29	30	32	33	35	36	38	39	
0.25	34	36	38	39	41	43	45	47	49	
0.3	41	43	45	47	50	52	54	56	59	

Compatibility
Do not administer through the same IV line as other drugs.

> **TREATMENT OF OVERDOSE/ANTIDOTE**
> Discontinue drug or decrease dosage. Initiate general supportive and resuscitative measures.

Pharmacokinetics

Route	Onset
IV	Immediate

Metabolism: Hepatic; $T_{1/2}$: 5 min
Excretion: Urine, feces

Adverse effects in *Italics* are most common; those in **Bold** are life-threatening

Adverse effects
▶ *CNS: Headache, flushing,* nervousness, anxiety, insomnia, dizziness
▶ *CV:* **Heart failure, myocardial infarction,** *hypotension,* postural hypotension, ST-T abnormalities, non-specific chest pain, extrasystoles, palpitations, bradycardia, ischemic heart disease, angina
▶ *Resp:* Dyspnea, upper respiratory disorder
▶ *GI: Nausea,* vomiting, abdominal pain/fullness, constipation, diarrhea
▶ *Hematologic:* Leukocytosis, bleeding
▶ *Misc:* Hypokalemia, injection site reaction, urinary tract infection, pyrexia, oliguria, limb cramps; elevated creatinine, BUN, serum glucose, transaminase, LDH

Clinically important drug–drug interactions
▶ Unexpected hypotension with beta-blockers

⬤ NURSING CONSIDERATIONS

Assessment
▶ *History:* Fenoldopam allergy, glaucoma, intraocular hypertension, sulfite sensitivity
▶ *Physical:* P, BP, R, ECG, I & O, IV site, weight, neurologic checks, intraocular pressure, skin assessment, cardiac auscultation, chest pain assessment, orthostatic BP, adventitious lung sounds, abdominal assessment, bowel sounds, serum electrolytes, liver and renal function tests, CBC, serum glucose

Implementation
▶ Exercise extreme caution when calculating and preparing doses. Fenoldopam is a very potent drug; small dosage errors can cause serious adverse effects.
▶ Aways administer through an IV infusion pump.
▶ Continuously monitor P, BP, R, and ECG during administration.
▶ Have dopamine and norepinephrine nearby in case of severe hypotensive reaction.
▶ Drug may produce potassium levels of < 3 mEq/L. Treat hypokalemia with IV or oral supplements.
▶ Administer infusion when patient is in a supine position.
▶ Change patient's position slowly to avoid postural hypotension.
▶ After dilution, solution is stable at room temperature for ≤ 24 h.

⬤ **fentanyl** *(fen' ta nil)* Duragesic, Sublimaze
Pregnancy Category B
C-II controlled substance

Adverse effects in *Italics* are most common; those in **Bold** are life-threatening

Drug class
Narcotic analgesic

Indications
▸ Analgesic action of short duration during anesthesia and in the immediate postoperative period
▸ Narcotic analgesic supplement in general or regional anesthesia
▸ Administration with a neuroleptic, such as droperidol, as an anesthetic premedication, for induction of anesthesia, and as an adjunct in maintenance of general and regional anesthesia
▸ Anesthetic agent with oxygen in selected high-risk patients
▸ Transdermal system: management of chronic pain in patients requiring opioid analgesia

Therapeutic actions
▸ Acts at specific opioid receptors in the CNS, causing analgesia, respiratory depression, physical depression, euphoria

Effects on hemodynamic parameters
▸ Decreased BP
▸ Decreased or unchanged HR
▸ Decreased RR to apnea

Contraindications/cautions
▸ **Contraindications:** allergy to fentanyl or other opioid narcotics; situations in which there is no opportunity to titrate proper dose (transdermal system); management of pain that can be controlled by lesser means (transdermal system)
▸ **Cautions:** head injury, brain tumor, increased ICP, coma, elderly or debilitated patients, cardiovascular disease, bradydysrhythmias, COPD, respiratory compromise, liver disease, kidney dysfunction, fever, drug abuse, alcoholism

Available forms
▸ *IV injection:* 50 mcg/mL
▸ *Transdermal:* 25, 50, 75, 100 mcg/h

IV/IM facts
Preparation
▸ **IV:** May be given undiluted or diluted in D5W or 0.9%NS.
▸ **IM:** Give undiluted.

Dosage and titration
▸ *Premedication:* 50–100 mcg IM 30–60 min before surgery.
▸ *Postoperatively:* 50–100 mcg IM; repeat in 1–2 h as needed.

Adverse effects in *Italics* are most common; those in **Bold** are life-threatening

- *Adjunct to general anesthesia:* **Low dose:** 2 mcg/kg IV. **Moderate dose:** 2–20 mcg/kg IV. Additional 25–100 mcg doses may be given as needed. **High dose:** 20–50 mcg/kg IV. Additional 25 mcg to 50% of initial loading dose may be given as needed.
- *Adjunct to regional anesthesia:* 50–100 mcg IV over 1 to 2 min.
- *General anesthesia:* 50–100 mcg/kg IV with oxygen and a muscle relaxant. May need to use up to 150 mcg/kg to produce desired effect.

Compatibility

Fentanyl may be given through the same IV line as atracurium, diltiazem, dobutamine, dopamine, enalaprilat, epinephrine, esmolol, etomidate, furosemide, heparin, hydrocortisone, hydromorphone, labetalol, midazolam, milrinone, morphine, nafcillin, nicardipine, nitroglycerin, norepinephrine, pancuronium, potassium chloride, propofol, ranitidine, sargramostim, thiopental, vecuronium, vitamin B complex with C.

Incompatibility

Do not administer through the same IV line as pentobarbital.

Transdermal dosage

- Apply to irritated and nonirradiated skin on a flat surface of the upper torso.
- Individualize dosage based on the patient's pain assessment, previous opioid drug use and dosage, opioid drug tolerance, and general condition. Use the lowest effective dose. Titrate dose up no more frequently than q3d after the initial dose and no more frequently than q6d thereafter.
- Apply dosage q48–72h. For large doses, use more than one transdermal system.

TREATMENT OF OVERDOSE/ANTIDOTE

Decrease dosage/infusion or remove transdermal patch. Initiate resuscitative measures as indicated. Treat respiratory depression by artifical ventilation, oxygen, and narcotic antagonists, such as naloxone. If depressed respiration is associated with muscular rigidity, an IV neuromuscular blocking agent may facilitate assisted or controlled respiration. Treat cardiovascular depression with IV fluids or pressor agents. Administer atropine for bradycardia.

Adverse effects in *Italics* are most common; those in **Bold** are life-threatening

Pharmacokinetics

Route	Onset	Peak	Duration
IV	Immediate	Several minutes	30–60 min
Transdermal	Gradual	24–72 h	72 h

Metabolism: Hepatic; $T_{1/2}$: 219 min (parenteral); 13–22 h (transdermal)
Excretion: Urine

Adverse effects

▸ *CNS:* **Convulsions,** *sedation, clamminess, sweating, vertigo, floating feeling, dizziness, lethargy, confusion, somnolence, lightheadedness,* headache, nervousness, unusual dreams, agitation, euphoria, hallucinations, delirium, insomnia, anxiety, fear, disorientation, impaired mental and physical performance, coma, mood changes, weakness, tremor, diplopia, blurred vision
▸ *CV:* **Cardiac arrest, shock,** palpitations, hypotension, hypertension, bradycardia, dysrhythmias
▸ *Resp:* **Apnea, bronchospasm;** slow, shallow respiration; suppressed cough reflex; laryngospasm; hypoventilation; dyspnea
▸ *GI:* *Nausea, vomiting, abdominal pain, constipation,* dry mouth, dyspepsia, anorexia, biliary tract spasm
▸ *GU:* Ureteral spasm, spasm of vesical sphincters, urinary retention or hesitancy, oliguria, antidiuretic effect, reduced libido or potency
▸ *Derm:* *Sweating,* rash, hives, pruritus, flushing, warmth, sensitivity to cold; local skin irritation with transdermal system; phlebitis at IV injection site
▸ *Musc/Skel:* Muscle rigidity
▸ *Dependence:* Physical tolerance and dependence, psychological dependence

Clinically important drug–drug interactions

▸ Enhanced effects with barbiturate anesthetics, tranquilizers, narcotics, general anesthetics
▸ Severe and unpredictable hypertension with MAO inhibitors
▸ Cardiovascular depression with diazepam
▸ Hypotension and decreased PAP with droperidol
▸ Increased CNS and respiratory depression with protease inhibitors

● NURSING CONSIDERATIONS

Assessment

▸ *History:* Fentanyl or narcotic allergy, physical dependence on a narcotic analgesic, drug abuse, COPD, respiratory depression, increased ICP, cardiovascular disease, biliary tract

Adverse effects in *Italics* are most common; those in **Bold** are life-threatening

surgery, renal or hepatic dysfunction, recent use of ETOH, age, debilitated status
▶ *Physical:* T, P, BP, R, ECG, I & O, SpO$_2$, IV site, weight, neurologic checks, vision assessment, level of sedation, respiratory status, pain assessment, adventitious lung sounds, bowel sounds, liver and renal function tests

Implementation
▶ Exercise extreme caution when calculating and preparing doses. Fentanyl is a very potent drug; small dosage errors can cause serious adverse effects.
▶ Always administer an infusion using an IV infusion pump.
▶ Use the smallest dose possible to achieve desired patient response.
▶ Monitor BP, R, ECG, and pain status closely during infusion to monitor effectiveness of therapy.
▶ Monitor for evidence of respiratory depression. Ensure oxygen, intubation equipment, and naloxone are available to treat respiratory depression.
▶ Use caution when giving IM injections to patients with hypotension or in shock; impaired perfusion may delay absorption. With repeated doses, an excessive amount may be absorbed when circulation is restored.
▶ Transdermal system: Prepare site by clipping (not shaving) hair at site; do not use soap, oils, lotions, alcohol; allow skin to dry completely before application. Apply immediately after removal from package. Do not cut or alter system. Firmly press the system in place with palm of hand for 30 s, ensuring that contact is complete. When removing a system, fold the system so that the adhesive adheres to itself, and flush down the toilet. Apply next dose to a different site.
▶ Implement additional nonpharmacologic measures to treat pain as indicated.
▶ Follow federal, state, and institutional policies for dispensing controlled substances.
▶ Protect ampules from light.

⬤ **filgrastim** (granulocyte colony stimulating factor, G-CSF) *(fill grass' stim)* Neupogen

Pregnancy Category C

Drug class
Colony-stimulating factor

Indications
▶ To decrease the incidence of infection in patients with non-myeloid malignancies who are receiving myelosuppressive

anticancer drugs associated with a significant incidence of severe neutropenia with fever
▸ To reduce the duration of neutropenia and neutropenia-related clinical sequelae in patients with nonmyeloid malignancies undergoing myeloablative chemotherapy and bone marrow transplant (BMT)
▸ To reduce severe neutropenia for patients undergoing induction and consolidation chemotherapy for acute myelogenous leukemia—reduces time for neutrophil recovery and duration of fever
▸ To treat severe chronic neutropenia
▸ To mobilize hematopoietic progenitor cells into the blood for leukapheresis collection
▸ Orphan drug uses: To treat AIDS with CMV retinitis being treated with ganciclovir; to reduce neutropenia, fever, antibiotic use, and hospitalization following induction and consolidation
▸ Unlabeled uses: to treat aplastic anemia, hairy cell leukemia, myelodysplasia, drug-induced and congenital agranulocytosis

Therapeutic actions
▸ Human G-CSF produced by recombinant DNA technology and in *Escherichia coli* bacteria
▸ Regulates production of neutrophils within the bone marrow
▸ Stimulates proliferation, differentiation, and some end-cell function activation of neutrophils with little effect on the production of other hematopoietic cells

Contraindications/cautions
▸ **Contraindications:** hypersensitivity to *E. coli* proteins, filgrastim, or product components
▸ **Caution:** hypothyroidism

Available form
▸ *Injection:* 300 mcg/mL

IV/SC facts
Preparation
▸ Prior to injection, may allow drug to reach room temperature for maximum of 24 h.
▸ Avoid shaking.
▸ Use only 1 dose per vial; do not re-enter vial.
▸ May be given undiluted or diluted in D5W to concentration ≥ 15 mcg/mL. If concentration is 5–15 mcg/mL, protect from adsorption to plastic materials by adding albumin (human) to

Adverse effects in *Italics* are most common; those in **Bold** are life-threatening

a final concentration of 2 mg/mL. Do not dilute to final concentration of < 5 mcg/mL.

Dosage

▶ *Myelosuppressive chemotherapy:* 5 mcg/kg/d as single daily injection given SC, IV over 15–30 min, or by continuous IV or SC infusion. May increase in increments of 5 mcg/kg for each chemotherapy cycle according to duration and severity of absolute neutrophil count (ANC) nadir.

▶ *Following BMT:* 10 mcg/kg/d as IV infusion of 4 or 24 h or as continuous 24-h SC. If ANC > 1000/mm³ for 3 d, reduce to 5 mcg/kg/d. If ANC > 1000/mm³ for 3 more d, discontinue drug. If ANC decreases to < 1000/mm³, resume drug at 5 mcg/kg/d.

▶ *Severe chronic neutropenia:* **Congenital neutropenia:** 6 mcg/kg SC bid. **Idiopathic or cyclic neutropenia:** 5 mcg/kg/d SC as a single injection.

▶ *Mobilization for harvesting:* 10 mcg/kg/d SC, as bolus or continuous infusion, at least 4 d before first leukapheresis; continue to last leukapheresis.

Compatibility

Filgrastim may be given through the same IV line as acyclovir, allopurinol, amikacin, aminophylline, ampicillin, ampicillin-sulbactam, aztreonam, bleomycin, bumetanide, buprenorphine, butorphanol, calcium gluconate, carboplatin, carmustine, cefazolin, cefotetan, ceftazidime, chlorpromazine, cimetidine, cisplatin, cyclophosphamide, cytarabine, dacarbazine, daunorubicin, dexamethasone, diphenhydramine, doxorubicin, doxycycline, droperidol, enalaprilat, famotidine, floxuridine, fluconazole, fludarabine, gallium, ganciclovir, granisetron, haloperidol, hydrocortisone, hydromorphone, hydroxyzine, idarubicin, ifosfamide, leucovorin, lorazepam, mechlorethamine, melphalan, meperidine, mesna, methotrexate, metoclopramide, miconazole, minocycline, mitoxantrone, morphine, nalbuphine, netilmicin, ondansetron, plicamycin, potassium chloride, promethazine, ranitidine, sodium bicarbonate, streptozocin, ticarcillin, ticarcillin-clavulanate, tobramycin, trimethoprim-sulfamethoxazole, vancomycin, vinblastine, vincristine, vinorelbine, zidovudine.

Incompatibility

Do not administer through the same IV line as amphotericin B, cefepime, cefonicid, cefoperazone, cefotaxime, cefoxitin, ceftizoxime, ceftriaxone, cefuroxime, clindamycin, dactinomycin, etoposide, fluorouracil, furosemide, heparin, mannitol, methylprednisolone, metronidazole, mezlocillin, mitomycin, piperacillin, prochlorperazine, thiotepa.

Adverse effects in *Italics* are most common; those in **Bold** are life-threatening

Pharmacokinetics

Route	Peak	Duration
SC	2–8 h	up to 7 d

$T_{1/2}$: 210–231 min

Adverse effects
▸ Most adverse experiences are sequelae of underlying malignancy or cytotoxic chemotherapy
▸ *CNS:* Headache, fever, generalized weakness, fatigue
▸ *CV:* **Dysrhythmias, AMI,** *hypertension,* chest pain
▸ *Resp:* **Adult respiratory distress syndrome (in septic patients),** dyspnea, cough
▸ *GI: Nausea, vomiting,* diarrhea, peritonitis, stomatitis, anorexia, constipation; increased lactic acid, LDH, alkaline phosphatase
▸ *GU:* Renal insufficiency
▸ *Derm: Rash,* alopecia, mucositis, vasculitis
▸ *Allergic:* Rash, facial edema, urticaria, wheezing, dyspnea, hypotension, tachycardia
▸ *Hematologic:* **Thrombocytopenia**
▸ *Misc: Bone pain,* generalized pain, sore throat, cough

Clinically important drug–drug interactions
▸ Use with caution with drugs, such as lithium, that may potentiate release of neutrophils

● NURSING CONSIDERATIONS

Assessment
▸ *History:* Hypersensitivity to *E. coli* proteins, filgrastim, or product components; hypothyroidism
▸ *Physical:* T, P, BP, R, ECG, I & O, skin and hair assessment, adventitious lung sounds, pain assessment, abdominal exam, mucous membrane assessment, CBC, liver and renal function tests

Implementation
▸ Obtain CBC and platelet count prior to and twice weekly during therapy.
▸ Do not give within 24 h before and after chemotherapy.
▸ Give daily for up to 2 wk until the neutrophil count is at least 10,000/mm³.

Adverse effects in *Italics* are most common; those in **Bold** are life-threatening

▸ To avoid excessive leukocytosis, discontinue therapy if ANC surpasses 10,000/mm^3 after the ANC nadir occurs. High ANC levels may not be more beneficial.

⬤ fluconazole *(floo kon' a zole)* Diflucan
Pregnancy Category C

Drug class
Antifungal

Indications
▸ Treatment of oropharyngeal and esophageal candidiasis
▸ Treatment of cryptococcal meningitis
▸ Treatment of candidal urinary tract infections, peritonitis, and systemic candidal infections, including candidemia, disseminated candidiasis, and pneumonia
▸ Prophylaxis to decrease incidence of candidiasis in bone marrow transplants

Therapeutic actions
▸ Inhibits fungal cytochrome and sterol synthesis
▸ Loss of normal sterols is associated with accumulation of other sterols in fungi and may cause fluconazole's fungistatic activity
▸ Has fungicidal or fungistatic effect depending on concentrations

Contraindications/cautions
▸ **Contraindication:** fluconazole allergy
▸ **Cautions:** abnormal liver function or liver function tests, renal impairment, allergy to other azoles

Available forms
▸ *Injection:* 2 mg/mL
▸ *Tablets:* 50, 100, 150, 200 mg
▸ *Powder for oral suspension:* 10, 40 mg/mL

IV facts
Preparation
▸ Do not remove overwrap until ready for use. Inner bag maintains sterility of product. Some opacity of plastic may occur, but this is normal and does not affect solution quality or safety. Check for minute leaks, squeezing bag firmly. Discard solution if any leaks are found.

Dosage and titration
▸ Individualize dosage based on patient's response.
▸ Infuse at a maximum rate of 200 mg/h.

Adverse effects in *Italics* are most common; those in **Bold** are life-threatening

- *Oropharyngeal candidiasis:* 200 mg IV first day, then 100 mg/d IV for 2 wk.
- *Esophageal candidiasis:* 200 mg IV first day, then 100 mg/d IV for at least 3 wk and for at least 2 wk following resolution of symptoms. Doses up to 400 mg/d may be used.
- *Candidiasis:* 50–200 mg/d IV. Doses up to 400 mg/d have been used.
- *Prevention of candidiasis in bone marrow transplant:* 400 mg/d IV several days before anticipated onset of neutropenia and continuing for 7 d after neutropenia.
- *Cryptococcal meningitis:* 400 mg IV first day, then 200–400 mg/d for 10–12 wk after cerebrospinal fluid becomes culture negative.
- *Suppression of cryptococcal meningitis in AIDS patients:* 200 mg/d IV.
- *Renal function impairment:* Initial dose of 50–400 mg IV. If creatinine clearance > 50 mL/min, use 100% recommended dose; if creatinine clearance 11–50 mL/min, use 50% of the recommended dose; if patient on hemodialysis, give one dose after each dialysis.

Compatibility

Fluconazole may be given through the same IV line as acyclovir, aldesleukin, allopurinol, amifostine, amikacin, aminophylline, ampicillin-sulbactam, aztreonam, benztropine, cefazolin, cefepime, cefotetan, cefoxitin, chlorpromazine, cimetidine, dexamethasone, diltiazem, diphenhydramine, dobutamine, dopamine, droperidol, famotidine, filgrastim, fludarabine, foscarnet, gallium, ganciclovir, gentamicin, granisetron, heparin, hydrocortisone, immune globulin, leucovorin, lorazepam, melphalan, meperidine, meropenem, metoclopramide, metronidazole, midazolam, morphine, nafcillin, nitroglycerin, ondansetron, oxacillin, paclitaxel, pancuronium, penicillin G potassium, phenytoin, piperacillin-tazobactam, prochlorperazine, promethazine, propofol, ranitidine, sargramostim, tacrolimus, teniposide, theophylline, thiotepa, ticarcillin-clavulanate, tobramycin, vancomycin, vecuronium, vinorelbine, zidovudine.

Incompatibility

Do not add supplementary medications to fluconazole. Do not administer through the same IV line as amphotericin B, ampicillin, calcium gluconate, cefotaxime, ceftazidime, ceftriaxone, cefuroxime, chloramphenicol, clindamycin, diazepam, digoxin, erythromycin, furosemide, haloperidol, hydroxyzine, imipenem-cilastatin, pentamidine, piperacillin, ticarcillin, trimethoprim-sulfamethoxazole.

Adverse effects in *Italics* are most common; those in **Bold** are life-threatening

F

Oral dosage
▶ Individualize dosage; because of rapid and almost complete absorption, oral dosage is same as IV dosage (see above).
▶ *Vaginal candidiasis:* 150 mg PO as a single dose.

> **TREATMENT OF OVERDOSE/ANTIDOTE**
> Discontinue drug or decrease dosage. Initiate general supportive and resuscitative measures. Initiate gastric lavage if indicated. Hemodialysis will decrease drug levels.

Pharmacokinetics

Route	Onset	Peak
IV	Rapid	1 h
Oral	Slow	1–2 h

$T_{1/2}$: 30 h
Excretion: Urine

Adverse effects
▶ *CNS: Headache,* dizziness, seizures
▶ *GI:* **Hepatic injury,** *nausea, vomiting, diarrhea, abdominal pain,* taste perversion
▶ *Derm:* **Stevens-Johnson syndrome, toxic epidermal necrolysis,** skin rash, alopecia
▶ *Allergic:* **Anaphylaxis, angioedema**
▶ *Misc:* **Thrombocytopenia, leukopenia,** hypercholesterolemia, hypertriglyceridemia, hypokalemia

Clinically important drug–drug interactions
▶ Decreased levels with cimetidine
▶ Reduced renal clearance and increased levels with hydrochlorothiazide
▶ Increased or decreased hormone levels of oral contraceptives
▶ Increased levels of zidovudine and sulfonylureas
▶ Increased serum levels and therefore therapeutic and toxic effects of cyclosporine, phenytoin, theophylline, oral hypoglycemics, warfarin
▶ Decreased half-life and serum levels with rifampin

● NURSING CONSIDERATIONS

Assessment
▶ *History:* Fluconazole allergy, renal impairment, allergy to other azoles
▶ *Physical:* T, P, R, BP, I & O, neurologic checks, skin assessment, respiratory effort, adventitious lung sounds, injection site, pain assessment, bowel sounds, renal and liver function tests, CBC, culture of area involved

Implementation
▶ Culture infection prior to therapy; begin treatment before lab results are returned.
▶ Infuse IV only; not intended for IM or SC use.
▶ Have emergency equipment (defibrillator, drugs, oxygen, intubation equipment) on standby in case anaphylaxis or adverse reaction occurs.
▶ Monitor liver and renal function tests; discontinue drug or decrease dosage at any sign of hepatic injury or renal toxicity.
▶ Monitor closely for a rash; discontinue drug if lesions progress.
▶ Shake oral suspension well before using.

⬤ fludrocortisone acetate *(floo droe kor' ti sone)*
Florinef

Pregnancy Category C

Drug classes
Corticosteroid
Mineralocorticoid

Indications
▶ Partial replacement therapy in primary and secondary cortical insufficiency and for the treatment of salt-losing adrenogenital syndrome (therapy must be accompanied by adequate doses of glucocorticoids)
▶ Unlabeled use: management of severe orthostatic hypotension

Therapeutic actions
▶ Acts on renal distal tubules to enhance reabsorption of sodium, leading to water retention
▶ Increases urinary excretion of potassium and hydrogen ions
▶ In larger doses, inhibits endogenous adrenal cortical secretion, thymic activity, and pituitary corticotropin excretion; promotes deposition of liver glycogen; and unless protein intake is adequate, induces negative nitrogen balance

Effects on hemodynamic parameters
▶ Increased BP

Contraindications/cautions
▶ **Contraindications:** fludrocortisone allergy, systemic fungal infections
▶ **Cautions:** Addison's disease, high sodium intake, infection, tuberculosis, hypothyroidism, cirrhosis, ocular herpes simplex, ulcerative colitis, diverticulitis, fresh intestinal anastomoses, active or latent peptic ulcer, renal insufficiency, hypertension, osteoporosis, myasthenia gravis, heart disease, CHF

Adverse effects in *Italics* are most common; those in **Bold** are life-threatening

F

Available form
▶ *Tablets:* 0.1 mg

Oral dosage
▶ *Addison's disease:* 0.1 mg/d PO (range 0.1 mg 3 times a wk to 0.2 mg/d). Reduce dose to 0.05 mg/d if transient hypertension develops. Administration with hydrocortisone (10–30 mg/d) or cortisone (10.0–37.5 mg/d) is preferable.
▶ *Salt-losing adrenogenital syndrome:* 0.1–0.2 mg/d PO.
▶ *Severe orthostatic hypotension:* 0.1–0.4 mg/d PO.

> **TREATMENT OF OVERDOSE/ANTIDOTE**
> Discontinue drug or decrease dosage. Initiate general supportive and resuscitative measures. Treat muscular weakness with potassium supplements.

Pharmacokinetics

Route	Onset	Peak	Duration
Oral	Gradual	1.7 h	18–36 h

Metabolism: Hepatic; $T_{1/2}$: 3.5 h

Adverse effects
▶ *CNS:* **Convulsions,** frontal and occipital headaches, arthralgia, increased intracranial pressure, dizziness, euphoria, mood swings, severe mental disturbances, insomnia
▶ *CV: Increased blood volume, edema, hypertension, CHF,* dysrhythmias, heart enlargement, syncope
▶ *GI:* **Peptic ulcer with perforation and hemorrhage, pancreatitis,** abdominal distention, ulcerative esophagitis
▶ *Derm:* Bruising, increased sweating, rash, impaired wound healing, thin fragile skin, petechiae, subcutaneous fat atrophy, purpura, striae, hyperpigmentation of skin and nails, hirsutism
▶ *Allergic:* **Anaphylaxis**
▶ *Musc/Skel:* Muscle weakness, steroid myopathy, loss of muscle mass, osteoporosis, vertebral compression fractures, pathologic fractures
▶ *Metabolic:* Hyperglycemia, hypokalemia, glycosuria, negative nitrogen balance
▶ *Ophthalmic:* Posterior subcapsular cataracts, increased intraocular pressure, glaucoma, exophthalmos
▶ *Misc:* Hypokalemic alkalosis, masking of infections, thrombophlebitis

Clinically important drug–drug interactions
▶ Decreased effects with barbiturates, phenytoin, rifampin
▶ Decreased serum levels and effectiveness of salicylates; increased ulcerogenic effect

Adverse effects in *Italics* are most common; those in **Bold** are life-threatening

- Enhanced hypokalemia with amphotericin B or potassium-depleting diuretics
- Increased dysrhythmias and digitalis toxicity related to hypokalemia
- Decreased PT levels with oral anticoagulants
- Decreased antidiabetic effect of antidiabetic drugs
- Increased edema with anabolic steroids

● NURSING CONSIDERATIONS

Assessment

- *History:* Fludrocortisone allergy, systemic fungal infections, Addison's disease, high sodium intake, infection, tuberculosis, hypothyroidism, cirrhosis, ocular herpes simplex, ulcerative colitis, diverticulitis, fresh intestinal anastomoses, active or latent peptic ulcer, renal insufficiency, hypertension, osteoporosis, myasthenia gravis, heart disease, CHF
- *Physical:* T, P, BP, R, ECG, I & O, weight, neurologic checks, skin assessment, eye assessment, intraocular pressure, adventitious lung sounds, heart sounds, JVD, edema, hydration status, skin turgor, muscle weakness, bone pain or deformity, serum electrolytes, liver function tests, CBC, nitrogen balance, serum glucose, stool and emesis guaiac

Implementation

- Use only in conjunction with glucocorticoid therapy and control of electrolytes and infection.
- Increase dosage during times of stress to prevent drug-induced adrenal insufficiency.
- Monitor BP and serum electrolytes regularly to prevent overdosage.
- Have emergency equipment (defibrillator, drugs, oxygen, intubation equipment) on standby in case anaphylaxis or adverse reaction occurs.
- Discontinue if signs of overdosage (hypertension, edema, excessive weight gain, increased heart size) appear.
- Evaluate for hypokalemia as evidenced by muscle weakness, fatigue, paralytic ileus, ECG changes, anorexia, nausea, vomiting, abdominal distention, dizziness, or polyuria.
- Assess for evidence of infection.
- Treat muscle weakness due to excessive K^+ loss with supplements.
- Restrict sodium intake if edema develops.
- Withdraw drug gradually when possible.

⬤ flumazenil *(floo maz' eh nill)* Anexate (CAN), Romazicon

F

Pregnancy Category C

Drug classes
Antidote
Benzodiazepine receptor antagonist

Indications
▶ Complete or partial reversal of the sedative effects of benzodiazepines when general anesthesia has been induced or maintained with them and when sedation has been produced for diagnostic and therapeutic procedures
▶ Management of benzodiazepine overdose

Therapeutic actions
▶ Antagonizes the actions of benzodiazepines on the CNS and inhibits activity at GABA/benzodiazepine receptor sites
▶ Does **not** antagonize opioid analgesics, alcohol, barbiturates, or general anesthetics

Contraindications/cautions
▶ **Contraindications:** flumazenil or benzodiazepine allergy, patients who have been given a benzodiazepine for control of a potentially life-threatening condition, patients who show signs of serious cyclic antidepressant overdose
▶ **Cautions:** head injury, respiratory depression, neuromuscular blockade, psychiatric illness, liver disease, alcohol or drug dependency, benzodiazepine abstinence syndromes

Available form
▶ *Injection:* 0.1 mg/mL

IV facts
Preparation
▶ May be given undiluted or diluted in D5W; LR; or 0.9%NS.
▶ Do not remove from vial until ready to use.

Dosage
▶ *Reversal of conscious sedation:* Initial dose of 0.2 mg (2 mL) IV over 15 s. Wait 45 s. If drug is not effective, repeat dose at 60-s intervals. Maximum dose 1 mg (10 mL). Usual dose 0.6 to 1 mg. If patient becomes resedated, give repeated doses at 20-min intervals as needed. For repeat treatment, administer no more than 1 mg IV at any one time and no more than 3 mg in any hour.
▶ *Management of suspected benzodiazepine overdose:* Initial

Adverse effects in *Italics* are most common; those in **Bold** are life-threatening

dose of 0.2 mg IV over 30 s. Wait 30 s. If drug is not effective, give 0.3 mg (3 mL) over 30 s. Further doses of 0.5 mg (5 mL) can be given over 30 s at 1-min intervals up to a cumulative dose of 3 mg.

Compatibility

Do not mix or infuse with other drugs.

> **TREATMENT OF OVERDOSE/ANTIDOTE**
> Discontinue drug or decrease dosage. Initiate general supportive and resuscitative measures. Treat convulsions with barbiturates, benzodiazepines, and phenytoin.

Pharmacokinetics

Route	Onset	Peak	Duration
IV	1–2 min	6–10 min	Variable depending on plasma concentration of benzodiazepine and dose of flumazenil

Metabolism: Hepatic; $T_{1/2}$: 41–79 min
Excretion: Metabolites excreted in urine

Adverse effects

▸ *CNS:* **Convulsions,** *dizziness, headache, blurred vision, diplopia, visual field defect,* speech disorder, confusion, somnolence, paresthesia, headache, emotional lability
▸ *CV:* Vasodilation, flushing, dysrhythmias, bradycardia, tachycardia, chest pain, hypertension
▸ *Resp:* *Hyperventilation,* dyspnea
▸ *GI:* *Nausea, vomiting,* hiccups
▸ *Derm:* *Pain at injection site*
▸ *Allergic:* **Anaphylaxis**
▸ *Misc:* Fatigue, rigors, shivering

Clinically important drug–drug interactions

▸ Convulsions and dysrhythmias when given in cases of mixed drug overdose

● NURSING CONSIDERATIONS

Assessment

▸ *History:* Flumazenil or benzodiazepine allergy, use of benzodiazepines for control of a potentially life-threatening condition, signs of serious cyclic antidepressant overdose, head injury, respiratory depression, neuromuscular blockade, psychiatric illness, liver disease, alcohol or drug dependency, benzodiazepine abstinence syndromes

---

Adverse effects in *Italics* are most common; those in **Bold** are life-threatening

▸ *Physical:* T, P, BP, R, ECG, I & O, IV site, neurologic checks, peripheral perfusion, degree of sedation, adventitious lung sounds, renal and liver function tests, serum drug levels

Implementation
▸ Carefully monitor T, P, BP, R, ECG, and neurologic status during administration.
▸ Maintain life-support equipment and emergency drugs on standby.
▸ Initiate seizure precautions.
▸ Secure patient's airway and ensure adequate ventilation before giving drug. Upon arousal, patients may attempt to remove endotracheal tubes or IV lines related to confusion and agitation.
▸ Recommend that drug be given as a series of small injections (not as a single bolus) to wake patient gradually. Do not rush the administration of this drug.
▸ Monitor clinical response carefully to determine effects of drug and need for repeated doses.
▸ To minimize pain and inflammation at IV site, insert IV into a large vein, and inject drug into a free-flowing IV infusion.
▸ Monitor for resedation or respiratory depression. Resedation is not likely to occur > 2 h after a 1-mg dose of flumazenil.
▸ If drug is mixed with any solution or drawn up in a syringe, use within 24 h or discard.

● **foscarnet sodium** *(foss kar' net)* Foscavir
Pregnancy Category C

Drug class
Antiviral

Indications
▸ Treatment of CMV retinitis in patients with AIDS
▸ Combination therapy with ganciclovir for patients who have relapsed after monotherapy with either drug
▸ Treatment of acyclovir-resistant mucocutaneous HSV infections in immunocompromised patients

Therapeutic actions
▸ Inhibits replications of all known herpes viruses by selectively inhibiting the pyrophosphate binding sites on DNA and reverse transcriptases

Adverse effects in *Italics* are most common; those in **Bold** are life-threatening

Contraindications/cautions
▸ **Contraindication:** foscarnet allergy
▸ **Cautions:** renal function impairment, hypovolemia, anemia, elderly patients, electrolyte imbalances

Available form
▸ *Injection:* 24 mg/mL

IV facts
Preparation
▸ May be given undiluted into a central line.
▸ If giving through a peripheral vein, dilute in D5W or 0.9%NS to make a 12 mg/mL solution.

Dosage
▸ Avoid IV bolus or rapid IV administration.
▸ *CMV retinitis:* 90 mg/kg IV (1.5- to 2-h infusion) q12h or 60 mg/kg IV (1-h infusion) q8h for 2–3 wk.
▸ *HSV infections:* 40 mg/kg IV (1-h infusion) q8–12h for 2–3 wk or until healed.
▸ *Maintenance dose:* 90–120 mg/kg/d IV given over 2 h.
▸ *Renal function impairment:* Individualize dosage according to patient's renal function. If creatinine clearance falls below 0.4 mL/min/kg, discontinue therapy.

Compatibility
Do not give other drugs concurrently through the same IV line.

Incompatibility
Do not administer through the same IV as 30% dextrose, acyclovir, amphotericin B, calcium solutions, diazepam, digoxin, diphenhydramine, dobutamine, droperidol, ganciclovir, gentamicin, haloperidol, leucovorin, LR, midazolam, morphine, pentamidine, phenytoin, prochlorperazine, promethazine, trimethoprim/sulfamethoxazole, trimetrexate, vancomycin.

TREATMENT OF OVERDOSE/ANTIDOTE
Discontinue drug or decrease dosage. Initiate general supportive and resuscitative measures. Hemodialysis and hydration may reduce drug plasma levels.

Pharmacokinetics
Route	Onset
IV	Immediate

$T_{1/2}$: 3.3–4 h (increased with impaired renal function)
Excretion: Urine

Adverse effects in *Italics* are most common; those in **Bold** are life-threatening

Adverse effects

▶ *CNS: **Seizures**, **death**, headache, dizziness, involuntary muscle contractions, vision abnormalities, neuropathy,* tremor, ataxia, dementia, stupor, meningitis, aphasia, abnormal coordination, EEG abnormalities, depression, confusion, anxiety, insomnia, somnolence, nervousness, cerebrovascular disorder, agitation

▶ *CV: **Cardiac arrest**,* hypertension, palpitations, tachycardia, first-degree AV block, nonspecific ST-T changes on ECG, hypotension, dysrhythmias

▶ *Resp: **Bronchospasm**, cough, dyspnea,* pneumonia, sinusitis, pharyngitis, rhinitis, respiratory insufficiency, pulmonary infiltration

▶ *GI: **Pancreatitis**, nausea, vomiting, diarrhea,* anorexia, abdominal pain, constipation, dysphagia, dyspepsia, rectal hemorrhage, dry mouth, melena, flatulence, ulcerative stomatitis, altered taste, thirst

▶ *GU: **Acute renal failure**, **abnormal renal function**, **nephrotoxicity**,* albuminuria, dysuria, polyuria, increased BUN, increased creatine phosphokinase, urethral disorder, urinary retention, urinary tract infection, nocturia

▶ *Derm:* Rash, injection site pain or inflammation, increased sweating, pruritus, skin ulceration, seborrhea

▶ *Hematologic: Anemia,* granulocytopenia, leukopenia, thrombocytopenia, platelet abnormalities, thrombosis

▶ *Metabolic: Hypokalemia, hypocalcemia, hypomagnesemia, hypophosphatemia or hyperphosphatemia, hyponatremia,* decreased weight

▶ *Misc: **Sepsis**,* fever, rigors, arthralgia, myalgia, malaise, pain, edema, lymphoma-like disorder, sarcoma

Clinically important drug–drug interactions

▶ Increased renal impairment with other nephrotoxic drugs
▶ Hypocalcemia with pentamidine

⬤ NURSING CONSIDERATIONS

Assessment

▶ *History:* Foscarnet allergy, renal function impairment, hypovolemia, anemia, age
▶ *Physical:* T, P, BP, R, ECG, I & O, IV site, weight, neurologic checks, skin assessment, cardiac auscultation, peripheral perfusion, edema, respiratory effort, adventitious lung sounds, presence of lesions, electrolyte levels, renal function tests, CBC, UA, specimens for culture and sensitivity

Adverse effects in *Italics* are most common; those in **Bold** are life-threatening

Implementation
- Always administer IV infusions using an IV infusion pump.
- Ensure patient is adequately hydrated; to prevent precipitation in renal tubules, recommended urine output is ≥ 500 mL/g of drug infused, especially during first 2 h after infusion.
- Carefully monitor renal function, electrolytes, and hydration status before and during therapy.
- Ensure adequate hydration during treatment. To reduce nephrotoxicity, give 500–1000 mL of NS or D5W prior to foscarnet infusions.
- Accidental skin or eye contact with foscarnet solution may cause local irritation and burning sensation. Flush exposed area with water.
- Stop infusion immediately at any report of tingling, paresthesias, numbness.
- Carefully assess IV site for phlebitis or infiltration.
- When diluted in NS to 12 mg/mL and stored at 5°C, drug is stable for 30 d. Do not freeze solution.

⬤ **fosphenytoin sodium** *(faws fen' i toe in)*
Cerebyx

Pregnancy Category D

Drug classes
Anticonvulsant agent
Hydantoin

Indications
- Short-term control of general convulsive status epilepticus
- Prevention and treatment of seizures occurring during or following neurosurgery
- Short-term substitute for oral phenytoin

Therapeutic actions
- Is converted to phenytoin after administration
- Is similar to anticonvulsant action of phenytoin
- Cellular mechanisms thought to be responsible for its anticonvulsant actions include modulation of voltage-dependent sodium and calcium channels of neurons, inhibition of calcium flux across neuronal membranes, and enhancement of sodium-potassium ATPase activity of neurons and glial cells

Contraindications/cautions
- **Contraindications:** hypersensitivity to hydantoins, sinus bradycardia, sinoatrial block, second- or third-degree AV heart block, Adams-Stokes syndrome

(contraindications continued on next page)

Adverse effects in *Italics* are most common; those in **Bold** are life-threatening

▶ *Physical:* T, BP, P, R, ECG, EEG, I & O, IV site, weight, neurologic checks, presence and type of seizure activity, skin assessment, vision exam, adventitious lung sounds, respiratory effort, bowel sounds, liver evaluation, liver and renal function tests, UA, CBC, blood and urine glucose; phosphate, phenytoin, and albumin levels

Implementation
▶ Continually monitor ECG, BP, and respiratory function during IV administration; continue for at least 10–20 min after infusion.
▶ Continue supportive measures, including use of an IV benzodiazepine, until drug becomes effective against seizures.
▶ Monitor infusion site carefully; drug solutions are very alkaline and irritating.
▶ Assess phenytoin blood levels 2 h after IV administration or 4 h after IM administration.
▶ Unbound phenytoin levels may be increased in patients with renal or hepatic disease or hypoalbuminemia; interpret values with caution. After IV doses, fosphenytoin conversion to phenytoin may be increased without a similar increase in phenytoin clearance, leading to the potential for increased frequency and severity of adverse reactions.
▶ This drug is recommended for short-term use only (up to 5 d); switch to oral phenytoin as soon as possible.
▶ Refrigerate drug; stable at room temperature for < 48 h.

⬤ **furosemide** *(fur ob' se mide)* Apo-Furosemide (CAN), Lasix

Pregnancy Category C

Drug class
Loop diuretic

Indications
▶ Edema associated with CHF, cirrhosis, renal disease (including nephrotic syndrome)
▶ Acute pulmonary edema (IV)
▶ Hypertension (oral)

Therapeutic action
▶ Inhibits the reabsorption of sodium and chloride from proximal and distal tubules and loop of Henle

Adverse effects in *Italics* are most common; those in **Bold** are life-threatening

Contraindications/cautions

▸ **Contraindications:** furosemide or sulfonamide allergy; tartrazine allergy (in oral solution), anuria, severe renal failure, untreated hepatic coma, increasing azotemia, electrolyte depletion

▸ **Cautions:** systemic lupus erythematosus (SLE), gout, diabetes, hypercholesteremia

Available forms

▸ *Injection:* 10 mg/mL
▸ *Tablets:* 20, 40, 80 mg
▸ *Oral elixir:* 10 mg/mL; 40 mg/5 mL

IV/IM facts
Preparation

▸ May be given undiluted or diluted in D5LR; D5W/0.9%NS; D5W; D10W; LR; Mannitol 20%; 3%NS; 0.9%NS; or Sodium Lactate (1/6 Molar) Injection.

Dosage

▸ *Edema:* 20–40 mg IV over 1–2 min or IM. May increase in increments of 20 mg in 2-h intervals until desired diuresis is achieved. Give this dose qd or bid. Give high-dose therapy as infusion at rate ≤ 4 mg/min.

▸ *Acute pulmonary edema:* 40 mg IV over 1–2 min. If response is not satisfactory within 1 h, increase to 80 mg IV over 1–2 min.

▸ *CHF and chronic renal failure:* IV bolus injection should not exceed 1 g/d given over 30 min.

Compatibility

Furosemide may be given through the same IV line as allopurinol, amifostine, amikacin, aztreonam, bleomycin, cefepime, cefmetazole, cisplatin, cladribine, cyclophosphamide, cytarabine, epinephrine, fentanyl, fludarabine, fluorouracil, foscarnet, gallium, granisetron, heparin, hydrocortisone, hydromorphone, indomethacin, kanamycin, leucovorin, lorazepam, melphalan, meropenem, methotrexate, mitomycin, nitroglycerin, norepinephrine, paclitaxel, piperacillin-tazobactam, potassium chloride, propofol, ranitidine, sargramostim, tacrolimus, teniposide, thiotepa, tobramycin, tolazoline, vitamin B complex with C.

Incompatibility

Do not administer through the same IV line as amsacrine, ciprofloxacin, diltiazem, droperidol, esmolol, filgrastim, fluconazole, gentamicin, hydralazine, idarubicin, metoclopramide, midazolam, milrinone, netilmicin, nicardipine, on-

Adverse effects in *Italics* are most common; those in **Bold** are life-threatening

dansetron, quinidine, thiopental, vecuronium, vinblastine, vincristine, vinorelbine.

Oral dosage
▸ *Edema:* 20–80 mg/d PO as a single dose. Depending on response, give second dose 6–8 h later. If response not satisfactory, increase by 20–40 mg no sooner than 6–8 h after previous dose. Give this dose qd or bid. Give up to 600 mg/d for patients with severe edema. Intermittent dosage schedule: give drug 2 to 4 consecutive d each wk; may be safer and more efficient.
▸ *Hypertension:* 40 mg PO bid adjusted according to patient response.
▸ *CHF and chronic renal failure:* Doses up to 2–2.5 g/d PO are well-tolerated and effective.

> **TREATMENT OF OVERDOSE/ANTIDOTE**
> Discontinue drug or decrease dosage. Initiate general supportive and resuscitative measures. Replace fluid and electrolyte losses. Carefully monitor urine and electrolyte output and serum electrolyte levels. Charcoal can reduce absorption of oral furosemide.

Pharmacokinetics

Route	Onset	Peak	Duration
IV/IM	Within 5 min	30 min	2 h
Oral	Within 60 min	60–120 min	6–8 h

Metabolism: Liver; $T_{1/2}$: 120 min (prolonged in renal failure, uremia)
Excretion: Urine

Adverse effects
▸ *CNS: Vertigo, dizziness, xanthopsia, paresthesias, weakness,* headache, blurred vision, tinnitus and hearing loss, restlessness
▸ *CV:* **Circulatory collapse,** *orthostatic hypotension, thrombophlebitis,* dehydration, dysrhythmias, hypotension, chronic aortitis
▸ *GI: Anorexia, nausea, vomiting, diarrhea, oral and gastric irritation, constipation,* cramping, pancreatitis, jaundice, ischemic hepatitis
▸ *GU:* **Renal failure,** frequency, glycosuria, urinary bladder spasm, hyperuricemia; increased BUN and creatinine
▸ *Derm: Photosensitivity, rash, urticaria, pruritus,* exfoliative dermatitis, erythema multiforme, local pain and irritation with IV use

Adverse effects in *Italics* are most common; those in **Bold** are life-threatening

▸ *Allergic:* Necrotizing angiitis, interstitial nephritis, systemic vasculitis
▸ *Hematologic: **Thrombocytopenia, leukopenia, anemia, agranulocytosis,*** purpura
▸ *Fluid/electrolytes: Hypochloremia, hypokalemia, hyponatremia, hypomagnesemia, hypocalcemia*
▸ *Misc: Muscle cramps/spasm,* metabolic alkalosis, fever, hyperglycemia

Clinically important drug–drug interactions
▸ Increased salicylate toxicity
▸ Antagonized skeletal muscle relaxing effects of tubocurarine and enhanced action of succinylcholine
▸ Increased plasma levels of propranolol
▸ Decreased arterial responsiveness to norepinephrine
▸ Decreased diuresis and natriuresis with NSAIDs
▸ Increased cardiac glycoside toxicity (secondary to hypokalemia)
▸ Aggravated postural hypotension with alcohol, barbiturates, narcotics
▸ Increased ototoxicity if taken with aminoglycoside antibiotics, cisplatin
▸ Increased lithium toxicity
▸ Reduced natriuretic and antihypertensive effects with probenecid
▸ Decreased urine and sodium excretion with indomethacin
▸ Increased profound diuresis and serious electrolyte abnormalities with thiazide diuretics
▸ Exaggerated diuresis with clofibrate
▸ Reduced diuretic effects with hydantoins (phenytoin)

◉ NURSING CONSIDERATIONS

Assessment
▸ *History:* Furosemide or sulfonamide allergy, tartrazine allergy (in oral solution), anuria, severe renal failure, untreated hepatic coma, increasing azotemia, electrolyte depletion, SLE, gout, diabetes mellitus, hypercholesteremia
▸ *Physical:* T, P, R, BP, I & O, ECG, IV site, weight, neurologic checks, skin assessment, skin turgor, mucous membranes, eighth cranial nerve function, hearing, peripheral perfusion, orthostatic BP, respiratory effort, adventitious lung sounds, liver evaluation, bowel sounds, CBC, serum electrolytes (including magnesium and calcium), serum glucose, liver and renal function tests, serum uric acid, UA, urine electrolytes

Implementation
▸ Closely monitor serum electrolytes, liver function, and CBC.

Adverse effects in *Italics* are most common; those in **Bold** are life-threatening

- Give with food or milk to prevent GI upset.
- Give single dose early in day so increased urination will not disturb sleep.
- Weigh patient daily to monitor fluid changes.
- Minimize postoral hypotension by helping the patient slowly change positions.
- Reduce dosage if given with other antihypertensives; readjust dosages gradually as BP responds.
- Evaluate for hypokalemia as evidenced by muscle weakness, fatigue, paralytic ileus, ECG changes (flat or inverted T wave, U wave, ST segment depression, atrial and ventricular dysrhythmias), anorexia, nausea, vomiting, abdominal distention, dizziness, and polyuria.
- Carefully assess fluid balance. Too frequent administration may lead to profound water loss, electrolyte depletion, dehydration, reduced blood volume, and circulatory collapse with possibility of vascular thrombosis and embolism.
- Provide diet rich in potassium or supplemental potassium.
- Protect drug from light, which may discolor tablets or solution; do not use discolored drug or solution.

G

● **ganciclovir sodium** *(gan sye' kloe vir)* DHPG
Cytovene

Pregnancy Category C

Drug class
Antiviral

Indications
- Treatment of cytomegalovirus (CMV) retinitis in immunocompromised patients, including patients with AIDS (parenteral)
- Prevention of CMV disease in transplant recipients at risk for CMV disease (parenteral)
- Alternative to IV for maintenance treatment of CMV retinitis (oral)
- Prevention of CMV disease in individuals with advanced HIV infection who are at risk of developing CMV disease (oral)
- Unlabeled use: Treatment of other CMV infections in immunocompromised patients

Therapeutic actions
- Antiviral activity; inhibits viral DNA replication in CMV

Adverse effects in *Italics* are most common; those in **Bold** are life-threatening

> ## Contraindications/cautions
> ▸ **Contraindications:** ganciclovir or acyclovir allergy
> ▸ **Cautions:** renal function impairment, retinal pathology, preexisting cytopenias; cytopenic reaction to drugs, chemicals, or irradiation; elderly, hypovolemia

Available forms
▸ *Powder for injection:* 500 mg/vial
▸ *Capsules:* 250, 500 mg

IV facts
Preparation
▸ Wear gloves when reconstituting or handling drug.
▸ Reconstitute powder by injecting 10 mL of Sterile Water for Injection into vial. Do not use Bacteriostatic Water for Injection because it will precipitate. Shake vial to dissolve drug. Discard vial if any particulate matter or discoloration is seen. Reconstituted solution in vial is stable at room temperature for 12 h. Do not refrigerate reconstituted solution.
▸ Add appropriate amount to 100 mL D5W; LR; 0.9%NS; or Ringer's Injection to achieve a concentration ≤ 10 mg/mL.

Dosage
▸ Avoid IV bolus or rapid IV administration.
▸ *CMV retinitis:* **Induction:** 5 mg/kg IV over 1 h q12h for 14–21 d. **Maintenance:** 5 mg/kg/d IV over 1 h 7 d/wk or 6 mg/kg/d 5 d/wk.
▸ *Prevention of CMV disease in transplant recipients:* 5 mg/kg IV over 1 h q12h for 7–14 d, followed by 5 mg/kg/d once daily for 7 d/wk or 6 mg/kg/d for 5 d/wk.
▸ *Renal function impairment:* Decrease dosage and increase dosing interval. Dosage for patients undergoing hemodialysis should not exceed 1.25 mg/kg 3 times/week following each hemodialysis session.

Compatibility
Ganciclovir may be given through the same IV line as allopurinol, cisplatin, cyclophosphamide, enalaprilat, filgrastim, fluconazole, granisetron, melphalan, methotrexate, paclitaxel, propofol, tacrolimus, teniposide, thiotepa.

Incompatibility
Do not administer through the same IV line as aldesleukin, amifostine, amsacrine, aztreonam, cefepime, cytarabine, doxorubicin, fludarabine, foscarnet, ondansetron, piperacillin-tazobactam, sargramostim, vinorelbine.

Adverse effects in *Italics* are most common; those in **Bold** are life-threatening

Oral dosage
▶ Oral ganciclovir is associated with a faster rate of CMV retinitis progression.
▶ *CMV retinitis:* After IV induction treatment, 1000 mg PO tid with food or 500 mg PO 6 times a day q3h with food while awake.
▶ *Prevention of CMV disease in patients with advanced HIV infection:* 1000 mg PO tid with food.

> **TREATMENT OF OVERDOSE/ANTIDOTE**
> Discontinue drug or decrease dosage. Initiate general supportive and resuscitative measures. Hemodialysis may reduce drug plasma levels. Maintain adequate hydration. Consider use of hematopoietic growth factors.

Pharmacokinetics

Route	Onset	Duration
IV	Immediate	1 h
PO	Slow	2–4 h

$T_{1/2}$: 3.5 h (IV); 4.8 h (PO)
Excretion: Urine

Adverse effects
▶ *CNS:* Dreams, ataxia, coma, confusion, dizziness, headache, agitation, amnesia, anxiety, confusion, depression, emotional lability
▶ *CV:* Dysrhythmias, hypertension, hypotension, vasodilation, chest pain, edema
▶ *Resp:* Cough, dyspnea, pharyngitis
▶ *GI:* **Pancreatitis, hemorrhage,** nausea, vomiting, dyspepsia, esophagitis, abnormal liver function tests, hepatitis, melena
▶ *GU:* Abnormal creatinine clearance, increased BUN, kidney failure, urinary frequency, UTI
▶ *Derm: Injection site inflammation,* acne, alopecia, dry skin, fixed eruption, herpes simplex, rash, skin discoloration, urticaria
▶ *Hematologic:* **Granulocytopenia, thrombocytopenia, anemia, leukopenia**
▶ *Musc/Skel:* Arthralgia, bone pain, leg cramps, myalgia
▶ *Metabolic:* **Sepsis, multiple organ failure,** weight loss, hypoglycemia
▶ *Misc: Fever,* asthenia, chills, retinal detachment

Clinically important drug–drug interactions
▶ Increased toxicity with dapsone, pentamidine, flucytosine, vincristine, vinblastine, adriamycin, amphotericin B,

Adverse effects in *Italics* are most common; those in **Bold** are life-threatening

trimethoprim/sulfamethoxazole combinations, nucleoside analogs
- Increased seizures with imipenem-cilastatin
- Increased serum creatinine with cyclosporine, amphotericin B
- Increased granulocytopenia and anemia with zidovudine
- Decreased renal clearance with probenecid

● NURSING CONSIDERATIONS

Assessment

- *History:* Ganciclovir or acyclovir allergy, renal function impairment, retinal pathology, preexisting cytopenias, cytopenic reaction to drugs, chemicals, irradiation; age, hypovolemia
- *Physical:* T, P, BP, R, ECG, I & O, IV site, weight, neurologic checks, ophthalmologic exam, cardiac auscultation, peripheral perfusion, edema, adventitious lung sounds, skin color, presence of lesions, electrolyte levels, renal and liver function tests, CBC, UA, specimens for culture and sensitivity

Implementation

- Always administer IV infusions using an IV infusion pump.
- Carefully monitor renal function, hematologic, electrolytes, and hydration status before and during therapy.
- Ensure adequate hydration to prevent kidney damage.
- Ganciclovir has caused cancer, chromosome damage, and suppressed fertility in animals.
- Carefully assess IV site for phlebitis or infiltration; avoid IM or SC administration.
- Administer drug with food to increase bioavailability.
- Avoid direct contact of drug to skin or mucous membranes. If contact occurs, wash thoroughly with soap and water; rinse eyes with water. Do not open or crush capsules.
- Follow institutional guidelines for disposal of antineoplastic drugs.
- Use infusion within 24 h of dilution.
- Do not freeze solution.

● **gentamicin sulfate** *(jen ta mye' sin)* **Parenteral, intrathecal:** Alcomicin (CAN), Cidomycin (CAN), Garamycin; **Topical dermatologic cream, ointment:** Garamycin; G-myticin; **Ophthalmic:** Garamycin, Gentak, Gentacidin, Genoptic S.O.P.; **Gentamicin-impregnated PMMA beads:** Septopal; **Gentamicin liposome injection:** Maitec

Pregnancy Category D

Drug class
Aminoglycoside

Adverse effects in *Italics* are most common; those in **Bold** are life-threatening

Indications
Parenteral
▸ Treatment of serious infections caused by susceptible strains of *Pseudomonas aeruginosa, Proteus* species, *Escherichia coli, Klebsiella* species, *Enterobacter* species, *Serratia* species, *Citrobacter* species, *Staphylococcus* species
▸ Effective in bacterial septicemia and serious bacterial infections of the CNS, urinary tract, respiratory tract, GI tract, skin, bone, and soft tissue
▸ Treatment of serious infections when causative organisms are not known (often in conjunction with a penicillin or cephalosporin)
▸ Used with carbenicillin for treatment of life-threatening infections caused by *P. aeruginosa;* used with penicillin for treatment of endocarditis caused by group D streptococci
▸ Unlabeled use: with clindamycin as an alternative regimen in pelvic inflammatory disease (PID)
Intrathecal
▸ For serious CNS infections caused by susceptible *Pseudomonas* species
Ophthalmic preparations
▸ Treatment of superficial ocular infections due to strains of microorganisms susceptible to gentamicin
Topical dermatologic preparation
▸ Treatment of infection due to susceptible organisms amenable to local treatment; prophylaxis of infection with minor cuts, wounds, burns, and skin abrasions; aid to healing
Gentamicin-impregnated PMAA beads on surgical wire
▸ Orphan drug use: treatment of chronic osteomyelitis of post-traumatic, postoperative, or hematogenous origin
Gentamicin liposome injection
▸ Orphan drug use: treatment of disseminated *Mycobacterium avium-intracellulare* infection

Therapeutic actions
▸ Bactericidal: inhibits protein synthesis in susceptible strains of gram-negative bacteria; binds to the 30S subunit of bacterial ribosomes, blocking the recognition step in protein synthesis, causing misreading of the genetic code; ribosomes separate from messenger RNA, leading to cell death

Contraindications/cautions
▸ **Contraindications:** allergy to any aminoglycoside; epithelial herpes simplex keratitis, vaccinia, varicella, fungal
(contraindications continued on next page)

Adverse effects in *Italics* are most common; those in **Bold** are life-threatening

infections of ocular structures, mycobacterial infections of the eye (ophthalmic preparations)
• **Cautions:** renal dysfunction, sulfite sensitivity, preexisting hearing loss, extensive burns, neuromuscular disorders (myasthenia gravis, parkinsonism), dehydration, elderly patients, concurrent use of other nephrotoxic drugs

Available forms
• *Injection:* 10, 40 mg/mL
• *Ophthalmic solution:* 3 mg/mL
• *Ophthalmic ointment:* 3 mg/g
• *Topical ointment:* 0.1%
• *Topical cream:* 0.1%
• *Ointment:* 1 mg
• *Cream:* 1 mg

IV/IM/Intrathecal facts
Preparation
• **IV:** Dilute single dose in 50–200 mL of D5W; D10W; Fructose 5% in water; Invert Sugar 7.5% with electrolytes; Mannitol 20%; 0.9%NS; or Ringer's Injection. Do not mix with any other drugs.
• **IM:** Give undiluted.
• **Intrathecal:** Use only 2 mg/mL intrathecal preparation without preservatives. Allow about 10% of the estimated total CSF volume to flow into the syringe and mix with the gentamicin.

Dosage
• *Loading dose:* A 1- to 2-mg/kg IV loading dose may be given over 0.5–2 h followed by a maintenance dose.
• *Serious infections, normal renal function:* 3 mg/kg/d IV over 0.5–2 h or IM in 3 equal doses q8h.
• *Life-threatening infections:* Up to 5 mg/kg/d IV over 0.5–2 h or IM in 3–4 equal doses. Reduce to 3 mg/kg/d when clinically indicated.
• *Prevention of bacterial endocarditis:* 1.5 mg/kg (not to exceed 80 mg) IV or IM 0.5 h before dental, oral, or GU, GI, or upper respiratory tract procedures. Usually given with ampicillin.
• *PID:* 2 mg/kg IV followed by 1.5 mg/kg IV tid. Also give clindamycin as ordered. Continue for at least 4 d and at least 48 h after patient improves, then continue clindamycin.
• *Intrathecal:* 4–8 mg/d over 3–5 min with the bevel of the needle directed upward.
• *"Once-daily dosing":* 5 or 7 mg/kg (using ideal body weight) IV over 60 min. Obtain serum drug concentration 8–10 h after starting the infusion. Use the 5- or 7-mg nomogram to determine the dosing interval (usually q24h, q36h, or q48h).
• *Renal function impairment:* Adjust dosage based on degree

Adverse effects in *Italics* are most common; those in **Bold** are life-threatening

G

of renal impairment, serum creatinine clearance, and peak and trough gentamicin concentrations. Give smaller dosage or adjust the interval between doses.

Therapeutic serum levels
▶ **Trough:** 0.5–2 mcg/mL
▶ **Peak:** 5–10 mcg/mL

Compatibility
Gentamicin may be given through the same IV line as acyclovir, amifostine, amiodarone, amsacrine, atracurium, aztreonam, ciprofloxacin, cyclophosphamide, cytarabine, diltiazem, enalaprilat, esmolol, famotidine, fluconazole, fludarabine, foscarnet, granisetron, hydromorphone, IL-2, insulin, labetalol, lorazepam, magnesium sulfate, melphalan, meperidine, meropenem, midazolam, morphine, multivitamins, ondansetron, paclitaxel, pancuronium, perphenazine, sargramostim, tacrolimus, teniposide, theophylline, thiotepa, tolazoline, vecuronium, vinorelbine, vitamin B complex with C, zidovudine.

Incompatibility
Do not administer through the same IV line as allopurinol, furosemide, heparin, hetastarch, idarubicin, indomethacin, iodipamide, propofol, warfarin.

Other dosages
▶ *Ophthalmic solution:* 1–2 drops into affected eye(s) q4h; up to 2 drops hourly for severe infections.
▶ *Ophthalmic ointment:* Apply small amount to affected eye(s) bid to tid.
▶ *Dermatologic preparations:* Apply tid–qid to affected area. Cover with sterile bandage if desired.

TREATMENT OF OVERDOSE/ANTIDOTE
Discontinue drug or decrease dosage. Initiate general supportive and resuscitative measures. Support respiration because neuromuscular blockade or respiratory paralysis may occur. Adequately hydrate patient, and carefully monitor fluid balance, creatinine clearance, and drug levels. Peritoneal dialysis and hemodialysis will remove the drug from the blood. Complexation with ticarcillin or carbenicillin may lower high serum concentrations.

Pharmacokinetics
Route	Onset	Peak
IV	Immediate	End of infusion
IM	Rapid	1 h

$T_{1/2}$: 2 h normal renal function; 24–60 h end-stage renal disease
Excretion: Urine

Adverse effects in *Italics* are most common; those in **Bold** are life-threatening

Adverse effects

‣ *CNS:* **Neuromuscular blockade, ototoxicity, auditory and vestibular toxicity, encephalopathy, convulsions,** acute organic brain syndrome, depression, pseudotumor cerebri, headache, confusion, lethargy, muscle twitching, myasthenia gravis-like syndrome, numbness, peripheral neuropathy, skin tingling

‣ *CV:* Hypotension, hypertension

‣ *Resp:* **Respiratory depression, apnea, laryngeal edema**

‣ *GI:* Nausea, vomiting, anorexia, weight loss, stomatitis, splenomegaly, transient hepatomegaly, hypersalivation; increased AST, ALT, bilirubin, LDH

‣ *GU:* **Nephrotoxicity,** proteinuria, increased creatinine and BUN, casts in urine, oliguria

‣ *Derm: Pain, irritation, and arachnoiditis at intrathecal injection sites*

‣ *Allergic:* **Anaphylaxis,** purpura, rash, urticaria, itching

‣ *Hematologic:* **Granulocytopenia, leukopenia, leukocytosis, thrombocytopenia, eosinophilia, pancytopenia, anemia,** hemolytic anemia, increased or decreased reticulocyte count; decreased serum calcium, sodium, potassium, and magnesium

‣ *Misc: Superinfections,* fever, joint pain, leg cramps

Ophthalmic Preparations

‣ *Derm:* Local transient irritation, burning, stinging, itching, angioneurotic edema, urticaria, vesicular and maculopapular dermatitis

Topical Dermatologic Preparations

‣ *Derm:* Possible photosensitization, superinfections

Clinically important drug–drug interactions

‣ Increased ototoxic, nephrotoxic, and neurotoxic effects with other aminoglycosides, cephalosporins, loop diuretics, enflurane, methoxyflurane, vancomycin

‣ Increased neuromuscular blockade and muscular paralysis with depolarizing and nondepolarizing blocking agents

‣ Inactivation of both drugs if mixed with beta-lactam-type antibiotics (space doses with concomitant therapy)

‣ Increased bactericidal effect with penicillins, cephalosporins, carbenicillin, ticarcillin

‣ Increased respiratory paralysis and renal dysfunction with polypeptide antibiotics

Adverse effects in *Italics* are most common; those in **Bold** are life-threatening

● NURSING CONSIDERATIONS

Assessment

▸ *History:* Allergy to any aminoglycoside; epithelial herpes simplex keratitis, vaccinia, varicella, fungal infections of ocular structures; mycobacterial infections of the eye, renal dysfunction, sulfite sensitivity, preexisting hearing loss, extensive burns, neuromuscular disorders (myasthenia gravis, parkinsonism), hypovolemia, age, concurrent use of other nephrotoxic drugs

▸ *Physical:* T, P, R, BP, I & O, weight, neurologic checks, eighth cranial nerve function, skin assessment, adventitious lung sounds, bowel sounds, liver evaluation, UA, serum electrolytes, liver and renal function tests, CBC, culture and sensitivity tests of infected area

Implementation

▸ Obtain specimens for culture and sensitivity of infected area before beginning therapy. May begin drug before results are available.

▸ Have emergency equipment (defibrillator, drugs, oxygen, intubation equipment) on standby in case anaphylactic reaction occurs.

▸ Assess for evidence of anaphylaxis; if suspected, discontinue drug immediately and notify provider.

▸ Monitor for occurrence of superinfections; treat as appropriate.

▸ Separate administration of other antibiotics by at least 1 h.

▸ Cleanse area before applying dermatologic preparations.

▸ Ensure adequate hydration of patient before and during therapy.

▸ Monitor renal function tests, complete blood counts, and serum drug levels during therapy. Adjust dosage as indicated.

▸ Febrile and anemic patients may have shorter drug half-life. Severely burned patients may have a significantly decreased half-life and lower serum drug concentrations.

▸ Solution for injection is colorless to slightly yellow.

● **glycopyrrolate** *(glye koe pye' roe late)* Robinul, Robinul Forte

Pregnancy Category C (parenteral)

Pregnancy Category B

Drug classes
Anticholinergic (quaternary)
Antimuscarinic agent
Antispasmodic

Indications
▸ To reduce salivary, tracheobronchial, and pharyngeal secretions preoperatively (parenteral)
▸ To reduce the volume and free acidity of gastric secretions (parenteral)
▸ To block cardiac vagal inhibitory reflexes during intubation (parenteral)
▸ To protect against the peripheral muscarinic effects (eg, bradycardia, excessive secretions) of cholinergic agents (neostigmine, pyridostigmine) that are used to reverse the neuromuscular blockade produced by nondepolarizing neuromuscular junction blockers (parenteral)
▸ Adjunctive therapy in the treatment of peptic ulcer (oral)
▸ Unlabeled use: bronchial asthma

Therapeutic actions
▸ Inhibits the action of acetylcholine on structures innervated by postganglionic cholinergic nerves and on smooth muscles that respond to acetylcholine but lack cholinergic innervation; diminishes volume and free acidity of gastric secretions and controls excessive pharyngeal, tracheal, and bronchial secretions
▸ Antagonizes muscarinic symptoms (bronchorrhea, bronchospasm, bradycardia, intestinal hypermotility) induced by cholinergic drugs

Contraindications/cautions
▸ **Contraindications:** glycopyrrolate allergy, glaucoma, obstructive uropathy, obstructive disease of the gastrointestinal tract, paralytic ileus, intestinal atony of the elderly or debilitated patient, unstable cardiovascular status in acute hemorrhage, severe ulcerative colitis, toxic megacolon complicating ulcerative colitis, myasthenia gravis
▸ **Cautions:** asthma, diarrhea, tachycardia, coronary artery disease, CHF, dysrhythmias, hypertension, hyperthyroidism, autonomic neuropathy, hepatic or renal disease, ulcerative colitis, prostatic hypertrophy, hiatal hernia, elderly patients

Available forms
▸ *Injection:* 0.2 mg/mL
▸ *Tablets:* 1, 2 mg

IV/IM facts
Preparation
▸ May be given undiluted or diluted in D5W; D5W/0.45%NS; 0.9%NS; or Ringer's injection. If diluted in LR, use solution immediately.

Adverse effects in *Italics* are most common; those in **Bold** are life-threatening

Dosage
▶ *Peptic ulcer:* 0.1–0.2 mg IV or IM tid to qid. Give each 0.2 mg over 1–2 min. Adjust dose and frequency according to patient's response.
▶ *Reversal of neuromuscular blockade:* 0.2 mg IV for each 1.0 mg neostigmine or 5.0 mg of pyridostigmine. May mix these drugs in the same syringe and administer simultaneously. Give each 0.2 mg over 1–2 min.
▶ *Preanesthetic medication:* 0.004 mg/kg (0.002 mg/lb) IM 30–60 min prior to anesthesia.

Compatibility
Glycopyrrolate may be given through the same IV line as propofol.

Incompatibility
Drug is incompatible with drugs or solutions with a pH > 6.

Oral dosage
▶ **Initial:** 1 mg PO tid or 2 mg PO bid to tid. **Maintenance:** 1 mg PO bid.

TREATMENT OF OVERDOSE/ANTIDOTE
Discontinue drug or decrease dosage. Initiate general supportive and resuscitative measures. Treat peripheral anticholinergic effects with neostigmine 0.25 mg IV. Repeat q5–10min until anticholinergic overactivity is reversed or up to 2.5 mg. If CNS symptoms of excitement, restlessness, convulsion, or psychotic behavior occur, give physostigmine 0.5–2 mg IV and repeat as needed up to 5 mg. Treat fever symptomatically.

Pharmacokinetics

Route	Onset	Peak	Duration
IV	1 min		
IM		30–45 min	2–7 h
Oral		60 min	8–12 h

Metabolism: Hepatic; $T_{1/2}$: 2.5 h
Excretion: Feces, urine

Adverse effects
▶ *CNS: Blurred vision,* drowsiness, mydriasis, cycloplegia, photophobia, pupil dilation, increased intraocular pressure, headache, nervousness, weakness, dizziness, insomnia, confusion
▶ *CV:* Palpitations, tachycardia
▶ *GI: Dry mouth,* altered taste perception, nausea, vomiting, dysphagia, constipation, bloated feeling, paralytic ileus, xerostomia

Adverse effects in *Italics* are most common; those in **Bold** are life-threatening

▸ *GU: Urinary hesitancy and retention,* impotence
▸ *Allergic:* **Anaphylaxis,** urticaria
▸ *Misc:* Decreased sweating and predisposition to heat prostration; fever, nasal congestion

Clinically important drug–drug interactions
▸ Decreased antipsychotic effectiveness of phenothiazines; increased anticholinergic side effects

● NURSING CONSIDERATIONS

Assessment
▸ *History:* Glycopyrrolate allergy, glaucoma, obstructive uropathy, obstructive disease of the gastrointestinal tract, paralytic ileus, intestinal atony of the elderly or debilitated patient, unstable cardiovascular status in acute hemorrhage, severe ulcerative colitis, toxic megacolon complicating ulcerative colitis, myasthenia gravis, asthma, diarrhea, coronary artery disease, CHF, hypertension, hyperthyroidism, autonomic neuropathy, hepatic or renal disease, ulcerative colitis, prostatic hypertrophy, hiatal hernia, age
▸ *Physical:* T, P, BP, R, I & O, weight, neurologic checks, skin assessment, intraocular pressure, vision, hydration status, adventitious lung sounds, respiratory effort, abdominal assessment, pain assessment, liver assessment, prostate palpation, liver and renal function tests

Implementation
▸ Assess T, P, R, and BP frequently during parenteral therapy.
▸ Have emergency equipment (defibrillator, drugs, oxygen, intubation equipment) on standby in case anaphylaxis or adverse reaction occurs.
▸ Monitor frequency and type of bowel movements.
▸ Ensure adequate hydration; provide environmental control (temperature) to prevent hyperpyrexia.
▸ Have patient void before each dose if urinary retention is a problem.

H

● **haloperidol**

● **haloperidol decanoate** *(ha loe per' i dole)*

Apo-Haloperidol (CAN), Haldol, Haldol Decanoate 50, Haldol Decanoate 100, Haldol LA (CAN),

Adverse effects in *Italics* are most common; those in **Bold** are life-threatening

Novo-Peridol (CAN), Peridol (CAN),
PMS-Haloperidol LA (CAN)

⬤ **haloperidol lactate** Haldol
Pregnancy Category C

Drug classes
Antipsychotic drug
Butyrophenone

Indications
▶ Management of manifestations of psychotic disorders
▶ Control of tics and vocalizations in Gilles de la Tourette's syndrome
▶ Prolonged parenteral therapy of chronic schizophrenia (haloperidol decanoate)
▶ Unlabeled uses: control of nausea and vomiting; control of acute psychiatric situations (parenteral); treat intractable hiccoughs

Therapeutic actions
▶ Mechanism not fully understood; blocks effects of dopamine and increases its turnover rate
▶ Produces sedative, anticholinergic effects; may contribute to orthostatic hypotension and extrapyramidal symptoms

Contraindications/cautions
▶ **Contraindications:** haloperidol allergy, coma or severe CNS depression, Parkinson's disease
▶ **Cautions:** severe CV disorders, concurrent use of anticonvulsant or anticoagulant medications, seizures, EEG abnormalities, thyrotoxicosis, respiratory impairment, glaucoma, prostatic hypertrophy, epilepsy or history of epilepsy, breast cancer, decreased renal function, allergy to aspirin if giving the 1-, 2-, 5-, or 10-mg tablets (these tablets contain tartrazine)

Available forms
▶ *Injection:* 5 mg/mL (lactate); 50, 100 mg/mL (decanoate)
▶ *Tablets:* 0.5, 1, 2, 5, 10, 20 mg
▶ *Concentrate:* 2 mg/mL

IV/IM facts
Preparation
▶ Check label carefully; use only haloperidol lactate.
▶ For direct IV or IM injection, give undiluted.
▶ For intermittent IV infusion, dilute drug in D5W.

Adverse effects in *Italics* are most common; those in **Bold** are life-threatening

Dosage

▸ Not approved for IV use; IV use is unlabeled.
▸ *Acute psychiatric situations:* 2–30 mg IV q1h at a rate of 5 mg/min. Adjust dosage based on patient's response.
▸ *Intractable hiccoughs:* 3–15 mg IV in divided doses.
▸ *IM (haloperidol lactate):* 2–5 mg (up to 10–30 mg) q60min or q4–8h IM as needed to control promptly acutely agitated patients with severe symptoms. Switch to oral dosage as soon as feasible, using total IM dosage in previous 24 h as a guide to total daily oral dosage. Give first oral dose 12–24 h after last parenteral dose.
▸ *IM (haloperidol decanoate):* 10–15 times the daily oral dose; repeat at 4-wk intervals. Give by deep IM injection with a 21-gauge needle. Do not inject > 3 mL/site.

Compatibility

Haloperidol may be given through the same IV line as amifostine, amsacrine, aztreonam, cimetidine, cladribine, dobutamine, dopamine, famotidine, filgrastim, fludarabine, granisetron, lidocaine, lorazepam, melphalan, midazolam, nitroglycerin, norepinephrine, ondansetron, paclitaxel, phenylephrine, propofol, sufentanil, tacrolimus, teniposide, theophylline, thiotepa, vinorelbine.

Incompatibility

Do not administer through the same IV line as allopurinol, cefepime, cefmetazole, fluconazole, foscarnet, gallium, heparin, piperacillin-tazobactam, sargramostim.

Oral dosage

▸ Full clinical effects may require 6 wk–6 mo of therapy. Individualize dosage according to the needs and response of each patient. Debilitated and geriatric patients and patients with a history of adverse reactions to neuroleptic drugs may require lower dosage.
▸ *Initial oral dosage range:* 0.5–2 mg PO bid–tid with moderate symptoms. 3–5 mg PO bid–tid for more resistant patients. 0.5–2 mg PO bid or tid for elderly or debilitated patients. 3–5 mg PO bid or tid for chronic or resistant patients. Daily dosages up to 100 mg/d (or more) have been used, but safety of prolonged use has not been demonstrated. For maintenance, reduce dosage to lowest effective level.

TREATMENT OF OVERDOSE/ANTIDOTE

Discontinue drug or decrease dosage. Initiate general supportive and resuscitative measures. For oral overdosage, initiate gastric lavage or emesis and give activated charcoal.

(treatment continued on next page)

Adverse effects in *Italics* are most common; those in **Bold** are life-threatening

Treat hypotension and circulatory collapse with IV fluids, plasma, albumin, and vasopressors. Avoid epinephrine. Treat severe extrapyramidal reactions with antiparkinson drugs. Closely monitor ECG for dysrhythmias and prolonged QT. Treat dysrhythmias with antidysrhythmics.

Pharmacokinetics

Route	Onset	Peak
IM	Rapid	20 min
IM, decanoate	Slow	6 d
Oral	Varies	3–5 h

Metabolism: Hepatic; $T_{1/2}$: 21–24 h, 3 wk for decanoate
Excretion: Urine, bile

Adverse effects

▶ *CNS:* **Neuroleptic malignant syndrome** (extrapyramidal symptoms, hyperthermia, autonomic disturbances, elevated CPK, rhabdomyolysis, acute renal failure); *drowsiness; extrapyramidal syndromes (pseudoparkinsonism, dystonia, akathisia);* insomnia, restlessness, anxiety, euphoria, agitation, depression, lethargy, headache, confusion, exacerbation of psychotic symptoms, vertigo, headache, blurred vision
▶ *CV:* Hypotension, postural hypotension, hypertension, tachycardia, prolonged QT interval
▶ *Resp:* **Bronchospasm, laryngospasm,** respiratory depression, increased depth of respiration
▶ *GI:* Anorexia, constipation, diarrhea, hypersalivation, dyspepsia, nausea, vomiting, dry mouth, impaired liver function, jaundice
▶ *Allergic:* **Anaphylaxis,** jaundice, urticaria, angioneurotic edema, laryngeal edema, photosensitivity, eczema, asthma, exfoliative dermatitis
▶ *Hematologic:* Mild leukopenia and leukocytosis, anemia
▶ *Endocrine:* Breast engorgement in females, mastalgia, menstrual irregularities, gynecomastia, impotence, increased libido, hyperglycemia, hypoglycemia, hyponatremia
▶ *Misc:* Urinary retention, diaphoresis, priapism

Clinically important drug–drug interactions

▶ Decreased plasma levels with barbiturates, carbamazepine, phenytoin
▶ Potentiates CNS depressants, anesthetics, opiates, alcohol
▶ Severe extrapyramidal reactions and toxic effects with fluoxetine, lithium, methyldopa

Adverse effects in *Italics* are most common; those in **Bold** are life-threatening

● NURSING CONSIDERATIONS

Assessment
▸ *History:* Haloperidol or aspirin allergy, coma or severe CNS depression, Parkinson's disease, severe CV disorders, concurrent use of anticonvulsant or anticoagulant medications, seizures, EEG abnormalities, thyrotoxicosis, respiratory impairment, glaucoma, prostatic hypertrophy, epilepsy or history of epilepsy, breast cancer, decreased renal function
▸ *Physical:* T, R, P, BP, I & O, ECG, neurologic checks, behavior, mental status, intraocular pressure, orthostatic BP, adventitious lung sounds, bowel sounds, presence of nausea or vomiting, liver evaluation, prostate size, CBC, UA; thyroid, liver and kidney function tests

Implementation
▸ Haloperidol decanoate is not for IV use.
▸ Assess for evidence of extrapyramidal symptoms, tardive dyskinesia, and neuroleptic malignant syndrome.
▸ Monitor patient response; adjust dosage to lowest effective dose.
▸ Have emergency equipment (defibrillator, drugs, oxygen, intubation equipment) on standby in case anaphylaxis or adverse reaction occurs.
▸ Initiate fall precautions; assist patient if he or she is out of bed.
▸ Minimize postural hypotension by helping the patient change positions slowly.
▸ Withdraw drug gradually when patient has been on maintenance therapy to avoid withdrawal-emergent dyskinesias.
▸ Discontinue drug if serum creatinine or BUN becomes abnormal or if WBC count is depressed.
▸ Monitor elderly patients for dehydration; institute remedial measures promptly; sedation and decreased thirst related to CNS effects can lead to severe dehydration.
▸ Consult provider about dosage reduction and use of anticholinergic antiparkinsonian drugs (controversial) if extrapyramidal effects occur.

● **heparin** *(hep' ah rin)*

● **heparin sodium injection** Hepalean (CAN), Heparin Leo (CAN)

● **heparin sodium and 0.9% sodium chloride**

● heparin sodium and 0.45% sodium chloride   H

● heparin sodium lock flush solution
Heparin Lock Flush, Hep-Lock, Hepalean-Lok (CAN)

Pregnancy Category C

Drug class
Anticoagulant

Indications
▶ Prevention and treatment of venous thrombosis, pulmonary embolism, peripheral arterial embolism, and atrial fibrillation with embolization
▶ Diagnosis and treatment of disseminated intravascular coagulation (DIC)
▶ Prevention of clotting in arterial and heart surgery, blood transfusions, extracorporeal circulation, dialysis procedures, and blood samples
▶ Maintenance of patency of IV catheters
▶ Unlabeled uses: adjunct in therapy of coronary occlusion with acute MI, prevention of left ventricular thrombi and CVA post-MI, treatment of myocardial ischemia in USA refractory to conventional treatment, prevention of cerebral thrombosis in the evolving stroke

Therapeutic actions
▶ Small amounts of heparin in combination with antithrombin III inhibit thrombosis by inactivating Factor Xa and inhibiting the conversion of prothrombin to thrombin
▶ Once active thrombosis has developed, larger amounts of heparin inhibit further clotting by inactivating thrombin and preventing conversion of fibrinogen to fibrin
▶ Does not lyse existing clots but can prevent extension of existing clots
▶ Enhances lipoprotein lipase release, increases circulating free fatty acids, and reduces lipoprotein levels

Contraindications/cautions
▶ **Contraindications:** heparin, beef, or pig protein allergy (except in life-threatening conditions); severe thrombocytopenia; uncontrolled bleeding (except with DIC); any patient who cannot be monitored regularly with blood coagulation tests

(contraindications continued on next page)

Adverse effects in *Italics* are most common; those in **Bold** are life-threatening

- **Cautions:** women > 60 y at high risk for hemorrhage; dysbetalipoproteinemia; recent surgery or injury; subacute bacterial endocarditis; severe hypertension; during and immediately after spinal tap, spinal anesthesia, or major surgery (especially of brain, spinal cord, or eye); hemophilia; vascular purpuras; thrombocytopenia; ulcerative lesions; diverticulitis; ulcerative colitis; continuous tube drainage of stomach or small intestine; menstruation; liver disease with impaired hemostasis; severe renal disease, diabetes, hypoaldosteronism, hyperkalemia

Available forms
- *Injection:* 1000, 2000, 2500, 5000, 10,000, 20,000, 40,000 U/mL
- *Single dose:* 1000, 5000, 10,000, 20,000, 40,000 U/mL
- *Unit dose:* 1000, 2500, 5000, 7500, 10,000, 20,000 U/dose
- *Premixed IV infusion:* 1000 U/500 mL, 2000 U/1000 mL, 12,500 U/250 mL, 25,000 U/250 and 500 mL
- *Heparin Lock Flush:* 10, 100 U/mL

IV/SC facts
Preparation
- Withdraw appropriate dose from container.
- Direct injection may be given undiluted or diluted in 50 to 100 mL 0.9%NS.
- For a heparin infusion, use a premixed IV infusion or dilute 1,000 to 25,000 U in 250 to 500 mL D25W; Dextran 6% in 0.9%NS or D5W; Dextrose-Lactated Ringer's combinations; Dextrose-Ringer's injection combinations; Dextrose-saline combinations; Fat Emulsion 10%; Invert sugar 5% or 10% in 0.9%NS or water; Ionosol; Normosol R; 0.45%NS; 0.9%NS; or Ringer's injection. After dilution, invert container ≥ six times to ensure drug is adequately mixed.
- Select a concentrated solution (20,000–40,000 U/mL) for SC injection.

Dosage
- Adjust dosage according to coagulation tests. Dosage is adequate when the APTT is 1.5–2 times normal.
- *General anticoagulation:* **IV infusion:** 5000 U IV bolus dose followed by continuous infusion of 20,000–40,000 U/d IV. **Intermittent IV injection:** 10,000 U IV then 5000–10,000 U IV q4–6h. **SC:** First give 5000 U IV. Immediately follow with 10,000–20,000 U SC. Then give 8000–10,000 U SC q8h or 15,000–20,000 U SC q12h.
- *Prophylaxis of postoperative thromboembolism:* 5000 U by deep SC injection 2 h before surgery and q8–12h thereafter for 7 d or until patient is fully ambulatory.

Adverse effects in *Italics* are most common; those in **Bold** are life-threatening

- *Surgery of heart and blood vessels:* Not less than 150 U/kg; often 300 U/kg is used for procedures < 60 min and 400 U/kg for procedures > 60 min.
- *Blood transfusion:* 400–600 U/100 mL whole blood. Add 7500 U to 100 mL 0.9%NS; from this sterile solution, add 6–8 mL/100 mL of whole blood.
- *Clot prevention in blood samples:* Add 70–150 U to 10–20 mL of whole blood.
- *Extracorporal dialysis:* Follow equipment manufacturers' instructions.
- *Clearing of intermittent infusion sets:* 10–100 U injected to fill entire set to needle tip.

Titration Guide

heparin							
25,000 U in 250 mL							
U/h	mL/h	U/h	mL/h	U/h	mL/h	U/h	mL/h
500	5	900	9	1300	13	1700	17
600	6	1000	10	1400	14	1800	18
700	7	1100	11	1500	15	1900	19
800	8	1200	12	1600	16	2000	20

Compatibility

Heparin may be given through the same IV line as acyclovir, aldesleukin, allopurinol, amifostine, aminophylline, ampicillin, ampicillin-sulbactam, atracurium, atropine, aztreonam, betamethasone, bleomycin, calcium gluconate, cefazolin, cefotetan, ceftazidime, ceftriaxone, cephalothin, cephapirin, chlordiazepoxide, chlorpromazine, cimetidine, cisplatin, cladribine, clindamycin, cyanocobalamin, cyclophosphamide, cytarabine, dexamethasone, digoxin, diphenhydramine, dopamine, edrophonium, enalaprilat, epinephrine, erythromycin, esmolol, estrogens (conjugated), ethacrynate, famotidine, fentanyl, fluconazole, fludarabine, fluorouracil, foscarnet, furosemide, gallium, granisetron, hydralazine, hydrocortisone, hydromorphone, insulin (regular), isoproterenol, kanamycin, leucovorin, lidocaine, lorazepam, magnesium sulfate, melphalan, menadiol, meperidine, meropenem, methicillin, methotrexate, methoxamine, methyldopate, methylergonovine, metoclopramide, metronidazole, midazolam, milrinone, minocycline, mitomycin, morphine, nafcillin, neostigmine, nitroglycerin, nitroprusside sodium, norepinephrine, ondansetron, oxacillin, oxytocin, paclitaxel, pancuronium, penicillin G potassium, pentazocine, phytonadione, piperacillin, piperacillin-tazobactam, potassium chloride, prednisolone, procainamide, prochlor-

Adverse effects in *Italics* are most common; those in **Bold** are life-threatening

perazine, propofol, propranolol, pyridostigmine, ranitidine, sargramostim, scopolamine, sodium bicarbonate, streptokinase, succinylcholine, tacrolimus, teniposide, theophylline, thiotepa, ticarcillin, ticarcillin-clavulanate, trimethobenzamide, trimethaphan, vecuronium, vinblastine, vincristine, vinorelbine, warfarin, zidovudine.

Incompatibility

Do not administer through the same IV line as alteplase, amiodarone, amsacrine, ciprofloxacin, diazepam, doxycycline, ergotamine, filgrastim, gentamicin, haloperidol, idarubicin, methotrimeprazine, nicardipine, phenytoin, tobramycin, triflupromazine, vancomycin.

> **TREATMENT OF OVERDOSE/ANTIDOTE**
> Discontinue drug or decrease dosage. Initiate general supportive and resuscitative measures. Protamine sulfate (1% solution) will reverse effects of heparin. Each mg of protamine neutralizes about 100 USP heparin units. Give protamine IV over 10 min. Be aware that protamine sulfate may cause hypotension or anaphylactic reactions.

Pharmacokinetics

Route	Onset	Peak	Duration
IV	Immediate	Minutes	2–6 h
SC	20–60 min	2–4 h	8–12 h

Metabolism: Liver, reticuloendothelial system; $T_{1/2}$: 30–150 min
Excretion: Urine

Adverse effects

▸ ***Derm:*** Transient alopecia, local reactions at SC site (irritation, erythema, mild pain, hematoma, ulceration, SC and cutaneous necrosis)
▸ ***Allergic:*** **Anaphylaxis,** chills, fever, urticaria, asthma, headache, nausea, vomiting, rhinitis, allergic vasospastic reaction (painful, ischemic, cyanotic limbs)
▸ ***Hematologic: Hemorrhage (at any site);* thrombocytopenia;** *bruising;* elevated AST, ALT levels, white clot syndrome
▸ ***Misc:*** Osteoporosis, rebound hyperlipidemia, heparin resistance, hyperkalemia, suppressed aldosterone synthesis, priapism

Clinically important drug–drug interactions

▸ Increased bleeding tendencies with oral anticoagulants, antiplatelet drugs, NSAIDs, salicylates, penicillins, cephalosporins
▸ Decreased anticoagulation effects with nitroglycerin

Adverse effects in *Italics* are most common; those in **Bold** are life-threatening

H

- Heparin resistance with streptokinase
- Counteracted anticoagulation effects with digitalis, tetracyclines, nicotine, antihistamines

⬤ NURSING CONSIDERATIONS

Assessment

- *History:* Heparin, beef, or pig protein allergy; severe thrombocytopenia, uncontrolled bleeding (except with DIC); any patient who cannot be monitored regularly with blood coagulation tests; sex, age, dysbetalipoproteinemia, recent surgery or injury, subacute bacterial endocarditis, severe hypertension; during and immediately after spinal tap, spinal anesthesia, or major surgery; hemophilia, vascular purpuras, thrombocytopenia, ulcerative lesions, diverticulitis, ulcerative colitis, continuous tube drainage of stomach or small intestine; menstruation; liver disease with impaired hemostasis; severe renal disease, diabetes, hypoaldosteronism, hyperkalemia
- *Physical:* T, P, BP, R, ECG, weight, IV site, neurologic checks, skin assessment, presence of bleeding, injection site assessment, peripheral perfusion, APTT, CBC, serum electrolytes, kidney and liver function tests, serum cholesterol; urine, stool, emesis guaiac

Implementation

- Administer heparin infusion using an IV infusion pump.
- Adjust dose according to coagulation test results performed just before injection (30 min before each intermittent dose or q4h if continuous IV dose). Therapeutic range: 1.5–2.5 times control.
- Give deep SC above iliac crest of abdominal fat layer. *Do not* give heparin by IM injection, which may cause hematoma formation.
- Use saline or heparin lock to avoid repeated injections.
- Monitor for evidence of hemorrhage/bleeding (bleeding gums, epistaxis, bruising, black tarry stools, hematuria, hematemesis, decreased Hgb/Hct, hypotension, pain, neurologic changes).
- Guaiac urine, feces, and emesis.
- Apply pressure to all injection sites after needle is withdrawn; inspect injection sites for signs of hematoma; do not massage injection sites.
- Provide for safety measures (electric razor, soft toothbrush) to prevent injury from bleeding.
- Have emergency equipment (defibrillator, drugs, oxygen, intubation equipment) on standby in case anaphylaxis or adverse reaction occurs.

Adverse effects in *Italics* are most common; those in **Bold** are life-threatening

- Assess for allergic reactions (chills, fever, urticaria, asthma, headache, nausea, vomiting).
- Alert all health care providers of heparin use.

● hyaluronidase *(hye al yoor on' i dase)* Wydase

Pregnancy Category C

Drug class
Protein enzyme

Indications
- Adjuvant to increase absorption and dispersion of injected drugs
- Hypodermoclysis

Therapeutic actions
- A spreading or diffusing substance that modifies the permeability of connective tissue through the hydrolysis of hyaluronic acid; this decreases the viscosity of the cellular cement and promotes diffusion of injected fluids, transudates, and exudates and facilitates their absorption

Contraindications
- **Contraindications:** hyaluronidase allergy, acutely inflamed or cancerous areas

Available forms
- *Powder for injection:* 150, 1500 U/vial
- *Solution for injection:* 150 U/mL

SC facts
Preparation
- To reconstitute the powder for injection, add 1 mL of 0.9%NS to the 150-U vial or 10 mL of 0.9%NS to the 1500-U vial.

Dosage
- *Absorption and dispersion of injected drugs:* Add 150 U to the injection solution. To prepare a solution containing epinephrine, add 0.5 mL epinephrine (1:1000) to the above solution.
- *Hypodermoclysis:* Inject hyaluronidase solution into rubber tubing close to needle inserted between skin and muscle, *or* inject hyaluronidase SC before clysis. 150 U will facilitate absorption of 1000 mL or more of solution. Individualize dose, rate of injection, and type of solution (saline, glucose, Ringer's).

Adverse effects in *Italics* are most common; those in **Bold** are life-threatening

TREATMENT OF OVERDOSE/ANTIDOTE
Discontinue drug or decrease dosage. Initiate general supportive and resuscitative measures. Keep epinephrine, corticosteroids, and antihistamines available for emergency treatment.

Pharmacokinetics

Route	Onset	Peak
SC	Rapid	36–40 h

Metabolism: Tissue

Adverse effects

⯈ *Allergic:* **Anaphylaxis,** urticaria
⯈ *Misc:* Hypovolemia (if solutions devoid of inorganic electrolytes are given by hypodermoclysis)

⬤ NURSING CONSIDERATIONS

Assessment

⯈ *History:* Hyaluronidase allergy, acutely inflamed or cancerous areas
⯈ *Physical:* T, P, BP, R, CVP, I & O, peripheral perfusion, skin assessment, skin turgor, hydration status, JVD, adventitious lung sounds

Implementation

⯈ Perform a preliminary skin test for sensitivity to hyaluronidase. Give an intradermal injection of 0.02 mL of solution. A positive reaction consists of a wheal with pseudopods appearing within 5 min and persisting for 20–30 min with itching. Transient vasodilation at the site is not a positive reaction.
⯈ Monitor for hypovolemia; correct with a solution change.
⯈ If given with epinephrine, assess for the systemic effects of epinephrine.
⯈ Store solution in refrigerator. Reconstituted solution may be stored for 2 wk.

⬤ hydralazine hydrochloride

(hye dral' a zeen) Apo-Hydralazine (CAN), Apresoline, Novo-Hylazin (CAN), Nu-Hydral (CAN)

Pregnancy Category C

Drug classes

Antihypertensive
Vasodilator

Indications
▸ Severe essential hypertension when the drug cannot be given orally or when need to lower blood pressure is urgent (parenteral)
▸ Essential hypertension, alone or in combination with other drugs (oral)
▸ Unlabeled uses: afterload reduction in the treatment of CHF, severe aortic insufficiency, and after valve replacement

Therapeutic actions
▸ Exerts a peripheral vasodilating effect through a direct relaxation of vascular smooth muscle
▸ Interferes with calcium movements in vascular smooth muscle that initiate and maintain a contractile state
▸ Increases the renin activity in plasma, leading to production of angiotensin II, which causes stimulation of aldosterone and sodium reabsorption
▸ Maintains or increases renal and cerebral blood flow

Effects on hemodynamic parameters
▸ Decreased BP (diastolic > systolic)
▸ Decreased SVR
▸ Increased HR
▸ Increased CO
▸ Decreased or unchanged CVP

Contraindications/cautions
▸ **Contraindications:** hydralazine allergy, coronary artery disease (CAD), mitral valvular rheumatic heart disease
▸ **Cautions:** advanced renal damage, cerebral vascular accident, increased intracranial pressure, pulmonary hypertension, peripheral neuritis, mitral valve disease

Available forms
▸ *Injection:* 20 mg/mL
▸ *Tablets:* 10, 25, 50, 100 mg

IV/IM facts
Preparation
▸ Use drug immediately after stopper is punctured.
▸ Administer undiluted; do not add hydralazine to infusion solutions.
▸ Hydralazine changes color after contact with a metal filter; avoid contact with metal.

Dosage
▸ Use IV or IM route only when drug cannot be taken orally.
▸ 20–40 mg IV, repeated as needed. Give at rate of 10 mg/min. Monitor blood pressure frequently.

Adverse effects in *Italics* are most common; those in **Bold** are life-threatening

◗ Most patients can be transferred to oral hydralazine within 24–48 h.

Compatibility
Hydralazine may be given through the same IV line as heparin, hydrocortisone, potassium chloride, verapamil, vitamin B complex with C.

Incompatibility
Do not administer through the same IV line as aminophylline, ampicillin, diazoxide, furosemide.

Oral dosage
◗ *Initial dose:* 10 mg PO qid for 2–4 d; increase to 25 mg PO qid for rest of week.
◗ *Second and subsequent weeks:* 50 mg PO qid.
◗ *Maintenance:* Adjust dosage to lowest effective level. Twice daily dosing may be adequate. Some patients may require up to 300 mg/d. Incidence of toxic reactions, particularly the lupus erythematosus syndrome, is high in patients receiving large doses.

TREATMENT OF OVERDOSE/ANTIDOTE
Discontinue drug or decrease dosage. Initiate general supportive and resuscitative measures. Evacuate gastric contents, prevent aspiration, and protect the airway. Administer activated charcoal if possible. Treat shock using volume expanders without vasopressors. If needed, use a vasopressor that is less likely to precipitate or aggravate dysrhythmias. Treat tachycardia with beta-blockers; digitalization may be necessary. Monitor renal function.

Pharmacokinetics

Route	Onset	Peak	Duration
IV	10–20 min	10–80 min	2–4 h
Oral	Rapid	1–2 h	6–12 h

Metabolism: Hepatic; $T_{1/2}$: 3–7 h
Excretion: Urine

Adverse effects
◗ *CNS: Headache,* peripheral neuritis, dizziness, tremors, psychotic reactions characterized by depression, disorientation, or anxiety
◗ *CV:* **Acute myocardial infarction,** *tachycardia, angina, palpitations,* ECG changes of myocardial ischemia, edema, hypotension, paradoxical pressor response

Adverse effects in *Italics* are most common; those in **Bold** are life-threatening

- ▸ **_Resp:_** Nasal congestion, dyspnea
- ▸ **_GI:_** _Nausea, vomiting, diarrhea,_ constipation, paralytic ileus
- ▸ **_GU:_** Urination difficulty
- ▸ **_Allergic:_** Rash, urticaria, pruritus, fever, chills, arthralgia, eosinophilia, hepatitis
- ▸ **_Hematologic:_** Blood dyscrasias consisting of reduced hemoglobin and RBC, leukopenia, agranulocytosis, purpura
- ▸ **_Misc:_** _Lupus-like syndrome,_ conjunctivitis, lacrimation

Clinically important drug–drug interactions

- ▸ Increased serum levels of either drug with metoprolol or propranolol
- ▸ Decreased effects with indomethacin
- ▸ Excessive hypotension with other potent parenteral antihypertensive drugs
- ▸ Enhanced by MAO inhibitors
- ▸ Reduced pressor response of epinephrine

◉ NURSING CONSIDERATIONS

Assessment

- ▸ _History:_ Hydralazine allergy, CAD, mitral valvular rheumatic heart disease, advanced renal damage, cerebral vascular accident, increased intracranial pressure, pulmonary hypertension, peripheral neuritis, mitral valve disease
- ▸ _Physical:_ T, P, BP, R, ECG, CVP, SVR, I & O, weight, neurologic checks, reflexes, vision, cardiac auscultation, edema, orthostatic BP, adventitious lung sounds, bowel sounds, skin condition, status of nasal mucous membranes, voiding pattern, lymph node palpation, serum electrolytes, LE cell preparations, antinuclear antibody (ANA) determinations, renal and hepatic function tests, UA

Implementation

- ▸ Exercise extreme caution when calculating and preparing doses. Hydralazine is a very potent drug; small dosage errors can cause serious adverse effects.
- ▸ Carefully monitor P, BP, R, and ECG during IV administration.
- ▸ Have emergency equipment (defibrillator, drugs, oxygen) on standby in case allergic or adverse reaction occurs.
- ▸ Give oral drug with food to increase bioavailability (give drug in a consistent relationship to ingestion of food for consistent response to therapy).
- ▸ Drug causes reflex tachycardia; beta-blockers are often prescribed.
- ▸ Discard drug if it changes color.
- ▸ Change patient's position slowly to avoid postural hypotension.

Adverse effects in _Italics_ are most common; those in **Bold** are life-threatening

H

- Withdraw drug gradually, especially from patients who have experienced marked blood pressure reduction. Rapid withdrawal may cause a sudden increase in BP.
- Assess CBC, LE cell preparations, and ANA titers before and periodically during prolonged therapy, even for asymptomatic patients. Discontinue if blood dyscrasias occur. Re–evaluate therapy if ANA or LE tests are positive.
- Discontinue or re–evaluate therapy if patient develops arthralgia, fever, chest pain, or continued malaise.
- Arrange for pyridoxine therapy if patient develops symptoms of peripheral neuritis.
- Stop drug immediately if patient develops jaundice or laboratory evidence of liver injury.
- Administer injection/infusion to patient while supine. Keep patient in supine position for at least 3 h after hydralazine injection is given.
- Do not discontinue drug abruptly after chronic therapy. (Hypersensitivity to catecholamines may have developed, causing exacerbation of angina, MI, and ventricular dysrhythmias.) Taper drug gradually over 2 wk with monitoring.
- Consult provider about withdrawing drug if patient is to undergo surgery (withdrawal is controversial).

● **hydrocortisone sodium succinate**
(*hye droe kor' ti zone*) A-Hydrocort, Solu-Cortef
Pregnancy Category C

Drug classes
Corticosteroid
Glucocorticoid, short-acting
Mineralocorticoid
Hormonal agent

Indications
- Used to manage a wide variety of endocrine, rheumatic, collagen, dermatologic, allergic, gastrointestinal, respiratory, hematologic, neoplastic, and edematous disorders
- Used as replacement therapy in adrenocortical insufficiency

Therapeutic actions
- Suppresses inflammation and normal immune response
- Causes profound and varied metabolic effects
- Is a potent mineralocorticoid that leads to salt retention
- Suppresses adrenal function with long-term use

Adverse effects in *Italics* are most common; those in **Bold** are life-threatening

Contraindications/cautions
▸ **Contraindications:** hydrocortisone allergy; systemic infections, especially tuberculosis, fungal infections, amebiasis, vaccinia and varicella, and antibiotic-resistant infections
▸ **Cautions:** renal or hepatic disease, cerebral malaria, hypothyroidism; ulcerative colitis with impending perforation; diverticulitis, active or latent peptic ulcer; inflammatory bowel disease, fresh intestinal anastomoses, psychotic tendencies, hypertension, metastatic carcinoma, thromboembolic disorders, osteoporosis, convulsive disorders, myasthenia gravis, diabetes, CHF, Cushing's syndrome, recent acute myocardial infarction (AMI), elderly patients

Available forms
▸ *Injection:* 100, 250, 500, 1000 mg/vial

IV facts
Preparation
▸ Reconstitute vial with 2 mL of bacteriostatic Water for Injection or Bacteriostatic Sodium Chloride Injection.
▸ If using Act-O-Vial container, press the plastic activator down to force the diluent into the lower chamber. Agitate gently to dissolve drug.
▸ May be given as reconstituted or added to a volume of D5W/0.9%NS; D5W; or 0.9%NS to yield a concentration of 0.1–1 mg/mL.

Dosage
▸ Dosage requirements vary; individualize dosage based on the disease and the patient's response. Use smallest effective dose.
▸ *Usual dosage:* 100–500 mg IV. Give each 100 mg over 30 s. Infuse ≥ 500 mg doses over 10 min. Repeat dose at 2-, 4-, or 6-h intervals. Up to 8 g daily has been given.
▸ *Severe shock:* 0.5–2 g IV q2–6h or 50 mg/kg IV repeated in 4 h or q24h. Discontinue high-dose therapy within 48–72 h.
▸ *Maintenance therapy:* Reduce initial dose in small increments at intervals until lowest clinically satisfactory dose is reached.

Compatibility
Hydrocortisone may be given through the same IV line as acyclovir, allopurinol, amifostine, aminophylline, ampicillin, amrinone, amsacrine, atracurium, atropine, aztreonam, betamethasone, calcium gluconate, cefepime, cefmetazole, cephalothin, cephapirin, chlordiazepoxide, chlorpromazine, cladribine, cyanocobalamin, cytarabine, dexamethasone, digoxin, diphenhydramine, dopamine, droperidol, edrophonium, enalaprilat,

epinephrine, esmolol, estrogens (conjugated), ethacrynate, famotidine, fentanyl, filgrastim, fludarabine, fluorouracil, foscarnet, furosemide, gallium, granisetron, heparin, hydralazine, insulin (regular), isoproterenol, kanamycin, lidocaine, lorazepam, magnesium sulfate, melphalan, menadiol, meperidine, methicillin, methoxamine, methylergonovine, minocycline, morphine, neostigmine, norepinephrine, ondansetron, oxacillin, oxytocin, paclitaxel, pancuronium, penicillin G potassium, pentazocine, phytonadione, piperacillin-tazobactam, prednisolone, procainamide, prochlorperazine, propofol, propranolol, pyridostigmine, scopolamine, sodium bicarbonate, succinylcholine, tacrolimus, teniposide, theophylline, thiotepa, trimethaphan, trimethobenzamide, vecuronium, vinorelbine.

Incompatibility
Do not administer through the same IV line as ciprofloxacin, diazepam, ergotamine, idarubicin, midazolam, phenytoin, sargramostim.

> **TREATMENT OF OVERDOSE/ANTIDOTE**
> Discontinue drug or decrease dosage. Initiate general supportive and resuscitative measures.

Pharmacokinetics

Route	Onset	Duration
IV	Rapid	1–1.5 d

Metabolism: Hepatic; $T_{1/2}$: 80–120 min
Excretion: Urine

Adverse effects
◗ Most occur with chronic therapy.
◗ *CNS:* **Convulsions,** *depression,* mood swings, increased intracranial pressure, vertigo, headache, psychosis
◗ *CV:* **Myocardial rupture after recent AMI, fat embolism,** hypertension, hypotension, CHF secondary to fluid retention, thromboembolism, thrombophlebitis, dysrhythmias secondary to electrolyte imbalances
◗ *GI:* Peptic ulcer, bowel perforation, pancreatitis, abdominal distention, ulcerative esophagitis, nausea, hiccups, increased appetite, weight gain
◗ *Derm:* *Impaired wound healing, petechiae, ecchymoses, thin and fragile skin,* acne, burning or tingling after IV injection, increased sweating, allergic dermatitis, urticaria, angioneurotic edema
◗ *Allergic:* **Anaphylaxis**

Adverse effects in *Italics* are most common; those in **Bold** are life-threatening

- *Fluid/Electrolytes: Sodium and fluid retention, hypokalemia,* hypokalemic alkalosis, metabolic alkalosis, hypocalcemia
- *Musc/Skel: Muscle weakness,* steroid myopathy, muscle mass loss, osteoporosis, vertebral compression fractures, pathologic fractures, tendon rupture
- *Endocrine: Secondary adrenocortical and pituitary unresponsiveness,* decreased carbohydrate tolerance, diabetes mellitus, cushingoid state, menstrual irregularities, negative nitrogen balance, hirsutism
- *Ophthalmic:* Cataracts, increased intraocular pressure, glaucoma
- *Misc: Increased susceptibility to infection, masking of signs of infection,* subcutaneous fat atrophy

Clinically important drug–drug interactions
- Increased blood levels with oral contraceptives, estrogens, ketoconazole
- Decreased blood levels with phenytoin, phenobarbital, rifampin, cholestyramine
- Decreased serum level of salicylates
- Decreased effectiveness of anticholinesterases (ambenonium, edrophonium, neostigmine, pyridostigmine) in myasthenia gravis
- Increased digitalis toxicity related to hypokalemia
- Altered response to coumarin anticoagulants, such as warfarin
- Increased hypokalemia with potassium-depleting diuretics
- Increased requirements for insulin, sulfonylurea drugs
- Decreased serum concentrations of isoniazid
- Increased cyclosporine toxicity
- Decreased effectiveness with barbiturates

● NURSING CONSIDERATIONS

Assessment
- *History:* Hydrocortisone allergy; systemic infections, especially tuberculosis, fungal infections, amebiasis, vaccinia and varicella, and antibiotic-resistant infections; renal or hepatic disease, cerebral malaria, hypothyroidism; ulcerative colitis with impending perforation; diverticulitis, active or latent peptic ulcer, inflammatory bowel disease, fresh intestinal anastomoses, psychotic tendencies, hypertension, metastatic carcinoma, thromboembolic disorders, osteoporosis, convulsive disorders, myasthenia gravis, diabetes, CHF, Cushing's syndrome; recent AMI; age
- *Physical:* T, P, R, BP, ECG, I & O, IV site, weight, ophthalmologic exam, neurologic checks, skin assessment, muscle

Adverse effects in *Italics* are most common; those in **Bold** are life-threatening

H

strength, peripheral perfusion, adventitious lung sounds, chest x-ray, upper GI x-ray (history or symptoms of peptic ulcer), abdominal assessment, presence of infection, CBC, serum electrolytes, 2-h postprandial blood glucose, serum glucose, UA, adrenal function tests, serum cholesterol, liver and renal function tests

Implementation

- Carefully monitor for evidence of fluid overload (I & O, daily weight, edema, lung sounds, JVD).
- Evaluate for hypokalemia as evidenced by muscle weakness, fatigue, paralytic ileus, ECG changes, anorexia, nausea, vomiting, abdominal distention, dizziness, or polyuria.
- Assess for hypocalcemia as evidenced by Chvostek's or Trousseau's signs, muscle twitching, laryngospasm, or paresthesias.
- Have emergency equipment (defibrillator, drugs, oxygen, intubation equipment) on standby in case anaphylaxis or adverse reaction occurs.
- Give daily doses before 9:00 AM to mimic normal peak corticosteroid blood levels.
- Increase dosage when patient is subject to stress.
- Patient is at higher risk of infection; initiate interventions to prevent infection. Drug may mask evidence of infection.
- Taper doses when discontinuing high-dose or long-term therapy. Symptoms of adrenal insufficiency from too-rapid withdrawal include nausea, fatigue, anorexia, dyspnea, hypotension, hypoglycemia, myalgia, fever, malaise, arthralgia, dizziness, desquamation of skin, and fainting.
- Do not give live virus vaccines with immunosuppressive doses of corticosteroids.
- Use minimal doses for minimal duration to minimize adverse effects.

⬤ hydromorphone hydrochloride

(hye droe mor' fone) Dilaudid, Dilaudid-HP, Dilaudid-5, Hydromorph Contin (CAN), PMS-Hydromorphone (CAN)

Pregnancy Category C

C-II controlled substance

Drug class
Narcotic agonist analgesic

Indication
- Relief of moderate to severe pain

Adverse effects in *Italics* are most common; those in **Bold** are life-threatening

Therapeutic actions

▶ Opium alkaloid; acts as agonist at specific opioid receptors in the CNS to produce analgesia, euphoria, sedation, and respiratory and physical depression

Contraindications/cautions

▶ **Contraindications:** hypersensitivity to hydromorphone or its components, physical dependence on a narcotic analgesic (drug may precipitate withdrawal), increased intracranial pressure, depressed ventilatory function, upper airway obstruction, COPD, cor pulmonale, emphysema, kyphoscoliosis, status asthmaticus; IV form contraindicated for patients who are not already receiving large amounts of parenteral narcotics

▶ **Cautions:** elderly or debilitated patients, impaired renal or hepatic function, hypothyroidism, myxedema, Addison's disease, prostatic hypertrophy, urethral stricture, pulmonary or cardiovascular disease, postoperative patients, hypotension, hypovolemia, circulatory shock, acute abdominal conditions, CNS depression, coma, toxic psychoses, gallbladder disease, acute alcoholism, delirium tremens, recent gastrointestinal surgery

Available forms

▶ *Injection:* 1, 2, 4, 10 mg/mL
▶ *Powder for injection:* 250 mg
▶ *Tablets:* 1, 2, 3, 4, 8 mg
▶ *Liquid:* 5 mg/5 mL
▶ *Suppositories:* 3 mg

IV/IM/SC facts
Preparation

▶ May be given undiluted or diluted in D5W/LR; D5W/0.45%NS; D5W/0.9%NS; D5W; D5W/Ringer's Injection; Fructose 10% in Water; LR; 0.45%NS; 0.9%NS; Ringer's Injection; Sodium Lactate (1/6 Molar) Injection; or Sterile Water for Injection.
▶ Use high-potency forms only for patients who are tolerant to other narcotics.
▶ Drug may have slight yellow discoloration, which does not affect its potency.

Dosage

▶ 1–2 mg IV (over 2–3 min), IM, or SC q4–6h as needed. For severe pain, give 3–4 mg q4–6h. Individualize dosage amount and frequency based on patient's pain level and response to therapy. Up to 14 mg has been given IM or SC.
▶ *Elderly/debilitated/high-risk patients:* Reduce dosage; use

Adverse effects in *Italics* are most common; those in **Bold** are life-threatening

with caution to prevent respiratory depression and adverse
reactions.

Compatibility

Hydromorphone may be given through the same IV line as
acyclovir, allopurinol, amifostine, amikacin, amsacrine, aztreonam, cefamandole, cefepime, cefmetazole, cefoperazone, cefotaxime, cefoxitin, ceftazidime, ceftizoxime, cefuroxime,
cephalothin, cephapirin, chloramphenicol, cisplatin, cladribine, clindamycin, cyclophosphamide, cytarabine, diltiazem,
dobutamine, dopamine, doxorubicin, doxycycline, epinephrine, erythromycin, famotidine, fentanyl, filgrastim, fludarabine, foscarnet, furosemide, gentamicin, granisetron, heparin,
kanamycin, magnesium sulfate, melphalan, methotrexate,
metronidazole, mezlocillin, midazolam, morphine, moxalactam, nafcillin, nicardipine, nitroglycerin, norepinephrine,
ondansetron, oxacillin, paclitaxel, penicillin G potassium,
piperacillin, piperacillin-tazobactam, propofol, ranitidine, teniposide, thiotepa, ticarcillin, tobramycin, trimethoprim-sulfamethoxazole, vancomycin, vecuronium, vinorelbine.

Incompatibility

Do not administer through the same IV line as diazepam, gallium, minocycline, phenobarbital, phenytoin, sargramostim,
thiopental.

Oral/rectal dosage

◗ *Oral:* 2–4 mg PO q4–6h. Give ≥ 4 mg q4–6h for more severe
pain. If using liquid form, give 2.5–10mg q4–6h. Individualize
dosage amount and frequency based on patient's pain level
and response to therapy.
◗ *Rectal:* 3 mg q6–8h.

TREATMENT OF OVERDOSE/ANTIDOTE

Discontinue drug or decrease dose. Initiate general supportive and resuscitative measures. Administer the antidote
naloxone 0.4–2 mg IV. Repeat at 2- to 3-min intervals if
needed to reverse respiratory depression. Gastric lavage or
induced emesis may remove oral hydromorphone.

Pharmacokinetics

Route	Onset	Peak	Duration
IV	Rapid	15–30 min	2–3 h
IM	15–30 min	30–60 min	4–5 h
Oral	30 min	60–120 min	4–5 h

Metabolism: Hepatic; $T_{1/2}$: 2–3 h
Excretion: Urine

Adverse effects in *Italics* are most common; those in **Bold** are life-threatening

Adverse effects

▸ *CNS: Lightheadedness, dizziness, sedation,* euphoria, dysphoria, delirium, insomnia, agitation, anxiety, fear, hallucinations, disorientation, drowsiness, lethargy, impaired mental and physical performance, coma, mood changes, weakness, headache, tremor, miosis, visual disturbances

▸ *CV:* **Circulatory depression, shock, cardiac arrest,** facial flushing, tachycardia, bradycardia, dysrhythmias, palpitations, chest wall rigidity, hypertension, hypotension, orthostatic hypotension, syncope

▸ *Resp:* **Respiratory depression, apnea, respiratory arrest,** suppressed cough reflex

▸ *GI: Nausea, vomiting,* dry mouth, anorexia, constipation, biliary tract spasm, taste alterations, increased colonic motility in patients with chronic ulcerative colitis

▸ *GU:* Ureteral spasm, spasm of vesical sphincters, urinary retention or hesitancy, oliguria, antidiuretic effect, reduced libido or potency

▸ *Derm: Sweating,* pruritus, urticaria; phlebitis following IV injection; pain at injection site; tissue irritation and induration (SC injection)

▸ *Allergic:* **Anaphylaxis, laryngospasm, bronchospasm,** pruritus, urticaria, edema

▸ *Dependence:* Tolerance, physical and psychological dependence

Clinically important drug–drug interactions

▸ Increased respiratory depression, hypotension, profound sedation, or coma with barbiturate anesthetics, alcohol, sedatives, antihistamines, MAO inhibitors, phenothiazines, butyrophenones, TCAs

▸ Enhanced effects of neuromuscular blocking agents

◉ NURSING CONSIDERATIONS

Assessment

▸ *History:* Hypersensitivity to hydromorphone or its components, physical dependence on a narcotic analgesic, increased intracranial pressure, depressed ventilatory function, upper airway obstruction, chronic obstructive pulmonary disease, cor pulmonale, emphysema, kyphoscoliosis, status asthmaticus, age, debilitation, impaired renal or hepatic function, hypothyroidism, myxedema, Addison's disease, prostatic hypertrophy, urethral stricture, pulmonary or cardiovascular disease, recent surgery, hypotension, hypovolemia, circulatory shock, acute abdominal conditions, CNS depression, coma, toxic psychoses, gall bladder disease, acute al-

Adverse effects in *Italics* are most common; those in **Bold** are life-threatening

coholism, delirium tremens, recent gastrointestinal surgery, previous narcotic use
▸ *Physical:* T, BP, P, R, ECG, SpO$_2$, ABG, I & O, injection site, weight, neurologic checks, skin assessment, respiratory effort, pain assessment, orthostatic BP, adventitious lung sounds, bowel sounds, hydration status, prostate exam, voiding pattern; thyroid, liver, and kidney function tests

Implementation
▸ Exercise extreme caution when calculating and preparing doses. Hydromorphone is a potent drug; small dosage errors can cause serious adverse effects. Avoid inadvertent bolus of drug.
▸ Monitor vital signs frequently with IV administration.
▸ Have emergency equipment (defibrillator, drugs, intubation equipment, oxygen) on standby in case of allergic or adverse reaction.
▸ Assess for evidence of respiratory depression.
▸ Correct hypovolemia before administering drug; maintain adequate hydration.
▸ Prevent constipation; give stool softeners and laxatives as ordered.
▸ Assess pain status frequently; notify provider if patient does not receive adequate pain relief.
▸ Minimize postural hypotension by helping the patient change positions slowly.
▸ Administer parenteral forms when the patient is lying down.
▸ Use caution when giving SC or IM injections to patients with hypotension or in shock; impaired perfusion may delay absorption; with repeated doses, an excessive amount may be absorbed when circulation is restored.
▸ Reassure patient about addiction liability; most patients who receive opiates for medical reasons do not develop dependence syndromes.
▸ Follow federal, state, and institutional policies for dispensing controlled substances.
▸ Protect from light during storage; refrigerate rectal suppositories.

◉ hydroxyzine hydrochloride
(hye drox' i zeen) Atarax, Atarax 100, Multipax (CAN), Vistaril, Vistazine 50

◉ hydroxyzine pamoate Vistaril
Pregnancy Category C

Drug classes
Antianxiety drug

Adverse effects in *Italics* are most common; those in **Bold** are life-threatening

Antihistamine
Antiemetic

Indications

▸ Symptomatic relief of anxiety and tension associated with psychoneurosis; adjunct in organic disease states in which anxiety is manifested; allergic conditions with strong emotional overlay (chronic urticaria and pruritus); alcoholism; asthma
▸ Management of pruritus due to allergic conditions, such as chronic urticaria, atopic and contact dermatosis, and in histamine-mediated pruritus
▸ Sedation when used as premedication and following general anesthesia (oral only)
▸ Management of the acutely disturbed or hysterical patient and the acute or chronic alcoholic with anxiety withdrawal symptoms or delirium tremens (parenteral)
▸ Preoperative and postoperative adjunctive medication to reduce narcotic dosage, allay anxiety, and control emesis (parenteral)

Therapeutic actions

▸ Mechanisms of action not understood; actions may be due to suppression of subcortical areas of the CNS
▸ Has clinically demonstrated antihistaminic, analgesic, antispasmodic, antiemetic, mild antisecretory, and bronchodilator activity

Contraindications

▸ **Contraindications:** allergy to hydroxyzine or cetirizine, porphyria

Available forms

▸ *Injection:* 25, 50 mg/mL
▸ *Tablets:* 10, 25, 50, 100 mg
▸ *Capsules:* 25, 50, 100 mg
▸ *Syrup:* 10 mg/5 mL
▸ *Oral suspension:* 25 mg/5 mL

IM facts
Preparation
▸ May give IM undiluted.

Dosage

▸ Start patients on IM therapy; maintain on oral therapy whenever practical. Adjust dosage to patient's response.
▸ Inject well within the body of a large muscle. Preferred site is the upper outer quadrant of the buttock or midlateral thigh.

Adverse effects in *Italics* are most common; those in **Bold** are life-threatening

H

Use deltoid area only if well developed, and then only with caution to avoid radial nerve injury. Do not inject into the lower two thirds of the upper arm.

‣ *Antiemetic/analgesic, adjunctive therapy:* 25–100 mg IM to permit narcotic dosage reduction.
‣ *Sedative (preoperative and postoperative):* 50–100 mg IM.
‣ *Pruritus:* 25 mg IM tid–qid.
‣ *Psychiatric/emotional emergencies, acute alcoholism, anxiety:* 50–100 mg IM STAT, then q4–6h PRN.

Oral dosage
‣ *Anxiety:* 50–100 mg PO qid.
‣ *Pruritus:* 25 mg PO tid to qid.
‣ *Sedative (preoperative and postoperative):* 50–100 mg PO.

> **TREATMENT OF OVERDOSE/ANTIDOTE**
> Discontinue drug or decrease dosage. Initiate general supportive and resuscitative measures. For oral overdosage, induce vomiting and initiate gastric lavage. Treat hypotension with IV fluids and vasopressors. Do not use epinephrine; hydroxyzine counteracts epinephrine's pressor effects.

Pharmacokinetics

Route	Onset	Peak	Duration
Oral	15–30 min	3 h	4–6 h

Metabolism: Hepatic, $T_{1/2}$: 3 h
Excretion: Urine

Adverse effects
‣ ***CNS:*** *Drowsiness;* involuntary motor activity, including rare tremor and convulsions with higher doses than recommended
‣ ***GI:*** *Dry mouth*
‣ ***Allergic:*** Wheezing, dyspnea, chest tightness

Clinically important drug–drug interactions
‣ Enhanced effects with alcohol, other CNS depressants, barbiturates, narcotics, hypnotics, sedatives, tranquilizers; reduce dose of other CNS depressants by 50%

⬤ NURSING CONSIDERATIONS

Assessment
‣ *History:* Allergy to hydroxyzine or cetirizine, porphyria
‣ *Physical:* P, R, BP, neurologic checks, behavior, mental status, presence of anxiety, skin assessment, adventitious lung sounds, nausea/vomiting, ETOH level with acute alcoholism, renal and liver function tests

Adverse effects in *Italics* are most common; those in **Bold** are life-threatening

Implementation
▸ Determine and treat underlying cause of vomiting. Drug may mask signs and symptoms of serious conditions, such as brain tumor, intestinal obstruction, or appendicitis.
▸ Do not administer parenteral solution SC, IV, or intra-arterially; significant tissue necrosis has occurred with SC and intra-arterial injection; hemolysis occurs with IV injection.
▸ Do not crush capsules or coated tablets; may crush scored tablets. Shake oral suspension vigorously until product is completely resuspended.
▸ Initiate fall precautions; assist patient if he or she is out of bed.

I

● **ibutilide fumarate** *(eye byu' ti lyed)* Corvert
Pregnancy Category C

Drug class
Antidysrhythmic

Indication
▸ Rapid conversion of atrial fibrillation/flutter of recent onset to sinus rhythm; most effective in dysrhythmias of < 90 d duration

Therapeutic actions
▸ Prolongs cardiac action potential
▸ Increases atrial and ventricular refractoriness
▸ Delays repolarization by activation of a slow, inward current (predominantly sodium), rather than by blocking outward potassium currents
▸ Produces mild slowing of sinus rate and AV conduction; prolongs QT interval

Contraindications/cautions
▸ **Contraindications:** ibutilide allergy, prolonged QT interval
▸ **Cautions:** ventricular dysrhythmias, second- or third-degree heart block, hepatic dysfunction, CHF, low left ventricular ejection fraction

Available form
▸ *Solution:* 0.1 mg/mL

IV facts
Preparation
▸ May be given undiluted or diluted in 50 mL D5W or 0.9%NS.

Adverse effects in *Italics* are most common; those in **Bold** are life-threatening

Dosage
- *Patient weight > 60 kg:* 1 mg IV over 10 min. If dysrhythmia does not terminate within 10 min after the end of the initial infusion, give a second 10-min infusion of equal strength.
- *Patient weight < 60 kg:* 0.01 mg/kg IV over 10 min. If dysrhythmia does not terminate within 10 minutes after the end of the initial infusion, give a second 10-min infusion of equal strength.

Compatibility
Do not mix or administer with other drugs.

> **TREATMENT OF OVERDOSE/ANTIDOTE**
> Discontinue drug or decrease dosage. Initiate general supportive and resuscitative measures. Treat dysrhythmias with overdrive cardiac pacing, electrical cardioversion, or defibrillation. Correct potassium or magnesium imbalances. Magnesium sulfate infusions may be helpful. Generally avoid antidysrhythmic drugs.

Pharmacokinetics

Route	Onset	Peak
IV	Rapid	Unknown; 70% of patients who convert do so within 30 min of start of infusion; all patients who converted did so within 90 min after the start of the infusion

Metabolism: Hepatic; $T_{1/2}$: 2–12 h
Excretion: Urine, feces

Adverse effects
- *CNS:* Headache
- *CV:* **Ventricular arrhythmias (ventricular tachycardia, ventricular extrasystoles, idioventricular rhythm, torsades de pointes),** prolonged QT syndrome, tachycardia, hypotension, postural hypotension, bundle branch block, AV block, bradycardia, hypertension, palpitations, supraventricular extrasystoles, syncope
- *GI: Nausea*
- *GU:* Renal failure

Clinically important drug–drug interactions
- Supraventricular dysrhythmias may mask the cardiotoxicity associated with excessive digoxin levels
- Increased serious to life-threatening dysrhythmias with disopyramide, quinidine, procainamide, amiodarone, sotalol; do not give together or within 4 h postinfusion

Adverse effects in *Italics* are most common; those in **Bold** are life-threatening

▸ Increased prodysrhythmias with phenothiazines, TCAs, tetra-cyclic antidepressants, H$_1$ receptor antagonists

● NURSING CONSIDERATIONS

Assessment
▸ *History:* Ibutilide allergy, ventricular dysrhythmias, hepatic dysfunction, CHF, low left ventricular ejection fraction
▸ *Physical:* P, R, BP, ECG, QTc, I & O, weight, orthostatic BP, bowel sounds, electrolyte levels, liver function tests

Implementation
▸ Administer only if trained to identify and treat acute ventricular dysrhythmias. Monitor ECG continuously during and for at least 4 h after administration or until QTc returns to baseline. Be alert for possible life-threatening dysrhythmias, including ventricular tachycardia, torsades de pointes, PVCs, sinus tachycardia, sinus bradycardia, heart block.
▸ Have emergency equipment (defibrillator, pacemaker, drugs, oxygen, intubation equipment) on standby in case severe dysrhythmias occur.
▸ Determine time of onset of dysrhythmia and potential benefit of therapy before beginning therapy. Conversion is more likely in patients with dysrhythmias of short (< 90 d) duration.
▸ Correct hypokalemia and hypomagnesemia before using drug.
▸ Ensure that patient is adequately anticoagulated if atrial fibrillation is of > 2 to 3 d duration.
▸ Administer other antidysrhythmics as ordered to maintain sinus rhythm.
▸ After dilution, solution is good for 24 h at room temperature and for 48 h when refrigerated.

● imipenem-cilastatin
*(em ee **pen'** em sigh lah **stat'** in)* Primaxin I.V., Primaxin I.M.

Pregnancy Category C

Drug class
Antibiotic (carbapenem)

Indications
▸ IV: Treatment of serious lower respiratory tract, urinary tract, intra-abdominal, gynecologic, bacterial septicemia, bone and joint, skin and skin structure, endocarditis, and polymicrobic infections caused by susceptible organisms
▸ IM: Treatment of mild to moderately severe lower respiratory tract, intra-abdominal, skin and skin structure, and gynecologic infections caused by susceptible organisms

Therapeutic actions

◗ Bactericidal, broad-spectrum antibiotic that is effective for a wide range of gram-positive and gram-negative organisms
◗ Imipenem inhibits cell wall synthesis in susceptible bacteria; cilastatin inhibits the renal enzyme that metabolizes imipenem; these drugs are commercially available only in the combined form

Contraindications/cautions

◗ **Contraindications:** hypersensitivity to any component of the product; IV: meningitis; IM: hypersensitivity to local anesthetics of the amide type, severe shock, heart block
◗ **Cautions:** renal function impairment, CNS disorders, seizures, history of allergy to penicillin or other allergens

Available forms

◗ *IV:* 250 mg imipenem and 250 mg cilastatin per vial or infusion bottle, 500 mg imipenem and 500 mg cilastatin per vial or infusion bottle
◗ *IM:* 500 mg imipenem and 500 mg cilastatin per vial, 750 mg imipenem and 750 mg cilastatin per vial

IV/IM facts

Preparation

◗ **IV: Infusion bottle:** Reconstitute contents of infusion bottles with 100 mL D5W; D10W; D5W/0.225%NS; D5W/0.45%NS; D5W/0.9%NS; D5W/0.15% potassium chloride solution; D5W/0.02% Sodium Bicarbonate; Mannitol 2.5%, 5%, or 10%; Normosol M in dextrose 5%; or 0.9%NS. **Vial:** Using 10 mL from a compatible diluent (see above) container, reconstitute each 250-mg or 500-mg vial. Shake well to ensure adequate mixing. Withdraw solution and add to not less than 100 mL infusion diluent. Repeat the procedure by adding an additional 10 mL diluent to each previously reconstituted vial to ensure that all medication is used. Transfer these remaining contents to the infusion diluent. **ADD-Vantage:** Activate ADD-Vantage vial by pulling the inner cap from the drug vial. Allow drug and diluent to mix. Drug appears colorless to yellow.
◗ **IM:** Prepare with 1% lidocaine HCl solution (with epinephrine). Add 2 mL lidocaine to 500-mg vial or 3 mL to 750-mg vial. Suspension appears white to light tan; discard if suspension darkens to brown.

Dosage

◗ Base dosage on type or severity of infection. Do not exceed IV doses of 50 mg/kg/d or 4 g/d, whichever is lower. Do not exceed IM doses of 1500 mg/d.

Adverse effects in *Italics* are most common; those in **Bold** are life-threatening

- Give 125–500 mg doses IV over 20–30 min; 750–1000 mg doses over 40–60 min. Slow infusion rate if nausea develops.
- Give by deep IM injection into a large muscle with a 21-gauge 2-inch needle. Aspirate to avoid inadvertent injection into a blood vessel.
- *IV:* **Mild infections:** 250–500 mg IV q6h. **Moderate infections:** 500 mg IV q6–8h or up to 1000 mg q8h. **Severe, life-threatening infections:** 500 to 1000 mg IV q6h or 1000 mg q8h. **Uncomplicated UTI:** 250 mg IV q6h. **Complicated UTI:** 500 mg IV q6h.
- *IM:* **Lower respiratory tract, skin and skin structure, gynecologic infections:** 500–750 mg IM q12h. **Intra-abdominal infections:** 750 mg IM q12h.
- *Renal function impairment (creatinine clearance < 70 mL/min) or weight < 70 kg:* Adjust dosage amount or frequency based on creatinine clearance, weight, type of infection, and organism.

Compatibility
Imipenem-cilastatin may be given through the same IV line as acyclovir, amifostine, aztreonam, cefepime, diltiazem, famotidine, fludarabine, foscarnet, granisetron, idarubicin, insulin (regular), melphalan, methotrexate, ondansetron, propofol, tacrolimus, teniposide, thiotepa, vinorelbine, zidovudine.

Incompatibility
Do not administer through the same IV line as allopurinol, fluconazole, gallium, lorazepam, meperidine, midazolam, sargramostim, sodium bicarbonate.

> TREATMENT OF OVERDOSE/ANTIDOTE
> Discontinue drug or decrease dosage. Initiate general supportive and resuscitative measures. Imipenem-cilastatin is hemodialyzable.

Pharmacokinetics

Route	Onset	Peak
IV	Immediate	End of infusion
IM	Rapid	2 h

Metabolism: Kidneys; $T_{1/2}$: 1 h (IV); 2–3 h (IM)
Excretion: Urine

Adverse effects
- *CNS:* **Seizures,** dizziness, somnolence, tremor, weakness, confusion, myoclonus, paresthesia, headache, psychic disturbances, hallucinations

Adverse effects in *Italics* are most common; those in **Bold** are life-threatening

- *CV:* Hypotension, palpitations, tachycardia
- *Resp:* Chest discomfort, dyspnea, hyperventilation
- *GI:* **Pseudomembranous or hemorrhagic colitis, hepatitis,** *nausea, vomiting, diarrhea,* staining of teeth or tongue, abdominal pain, gastroenteritis, glossitis, heartburn, pharyngeal pain, increased salivation, taste perversion, increased liver transaminases, increased BUN and creatinine
- *GU:* **Acute renal failure,** polyuria, oliguria/anuria, urine discoloration; presence of RBCs, WBCs, casts, and bacteria in urine
- *Derm:* **Stevens-Johnson syndrome, toxic epidermal necrolysis,** angioneurotic edema, rash, pruritus, erythema multiforme, flushing, cyanosis, skin texture changes; pain and erythema at injection site, vein induration, infused vein infection
- *Allergic:* **Anaphylaxis**
- *Hematologic:* Increased eosinophils, monocytes, lymphocytes, basophils; decreased neutrophils, granulocytes, Hgb, Hct; abnormal PT, positive Coombs' test, increased or decreased WBCs and platelets
- *Misc:* *Phlebitis,* drug fever, hearing loss, tinnitus, polyarthralgia, superinfections

Clinically important drug–drug interactions

- Increased imipenem levels and half-life with probenecid; do not give concurrently
- Increased CNS side effects of either imipenem-cilastatin or cyclosporine when used together
- Increased seizures with ganciclovir

◉ NURSING CONSIDERATIONS

Assessment

- *History:* Hypersensitivity to any component of the product, meningitis, hypersensitivity to local anesthetics of the amide type, severe shock, renal function impairment, CNS disorders, seizures, history of allergy to penicillin or other allergens
- *Physical:* T, P, R, BP, ECG, I & O, IV site, SpO_2, neurologic checks, skin assessment, respiratory effort, adventitious lung sounds, edema, bowel sounds, abdominal exam, renal and liver function tests, CBC, culture and sensitivity of infection site, stool and emesis guaiac, PT, PTT

Implementation

- Obtain specimens for culture and sensitivity of infected area before beginning therapy. May begin drug before results are available.

Adverse effects in *Italics* are most common; those in **Bold** are life-threatening

- Have emergency equipment (defibrillator, drugs, oxygen, intubation equipment) on standby in case anaphylaxis or adverse reaction occurs.
- Assess for evidence of anaphylaxis; if suspected, discontinue drug immediately and notify provider.
- Monitor renal, hepatic, and hematopoietic function.
- Initiate seizure precautions for patients at increased risk for seizures.
- Monitor for occurrence of superinfections; treat as appropriate.
- Discontinue drug at any sign of colitis; initiate appropriate supportive treatment.
- Solution is stable for 4 h at room temperature and 24 h when refrigerated. Do not freeze.

● immune globulin intravenous (IVIG) *(im myoun' glob' you lin)* Gamimune N, Gammagard S/D, Polygam S/D, Sandoglobulin, Venoglobulin-I, Venoglobulin-S, Gammar-P IV, Iveegam, Polygam

Pregnancy Category C

Drug class
Immune serum

Indications
- For maintenance treatment of patients with immunodeficiency syndromes, such as congenital agammaglobulinemia, common variable hypogammaglobulinemia, x-linked immunodeficiency with or without hyper-IgM, Wiskott-Aldrich syndrome, and combined immunodeficiency, who are unable to produce sufficient IgG antibodies
- Treatment of idiopathic thrombocytopenic purpura (Gamimune N, Gammagard S/D, Polygam S/D, Sandoglobulin, Venoglobulin-I, Venoglobulin-S)
- Prevention of bacterial infections in patients with hypogammaglobulinemia or recurrent bacterial infections associated with B-cell chronic lymphocytic leukemia (CLL) (Gammagard S/D, Polygam S/D)
- Treatment of Kawasaki syndrome in conjunction with aspirin (Iveegam)
- Prevention of systemic and local infections, interstitial pneumonia of infectious and idiopathic etiologies, and acute graft-

versus-host disease in bone marrow transplant patients (Gamimune N)
▸ Unlabeled use: Chronic fatigue syndrome, quinidine-induced thrombocytopenia

Therapeutic actions
▸ Contains 5% immune globulins
▸ Provides immediate antibody levels and provides passive immunity against infection
▸ Some forms cause a rapid but temporary increase in platelet counts

Contraindications/cautions
▸ **Contraindications:** allergic response to gamma globulin, anti-immunoglobulin A (IgA) antibodies, thimerosal, or component of individual drug; isolated IgA deficiency
▸ **Cautions:** prior systemic allergic reactions after administration of human immunoglobulin preparations

Available forms
▸ *Injection:* 5%, 10%
▸ *Powder for injection:* 50 mg/mL; 1, 3, 6, 12 g

IV facts
Preparation
▸ **Sandoglobulin:** Store at room temperature. Reconstitute with supplied diluent or 0.9%NS to a 3% to 12% solution. Carefully rotate bottle; *do not* shake. When using the supplied diluent, use the transfer device to add the diluent to the bottle containing the drug. The following table lists the required diluent volumes:

Required Diluent Volume			
Concentration	1-g Vial	3-g Vial	6-g Vial	12-g Vial
---	---	---	---	---
3%	33.0 mL	100 mL	200 mL	
6%	16.5 mL	50 mL	100 mL	200 mL
9%	11.0 mL	33 mL	66 mL	132 mL
12%	8.3 mL	25 mL	50 mL	100 mL

▸ **Gammagard S/D:** Store at ≤ 77°F; do not freeze. Begin administration ≤ 2 h after reconstitution. Reconstitute with supplied Sterile Water for Injection using provided transfer device. Gently rotate to dissolve the drug. The following table lists the required diluent volumes:

Required Diluent Volume			
Concentration	2.5-g Bottle	5-g Bottle	10-g Bottle
5%	50 mL	96 mL	192 mL
10%	25 mL	48 mL	96 mL

▸ **Gammar-P IV:** Store at ≤ 77°F; do not freeze. Reconstitute with supplied diluent and transfer spike.

▸ **Venoglobulin-I:** Store at ≤ 86°F. Reconstitute with supplied diluent or Sterile Water for Injection.

▸ **Gamimune N:** Store at 36°–46°F; do not freeze. May be given undiluted or diluted with D5W.

▸ **Iveegam:** Store at 36°–46°F; do not freeze. Reconstitute with supplied diluent using double-ended spike. May be further diluted with D5W or 0.9%NS.

▸ **Polygam S/D:** Store at ≤ 77°F; do not freeze. Begin administration ≤ 2 h after reconstitution. Reconstitute according to manufacturer's directions.

▸ **Venoglobulin-S:** Store at ≤ 77°F; do not freeze. Further prepare according to manufacturer's directions.

Dosage

▸ *Immunodeficiency syndrome*

▸ **Sandoglobulin:** Give only if solution is at room temperature. For first infusion, use a 3% solution. Give 200 mg/kg/mo IV beginning with 0.5–1 mL/min. After 15–30 min, increase rate to 1.5–2.5 mL/min. If clinical response or IgG level is insufficient, increase to 300 mg/kg/mo or give more frequently. If patient tolerates the first infusion, may administer subsequent infusions at a higher rate or concentration.

▸ **Gammagard S/D:** 200–400 mg/kg IV at 0.5 mL/kg/h. If patient tolerates it, increase rate gradually but not to exceed 4 mL/kg/h. Monthly doses of ≥ 100 mg/kg are recommended.

▸ **Gammar-P IV:** 200–400 mg/kg IV q3–4wk. Begin with 0.01 mL/kg/min; increase to 0.02 mL/kg/min after 15–30 min. Most patients tolerate a gradual increase to 0.03–0.06 mL/kg/min.

▸ **Venoglobulin-I:** 200 mg/kg/mo IV beginning with 0.01–0.02 mL/kg/min for the first 30 min. If patient is without distress, increase to 0.04 mL/kg/min. Subsequent infusions may be given at a higher rate. If clinical response of IgG level is insufficient, increase to 300–400 mg/kg/mo or give more frequently.

▸ **Gamimune N:** 100–200 mg/kg/mo IV beginning with 0.01–0.02 mL/kg/min for 30 min. If patient does not experience discomfort, increase rate to a maximum of 0.08 mL/kg/min. If clinical response or IgG level is insufficient, increase to 400 mg/kg/mo or give more frequently.

▶ **Iveegam:** 200 mg/kg/mo IV at 1–2 mL/min for a 5% solution. If clinical response or IgG level is insufficient, increase dosage up to 800 mg/kg or give more frequently.

▶ **Polygam S/D:** 100 mg/kg/mo IV beginning with 0.5 mL/kg/h. An initial dose of 200–400 mg/kg may be given. If patient tolerates it, gradually increase rate up to 4 mL/kg/h. Patients who tolerate this higher rate can receive a 10% solution starting at 0.5 mL/kg/h.

▶ **Venoglobulin-S:** 200 mg/kg/mo IV beginning with 0.01–0.02 mL/kg/min. If patient does not experience discomfort, increase rate of 5% solution to 0.04 mL/kg/min or increase rate of 10% solution to 0.05 mL/kg/min. If clinical response or IgG level is insufficient, increase to 300–400 mg/kg/mo or give more frequently.

▶ *Idiopathic thrombocytopenic purpura*

▶ **Sandoglobulin:** 400 mg/kg IV for 2–5 d. See above for administration rates.

▶ **Gammagard S/D:** 1000 mg/kg IV. Determine need for additional doses based on clinical response and platelet count. If needed, give up to 3 doses on alternate days. See above for administration rates.

▶ **Venoglobulin-I: Induction:** Up to 2000 mg/kg/d IV over 2–7 d. **Acute:** If patient responds to induction therapy by manifesting a platelet count of 30,000 to 50,000/mm^3, discontinue after 2–7 daily doses. **Maintenance:** If platelet count < 30,000/mm^3 or clinically significant bleeding occurs, give up to a single 2000 mg/kg infusion q2wk or less as needed to maintain a platelet count > 20,000/mm^3. See above for administration rates.

▶ **Gamimune N:** 400 mg/kg for 5 d or 1000 mg/kg/d for 1–2 d. If platelet count < 30,000/mm^3 or clinically significant bleeding occurs, give 400 mg/kg as a single infusion. If response is inadequate, increase to 800–1000 mg/kg as a single infusion. Give intermittent infusions as needed to maintain a platelet count > 30,000/mm^3. See above for administration rates.

▶ **Polygam S/D:** 1 g/kg IV. Determine need for additional doses based on patient's response. Give up to 3 separate doses on alternate days if needed. See above for administration rates.

▶ **Venoglobulin-S: Induction:** 2000 mg/kg IV over ≤ 5 d. **Maintenance:** 1000 mg/kg as needed to maintain platelet

counts of 20,000/mm^3 or to prevent bleeding episodes between infusions. See above for administration rates.
▸ *B-Cell CLL*
  ▸ **Gammagard S/D:** 400 mg/kg IV q3–4wk.
  ▸ **Polygam S/D:** 400 mg/kg IV q3–4wk.
▸ *BMT*
  ▸ **Gamimune N:** 500 mg/kg IV beginning on days 7 and 2 pretransplant or at the time conditioning therapy for transplantation is begun. Continue weekly through the 90-d post-transplant period.
▸ *Kawasaki syndrome*
  ▸ **Iveegam:** 400 mg/kg/d IV for 4 d or a single dose of 2000 mg/kg over 10 h. Begin treatment within 10 d of disease onset.

Compatibility
Do not mix or give with other drugs.

TREATMENT OF OVERDOSE/ANTIDOTE
Discontinue drug or decrease dosage. Initiate general supportive and resuscitative measures. Treat anaphylaxis with epinephrine.

Pharmacokinetics

Route	Onset
IV	Immediate

$T_{1/2}$: 3 wk

Adverse effects
▸ *CNS:* Lethargy, headache, feeling of faintness
▸ *CV:* Chest tightness, chest pain
▸ *GI:* Emesis, nausea
▸ *GU:* Nephrotic syndrome
▸ *Derm:* Pruritus, rash, hives, local inflammation/discomfort at injection site
▸ *Allergic:* **Angioedema, anaphylaxis**
▸ *Misc:* Fever, chills

Clinically important drug–drug interactions
▸ Interferes with response to live viral vaccines, such as measles, mumps, rubella; do not give these vaccines until about 6 mo after immune globulin

● NURSING CONSIDERATIONS

Assessment
▸ *History:* Allergic response to gamma globulin, anti-IgA antibodies, thimerosal, or component of individual drug; isolated

Adverse effects in *Italics* are most common; those in **Bold** are life-threatening

IgA deficiency; prior systemic allergic reactions after administration of human immunoglobulin preparations
▸ *Physical:* P, BP, R, I & O, IV site, weight, neurologic checks, adventitious lung sounds, skin condition, abdominal exam, bowel sounds, IgG level, platelet count

Implementation
▸ Administer using an IV infusion pump. Most adverse reactions are related to a too-rapid administration rate.
▸ Continuously monitor vital signs during infusion.
▸ Have emergency equipment (defibrillator, drugs, oxygen, intubation equipment) on standby in case anaphylaxis or adverse reaction occurs.
▸ Discard partially used vials.

insulin *(in' su lin)* ***Insulin injection:*** Humulin R, Iletin II (CAN), Novolin ge Toronto (CAN), Novolin R, Regular Iletin I, Regular Iletin II, Regular Purified Pork Insulin, Velosulin Human BR
Insulin analog injection: Humalog
Isophane insulin suspension (NPH) and insulin injection: Humulin 70/30, Novolin 70/30, Humulin 30/70 (CAN), Novolin ge (CAN)
Isophane insulin suspension and insulin injection: Humulin 50/50, Novolin ge (CAN)
Isophane insulin suspension (NPH): Humulin N, Novolin N, NPH Iletin II, NPH Iletin I, Novolin ge NPH (CAN), NPH-N
Insulin zinc suspension (Lente): Humulin L, Humulin-L (CAN), Lente Iletin I, Lente Iletin II, Lente L, Novolin ge Lente (CAN), Novolin L
Insulin zinc suspension, extended (Ultralente): Humulin U Ultralente, Novolin ge Ultralente (CAN)
Insulin injection concentrated: Regular (concentrated) Iletin II

Pregnancy Category B

Drug classes
Antidiabetic agent
Hormone

Indications
▸ Treatment of diabetes mellitus type 1
▸ Treatment of diabetes mellitus type 2 that cannot be controlled by diet, exercise, or weight reduction
▸ Treatment of severe ketoacidosis or diabetic coma (regular insulin injection IV or IM)

Adverse effects in *Italics* are most common; those in **Bold** are life-threatening

- Treatment of hyperkalemia with infusion of glucose to produce a shift of potassium into the cells (IV)
- Highly purified and human insulins: local insulin allergy, immunologic insulin resistance, injection site lipodystrophy, temporary insulin use (eg, surgery, acute stress type 2 diabetes), newly diagnosed diabetics
- Insulin injection concentrated: treatment of diabetic patients with marked insulin resistance (requirements > 200 U/d)

Therapeutic actions
- Stimulates carbohydrate metabolism by increasing glucose transport across the cell membrane in muscle and fat, increasing glycogenesis, and inhibiting gluconeogenesis
- Stimulates protein metabolism by increasing amino acid transport across the cell membrane, increasing protein synthesis, and decreasing protein catabolism
- Stimulates fat metabolism by increasing triglyceride synthesis, increasing fatty acid transport across the cell membrane, and inhibiting lipolysis
- Promotes the entry of potassium and magnesium into the cells, lowering the extracellular levels of these electrolytes

Contraindications/cautions
- **Contraindications:** hypoglycemia, allergy to any ingredient of the product (varies with preparations)
- **Cautions:** renal or hepatic function impairment, hyperthyroidism, hypothyroidism, hypokalemia

Available form
- *Injection:* 100 U/mL
- *Concentrated injection:* 500 U/mL

IV/IM/SC facts
Preparation
- *Direct IV, IM, or SC:* Give undiluted.
- *IV infusion:* Add 100 U regular insulin to 100 mL 0.9%NS.

Dosage
- The number and size of daily doses, times of administration, and type of insulin preparation are determined after close medical scrutiny of the patient's blood and urine glucose, diet, exercise, infections, and other stresses. Usually given SC. Regular insulin may be given IV or IM in diabetic coma, ketoacidosis, or hyperkalemia. Give insulin injection concentrated SC or IM, not IV.
- SC doses are usually given 15–30 min before meals and at hs.
- *Severe diabetic acidosis and coma:* 100–200 U in two equal portions (one IV; one SC). Give additional doses based on

the patient's response, blood glucose, acetone, or ketone determinations. Or loading dose of 2.4–7.2 U IV followed by a continuous infusion of 2.4–7.2 U/h. Or 0.22 U/kg IM followed by 5 U/h IM.

◗ *Initial therapy:* 5–10 U SC 15–30 min before meals and at hs.

Normal fasting serum glucose level
◗ 60–115 mg/dL

Compatibility
Insulin may be given through the same IV line as amiodarone, ampicillin, ampicillin-sulbactam, aztreonam, cefazolin, cefotetan, dobutamine, esmolol, famotidine, gentamicin, heparin, heparin with hydrocortisone, imipenem-cilastatin, indomethacin, magnesium sulfate, meperidine, meropenem, midazolam, morphine, nitroglycerin, nitroprusside sodium, oxytocin, pentobarbital, potassium chloride, propofol, ritodrine, sodium bicarbonate, tacrolimus, terbutaline, ticarcillin, ticarcillin-clavulanate, tobramycin, vancomycin, vitamin B complex with C.

Incompatibility
Do not administer through the same IV line as dopamine, nafcillin, norepinephrine.

TREATMENT OF OVERDOSE/ANTIDOTE
Discontinue drug or decrease dosage. Initiate general supportive and resuscitative measures. Treat mild hypoglycemia with oral glucose. Treat more severe hypoglycemia with IM/SC glucagon or concentrated IV glucose. Sustained carbohydrate intake and observation may be necessary because hypoglycemia may recur after apparent clinical recovery.

Pharmacokinetics

Type	Onset	Peak	Duration
Regular	0.5–1 h	15–30 min (IV)	8–12 h
NPH	1.1–5 h	4–12 h	24 h
Lente	1–2.5 h	7–15 h	24 h
Ultralente	4–8 h	10–30 h	> 36 h

Metabolism: Liver, kidney, muscle; $T_{1/2}$: varies with preparation

Adverse effects
◗ *CNS:* Blurred vision, headache, drowsiness
◗ *Derm:* Redness, swelling, itching, lipoatrophy at injection site; usually resolves in a few days to a few weeks; a change in type or species source of insulin may be tried
◗ *Allergic:* **Anaphylaxis, angioedema,** rash, shortness of breath, tachycardia, hypotension, sweating

Adverse effects in *Italics* are most common; those in **Bold** are life-threatening

‣ *Metabolic:* Hypoglycemia, rebound hyperglycemia, ketoacidosis

Clinically important drug–drug interactions

‣ Increased hypoglycemic effects with ACE inhibitors, alcohol, anabolic steroids, beta-blockers, calcium, chloroquine, clofibrate, fenfluramine, guanethidine, lithium, monoamine oxidase inhibitors, mebendazole, octreotide, pentamidine, phenylbutazone, pyridoxine, salicylates, sulfinpyrazone, sulfonamides, tetracyclines

‣ Decreased hypoglycemic effects with acetazolamide, AIDS antivirals, asparaginase, calcitonin, contraceptives (oral), corticosteroids, cyclophosphamide, dextrothyroxine, diazoxide, diltiazem, diuretics, dobutamine, epinephrine, estrogens, ethacrynic acid, isoniazid, lithium, morphine, niacin, phenothiazines, phenytoin, nicotine, thiazide diuretics, thyroid drugs

● NURSING CONSIDERATIONS

Assessment

‣ *History:* Hypoglycemia, allergy to any ingredient of the product, renal or hepatic function impairment, hyperthyroidism, hypothyroidism

‣ *Physical:* P, R, BP, I & O, weight, injection site, neurologic checks, skin assessment, mucous membranes, eyeball turgor, peripheral sensation, adventitious lung sounds, hydration status, UA, serum and urine glucose, serum electrolytes, serum and urine ketones, ABG, hemoglobin A1C

Implementation

‣ Always administer an infusion using an IV pump.

‣ Ensure uniform dispersion of insulin suspensions by rolling the vial gently between hands; avoid vigorous shaking.

‣ Have emergency equipment (defibrillator, drugs, oxygen, intubation equipment) on standby in case anaphylaxis or hypoglycemia occurs.

‣ Use only an insulin syringe to draw up the dose. Carefully verify the type, dose, and expiration date of the insulin.

‣ Give maintenance doses SC; rotate injection sites regularly to decrease incidence of lipodystrophy.

‣ When treating hyperglycemia with IV insulin, decrease or discontinue insulin infusion when serum glucose is 250–300 mg/dL and add D5W to the IV infusion.

‣ Carefully assess the patient for response to therapy and for hypoglycemia (headache, fatigue, irritability, pale skin, tremors, hunger, altered responsiveness, cool and clammy skin, tachycardia, coma, nausea) or hyperglycemia (flushed

Adverse effects in *Italics* are most common; those in **Bold** are life-threatening

skin, dry mucous membranes, tachycardia, hypotension, fruity breath, polyuria, unusual thirst, diminished consciousness, tachypnea, Kussmaul respirations, vomiting, anorexia, decreased skin turgor).

▸ Carefully monitor patients receiving IV insulin; plastic IV infusion sets have been reported to remove 20%–80% of the insulin; dosage delivered to the patient will vary.

▸ Do not give insulin injection concentrated IV; severe anaphylactic reactions can occur.

▸ Use caution when mixing two types of insulin; always draw the clear regular insulin into the syringe first; use mixtures of regular and lente insulins within 5 min of combining them.

▸ Carefully monitor patients being switched from one type of insulin to another; dosage adjustments are often needed. Human insulins often require smaller doses than beef or pork insulin.

▸ Store insulin in a cool place away from direct sunlight. Refrigeration is preferred. Do not freeze insulin.

⬤ ipecac syrup (ip' e kak)
Pregnancy Category C

Drug class
Antidote

Indications
▸ Treatment of drug overdose and certain poisonings

Therapeutic actions
▸ Produces vomiting by a local GI mucosa irritant effect and a central medullary effect (stimulation of chemoreceptor trigger zone)

Contraindications/cautions
▸ **Contraindications:** semiconscious or unconscious patients, convulsive states; ingestion of strychnine, corrosives such as alkalies and strong acids, or petroleum distillates
▸ **Caution:** cardiovascular disease

Available forms
▸ *Syrup:* 1.5–1.75%, 2% alcohol

Oral dosage
▸ 15–30 mL PO followed by 3–4 glasses of water.
▸ Repeat dose of 15 mL PO if vomiting does not occur within 20–30 min.

Adverse effects in *Italics* are most common; those in **Bold** are life-threatening

> **TREATMENT OF OVERDOSE/ANTIDOTE**
> Discontinue drug or decrease dosage. Initiate general supportive and resuscitative measures. Activated charcoal may adsorb ipecac syrup. Perform gastric lavage.

Pharmacokinetics

Route	Onset
Oral	20–30 min

Adverse effects

▸ *CNS:* Mild CNS depression
▸ *CV:* If drug is absorbed: **cardiotoxicity, fatal myocarditis, hypotension conduction disturbances, dysrhythmias,** bradycardia, atrial fibrillation
▸ *GI:* Diarrhea, GI upset

⬤ NURSING CONSIDERATIONS

Assessment

▸ *History:* Semiconscious or unconscious patients, convulsive states, cardiovascular disease, substance ingested
▸ *Physical:* BP, P, R, ECG, I & O, SpO_2, neurologic checks, skin assessment, adventitious lung sounds, cardiac assessment, serum drug levels for agent ingested

Implementation

▸ Consult a Poison Control Center if in doubt about whether to use ipecac.
▸ Give only to conscious patients.
▸ Give as soon after poisoning as possible.
▸ Before giving drug, have patient sit upright with head forward.
▸ Give with water; do not use milk or carbonated beverages.
▸ Have emergency equipment (defibrillator, drugs, oxygen, intubation equipment) on standby in case ipecac is not effective in treating the overdose/poisoning.
▸ Use activated charcoal if vomiting of ipecac does not occur.
▸ Assess emesis for pill fragments or evidence of ingested substance.
▸ Do not confuse ipecac syrup with ipecac fluid extract, which is 14 times stronger and has caused deaths.

⬤ **ipratropium bromide** *(i pra troe' pee um)*
Alti-Ipratropium (CAN), Apo-Ipravent (CAN), Atrovent, Novo-Ipramide (CAN)

Adverse effects in *Italics* are most common; those in **Bold** are life-threatening

Pregnancy Category B

Drug class
Anticholinergic
Antimuscarinic agent
Parasympatholytic

Indications
▸ Bronchodilator for maintenance treatment of bronchospasm associated with chronic obstructive pulmonary disease, including chronic bronchitis and emphysema (solution, aerosol)
▸ Symptomatic relief of rhinorrhea associated with perennial rhinitis, common cold (nasal spray)

Therapeutic actions
▸ Anticholinergic, chemically related to atropine, which blocks vagally mediated reflexes by antagonizing the action of acetylcholine
▸ Inhibits secretions from serous, seromucous glands lining nasal mucosa
▸ Localized bronchodilation

Contraindications/cautions
▸ **Contraindications:** allergy to ipratropium, atropine or its derivatives, acute episodes of bronchospasm, allergy to soya lecithin or related food products, such as soybeans, peanuts
▸ **Cautions:** narrow-angle glaucoma, prostatic hypertrophy, bladder neck obstruction

Available forms
▸ *Aerosol:* 18 mcg/actuation
▸ *Solution for inhalation:* 0.02%
▸ *Nasal spray:* 0.03% (21 mcg/spray), 0.06% (42 mcg/spray)

Dosage
▸ **Inhalation:** Usual dosage is 2 inhalations (36 mcg) qid. Give additional inhalations as required. Do not exceed 12 inhalations/24 h. Solution for inhalation: 500 mcg, tid to qid with doses 6–8 h apart.
▸ **Nasal spray:** 2 sprays 0.03% per nostril bid to tid or 2 sprays 0.06% per nostril tid–qid.

TREATMENT OF OVERDOSE/ANTIDOTE
Discontinue drug or decrease dosage. Initiate general supportive and resuscitative measures.

Adverse effects in *Italics* are most common; those in **Bold** are life-threatening

Pharmacokinetics

Route	Onset	Peak	Duration
Inhalation	15 min	1–2 h	3–5 h

Minimal systemic absorption; $T_{1/2}$: 2 h
Elimination: Feces

Adverse effects

▸ *CNS: Nervousness, dizziness, headache, blurred vision,* fatigue, insomnia
▸ *Resp: Cough,* exacerbation of symptoms, hoarseness
▸ *GI: Nausea, dry mouth,* GI distress
▸ *Allergic:* **Angioedema, bronchospasm, oropharyngeal edema,** urticaria, rash
▸ *Misc:* Palpitations, rash, pain, nasal dryness, epistaxis

Clinically important drug–drug interactions

▸ Enhanced by other anticholinergic drugs

◉ NURSING CONSIDERATIONS

Assessment

▸ *History:* Allergy to ipratropium, atropine, soya lecithin, or related food products; acute bronchospasm, narrow-angle glaucoma, prostatic hypertrophy, bladder neck obstruction
▸ *Physical:* P, BP, R, I & O, SpO_2, neurologic checks, skin assessment, respiratory effort, adventitious lung sounds, ophthalmic exam, bowel sounds, prostate palpation, ABG, peak flow test, pulmonary function tests

Implementation

▸ Drug may be mixed in nebulizer with albuterol if used within 1 h.
▸ Ensure adequate hydration, provide environmental control (temperature) to prevent hyperpyrexia.
▸ Have patient void before taking medication to prevent urinary retention.
▸ Initial nasal spray pump priming requires seven actuations of the pump. If not used for > 24 h, reprime with two actuations.
▸ Teach patient proper use of inhaler.
▸ Store drug at room temperature; protect solution for inhalation from light.

◉ isoproterenol *(eye soe proe ter' e nole)*

◉ isoproterenol hydrochloride
Isuprel, Isuprel Mistometer

◉ isoproterenol sulfate Medihaler-Iso

Adverse effects in *Italics* are most common; those in **Bold** are life-threatening

Pregnancy Category C

Drug classes
Beta-adrenergic agonist
Inotropic agent
Sympathomimetic
Antidysrhythmic
Bronchodilator

Indications
▶ Mild or transient heart block that does not require electric shock or pacemaker therapy
▶ Serious heart block and Adams-Stokes attacks (except when caused by ventricular tachycardia or fibrillation)
▶ Cardiac arrest until electric shock or pacemaker treatment is available
▶ As an adjunct to fluid and electrolyte replacement therapy and other drugs in the treatment of hypovolemic, cardiogenic, and septic shock; low cardiac output states; and CHF
▶ Relief of reversible bronchospasm associated with acute and chronic asthma, chronic bronchitis, and emphysema

Therapeutic actions
▶ Effects are mediated by beta-1 and beta-2 adrenergic receptors
▶ Acts on beta-1 receptors in the heart to produce positive chronotropic and positive inotropic effects and increased automaticity
▶ Acts on beta-2 receptors in the bronchi to cause bronchodilation
▶ Acts on beta-2 receptors in smooth muscle walls of blood vessels in skeletal muscle and splanchnic beds to cause dilation

Effects on hemodynamic parameters
▶ Increased HR
▶ Decreased or unchanged SVR
▶ Decreased diastolic BP
▶ Unchanged or increased systolic BP (except with very high doses systolic BP drops related to decreased SVR)
▶ Decreased or unchanged PCWP
▶ Decreased or unchanged CVP
▶ Increased CO

Contraindications/cautions
▶ **Contraindications:** isoproterenol allergy, tachydysrhythmias; tachycardia or heart block caused by digitalis toxicity; angina pectoris, ventricular dysrhythmias that require inotropic therapy

(contraindications continued on next page)

Adverse effects in *Italics* are most common; those in **Bold** are life-threatening

> ▸ **Cautions:** acute myocardial infarction (AMI), organic disease of the AV node or its branches, sulfite or sympathomimetic amine sensitivity, coronary artery disease, cardiogenic shock, coronary insufficiency, hypovolemia, hypotension, hypertension, diabetes, hyperthyroidism, elderly patients

Available forms
▸ *IV injection:* 0.02, 0.2 mg/mL
▸ *Solution for inhalation:* 0.5%, 1%
▸ *Aerosol:* 103 mcg/dose; 80 mcg/actuation

IV facts
Preparation
▸ For a continuous infusion, add 1–2 mg isoproterenol to 250–500 mL of: D2.5W; D5W; D10W; Dextran 6% in D5W or 0.9%NS; Dextrose-LR combinations; Dextrose-Ringer's combinations; Dextrose-Saline combinations; Invert Sugar 5% or 10% in 0.9%NS or Water; Ionosol products; LR; Ringer's Injection; or Sodium Lactate (1/6 Molar) Injection.

Dosage and titration
▸ *Heart block, Adams-Stokes attacks, cardiac arrest (IV injection):* Dilute 0.2 mg in 10 mL with 0.9%NS or D5W. Administer 0.02–0.06 mg (1–3 mL) of diluted IV solution over 1 min. Repeat with 0.01–0.2 mg (0.5–10 mL) as indicated.
▸ *Heart block, Adams-Stokes attacks, cardiac arrest (IV infusion):* Usual dosage is 2–10 mcg/min. Initiate infusion at 5 mcg/min. Titrate up to 30 mcg/min to achieve desired HR, CVP, BP, and urine output.
▸ *Heart block, Adams-Stokes attacks, cardiac arrest (intracardiac injection):* In emergencies, give 0.02 mg undiluted.

Titration Guide

isoproterenol hydrochloride
1 mg in 250 mL

mcg/min	1	2	3	4	5	6	7
mL/h	15	30	45	60	75	90	105

mcg/min	8	9	10	12	14	16	18
mL/h	120	135	150	180	210	240	270

mcg/min	20	22	24	26	28	30
mL/h	300	330	360	390	420	450

Adverse effects in *Italics* are most common; those in **Bold** are life-threatening

Compatibility

Isoproterenol may be given through the same IV line as amiodarone, amrinone, atracurium, bretylium, famotidine, heparin, hydrocortisone, pancuronium, potassium chloride, ranitidine, tacrolimus, vecuronium, vitamin B complex with C.

Inhalation dosage

▸ *Acute bronchial asthma (metered-dose inhaler):* **Isoproterenol sulfate:** Give 1 inhalation. If no relief after 2–5 min, give a second inhalation. For daily maintenance, give 1–2 inhalations 4–6 times daily. Do not give > 2 inhalations at any one time or > 6 inhalations per hour. **Isoproterenol HCl:** Give 1 inhalation. Wait 1 min before giving a second a dose. May repeat up to 5 times daily if needed.

▸ *Bronchospasm in chronic obstructive lung disease:* **Nebulization by compressed air or oxygen and intermittent positive pressure breathing:** Dilute 0.5 mL of a 1:200 solution to 2–2.5 mL water or isotonic saline. Deliver over 15–20 min. May repeat up to 5 times daily. **Metered-dose inhaler:** 1–2 inhalations. Repeat at no less than 3- to 4-h intervals.

TREATMENT OF OVERDOSE/ANTIDOTE
Discontinue drug or decrease dosage. Initiate general supportive or resuscitative measures.

Pharmacokinetics

Route	Onset	Duration
IV	Immediate	<1 h
Inhalation	2–5 min	1–3 h

Metabolism: Tissue
Excretion: Urine

Adverse effects

▸ *CNS: Restlessness, apprehension, anxiety, fear,* headache, dizziness, nervousness, insomnia, tremor, drowsiness, irritability, weakness

▸ *CV:* **Cardiac arrest,** *dysrhythmias, tachycardia, palpitations,* angina, changes in BP; paradoxical precipitation of Adams-Stokes seizures during normal sinus rhythm or transient heart block; chest tightness, hypotension

▸ *Resp:* **Pulmonary edema, bronchospasm,** *respiratory difficulties, coughing, paradoxical airway resistance with repeated excessive use, throat dryness/irritation*

▸ *GI: Nausea, vomiting, heartburn,* unusual or bad taste, parotid gland swelling

▸ *Misc: Sweating, pallor,* flushing, muscle cramps

Adverse effects in *Italics* are most common; those in **Bold** are life-threatening

Clinically important drug–drug interactions

- Serious dysrhythmias with epinephrine; may be given alternately with epinephrine if proper interval has elapsed between doses
- Enhanced by bretylium; may cause dysrhythmias
- Enhanced pressor response with guanethidine, oxytocic drugs, TCAs

◯ NURSING CONSIDERATIONS

Assessment

- *History:* Isoproterenol allergy, angina pectoris, AMI, organic disease of the AV node or its branches, sulfite or sympathomimetic amine sensitivity, coronary artery disease, cardiogenic shock, coronary insufficiency, hypovolemia, hypotension, hypertension, diabetes, hyperthyroidism, digitalis toxicity, age
- *Physical:* T, P, BP, R, SVR, CVP, PCWP, CO, ECG, I & O, SpO_2, neurologic checks, respiratory status, chest pain assessment, skin color and turgor, adventitious lung sounds, blood and urine glucose, serum electrolytes, ABG, chest x-ray, peak flow test, pulmonary function tests

Implementation

- Exercise extreme caution when calculating and preparing doses. Isoproterenol is a very potent drug; small dosage errors can cause serious adverse effects.
- Always administer an infusion using an IV infusion pump.
- Administer into large veins of antecubital fossa rather than hand or ankle veins. Use a central line whenever possible.
- Use minimal doses for shortest time possible.
- Correct hypovolemia before administering isoproterenol.
- Maintain a beta-adrenergic blocker on standby in case cardiac dysrhythmias occur.
- Monitor ECG, BP, CO, and SVR closely during infusion. Adjust dose/rate accordingly.
- Discontinue drug if patient has chest pain or dysrhythmias.
- Do not use if solution is pink or brown or contains a precipitate.
- Do not exceed recommended dosage; administer pressurized inhalation drug forms during second half of inspiration, because the airways are open wider, and the aerosol distribution is more extensive.
- Store drug at room temperature; protect from light during storage.

Adverse effects in *Italics* are most common; those in **Bold** are life-threatening

◗ isosorbide dinitrate *(eye soe sor' bide)*
Apo-ISDN (CAN), Cedocard SR (CAN), Dilatrate SR,
Isordil, Isordil Tembids, Isordil Titradose, Sorbitrate

Pregnancy Category C

Drug classes
Antianginal agent
Nitrate

Indications
▸ Treatment and prevention of angina pectoris

Therapeutic actions
▸ Relaxes vascular smooth muscle
▸ Dilates both venous and arterial beds; venous effects predominate
▸ Dilates postcapillary vessels, including large veins
▸ Improves blood flow to ischemic myocardium
▸ Decreases myocardial oxygen consumption

Effects on hemodynamic parameters
▸ Decreased SVR/PVR (if previously elevated)
▸ Decreased LVEDP
▸ Decreased BP
▸ Decreased CVP (if previously elevated)
▸ Decreased PCWP (if previously elevated)
▸ Possible reflex tachycardia
▸ Unchanged, increased, or decreased CO

Contraindications/cautions
▸ **Contraindications:** allergy to nitrates, severe anemia, closed-angle glaucoma, postural hypotension, head trauma, cerebral hemorrhage
▸ **Cautions:** hypertrophic cardiomyopathy, glaucoma, hypotension, hypovolemia

Available Forms
▸ *Tablets:* 5, 10, 20, 30, 40 mg
▸ *SL tablets:* 2.5, 5, 10 mg
▸ *Chewable tablets:* 5, 10 mg
▸ *SR tablets:* 40 mg
▸ *SR capsules:* 40 mg

Oral dosage
▸ *Angina pectoris:* **Starting dose:** 2.5–5 mg sublingual, 5 mg chewable tablets, 5–20 mg PO oral tablets or capsules; 40 mg PO SR. **Maintenance:** 10–40 mg PO q6h oral tablets or capsules; 40–80 mg PO q8–12h SR.

Adverse effects in *Italics* are most common; those in **Bold** are life-threatening

▸ *Acute prophylaxis:* Initial dosage: 5–10 mg sublingual or chewable tablets q2–3h.

> **TREATMENT OF OVERDOSE/ANTIDOTE**
> Discontinue drug or decrease dosage. Initiate general supportive and resuscitative measures. For ingested nitrates, induce emesis, perform gastric lavage, and give charcoal. Keep patient warm and recumbent with legs elevated. Passive extremity movement may aid venous return. Monitor methemoglobin levels; treat methemoglobinemia. Treat severe hypotension and reflex tachycardia with IV fluids; consider phenylephrine or methoxamine. Epinephrine is ineffective and contraindicated for hypotension.

Pharmacokinetics

Route	Onset	Duration
Oral	20–40 min	4–6 h
Oral, SR	Up to 4 h	6–8 h
SL	2–5 min	1–3 h

Metabolism: Hepatic; $T_{1/2}$: 2–5 h

Adverse effects

▸ *CNS: Headache, dizziness,* agitation, anxiety, confusion, dyscoordination, hypoesthesia, hypokinesia, insomnia, nervousness, nightmares
▸ *CV:* **CV collapse,** tachycardia, palpitations, hypotension, postural hypotension, angina, dysrhythmias
▸ *Resp:* Bronchitis, pneumonia, upper respiratory tract infection
▸ *GI: Nausea, vomiting,* abdominal pain, diarrhea, dyspepsia, increased appetite
▸ *Derm:* Rash, cutaneous vasodilation with flushing, pruritus
▸ *Misc:* **Methemoglobinemia,** muscle twitching, pallor, perspiration, cold sweat, neck stiffness, blurred vision, arthralgia

Clinically important drug–drug interactions

▸ Increased hypotension with other vasodilators or alcohol
▸ Marked symptomatic postural hypotension with calcium channel-blockers, beta-blockers, organic nitrates
▸ Increased serum nitrate concentrations with aspirin
▸ Increased hypertension and decreased antianginal effect with ergot alkaloids

● NURSING CONSIDERATIONS

Assessment

▸ *History:* Allergy to nitrates, severe anemia, closed-angle glaucoma, postural hypotension, head trauma, cerebral hemor-

Adverse effects in *Italics* are most common; those in **Bold** are life-threatening

rhage, hypertrophic cardiomyopathy, glaucoma, hypotension, hypovolemia

▶ *Physical:* T, BP, R, P, ECG, I & O, neurologic checks, skin assessment, ophthalmic exam, adventitious lung sounds, orthostatic BP, chest pain assessment (type, location, intensity, duration, precipitating events, radiation, quality), hydration status, peripheral perfusion, liver evaluation, liver and renal function tests, CBC

Implementation

▶ Give sublingual preparations under the tongue or in the buccal pouch; encourage patient not to swallow.

▶ Give chewable tablets slowly, only 5 mg initially because severe hypotension can occur; ensure patient does not chew or crush sustained-release preparations.

▶ Give oral preparations on an empty stomach, 1 h before or 2 h after meals; take with meals if severe, uncontrolled headache occurs.

▶ Have emergency equipment (defibrillator, drugs, intubation equipment, oxygen) on standby in case an adverse reaction occurs.

▶ Monitor patient's response to therapy (vital signs, hemodynamic parameters, ECG, chest pain status).

▶ Correct hypovolemia before administering drug.

▶ Minimize postural hypotension by having the patient change positions slowly.

▶ Aspirin or acetaminophen may relieve headaches associated with nitroglycerin therapy.

▶ Gradually reduce dose if anginal treatment is being terminated; rapid discontinuation can lead to problems of withdrawal.

▶ Tolerance to these drugs may develop. Consider giving the short-acting forms bid or tid daily (last dose no later than 7 PM) and the sustained released forms qd or bid at 8 AM and 2 PM.

● isosorbide mononitrate *(eye soe sor' bide)*
Monoket, ISMO, Imdur, Isotrate ER

Pregnancy Category C

Drug classes
Antianginal agent
Nitrate

Indications
▶ Prevention of angina pectoris

Therapeutic actions
▶ Relaxes vascular smooth muscle
▶ Dilates both venous and arterial beds; venous effects predominate

Adverse effects in *Italics* are most common; those in **Bold** are life-threatening

- Dilates postcapillary vessels, including large veins
- Improves blood flow to ischemic myocardium
- Decreases myocardial oxygen consumption

Effects on hemodynamic parameters
- Decreased SVR/PVR (if previously elevated)
- Decreased LVEDP
- Decreased BP
- Decreased CVP (if previously elevated)
- Decreased PCWP (if previously elevated)
- Possible reflex tachycardia
- Unchanged, increased, or decreased CO

Contraindications/cautions
- **Contraindications:** allergy to nitrates, severe anemia, closed-angle glaucoma, postural hypotension, head trauma, cerebral hemorrhage, acute myocardial infarction (AMI), CHF
- **Cautions:** hypertrophic cardiomyopathy, glaucoma, hypotension, hypovolemia

Available Forms
- *Tablets:* 10, 20 mg
- *Extended release tablets:* 30, 60, 120 mg

Oral dosage
- *Tablets:* 20 mg PO bid with two doses given 7 h apart.
- *Extended-release tablets:* 30–60 mg/d PO (preferably in morning on arising). After several days, may increase to 120 mg/d PO. Up to 240 mg/d may be required.

TREATMENT OF OVERDOSE/ANTIDOTE
Discontinue drug or decrease dosage. Initiate general supportive and resuscitative measures. For ingested nitrates, induce emesis, perform gastric lavage, and give charcoal. Keep patient warm and recumbent with legs elevated. Passive extremity movement may aid venous return. Monitor methemoglobin levels; treat methemoglobinemia. Treat severe hypotension and reflex tachycardia with IV fluids; consider phenylephrine or methoxamine. Epinephrine is ineffective and contraindicated for hypotension.

Pharmacokinetics

Route	Onset	Peak
Oral	30–60 min	1–4 h

$T_{1/2}$: 5 h
Excretion: Urine

Adverse effects in *Italics* are most common; those in **Bold** are life-threatening

Adverse effects
- *CNS: Headache,* dizziness, anxiety, dyscoordination, depression, insomnia, nervousness, nightmares, restlessness
- *CV:* **AMI,** dysrhythmias, bradycardia, edema, hypertension, hypotension, pallor, palpitations, tachycardia, chest pain
- *Resp:* Asthma, dyspnea, sinusitis, upper respiratory tract infection, cough
- *GI:* Nausea, vomiting, anorexia, dry mouth, thirst, decreased weight, bitter taste
- *Derm:* Sweating, flushing, pruritus
- *Misc:* **Methemoglobinemia,** prostatic disorder, back pain, muscle cramps, paresthesia

Clinically important drug–drug interactions
- Increased hypotension with other vasodilators, alcohol
- Marked symptomatic postural hypotension with calcium channel-blockers, beta-blockers, organic nitrates

● NURSING CONSIDERATIONS
Assessment
- *History:* Allergy to nitrates, severe anemia, closed-angle glaucoma, postural hypotension, head trauma, cerebral hemorrhage, AMI, CHF, hypertrophic cardiomyopathy, glaucoma, hypotension, hypovolemia
- *Physical:* T, BP, R, P, ECG, I & O, neurologic checks, skin assessment, ophthalmic exam, adventitious lung sounds, orthostatic BP, chest pain assessment (type, location, intensity, duration, precipitating events, radiation, quality), hydration status, peripheral perfusion, liver evaluation, liver and renal function tests, CBC

Implementation
- By giving the two daily doses 7 h apart, the patient has a drug-free interval that may prevent tolerance to the drug.
- Give drug on an empty stomach.
- Have emergency equipment (defibrillator, drugs, intubation equipment, oxygen) on standby in case an adverse reaction occurs.
- Monitor patient's response to therapy (vital signs, hemodynamic parameters, ECG, chest pain status).
- Correct hypovolemia before administering drug.
- Minimize postural hypotension by having the patient change positions slowly.
- Aspirin or acetaminophen may relieve headaches associated with nitroglycerin therapy.

Adverse effects in *Italics* are most common; those in **Bold** are life-threatening

L

● labetalol hydrochloride *(la bet' a lol)*

Normodyne, Trandate

Pregnancy Category C

Drug classes
Alpha/Beta adrenergic blocker
Antihypertensive

Indications
▸ Hypertension, alone or with other oral agents, especially diuretics
▸ Severe hypertension (parenteral)
▸ Unlabeled uses: pheochromocytoma; clonidine withdrawal hypertension

Therapeutic actions
▸ Blocks α_1-, β_1-, and β_2-adrenergic receptors and has some sympathomimetic activity at β_2-receptors
▸ Beta blockade prevents reflex tachycardia seen with most alpha-blocking drugs and decreases plasma renin activity

Effects on hemodynamic parameters
▸ Decreased BP
▸ Decreased SVR
▸ Increased or unchanged CO
▸ Decreased or unchanged HR

Contraindications/cautions
▸ **Contraindications:** beta-blocker allergy, bronchial asthma, overt cardiac failure, second- or third-degree heart block, cardiogenic shock, severe bradycardia, recent CABG
▸ **Cautions:** well-compensated CHF, diabetes, hypoglycemia, liver dysfunction, elderly, pheochromocytoma, concurrent use of other antihypertensive drugs

Available forms
▸ *Injection:* 5 mg/mL
▸ *Tablets:* 100, 200, 300 mg

IV facts
Preparation
▸ For an infusion, add 200 mg to 160 mL of D5W/5%LR; D2.5%W/0.45%NS; D5W/0.2%NS; D5W/0.33%NS; D5W/

Adverse effects in *Italics* are most common; those in **Bold** are life-threatening

0.9%NS; D5W/Ringer's Injection; D5W; LR; 0.9%NS; Polysal in Dextrose 5%; or Ringer's Injection.

Dosage

▸ *Repeated IV injection:* 20 mg IV over 2 min. Individualize dosage using supine BP. Give additional doses of 40 or 80 mg at 10-min intervals until desired BP is achieved or total of 300 mg is given.

▸ *Continuous IV infusion:* Infuse at rate of 2 mg/min, adjusting rate according to BP response. Effective dose range is 50–200 mg, up to 300 mg. Continue until satisfactory response is obtained. Convert to oral dosing when supine diastolic BP begins to rise.

Titration Guide

labetalol hydrochloride			
200 mg in 160 mL			
mg/min	1	2	3
mL/h	60	120	180

Compatibility

Labetalol may be given through the same IV line as amikacin, aminophylline, amiodarone, ampicillin, butorphanol, calcium gluconate, cefazolin, ceftazidime, ceftizoxime, chloramphenicol, cimetidine, clindamycin, dobutamine, dopamine, enalaprilat, epinephrine, erythromycin, esmolol, famotidine, fentanyl, gentamicin, heparin, hydromorphone, lidocaine, lorazepam, magnesium sulfate, meperidine, metronidazole, midazolam, milrinone, morphine, nicardipine, nitroglycerin, nitroprusside sodium, norepinephrine, oxacillin, penicillin G potassium, piperacillin, potassium chloride, potassium phosphates, propofol, ranitidine, sodium acetate, tobramycin, trimethoprim-sulfamethoxazole, vancomycin, vecuronium.

Incompatibility

Do not administer through the same IV line as cefoperazone, ceftriaxone, nafcillin, warfarin.

Oral dosage

▸ *Initial dose:* 100 mg PO bid. After 2–3 d, using standing BP as an indicator, titrate dosage in increments of 100 mg PO bid q2–3d.

▸ *Maintenance dose:* 200–400 mg PO bid. Patients with severe HTN may require up to 2400 mg/d. If side effects occur with bid dosing, give same total dose in tid dosing.

Adverse effects in *Italics* are most common; those in **Bold** are life-threatening

TREATMENT OF OVERDOSE/ANTIDOTE

Discontinue drug or decrease dosage. Initiate general supportive and resuscitative measures. Initiate gastric lavage or induce emesis to remove drug after oral ingestion. Place patient in supine position with legs elevated. Treat bradycardia with atropine or epinephrine; cardiac failure with a digitalis glycoside, a diuretic, or dopamine, or dobutamine; PVCs with lidocaine; hypotension with vasopressors, such as norepinephrine; bronchospasm with epinephrine or an aerosolized β_2-agonist; and seizures with diazepam. Give glucagon (5–10 mg IV over 30 s, followed by infusion of 5 mg/h) for severe beta-blocker overdose.

Pharmacokinetics

Route	Onset	Peak	Duration
IV	Immediate	5 min	up to 16–18 h
Oral	Varies	1–2 h	8–12 h

Metabolism: Hepatic; $T_{1/2}$: 6–8 h (oral); 5.5 (parenteral)
Excretion: Urine, feces

Adverse effects

▸ *CNS: Headache, dizziness, numbness, tingling of scalp/skin,* drowsiness
▸ *CV:* **Ventricular dysrhythmias, congestive heart failure,** edema, postural hypotension, syncope, heart block
▸ *Resp:* **Bronchospasm,** wheezing, dyspnea, nasal stuffiness
▸ *GI:* **Hepatic necrosis,** *nausea, vomiting,* taste distortion, dyspepsia, hepatitis, elevated liver enzymes
▸ *GU:* Urinary retention, difficulty in micturition, impotence, ejaculation failure
▸ *Allergic:* **Anaphylaxis, angioedema,** rash, urticaria, pruritus, dyspnea
▸ *Musc/Skel:* Muscle cramps, toxic myopathy
▸ *Misc: Sweating,* systemic lupus erythematosus, fever, positive antinuclear factor

Clinically important drug–drug interactions

▸ Reduced bronchodilator effects of beta-adrenergic agonists for patients with bronchospasm
▸ Increased hypotension due to reduced reflex tachycardia of nitroglycerin
▸ Tremors with TCAs
▸ Oral forms enhanced by cimetidine
▸ Enhanced by calcium channel-blockers, other beta-blockers, quinidine, phenothiazines

Adverse effects in *Italics* are most common; those in **Bold** are life-threatening

▶ May potentiate, counteract, or have no effect on nondepolarizing muscle relaxants
▶ Reduced insulin release in response to hyperglycemia

● NURSING CONSIDERATIONS

Assessment

▶ *History:* Labetalol allergy, bronchial asthma, overt cardiac failure, cardiogenic shock, recent CABG, well-compensated CHF, diabetes, hypoglycemia, liver dysfunction, age, pheochromocytoma, concurrent use of other antihypertensive drugs, angina
▶ *Physical:* P, BP, R, SVR, CO, ECG, I & O, weight, neurologic checks, skin assessment, adventitious lung sounds, respiratory effort, cardiac auscultation, chest pain assessment, JVD, edema, serum electrolytes, thyroid and renal function tests, UA, serum glucose

Implementation

▶ Exercise extreme caution when calculating and preparing doses. Labetalol is a very potent drug; small dosage errors can cause serious adverse effects.
▶ Always administer an infusion using an IV infusion pump.
▶ Carefully monitor P, BP, R, and ECG during IV administration.
▶ Have emergency equipment (defibrillator, drugs, oxygen, intubation equipment) on standby in case anaphylaxis or adverse reaction occurs.
▶ Assess patients with depressed cardiac function closely; drug may lead to cardiac failure. If failure is suspected, discontinue drug and begin digitalis and/or diuretics.
▶ Decrease dose in patients with renal impairment.
▶ Monitor diabetic patients closely; drug may mask signs and symptoms of hypoglycemia.
▶ Stop drug immediately if patient develops jaundice or laboratory evidence of liver injury.
▶ Administer injection/infusion to patient while supine. Keep patient in supine position for at least 3 h after labetalol injection is given.
▶ Minimize postural hypotension by helping the patient change positions slowly.
▶ Do not discontinue drug abruptly after chronic therapy. (Hypersensitivity to catecholamines may have developed, causing exacerbation of angina, MI, and ventricular dysrhythmias.) Taper drug gradually over 2 wk with monitoring.
▶ Consult with provider about withdrawing drug if patient is to undergo surgery (withdrawal is controversial).

Adverse effects in *Italics* are most common; those in **Bold** are life-threatening

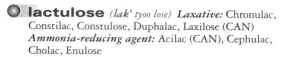

lactulose *(lak' tyoo lose)* **Laxative:** Chronulac, Constilac, Constulose, Duphalac, Laxilose (CAN) ***Ammonia-reducing agent:*** Acilac (CAN), Cephulac, Cholac, Enulose

Pregnancy Category B

Drug classes
Laxative
Ammonia-reduction agent

Indications
▸ Prevention and treatment of portal-systemic encephalopathy
▸ Treatment of constipation

Therapeutic actions
▸ Passes unchanged into the colon where bacteria break it down into organic acids and carbon dioxide; these products increase the colon's osmotic pressure and slightly acidify colonic contents, resulting in an increase in stool water content and stool softening; because colonic contents are more acidic than blood, ammonia migrates from blood into colon where it is trapped and expelled in the feces

Contraindications/cautions
▸ **Contraindications:** lactulose allergy, low-galactose diet
▸ **Cautions:** diabetes, elderly and debilitated patients

Available form
▸ *Syrup:* 10 g/15 mL

Oral dosage
▸ *Portal-systemic encephalopathy:* **Oral:** 30–45 mL PO tid or qid. Adjust dosage every 1–2 d to produce 2–3 soft stools qd. Initially, 30–45 mL/h may be used to induce rapid laxation. Return to standard dose as soon as possible. **Rectal:** Use rectal route during impending coma or coma when patient is at risk for aspiration or when endoscopic or intubation procedures interfere with oral administration. Give as a retention enema through a rectal balloon catheter. Retain enema for 30–60 min. May repeat q4–6h or immediately if inadvertently evacuated too promptly. Start oral drug as soon as feasible and before stopping enemas.
▸ *Laxative:* 15–30 mL/d PO; may increase to 60 mL/d as needed.

Adverse effects in *Italics* are most common; those in **Bold** are life-threatening

TREATMENT OF OVERDOSE/ANTIDOTE
Discontinue drug or decrease dosage. Initiate general supportive and resuscitative measures.

Pharmacokinetics

Route	Onset
Oral	24–48 h
Rectal	≤ 2 h

Poorly absorbed systemically

Adverse effects
▶ *GI: Transient flatulence, distention, intestinal cramps, belching,* diarrhea, nausea, vomiting
▶ *Metabolic:* Acid–base imbalance

Clinically important drug–drug interactions
▶ Desired decrease in colonic pH inhibited with nonabsorbable antacids
▶ Bacteria needed to degrade drug eliminated by neomycin, other anti-infectives; prevents acidification of colonic contents
▶ Acidifying effects counteracted by soap suds enemas, alkaline agents

● NURSING CONSIDERATIONS

Assessment
▶ *History:* Lactulose allergy, low-galactose diet, diabetes, age, debilitated status
▶ *Physical:* P, R, BP, I & O, neurologic checks, abdominal assessment, frequency/amount/consistency of stools, bowel sounds, stool pH; serum electrolytes, glucose, and ammonia levels

Implementation
▶ Monitor serum ammonia levels.
▶ Assess for potential electrolyte and acid–base imbalances.
▶ Give laxative syrup orally with fruit juice, water, or milk to increase palatability.
▶ Do not freeze laxative form. Extremely dark or cloudy syrup may be unsafe; do not use.
▶ Do not use cleansing enemas containing soap suds or other alkaline agents that counteract the effects of lactulose.
▶ Do not administer other laxatives while using lactulose.

Adverse effects in *Italics* are most common; those in **Bold** are life-threatening

● leucovorin calcium (citrovorum factor, folinic acid) *(loo koe vor' in)* Wellcovorin

Pregnancy Category C

Drug classes
Folic acid derivative
Antidote

Indications
▸ Leucovorin "rescue" after high-dose methotrexate therapy in osteosarcoma
▸ Antidote to diminish toxicity and counteract effects of impaired methotrexate elimination and folic acid antagonist overdosage
▸ Treatment of megaloblastic anemias due to sprue, nutritional deficiency, and pregnancy when oral folic acid therapy is not feasible (parenteral)
▸ With 5-fluorouracil for palliative treatment of advanced colorectal cancer (parenteral)

Therapeutic actions
▸ Chemically reduced form of folic acid
▸ Exogenous folate required for nucleoprotein synthesis and maintenance of normal erythropoiesis
▸ Counteracts effects of folic acid antagonists, such as methotrexate, by bypassing their site of action
▸ Enhances therapeutic and toxic effects of fluoropyrimidines, such as 5-fluorouracil, used in cancer therapy

Contraindications/cautions
▸ **Contraindications:** allergy to leucovorin on previous exposure, pernicious anemia or other megaloblastic anemias secondary to vitamin B_{12} deficiency
▸ **Cautions:** 5-fluorouracil therapy, elderly or debilitated patients with colorectal cancer

Available forms
▸ *Injection:* 3 mg/mL (as calcium)
▸ *Powder for injection:* 50, 100, 350 mg/vial (as calcium)
▸ *Tablets:* 5, 15, 25 mg (as calcium)

IV/IM Facts
Preparation
▸ Reconstitute powder for injection with Bacteriostatic Water for Injection or Sterile Water for Injection. Add 5 mL to 50-mg vial (10 mg/mL), 10 mL to 100-mg vial (10 mg/mL), or 17 mL to 350-mg vial (20 mg/mL).

▶ Both leucovorin in 1-mL ampules and Bacteriostatic Water for Injection contain benzyl alcohol; when doses > 10 mg/m^2 are administered, reconstitute drug with Sterile Water for Injection.

▶ If reconstituted with Sterile Water for Injection, use solution immediately; if reconstituted with Bacteriostatic Water for Injection, use solution within 7 d. Protect drug from light.

▶ May further dilute in D10W/0.9%NS; D5W; D10W; LR; or Ringer's Injection.

Dosage

▶ Because of this drug's calcium content, infuse IV doses slowly over 3–5 min. Do not give more than 160 mg/min.

▶ *Rescue after high-dose methotrexate therapy:* 15 mg IV or IM q6h for 10 doses, or until methotrexate level < 0.05 micromolar, starting 24 h after beginning methotrexate infusion. For delayed early methotrexate elimination or for evidence of acute renal injury, give 150 mg IV q3h until methotrexate level is < 1 micromolar; then give 15 mg IV q3h until methotrexate level is < 0.05 micromolar.

▶ *Impaired methotrexate elimination or inadvertent overdosage:* Begin ASAP after inadvertent overdosage and within 24 h of methotrexate administration when there is delayed excretion. Give 10 mg/m^2 IV or IM q6h until serum methotrexate level is < 10^{-8}M. If 24-h serum creatinine increases 50% over baseline or if the 24 or 28 h methotrexate level is > 5 × 10^{-6}M or > 9 × 10^{-7}M, respectively, increase leucovorin dose to 100 mg/m^2 IV q3h until methotrexate level is < 10^{-8}M.

▶ *Folic acid antagonist overdosage:* 5–15 mg/d.

▶ *Megaloblastic anemia:* Up to 1 mg/d.

▶ *Advanced colorectal cancer:* Give 200 mg/m^2 IV over 3 min, followed by 5-FU 370 mg/m^2 IV *or* give 20 mg/m^2 IV, followed by 5-FU 425 mg/m^2 IV. Repeat daily for 5 d; may be repeated at 4-wk intervals for 2 courses and then at 4- to 5-wk intervals if patient has completely recovered from toxic effects of prior treatment.

Compatibility

Leucovorin may be given through the same IV line as amifostine, aztreonam, bleomycin, cefepime, cisplatin, cladribine, cyclophosphamide, doxorubicin, filgrastim, fluconazole, fluorouracil, furosemide, granisetron, heparin, methotrexate, metoclopramide, mitomycin, piperacillin-tazobactam, tacrolimus, teniposide, thiotepa, vinblastine, vincristine.

Adverse effects in *Italics* are most common; those in **Bold** are life-threatening

Incompatibility

Do not administer through the same IV line as droperidol, foscarnet, sodium bicarbonate.

Oral dosage

- *Rescue after high-dose methotrexate therapy:* 15 mg PO q6h for 10 doses or until methotrexate level < 0.05 micromolar, starting 24 h after beginning methotrexate infusion.
- *Impaired methotrexate elimination or inadvertent overdosage:* Begin ASAP after inadvertent overdosage and within 24 h of methotrexate administration when there is delayed excretion. Give 10 mg/m² PO q6h until serum methotrexate level is < 10^{-8}M.
- *Folic acid antagonist overdosage:* 5–15 mg/d.
- *Megaloblastic anemia:* Up to 1 mg/d.
- Oral administration of doses > 25 mg is not recommended.

> ### TREATMENT OF OVERDOSE/ANTIDOTE
> Decrease dosage or discontinue drug. Initiate general supportive and resuscitative measures.

Pharmacokinetics

Route	Peak	Duration
IV	10 min	3–6 h
IM	52 min	3–6 h
Oral	2.3 h	3–6 h

Metabolism: Hepatic; $T_{1/2}$: 5.7–6.2 h
Excretion: Urine

Adverse effects

- *Allergic:* **Anaphylaxis,** wheezing, urticaria, rash, erythema

Clinically important drug–drug interactions

- Counteracts antiepileptic effect of phenobarbital, phenytoin, primidone
- Increased toxicity with 5-fluorouracil
- High doses reduce efficacy of intrathecally administered methotrexate

● NURSING CONSIDERATIONS

Assessment

- *History:* Leucovorin allergy, pernicious anemia or other megaloblastic anemias secondary to vitamin B_{12} deficiency, 5-fluorouracil therapy, age, debilitated status, colorectal cancer
- *Physical:* P, R, BP, I & O, neurologic checks, skin assessment, adventitious lung sounds, abdominal assessment, hy-

Adverse effects in *Italics* are most common; those in **Bold** are life-threatening

dration status, CBC, serum folate levels, creatinine, serum methotrexate concentration, serum electrolytes, liver function tests, UA

Implementation
▸ Begin leucovorin rescue within 24 h of methotrexate administration. Provide hydration therapy and urinary alkalinization with sodium bicarbonate to decrease methotrexate nephrotoxicity.
▸ When treating folic acid overdosage, begin leucovorin as promptly as possible.
▸ Monitor patient for allergic reactions.
▸ Give drug orally unless intolerance to oral route develops due to nausea and vomiting from chemotherapy or clinical condition. Switch to oral drug when feasible.
▸ Have emergency equipment (defibrillator, drugs, oxygen, intubation equipment) on standby in case anaphylaxis occurs.
▸ Delayed methotrexate excretion may be caused by third space fluid accumulation, renal insufficiency, or inadequate hydration. Higher drug doses or prolonged administration may be required.

⬤ **levofloxacin** *(lee voe flox' a sin)* Levaquin
Pregnancy Category C

Drug class
Fluoroquinolone

Indications
▸ Treatment of acute maxillary sinusitis caused by *Streptococcus pneumoniae, Haemophilus influenzae, Moraxella catarrhalis*
▸ Treatment of acute exacerbation of chronic bronchitis caused by *Staphylococcus aureus, S. pneumoniae, H. influenzae, Haemophilus parainfluenzae, M. catarrhalis*
▸ Treatment of community-acquired pneumonia caused by *S. aureus, S. pneumoniae, H. influenzae, H. parainfluenzae, Klebsiella pneumoniae, M. catarrhalis, Chlamydia pneumoniae, Legionella pneumophila, Mycoplasma pneumoniae*
▸ Treatment of uncomplicated skin and skin structure infections due to *S. aureus, Streptococcus pyogenes*
▸ Treatment of complicated UTIs caused by *Enterococcus faecalis, Enterobacter cloacae, Escherichia coli, K. pneumoniae, Proteus mirabilis, Pseudomonas aeruginosa*
▸ Treatment of uncomplicated UTIs in women caused by *E. coli, K. pneumoniae, Staphylococcus saprophyticus*
▸ Treatment of acute pyelonephritis caused by *E. coli*

Therapeutic actions
▸ Bactericidal: interferes with the enzyme DNA gyrase needed for the synthesis of bacterial DNA

Contraindications/cautions
▸ **Contraindications:** allergy to levofloxacin, quinolone antimicrobial agents, or any component of the product
▸ **Cautions:** renal dysfunction, seizures, dehydration, severe cerebral arteriosclerosis, epilepsy, diabetes

Available forms
▸ *Injection:* 500 mg/vial
▸ *Premixed injection:* 250, 500 mg
▸ *Tablets:* 250, 500 mg

IV facts
Preparation
▸ Obtain premixed bag or dilute drug in D5W/LR; D5W/0.45%NS with 0.15% Potassium Chloride Injection; D5W/0.9%NS; D5W; 0.9%NS; Plasma-Lyte 56/D5W; Sodium Lactate (1/6 Molar) Injection; or Sterile Water for Injection. The resulting diluted solution should be 5 mg/mL.

Dosage
▸ Give each IV dose over at least 60 min.
▸ *Bacterial exacerbation of chronic bronchitis:* 500 mg/d IV for 7 d.
▸ *Pneumonia:* 500 mg/d IV for 7–14 d.
▸ *Complicated UTI, pyelonephritis:* 250 mg/d IV for 10 d.
▸ *Uncomplicated UTI:* 250 mg/d IV for 3 d.
▸ *Sinusitis:* 500 mg/d IV for 10–14 d.
▸ *Skin and skin structure infections:* 500 mg/d IV for 7–10 d.
▸ *Renal impairment:* Patients with a UTI or pyelonephritis with a creatinine clearance ≥ 20 mL/min do not require a dosage adjustment; if creatinine clearance is 10–19 mL/min, give 250 mg q48h. Refer to the following table for patients with bronchitis, pneumonia, sinusitis, or skin and skin structure infections:

Creatinine Clearance (mL/min)	Dose
50–80	No adjustment
20–49	500 mg initially, then 250 mg/d
10–19	500 mg initially, then 250 mg q48h
Hemodialysis/chronic peritoneal dialysis	500 mg initially, then 250 mg q48h

Adverse effects in *Italics* are most common; those in **Bold** are life-threatening

L

Compatibility

Do not admix with other drugs or administer with other drugs through the same IV line.

Oral dosage

▶ *Bacterial exacerbation of chronic bronchitis:* 500 mg/d PO for 7 d.
▶ *Pneumonia:* 500 mg/d PO for 7–14 d.
▶ *Complicated UTI, pyelonephritis:* 250 mg/d PO for 10 d.
▶ *Uncomplicated UTI:* 250 mg/d PO for 3 d.
▶ *Sinusitis:* 500 mg/d PO for 10–14 d.
▶ *Skin and skin structure infections:* 500 mg/d PO for 7–10 d.
▶ *Renal impairment:* Patients with a UTI or pyelonephritis with a creatinine clearance ≥ 20 mL/min do not require a dosage adjustment; if creatinine clearance is 10–19 mL/min, give 250 mg q48h. Refer to the following table for patients with bronchitis, pneumonia, sinusitis, or skin and skin structure infections:

Creatinine Clearance (mL/min)	Dose
50–80	No adjustment
20–49	500 mg initially, then 250 mg/d
10–19	500 mg initially, then 250 mg q48h
Hemodialysis/chronic peritoneal dialysis	500 mg initially, then 250 mg q48h

TREATMENT OF OVERDOSE/ANTIDOTE

Discontinue drug or decrease dosage. Initiate general supportive and resuscitative measures. Induce emesis or perform gastric lavage to empty the stomach. Maintain hydration.

Pharmacokinetics

Route	Onset	Peak
IV	Immediate	End of infusion
Oral	Rapid	1–2 h

$T_{1/2}$: 6–8 h
Excretion: Urine

Adverse effects

▶ *CNS: Headache,* insomnia, dizziness, fatigue, somnolence, depression, blurred vision
▶ *GI:* **Pseudomembranous colitis,** *nausea, diarrhea, constipation,* vomiting, dry mouth, abdominal pain, flatulence
▶ *Allergic:* **Anaphylaxis,** pruritus, rash

Adverse effects in *Italics* are most common; those in **Bold** are life-threatening

- *Hematologic:* Elevated BUN, AST, ALT, serum creatinine, and alkaline phosphatase; decreased glucose and lymphocytes
- *Musc/Skel:* Tendon rupture
- *Misc:* **Stevens-Johnson syndrome,** *pain at injection site,* fever, vaginitis, back pain

Clinically important drug–drug interactions

- Decreased therapeutic effect with sucralfate, iron, zinc, antacids (separate by at least 2 h)
- Increased seizures with NSAIDs; avoid this combination
- Hypoglycemia or hyperglycemia with antidiabetic agents

● NURSING CONSIDERATIONS

Assessment

- *History:* Allergy to levofloxacin, quinolone antimicrobial agents, or any component of the product; renal dysfunction, seizures, dehydration, severe cerebral arteriosclerosis, epilepsy, diabetes
- *Physical:* T, P, R, BP, I & O, IV site, neurologic checks, skin assessment, respiratory status, abdominal assessment, bowel sounds, culture and sensitivity tests of infected area, renal and liver function tests, UA, CBC, serum glucose

Implementation

- Obtain specimens for culture and sensitivity of infected area before beginning therapy. May begin drug before results are available.
- Have emergency equipment (defibrillator, drugs, oxygen, intubation equipment) on standby in case anaphylactic reaction occurs.
- Assess for evidence of anaphylaxis; if suspected, discontinue drug immediately and notify provider.
- Monitor renal, hepatic, and hematopoietic function.
- Monitor for occurrence of superinfections; treat as appropriate.
- Discontinue drug at any sign of colitis; initiate appropriate supportive treatment.
- Give drug without regard to meals.
- Ensure that patient is well hydrated during course of therapy.
- Discontinue drug at complaint of tendon pain, inflammation, or rupture.
- When diluted to a concentration of 5 mg/mL, drug is stable for 72 h when stored ≤ 77°F or for 14 d when refrigerated.

● **levothyroxine sodium** (L-thyroxine, T_4)

(lee voe thye rox' een)   Eltroxin, Levo-T, Levothroid, Levoxine, Levoxyl, Synthroid

Pregnancy Category A

Adverse effects in *Italics* are most common; those in **Bold** are life-threatening

Drug class
Thyroid hormone

Indications
▶ Replacement therapy in hypothyroidism except transient hypothyroidism during recovery phase of subacute thyroiditis
▶ Pituitary TSH suppression in the treatment and prevention of euthyroid goiters and in the management of thyroid cancer
▶ Thyrotoxicosis in conjunction with antithyroid drugs and to prevent goitrogenesis, hypothyroidism, and thyrotoxicosis during pregnancy
▶ Treatment of myxedema coma

Therapeutic actions
▶ Effects exerted through control of DNA transcription and protein synthesis
▶ Exerts profound influence on every organ system; especially important in CNS development
▶ Increases the metabolic rate of body tissues, thereby increasing oxygen consumption
▶ Increases fat, protein, and carbohydrate metabolism; enzyme system activity; growth and maturation; GI tract motility; rapidity of cerebration

Effects on hemodynamic parameters
▶ Increased body temperature
▶ Increased CO
▶ Increased HR
▶ Increased blood volume
▶ Increased depth and quality of respiration
▶ Decreased SVR

Contraindications/cautions
▶ **Contraindications:** allergy to active or extraneous constituents of drug, thyrotoxicosis and acute MI uncomplicated by hypothyroidism, concurrent artificial rewarming of patient
▶ **Cautions:** Addison's disease (treat hypoadrenalism with corticosteroids before thyroid therapy), coronary artery disease (CAD), diabetes mellitus or insipidus, hypertension, elderly patients

Available forms
▶ *Powder for injection:* 200, 500 mcg/vial
▶ *Tablets:* 0.025, 0.05, 0.075, 0.088, 0.1, 0.112, 0.125, 0.137, 0.15, 0.175, 0.2, 0.3 mg
▶ 0.05–0.06 mg equals about 60 mg (1 grain) thyroid

Adverse effects in *Italics* are most common; those in **Bold** are life-threatening

IV/IM Facts
Preparation
▸ Reconstitute by adding 5 mL Bacteriostatic Sodium Chloride Injection, USP with Benzyl Alcohol or 0.9%NS only. Shake vial to mix. Use immediately. Do not add to other IV fluids.

Dosage
▸ Base dosage on continuous monitoring of the patient's clinical status and response.
▸ *Myxedema coma:* 0.4 mg IV. Give each 0.1 mg over 1 min. Follow with daily dose of 0.1–0.2 mg IV. Once T_4 levels are normal, continue IV dosing at reduced dose (usually 0.05–0.1 mg/d) until patient is able to take oral therapy.
▸ *Hypothyroidism:* 0.025 mg IV or IM qd. Give each 0.1 mg over 1 min IV. Increase in increments of 0.0125–0.025 mg q2–3wk. Use ≤ 0.025 mg for patients with long-standing hypothyroidism, especially with known or suspected cardiovascular impairment.

Compatibility
Information unavailable. Do not admix or administer with other drugs.

Oral dosage
▸ *Hypothyroidism:* **Initial dosage:** 0.05 mg PO with increasing increments of 0.025 mg q2–3wk. **Usual maintenance dosage:** Most patients require ≤ 0.2 mg/d.
▸ *TSH suppression in thyroid cancer, nodules, and euthyroid goiters:* Larger amounts than those used for replacement therapy are required.
▸ *Thyroid suppression therapy:* 2.6 mcg/kg/d PO for 7–10 d.

> ### TREATMENT OF OVERDOSE/ANTIDOTE
> Discontinue drug or decrease dosage. Initiate general supportive and resuscitative measures. Induce vomiting to prevent GI absorption. Cholestyramine and activated charcoal have been used to decrease drug absorption. Treat CHF with cardiac glycosides. Control fever, hypoglycemia, and fluid loss. Antiadrenergic agents, such as propranolol (1–3 mg IV over 10 min or 80–160 mg/d PO), have been successfully used to treat increased sympathetic activity. Glucocorticoids may be given to inhibit conversion of T_4 to T_3. May restart levothyroxine therapy at a lower dose.

Adverse effects in *Italics* are most common; those in **Bold** are life-threatening

Pharmacokinetics

Route	Onset	Peak
IV	6–8 h	24–48 h
Oral	Slow	1–3 wk

Metabolism: Hepatic; $T_{1/2}$: 6–7 d
Excretion: Feces through bile

Adverse effects

▸ *CNS: Tremors, irritability, insomnia,* nervousness, headache
▸ *CV:* **Cardiac arrest,** *palpitations, tachycardia,* dysrhythmias, angina, hypertension
▸ *GI:* Diarrhea, vomiting, increased bowel motility, changes in appetite, weight loss
▸ *Derm:* Sweating
▸ *Misc:* Menstrual irregularities, heat intolerance, fever, decreased bone density of hip and spine in premenopausal and postmenopausal women

Clinically important drug–drug interactions

▸ Increased bleeding with oral anticoagulants; reduce dosage of anticoagulant when T_4 is begun
▸ Decreased clearance of theophyllines if patient is in hypothyroid state; monitor response and adjust dosage as patient approaches euthyroid state
▸ Impaired effects of some beta-blockers when hypothyroid patient is converted to the euthyroid state
▸ Increased dysrhythmias with maprotiline
▸ Decreased absorption from GI tract with aluminum hydroxide, cholestyramine resin, colestipol hydrochloride, ferrous sulfate, sodium polystyrene sulfonate, sucralfate
▸ Increased dosage requirements of insulin, oral hypoglycemics
▸ Reduced therapeutic effects of digitalis; digitalis levels may be decreased in hyperthyroidism or when a hypothyroid patient becomes euthyroid
▸ Hypertension and tachycardia with ketamine
▸ Increased coronary insufficiency with sympathomimetics in patients with CAD
▸ Enhanced antidepressant activity, enhanced thyroid hormone activity, and transient dysrhythmias with TCAs

◉NURSING CONSIDERATIONS

Assessment

▸ *History:* Allergy to active or extraneous constituents of drug, thyrotoxicosis and acute MI uncomplicated by hypothyroidism, Addison's disease, CAD, diabetes mellitus or insipidus, hypertension, age

Adverse effects in *Italics* are most common; those in **Bold** are life-threatening

▸ *Physical:* T, P, BP, R, ECG, I & O, weight, neurologic checks, skin assessment, abdominal assessment, adventitious lung sounds, hydration status, serum glucose, thyroid function tests

Implementation
▸ Monitor patient response carefully at start of therapy, adjust dosage as indicated.
▸ Therapy for myxedema coma requires simultaneous administration of glucocorticoids.
▸ Obtain daily weight.
▸ Before therapy, rule out morphologic hypogonadism and nephrosis; correct any adrenal deficiency.
▸ Monitor for evidence of chronic excessive dosage as evidenced by headache, irritability, nervousness, sweating, tachycardia, increased bowel motility, menstrual irregularities, palpitations, vomiting, psychosis, seizure, fever, angina, CHF, shock, cardiac failure, dysrhythmias, thyroid storm.
▸ Monitor PT and INR frequently if patient is on oral anticoagulant therapy.
▸ Administer as a single daily dose before breakfast.
▸ Monitor thyroid function tests regularly.
▸ Monitor cardiac response (angina, palpitations, HR, BP, CHF, heart rhythm).
▸ Do not change from one brand to another; products may not be equivalent.

⬤ lidocaine hydrochloride *(lye' doe kane)*
For direct administration: Lidocaine HCl for Cardiac Arrhythmias, Xylocaine HCl IV for Cardiac Arrhythmias
For IV admixtures: Lidocaine HCl for Cardiac Arrhythmias, Xylocaine HCl IV for Cardiac Arrhythmias
For IV infusion: Lidocaine HCl in 5% Dextrose
For IM administration: LidoPen Auto-Injector
Local Anesthetic Injectable Preparations: Dilocaine, Duo-Trach Kit, Lidoject-1, Lidoject-2, Nervocaine 1%, Octocaine, Xylocaine HCl
Topical for Mucous Membranes: Anestacon, Lidocaine 2% Viscous, Xylocaine, Xylocaine 10%
Topical for Skin Disorders: Burn-O-Jel, DermaFlex, ELA-Max, Numby Stuff, Solarcaine Aloe Extra Burn Relief, Xylocaine, Zilactin-L

Pregnancy Category B

Drug classes
Antidysrhythmic
Local anesthetic

Adverse effects in *Italics* are most common; those in **Bold** are life-threatening

Indications

▸ As antidysrhythmic: management of acute ventricular dysrhythmias during cardiac surgery or MI (IV use); use single-dose IM injection when IV administration is not possible or when ECG monitoring is not available and the danger of ventricular dysrhythmias is great
▸ As anesthetic: infiltration anesthesia, peripheral and sympathetic nerve block, central nerve block, spinal and caudal anesthesia, retrobulbar and transtracheal injection, topical anesthetic for skin disorders and accessible mucous membranes

Therapeutic actions

▸ Type IB antidysrhythmic with local anesthetic properties
▸ Decreases phase 4 diastolic depolarization, decreases automaticity, and causes a decrease or no change in excitability and membrane responsiveness
▸ Decreases action, potential duration, and effective refractory period of Purkinje fibers and ventricular muscle
▸ May increase, decrease, or not affect AV nodal conduction time
▸ Increases the electrical stimulation threshold of the ventricle during diastole
▸ In therapeutic doses, does not change myocardial contractility, systolic arterial BP, or absolute refractory period
▸ As a local anesthetic, inhibits conduction of nerve impulses from sensory nerves by altering the cell membrane's permeability to ions, increasing the electrical excitation threshold, slowing nerve impulse propagation, and reducing the rate of rise of action potential; order of loss of nerve function is pain, temperature, touch, proprioception, and skeletal muscle tone

Contraindications/cautions

▸ **Contraindications:** allergy to lidocaine or amide-type local anesthetics, cardiogenic shock, second- or third-degree heart block (if no artificial pacemaker), Wolff-Parkinson-White syndrome, Adams-Stokes syndrome; spinal and caudal anesthesia in septicemia, neurologic disease, spinal deformities, and severe hypertension (local anesthetics)
▸ **Cautions:** hepatic or renal disease, reduced cardiac output, digitalis toxicity, CHF, hypovolemia, shock

Available forms

▸ *Direct IV injection:* 10, 20 mg/mL
▸ *For IV admixtures:* 40, 100, 200 mg/mL
▸ *IV infusion:* 2, 4, 8 mg/mL
▸ *IM injection:* 300 mg/3 mL
▸ *Injection for local anesthesia:* 0.5%, 1%, 1.5%, 2%, 4%

Adverse effects in *Italics* are most common; those in **Bold** are life-threatening

- *Topical liquid:* 2.5%, 5%
- *Topical ointment:* 2.5%, 5%
- *Topical cream:* 0.5%, 4%
- *Topical gel:* 0.5%, 2.5%
- *Topical spray:* 0.5%, 10%
- *Topical solution:* 2%, 4%
- *Topical jelly:* 2%

IV/IM/endotracheal facts
Preparation
- For an IV infusion, use a premixed bag or mix 1–2 g Lidocaine in 250–500 mL of D5W/LR; D5W/0.45%NS; D5W/0.9%NS; D5W; LR; 0.45%NS; or 0.9%NS.

Dosage
- For IV use, use only lidocaine injection without preservatives and clearly labeled for IV use.
- *IV bolus:* 50–100 mg IV at a rate of 25–50 mg/min. If the initial dose does not produce the desired clinical response, give a second bolus dose after 5 min. Do not exceed 200–300 mg/h.
- *IV continuous infusion:* Needed to maintain therapeutic plasma levels in patients whose dysrhythmias tend to recur and who cannot receive oral antidysrhythmic drugs. Give 1–4 mg/min (20–50 mcg/kg/min). Reassess infusion rate as soon as cardiac rhythm stabilizes or at the earliest signs of toxicity. Use lowest effective dose. Change to oral antidysrhythmics as soon as possible.
- *Cardiac arrest (endotracheal administration):* Give 2–2.5 times the IV dose diluted in 10 mL of sterile water or normal saline.
- *Patients with CHF, reduced cardiac output, liver disease, advanced age:* Reduce loading and maintenance doses.
- *IM:* 300 mg IM into the deltoid muscle using only the 10% solution for IM injection. Change to oral antidysrhythmic therapy as soon as possible. If needed, repeat IM injection after 60–90 min.

Titration Guide

| lidocaine hydrochloride |

2 g in 250 mL

mg/min	1	2	3	4
mL/h	8	15	23	30

Therapeutic serum level
- 1.5–6 mcg/mL

Adverse effects in *Italics* are most common; those in **Bold** are life-threatening

Compatibility
Lidocaine may be given through the same IV line as alteplase, amiodarone, amrinone, cefazolin, ciprofloxacin, diltiazem, dobutamine, dopamine, enalaprilat, etomidate, famotidine, haloperidol, heparin, labetalol, meperidine, morphine, nitroglycerin, nitroprusside sodium, potassium chloride, propofol, streptokinase, theophylline, vitamin B complex with C, warfarin.

Incompatibility
Do not administer through the same IV line as thiopental.

Anesthetic dosage
❱ Do not use preparations containing preservatives for spinal or epidural anesthesia. Drug concentration and diluent should be appropriate to particular local anesthetic use. Dosage varies with the area to be anesthetized and the reason for the anesthesia; use the lowest effective dose to achieve results. Use lower concentrations in debilitated and elderly patients and those with cardiac or liver disease.

TREATMENT OF OVERDOSE/ANTIDOTE
Discontinue drug or decrease dosage. Initiate general supportive and resuscitative measures. Treat severe convulsions with diazepam or thiopental. If these are not available, use pentobarbital or secobarbital. Treat hypotension with vasopressors.

Pharmacokinetics

Route	Onset	Peak	Duration
IV	Immediate	Immediate	10–20 min after bolus dose
IM	5–10 min	5–15 min	2 h
Topical	Rapid	2–5 min when applied to mucous membranes	15–45 min

Metabolism: Hepatic; $T_{1/2}$: 10 min, then 1.5 to 3 h
Excretion: Urine

Adverse effects
Lidocaine as Antidysrhythmic—Systemic Administration
❱ *CNS:* **Convulsions,** *dizziness/lightheadedness, drowsiness,* unconsciousness, dizziness, tremors, twitching, euphoria, mood changes, vision changes; sensation of heat, cold, or numbness, obtundation, coma

Adverse effects in *Italics* are most common; those in **Bold** are life-threatening

- *CV:* **Cardiac arrest, dysrhythmias,** hypotension, bradycardia, cardiovascular depression, decreased cardiac output
- *Resp:* **Respiratory depression and arrest**
- *GI:* Nausea, vomiting
- *Allergic:* **Anaphylaxis,** cutaneous lesions, urticaria, edema
- *Misc:* **Malignant hyperthermia,** fever, soreness at IM injection site, extravasation, venous thrombosis or phlebitis at injection site

Lidocaine as Injectable Local Anesthetic for Epidural or Caudal Anesthesia

- *CNS:* *Headache, backache,* restlessness, anxiety, tinnitus, blurred vision, arachnoiditis, palsies, cranial nerve palsies, septic meningitis; persistent sensory, motor, or autonomic deficit of lower spinal segments, sometimes with incomplete recovery
- *CV:* **Ventricular dysrhythmias, cardiac arrest, hypotension due to sympathetic block,** myocardial depression, heart block, syncope, bradycardia, decreased cardiac output
- *Resp:* **Respiratory paralysis or impairment**
- *GU:* *Urinary retention, urinary or fecal incontinence*
- *Derm:* **Angioneurotic edema,** cutaneous lesions, urticaria, pruritus, erythema, excessive sweating
- *Allergic:* **Anaphylaxis**

Lidocaine as Topical Local Anesthetic

- *Derm:* *Local burning, stinging, tenderness, swelling, tissue irritation,* tissue necrosis; contact dermatitis, urticaria, cutaneous lesions
- *Allergic:* **Anaphylaxis, bronchospasm, shock,** cutaneous lesions, urticaria, edema, contact dermatitis
- *Misc:* **Methemoglobinemia**

Clinically important drug–drug interactions

- Increased levels with beta-blockers (propranolol, metoprolol, nadolol, pindolol, atenolol), cimetidine
- Increased cardiodepressant action and conduction abnormalities with procainamide
- Increased adverse reactions with tocainide
- Prolonged neuromuscular blockade with succinylcholine

● NURSING CONSIDERATIONS

Assessment

- *History:* Allergy to lidocaine or amide-type local anesthetics, cardiogenic shock, presence of pacemaker, Wolff-Parkinson-White syndrome, Adams-Stokes syndrome, septicemia, neurologic disease, spinal deformities, severe hypertension, hepatic

Adverse effects in *Italics* are most common; those in **Bold** are life-threatening

or renal disease, reduced cardiac output, digitalis toxicity, CHF, hypovolemia, shock

▶ *Physical:* T, P, R, BP, ECG, I & O, SpO$_2$, IV site, weight, neurologic checks, presence of twitching or seizures, skin assessment, sensation and movement (local anesthetic), edema, respiratory effort, adventitious lung sounds, bowel sounds, liver evaluation, serum electrolytes, liver and renal function tests, serum lidocaine level, ABG

Implementation

▶ Exercise extreme caution when calculating and preparing doses. Lidocaine is a very potent drug; small dosage errors can cause serious adverse effects. Avoid inadvertent bolus of drug.

▶ Always administer a continuous lidocaine infusion using an IV infusion pump.

▶ When used as antidysrhythmic, monitor for safe and effective serum drug concentrations.

▶ Continuously monitor P, BP, and ECG when given as an antidysrhythmic.

▶ Continuously monitor PRI and QRS duration; notify physician if these exceed normal limits.

▶ Have emergency equipment (defibrillator, drugs, oxygen, intubation equipment) on standby in case anaphylaxis or adverse reaction occurs.

▶ Monitor for lidocaine toxicity as evidenced by drowsiness, dizziness, paresthesias, vertigo, tremors, twitching, impaired hearing, disorientation, convulsions, blurred or double vision, dyspnea, respiratory depression, nausea, vomiting, or bradycardia. Keep IV diazepam or thiopental on standby in case of convulsions.

▶ Establish safety precautions if CNS changes occur.

▶ Check drug concentration carefully; many concentrations are available.

▶ IM administration may increase CPK levels. Evaluate CPK-MB levels when assessing for AMI.

▶ Following local anesthetic administration, assess for malignant hyperthermia as evidenced by tachycardia, tachypnea, labile blood pressure, metabolic and respiratory acidosis, dysrhythmias, hyperkalemia, elevated CPK and myoglobinuria, skeletal rigidity, jaw muscle spasm, or high temperature. Keep IV dantrolen on standby.

▶ Ensure that patients who receive lidocaine as a spinal anesthetic are adequately hydrated to minimize risk of headache.

▶ Use caution to prevent aspiration and choking. Patient may

have difficulty swallowing following use of oral topical anesthetic. After using an oral topical anesthetic, do not give food or drink for 1 h and until patient has a positive gag reflex.
▸ Treat methemoglobinemia with 1% methylene blue, 1–2 mg/kg IV over 10 min.
▸ Apply lidocaine ointments or creams to a gauze or bandage before applying to the skin.

⬤ liothyronine sodium (T_3, triiodothyronine)
(lye' oh thye' roe neen) Cytomel, Triostat

Pregnancy Category A

Drug classes
Thyroid hormone

Indications
▸ Replacement therapy in hypothyroidism except transient hypothyroidism during recovery phase of subacute thyroiditis
▸ Pituitary TSH suppression in the treatment and prevention of euthyroid goiters and in the management of thyroid cancer
▸ Thyrotoxicosis in conjunction with antithyroid drugs and to prevent goitrogenesis, hypothyroidism, and thyrotoxicosis during pregnancy
▸ Synthetic hormone used with patients allergic to desiccated thyroid or thyroid extract derived from pork or beef
▸ Diagnostic use: T_3 suppression test to differentiate suspected hyperthyroidism from euthyroidism
▸ Orphan drug use: treatment of myxedema coma and precoma

Therapeutic actions
▸ Effects exerted through control of DNA transcription and protein synthesis
▸ Exerts profound influence on every organ system; especially important in CNS development
▸ Increases the metabolic rate of body tissues, thereby increasing oxygen consumption
▸ Increases fat, protein, and carbohydrate metabolism; enzyme system activity, growth and maturation, GI tract motility, rapidity of cerebration

Effects on hemodynamic parameters
▸ Increased body temperature
▸ Increased CO
▸ Increased HR
▸ Increased blood volume

Adverse effects in *Italics* are most common; those in **Bold** are life-threatening

L

▸ Increased depth and quality of respiration
▸ Decreased SVR

Contraindications/cautions
▸ **Contraindications:** allergy to active or extraneous constituents of drug, thyrotoxicosis and acute MI uncomplicated by hypothyroidism, concurrent artificial rewarming of patient
▸ **Cautions:** Addison's disease (treat hypoadrenalism with corticosteroids before thyroid therapy), coronary artery disease (CAD), diabetes mellitus or insipidus, hypertension, elderly patients

Available forms
▸ *Injection:* 10 mcg/mL
▸ *Tablets:* 5, 25, 50 mcg
▸ 15–37.5 mcg equals about 60 mg (1 grain) desiccated thyroid

IV Facts
Preparation
▸ May be given undiluted.

Dosage
▸ Base dosage on continuous monitoring of the patient's clinical status and response.
▸ *Myxedema coma:* 25–50 mcg IV. Give each 10 mcg or less over 1 min. Give doses 4–12 h apart. Initial doses of ≥ 65 mcg/d are associated with lower mortality. For patients with known or suspected cardiovascular disease, give 10–20 mcg IV. Change to oral therapy as soon as patient is stabilized and able to take oral medication. When changing to liothyronine tablets, discontinue injection, start oral therapy at a low dosage, and increase gradually according to patient's response. If oral levothyroxine is used, discontinue IV therapy gradually because levothyroxine oral therapy is not effective for several days.

Compatibility
Information unavailable. Do not admix or administer with other drugs.

Oral dosage
▸ *Hypothyroidism:* **Initial dosage:** 25 mcg/d PO. May increase dose q1–2wk in 12.5- or 25-mcg increments. **Usual maintenance dosage:** 25–75 mcg/d.
▸ *Myxedema:* **Initial dosage:** 5 mcg/d PO. Increase in 5- to 10-mcg increments every 1–2 wk. **Usual maintenance dosage:** 50–100 mcg/d.

Adverse effects in *Italics* are most common; those in **Bold** are life-threatening

- *Simple goiter:* **Initial dosage:** 5 mcg/d PO. May increase by 5- or 10-mcg increments every 1–2 wk. **Usual maintenance dosage:** 75 mcg/d.
- *T_3 suppression test:* 75–100 mcg/d PO for 7 d, then repeat I^{131} Thyroid Uptake test. A ≥ 50% suppression test indicates a normal thyroid-pituitary axis and rules out thyroid gland autonomy.
- *Elderly:* Start therapy with 5 mcg/d PO. Increase by 5-mcg increments; monitor patient response.

> **TREATMENT OF OVERDOSE/ANTIDOTE**
> Discontinue drug or decrease dosage. Initiate general supportive and resuscitative measures. Induce vomiting if GI absorption can be prevented and if patient is without contraindications, such as coma, convulsions, or absent gag reflex. Administer cardiac glycosides if CHF develops. Control fever, hypoglycemia, and fluid loss. Antiadrenergic agents, such as propranolol (1–3 mg IV over 10 min or 80–160 mg/d PO), have been successfully used to treat increased sympathetic activity. May restart liothyronine therapy at a lower dose.

Pharmacokinetics

Route	Onset	Peak	Duration
IV	2–4 h	Within 2 d	72 h
Oral	Rapid	2–3 d	3–4 d

Metabolism: Hepatic; $T_{1/2}$: 1–2 d
Excretion: Urine

Adverse effects

- **CNS:** *Tremors, headache, irritability, insomnia,* nervousness, psychosis
- **CV: Cardiac arrest,** *palpitations, tachycardia,* dysrhythmias, angina
- **GI:** Diarrhea, vomiting, increased bowel motility, changes in appetite, weight loss
- **Derm:** Allergic skin reactions, sweating
- **Misc:** Menstrual irregularities, heat intolerance, fever

Clinically important drug–drug interactions

- Decreased absorption with cholestyramine
- Increased bleeding with oral anticoagulants; reduce dosage of anticoagulant when T_3 is begun
- Decreased clearance of theophyllines if patient is in hy-

Adverse effects in *Italics* are most common; those in **Bold** are life-threatening

pothyroid state; monitor response and adjust dosage as patient approaches euthyroid state
- Impaired effects of some beta-blockers when hypothyroid patient is converted to the euthyroid state
- Increased dosage requirements of insulin, oral hypoglycemics
- Enhanced toxic effects of digitalis; increased metabolic rate may require increased digitalis dosage
- Hypertension and tachycardia with ketamine
- Increased coronary insufficiency with sympathomimetics in patients with CAD
- Enhanced antidepressant activity, enhanced thyroid hormone activity, and transient dysrhythmias with TCAs

⬤ NURSING CONSIDERATIONS

Assessment
- *History:* Allergy to active or extraneous constituents of drug, thyrotoxicosis and AMI uncomplicated by hypothyroidism, concurrent artificial rewarming of patient, Addison's disease, CAD, diabetes mellitus or insipidus, age
- *Physical:* T, P, BP, R, ECG, I & O, weight, neurologic checks, skin assessment, abdominal assessment, adventitious lung sounds, hydration status, serum glucose, thyroid function tests

Implementation
- Monitor patient response carefully at start of therapy; adjust dosage.
- Therapy for myxedema coma requires simultaneous administration of glucocorticoids.
- Monitor cardiac response (angina, palpitations, HR, BP, CHF, heart rhythm).
- Obtain daily weight.
- Before therapy, rule out morphologic hypogonadism and nephrosis; correct any adrenal deficiency.
- Monitor for evidence of chronic excessive dosage as evidenced by headache, irritability, nervousness, sweating, tachycardia, increased bowel motility, menstrual irregularities, palpitations, vomiting, psychosis, seizure, fever, angina, CHF, shock, cardiac failure, dysrhythmias, thyroid storm.
- Monitor exchange to T_3 from other forms of thyroid replacement. Discontinue the other medication, then begin this drug at a low dose with gradual increases based on the patient's response.
- Monitor PT and INR frequently if patient is on oral anticoagulant therapy.

Adverse effects in *Italics* are most common; those in **Bold** are life-threatening

- Administer as a single daily dose before breakfast.
- Monitor thyroid function tests regularly.
- Do not change from one brand to another; products may not be equivalent.

● lisinopril *(lyse in' oh pril)* Apo-Lisinopril (CAN), Prinivil, Zestril

Pregnancy Category C (first trimester) and D (second and third trimesters)

Drug classes
ACE inhibitor
Antihypertensive

Indications
- Treatment of hypertension alone or with thiazide diuretics
- Adjunctive therapy in CHF for patients unresponsive to diuretic and digitalis
- Treatment of stable patients within 24 h of AMI to improve survival

Therapeutic actions
- Blocks ACE from converting angiotensin I to angiotensin II, a powerful vasoconstrictor; leads to decreased blood pressure, decreased aldosterone secretion, a small increase in serum potassium levels, and sodium and fluid loss
- Increased prostaglandin synthesis also may be involved in the antihypertensive action

Effects on hemodynamic parameters
- Decreased BP
- Decreased SVR

Contraindications/cautions
- **Contraindications:** lisinopril allergy, angioedema related to previous treatment with an ACE inhibitor
- **Cautions:** elderly, neutropenia, agranulocytosis, salt/volume depletion, impaired renal function

Available forms
- *Tablets:* 2.5, 5, 10, 20, 40 mg

Oral dosage
- *Hypertension without diuretics:* 10 mg/d PO. Dose range is 20–40 mg/d as a single dose.
- *Hypertension with diuretics:* If possible, discontinue diuretic 2–3 d before lisinopril is initiated. If not possible to discon-

Adverse effects in *Italics* are most common; those in **Bold** are life-threatening

tinue diuretic, give initial dose of 5 mg PO and monitor for hypotension.

▸ *Hypertension with renal function impairment:* Initiate according to following chart. Titrate up to maximum of 40 mg/d.

Creatinine Clearance (mL/min)	Serum Creatinine (mg/dL)	Initial Dose (mg/d)
>30	≤3	10 mg
10–30	≥3	5 mg
<10	—	2.5 mg

▸ *CHF:* 5 mg/d PO with diuretics and digitalis. Usual dose range is 5–20 mg/d as a single dose. Give 2.5 mg/d PO if serum sodium < 130 mEq/L or if patient has renal failure.

▸ *AMI:* Start within 24 h of MI with 5 mg PO, followed by 5 mg after 24 h, 10 mg after 48 h, and then 10 mg/d for 6 wk. If patient is hypotensive, begin with 2.5-mg dose.

TREATMENT OF OVERDOSE/ANTIDOTE
Discontinue drug or decrease dose. Initiate general supportive and resuscitative measures. Initiate IV infusion of normal saline to treat hypotension. Treat anaphylaxis or angioedema with epinephrine and maintain a patent airway. May be removed by hemodialysis.

Pharmacokinetics

Route	Onset	Peak	Duration
Oral	60 min	7 h	24 h

$T_{1/2}$: 12 h
Excretion: Urine

Adverse effects

▸ *CNS:* **Stroke,** *headache, dizziness, fatigue, depression,* insomnia, sleep disturbances, paresthesias, somnolence, drowsiness, ataxia, confusion, malaise, nervousness, vertigo, memory impairment, tremor, irritability, peripheral neuropathy, transient ischemic attacks

▸ *CV:* **AMI, cardiac arrest, CVA,** *chest pain, hypotension, palpitations,* tachycardia, dysrhythmias, hypotension, worsening heart failure, chest sound abnormalities, pulmonary edema, postural hypotension

▸ *Resp:* *Cough, dyspnea, upper respiratory infection,* asthma, bronchitis, bronchospasm, sinusitis, hemoptysis, pulmonary

Adverse effects in *Italics* are most common; those in **Bold** are life-threatening

infiltrates, wheezing, orthopnea, painful respiration, epistaxis, laryngitis, rhinorrhea, pharyngeal pain
- **GI:** *Abdominal pain, vomiting, nausea, diarrhea,* flatulence, gastritis, heartburn, GI cramps, weight loss/gain, taste alterations, hepatocellular/cholestatic jaundice, increased salivation, constipation, dry mouth
- **GU:** *Proteinuria,* UTI, acute renal failure, oliguria, anuria, uremia, progressive azotemia, renal dysfunction, urinary frequency, nephrotic syndrome, pyelonephritis, dysuria, increased BUN and creatinine, impotence, decreased libido, pelvic pain
- **Derm:** **Toxic epidermal necrolysis,** *rash, pruritus,* alopecia, Stevens-Johnson syndrome, diaphoresis, erythema multiforme, flushing, photosensitivity, urticaria, herpes zoster
- **Allergic:** **Anaphylaxis, angioedema**
- **Hematologic:** **Neutropenia, agranulocytosis, thrombocytopenia,** pancytopenia, bone marrow depression, leukopenia, anemia
- **Misc:** *Asthenia, myalgia,* blurred vision, fever, chills, tinnitus, arthritis, vasculitis

Clinically important drug–drug interactions
- Decreased bioavailability if antacids given within 2 h
- Decreased hypotensive effects with indomethacin
- Increased effects with phenothiazines
- Increased digoxin, lithium toxicity
- Elevated serum potassium levels with potassium, potassium-sparing diuretics
- Severe hypotension when patient is on diuretic therapy, salt-restricted diet, dialysis
- Enhanced by vasodilator drugs, such as nitroglycerin or nitrates; if possible, discontinue these drugs before starting this drug

● NURSING CONSIDERATIONS

Assessment
- *History:* Lisinopril allergy, angioedema related to previous treatment with an ACE inhibitor, age, neutropenia, agranulocytosis, salt/volume depletion, impaired renal function
- *Physical:* T, P, BP, R, ECG, I & O, weight, neurologic checks, vision, skin assessment, cardiac auscultation, edema, JVD, adventitious lung sounds, orthostatic BP, bowel sounds, serum electrolytes, liver and renal function tests, UA, CBC

Implementation
- Change patient's position slowly to avoid postural hypotension.
- Have emergency equipment (defibrillator, drugs, oxygen) on standby in case anaphylaxis or adverse reaction occurs.

Adverse effects in *Italics* are most common; those in **Bold** are life-threatening

▶ Alert surgeon and mark patient's chart with notice that lisinopril is being taken; the angiotensin II formation subsequent to compensatory renin release during surgery will
  be blocked; hypotension may be reversed with volume
  expansion.
▶ Monitor patients on diuretic therapy for excessive hypotension following the first few doses of lisinopril.
▶ Monitor patients closely for conditions, such as excessive perspiration, vomiting, diarrhea, dehydration, that may lead to
  hypotension secondary to hypovolemia.

⬤ **lorazepam** *(lor a' ze pam)* Apo-Lorazepam (CAN),
  Ativan, Novo-Lorazem (CAN), Nu-Loraz (CAN)

Pregnancy Category D

C-IV controlled substance

Drug classes
Benzodiazepine
Antianxiety agent
Sedative/hypnotic

Indications
▶ Management of anxiety disorders or for short-term relief of
  symptoms of anxiety or anxiety associated with depression
▶ Preanesthetic medication to produce sedation, relieve anxiety, and decrease recall of events related to surgery
  (parenteral)
▶ Unlabeled use: *parenteral:* management of status epilepticus,
  chemotherapy induced nausea and vomiting, acute
  alcohol withdrawal, psychogenic catatonia; *oral:* chronic
  insomnia

Therapeutic actions
▶ Exact mechanisms are not understood; appears to produce
  CNS depression by potentiating GABA
▶ Activity may involve the spinal cord (muscle relaxation),
  brain stem (anticonvulsant properties), cerebellum (ataxia),
  limbic and cortical areas (emotional behavior)
▶ Anxiolytic effects occur at doses well below those necessary
  to cause sedation and ataxia

Contraindications/cautions
▶ **Contraindications:** hypersensitivity to benzodiazepines
  or their components (parenteral form with propylene glycol, polyethylene glycol, or benzyl alcohol), psychoses,
  (contraindications continued on next page)

Adverse effects in *Italics* are most common; those in **Bold** are life-threatening

acute narrow-angle glaucoma, shock, coma, acute alcoholic intoxication with depressed vital signs
▸ **Cautions:** impaired liver or kidney function, debilitation,
depression

Available forms
▸ *Injection:* 2, 4 mg/mL
▸ *Tablets:* 0.5, 1, 2 mg
▸ *Oral solution:* 2 mg/mL

IV/IM facts
Preparation
▸ *IV:* Immediately before use, dilute with an equal volume of
D5W; 0.9%NS; or Sterile Water for Injection.
▸ *IM:* Give undiluted.

Dosage
▸ *Preoperative sedation:* **IV:** 2 mg or 0.044 mg/kg IV, whichever
is smaller. Give 15–20 min before the procedure and directly
into a vein or into the tubing of a running IV infusion; do not
exceed 2 mg/min. Do not give larger doses to patients > 50
yr old. For other patients, may give doses as high as 0.05
mg/kg up to a total of 4 mg. **IM:** 0.05 mg/kg, up to 4 mg at
least 2 h before surgery. Inject deep into the muscle mass.

Compatibility
Lorazepam may be given through the same IV line as acyclovir,
albumin, allopurinol, amifostine, amikacin, amoxicillin, amoxicillin-clavulanate, amsacrine, atracurium, bumetanide, cefepime,
cefmetazole, cefotaxime, ciprofloxacin, cisplatin, cladribine, cyclophosphamide, cytarabine, dexamethasone, diltiazem, dobutamine, dopamine, doxorubicin, epinephrine, erythromycin, etomidate, famotidine, fentanyl, filgrastim, fluconazole, fludarabine,
furosemide, gentamicin, granisetron, haloperidol, heparin, hydrocortisone, hydromorphone, labetalol, melphalan, methotrexate, metronidazole, paclitaxel, pancuronium, piperacillin,
piperacillin-tazobactam, potassium chloride, propofol, ranitidine,
tacrolimus, teniposide, thiotepa, trimethoprim-sulfamethoxazole,
vancomycin, vecuronium, vinorelbine, zidovudine.

Incompatibility
Do not administer through the same IV line as aldesleukin,
aztreonam, floxacillin, gallium, idarubicin, imipenem-cilastatin,
omeprazole, ondansetron, sargramostim, sufentanil.

Oral dosage
▸ Use 2–6 mg/d (range 1–10 mg/d) PO in divided doses, the
largest dose at hs.

Adverse effects in *Italics* are most common; those in **Bold** are life-threatening

- *Anxiety:* 2–3 mg/d PO given 2–3 times qd.
- *Insomnia due to anxiety or transient situational stress:* 2–4 mg PO at hs.
- *Elderly or debilitated patients:* 1–2 mg/d PO in divided doses. Adjust as needed and tolerated.

TREATMENT OF OVERDOSE/ANTIDOTE

Discontinue drug or decrease dosage. Initiate general supportive and resuscitative measures. For oral overdosage, induce vomiting and give activated charcoal. With normal kidney function, forced diuresis with IV fluids and electrolytes may accelerate drug elimination. Osmotic diuretics, such as mannitol, may be effective. Treat hypotension with norepinephrine or metaraminol. Flumazenil may reverse lorazepam's effects. Renal dialysis and exchange blood transfusions may be indicated.

Pharmacokinetics

Route	Onset	Peak	Duration
IV	1–5 min	15–20 min	12–24 h
IM	15–30 min	60–90 min	12–24 h
Oral	Intermediate	2 h	12–24 h

Metabolism: Hepatic; $T_{1/2}$: 10–20 h
Excretion: Urine

Adverse effects

- *CNS: Excessive drowsiness and sleepiness, sedation, dizziness, weakness, unsteadiness,* disorientation, depression, headache, sleep disturbance, agitation, transient amnesia or memory impairment, restlessness, confusion, crying, delirium, hallucinations, diplopia, blurred vision
- *CV:* Hypertension, hypotension
- *Resp:* **Hypoxic cardiac arrest, airway obstruction,** respiratory depression
- *GI:* Nausea, change in appetite, vomiting
- *Derm:* Skin rash; pain, redness, and/or burning sensation at IV or IM injection site
- *Dependence:* Physical and psychological dependence

Clinically important drug–drug interactions

- Increased CNS depression with alcohol, barbiturates, MAO inhibitors, other antidepressants
- Increased sedation, hallucinations, and irrational behavior with scopolamine
- Increased clearance rate with oral contraceptives

Adverse effects in *Italics* are most common; those in **Bold** are life-threatening

● NURSING CONSIDERATIONS

Assessment
▸ *History:* Hypersensitivity to benzodiazepines or their components, psychoses, acute narrow-angle glaucoma, shock, coma, acute alcoholic intoxication, impaired liver or kidney function, debilitation, depression
▸ *Physical:* T, P, R, BP, I & O, IV site, SpO$_2$, weight, neurologic checks, presence of anxiety or insomnia, skin assessment, ophthalmologic exam, respiratory effort, adventitious lung sounds, liver evaluation, abdominal exam, bowel sounds, CBC, liver and renal function tests

Implementation
▸ Do not administer intra-arterially; arteriospasm and gangrene may result.
▸ Assess IV or IM sites frequently; avoid extravasation.
▸ Give IV forms when patient is lying down.
▸ Have emergency equipment (defibrillator, drugs, oxygen, intubation equipment) on standby in case of airway obstruction/compromise or adverse reaction.
▸ Monitor patient response; adjust dosage to lowest effective dose.
▸ Initiate fall precautions; assist patient if he or she is out of bed.
▸ Reduce dose of narcotic analgesics by at least half in patients who have received parenteral lorazepam.
▸ Taper dosage gradually after long-term therapy, especially in epileptic patients.
▸ Drug may produce drug dependence and has the potential for being abused. Psychic and physical dependence may develop with repeated administration.
▸ Follow federal, state, and institutional policies for dispensing controlled substances.
▸ Do not use solutions that are discolored or contain a precipitate. Protect drug from light; refrigerate solution.

M

● magnesium sulfate *(mag nee' zhum sul' fate)*
Pregnancy Category A

Drug classes
Electrolyte
Anticonvulsant
Antidysrhythmic

Adverse effects in *Italics* are most common; those in **Bold** are life-threatening

Indications
- Replacement therapy for hypomagnesemia
- Prevention or treatment of hypomagnesemia associated with total parenteral nutrition therapy
- Treatment of convulsions associated with low magnesium levels
- Prevention and control of convulsions and hypertension in severe preeclampsia and eclampsia
- Unlabeled uses: prevention of post-AMI hypomagnesemia and subsequent dysrhythmias; promotion of bronchodilation in asthmatic patients

Therapeutic actions
- Is a cofactor in many enzyme systems involved in neurochemical transmission and muscular excitability
- Prevents or controls convulsions by blocking neuromuscular transmission and decreasing acetylcholine release
- Exerts a depressant effect on the CNS
- Acts peripherally to produce vasodilation
- 1 g of magnesium sulfate provides 8.12 mEq of magnesium

Effects on hemodynamic parameters
- Decreased BP (large doses)
- Decreased SVR (large doses)

Contraindications/cautions
- **Contraindications:** magnesium allergy, hypermagnesemia, heart block, myocardial damage, impending (within 2 h) delivery
- **Caution:** renal function impairment, elderly patients

Available forms
- *Injection:* 0.8, 1, 4 mEq/mL

IV/IM facts
Preparation
- *Direct IV injection:* Administer 10% solution undiluted.
- *Intermittent/continuous infusion:* Dilute magnesium in D5W or 0.9%NS to a concentration of ≤ 20%.
- *IM:* Use undiluted 50% solution.

Dosage
- *Cardiac arrest:* **Ventricular tachycardia:** 1–2 g (2–4 mL of a 50% solution) diluted in 10 mL of D5W IV over 1–2 min. **Ventricular fibrillation:** 1–2 g IVP. **Torsades de pointes:** Up to 5–10 mg IV has been used.
- *Severe hypomagnesemia:* Up to 5 g IV over 3 h, or up to 2 mEq/kg (0.5 mL of 50% solution) IM within 4 h if needed.
- *Mild hypomagnesemia:* 1 g (2 mL of a 50% solution) IM q6h for 4 doses.

Adverse effects in *Italics* are most common; those in **Bold** are life-threatening

- *Hyperalimentation:* 8–24 mEq/d IV.
- *Convulsions/preeclampsia, eclampsia:* **IV:** 4 g of a 10%–20% solution, not exceeding 1.5 mL/min of a 10% solution. **IV infusion:** 4–5 g in 250 mL of D5W or 0.9%NS, not exceeding 3 mL/min. **IM:** 4–5 g of a 50% solution q4h as needed.
- *Elderly/renal impaired patients:* Reduce dose; do not exceed 20 g in 48 h.

Normal magnesium level
- 1.5–2.5 mEq/L

Therapeutic anticonvulsant level
- 2.5–7.5 mEq/L

Compatibility
Magnesium sulfate may be given through the same IV line as acyclovir, aldesleukin, amifostine, amikacin, ampicillin, aztreonam, cefamandole, cefazolin, cefmetazole, cefoperazone, cefotaxime, cefoxitin, cephalothin, cephapirin, chloramphenicol, ciprofloxacin, clindamycin, dobutamine, doxycycline, enalaprilat, erythromycin, esmolol, famotidine, fludarabine, gallium, gentamicin, granisetron, heparin, hydrocortisone, hydromorphone, idarubicin, insulin (regular), kanamycin, labetalol, meperidine, metronidazole, minocycline, morphine, moxalactam, nafcillin, ondansetron, oxacillin, paclitaxel, penicillin G potassium, pip-eracillin, piperacillin-tazobactam, potassium chloride, propofol, sargramostim, ticarcillin, thiotepa, tobramycin, trimethoprim-sulfamethoxazole, vancomycin, vitamin B complex with C.

Incompatibility
Do not administer magnesium sulfate through the same IV line as cefepime.

TREATMENT OF OVERDOSE/ANTIDOTE
Discontinue drug or decrease dose. Initiate general supportive and resuscitative measures. Calcium gluconate or chloride 5–10 mEq IV will usually antagonize the effects of magnesium. Physostigmine 0.5–1 mg SC may be helpful. Peritoneal dialysis and hemodialysis are also effective.

Pharmacokinetics

Route	Onset	Duration
IV	Immediate	30 min
IM	60 min	3–4 h

Excretion: Urine

Adverse effects in *Italics* are most common; those in **Bold** are life-threatening

M

Adverse effects

▸ *CV:* **Asystole,** palpitations; prolonged PRI, wide QRS, tall T waves, prolonged QT interval on ECG; bradycardia, heart block
▸ *Derm:* Flushing, sweating
▸ *Fluid/electrolytes:* *Magnesium intoxication*—flushing, sweating, hypotension, stupor, depressed reflexes, flaccid paralysis, hypothermia, **circulatory collapse,** cardiac and CNS depression leading to **respiratory paralysis;** hypocalcemia

Clinically important drug–drug interactions

▸ Increased neuromuscular blocking effects with nondepolarizing neuromuscular blocking agents; prolonged respiratory depression with extended apnea may occur
▸ Effects offset by calcium
▸ Increased heart block with digoxin

◉ NURSING CONSIDERATIONS

Assessment

▸ *History:* Magnesium allergy, heart block, myocardial damage, impending delivery, renal function impairment, age
▸ *Physical:* T, P, BP, R, I & O, ECG, weight, neurologic checks, deep tendon reflexes, adventitious lung sounds, bowel sounds, renal function tests, serum electrolytes, digoxin level

Implementation

▸ Always administer IV infusion using an IV pump.
▸ Carefully monitor HR, BP, and ECG during therapy.
▸ Monitor serum magnesium levels during therapy. Discontinue administration as soon as levels are within normal limits and desired clinical response is obtained.
▸ Monitor knee jerk reflex and respiratory rate before repeated administration. If respiratory rate < 16/min or knee jerk reflexes are suppressed, do not give magnesium because respiratory center failure may occur.
▸ Maintain urine output of 100 mL q4h.
▸ Keep calcium salts readily available in case of hypermagnesemia or adverse reactions.
▸ Monitor for hypermagnesemia as evidenced by hypotension, depressed deep tendon reflexes, flushing, nausea, vomiting, depression, drowsiness, bradycardia; tall T waves, widened QRS, prolonged PRI and QT intervals on ECG; hypoventilation, paralysis, coma, apnea, and arrest.

Adverse effects in *Italics* are most common; those in **Bold** are life-threatening

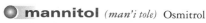 **mannitol** *(man'i tole)* Osmitrol

Pregnancy Category C

Drug class
Osmotic diuretic
Diagnostic agent

Indications
- Reduction of ICP and treatment of cerebral edema by reducing brain mass
- Promotion of diuresis to prevent or treat oliguric phase of acute renal failure before irreversible renal failure occurs
- Promotion of urinary excretion of toxic substances
- Prophylaxis of acute renal failure in conditions where glomerular filtration is greatly reduced
- Reduction of elevated intraocular pressure when pressure cannot be lowered by other means

Therapeutic actions
- Induces diuresis by elevating the osmolarity of the glomerular filtrate, inhibiting tubular reabsorption of water
- Increases sodium and chloride excretion
- Maintains flow of dilute urine, preventing damage to the nephron by toxic solutes
- In the eyes, creates an osmotic gradient between the plasma and ocular fluids

Effects on hemodynamic parameters
- Decreased ICP
- Decreased CVP (with diuresis)
- Increased CVP (with renal function impairment)
- Increased PAP and PCWP (with renal function impairment)

Contraindications/cautions
- **Contraindications:** mannitol allergy, anuria due to severe renal disease; severe pulmonary congestion or pulmonary edema; active intracranial bleeding except during craniotomy; severe dehydration; progressive renal damage or dysfunction after instituting mannitol therapy; increasing oliguria and azotemia; progressive heart failure or pulmonary edema after mannitol therapy
- **Cautions:** fluid/electrolyte imbalance, renal function impairment, CHF, hypovolemia, hemoconcentration

Available forms
- *Injection:* 5%, 10%, 15%, 20%, 25%

Adverse effects in *Italics* are most common; those in **Bold** are life-threatening

M

IV facts
Preparation
▶ If solution has crystallized, warm the bottle in hot water and shake vigorously. Do not administer drug if crystals remain. Cool solution to body temperature before administering.
▶ Add an in-line filter to IV tubing.

Dosage and titration
▶ *Reduction of intracranial pressure and brain mass:* 1.5–2 g/kg IV as a 15%–25% solution over 30–60 min.
▶ *Prevention of acute renal failure:* 50–100 g IV as a 5%–25% solution.
▶ *Treatment of oliguria:* 50–100 g IV of a 15%–25% solution.
▶ *Promote excretion of toxic substances:* Maximum of 200 g IV with other fluids and electrolytes. Concentration depends on patient's fluid requirements and urinary output.
▶ *Reduction of intraocular pressure:* 1.5–2 g/kg as a 15% or 20% solution IV over 30 min. When used preoperatively, give 1–1.5 h before surgery.
▶ *Test dose for patients with marked oliguria or inadequate renal function:* 0.2 g/kg IV (about 50 mL of a 25% solution, 75 mL of a 20% solution, or 100 mL of a 15% solution) over 3–5 min to produce urine flow of 30–50 mL/h. If urine output does not increase, repeat dose. If no response to second dose, reevaluate the patient.

Compatibility
Mannitol may be given through the same IV line as allopurinol, amifostine, aztreonam, cladribine, fludarabine, fluorouracil, gallium, idarubicin, melphalan, ondansetron, paclitaxel, piperacillin-tazobactam, propofol, sargramostim, teniposide, thiotepa, vinorelbine.

Incompatibility
Do not administer through the same IV line as cefepime or filgrastim. Do not give electrolyte-free mannitol solutions with blood. If giving blood simultaneously, add at least 20 mEq sodium chloride to each liter of mannitol solution to prevent pseudoagglutination.

> ### TREATMENT OF OVERDOSE/ANTIDOTE
> Discontinue drug or decrease dose. Initiate general supportive and resuscitative measures. Correct fluid and electrolyte imbalances. Hemodialysis will clear drug and reduce serum osmolality.

Adverse effects in *Italics* are most common; those in **Bold** are life-threatening

Pharmacokinetics

Route	Onset	Peak	Duration
IV	15–60 min	1 h	6–8 h

Metabolism: Liver (slightly); $T_{1/2}$: 15–100 min
Excretion: Urine

Adverse effects
- **CNS: Convulsions,** *dizziness,* headache, blurred vision
- **CV:** Hypotension, hypertension, edema, thrombophlebitis, tachycardia, chest pain, CHF
- **Resp:** Pulmonary congestion, rhinitis
- **GI:** *Nausea, dry mouth, thirst,* vomiting, diarrhea
- **GU:** *Diuresis,* urinary retention
- **Derm:** Urticaria, skin necrosis
- **Metabolic:** Fluid and electrolyte imbalances, dehydration, acidosis
- **Misc:** Fever, chills, pain

◉ NURSING CONSIDERATIONS

Assessment
- *History:* Mannitol allergy, anuria due to severe renal disease; pulmonary congestion, pulmonary edema, active intracranial bleeding, severe dehydration, increasing oliguria and azotemia; heart failure; fluid/electrolyte imbalance, renal function impairment, CHF, hypovolemia, hemoconcentration
- *Physical:* T, BP, P, R, CVP, ICP, CPP, PAP, I & O, IV site, weight, neurologic checks, vision, intraocular pressure, skin assessment, cardiac auscultation, JVD, edema, adventitious lung sounds, presence of pain, hydration status, CBC, serum electrolytes, UA, renal function tests

Implementation
- Always administer using an IV infusion pump.
- Frequently monitor I & O, CVP, PAP, ICP, and CPP.
- Monitor for evidence of dehydration (dry mucous membranes, dry skin, thirst, decreased skin turgor, tachycardia, flat neck veins, low-grade fever, postural hypotension, oliguria; decreased CVP, PAP, and ICP) or fluid overload (crackles, dyspnea, edema, JVD; increased urine output, weight, BP, CVP, PAP, and ICP).
- Carefully monitor electrolyte balance.
- Weigh patient daily.
- Carefully monitor IV site for evidence of infiltration.

⬤ **meperidine hydrochloride** *(me per' i deen)* Ⓜ
Demerol HCl

Pregnancy Category C

C-II controlled substance

Drug class
Narcotic agonist analgesic

Indications
▶ Relief of moderate to severe pain (oral, parenteral)
▶ Preoperative medication, support of anesthesia (parenteral)

Therapeutic actions
▶ Opium alkaloid; acts as agonist at specific opioid receptors in the CNS to produce analgesia, euphoria, sedation, and respiratory and physical depression

Contraindications/cautions
▶ **Contraindications:** hypersensitivity to narcotics, use of MAO inhibitors within previous 14 d, diarrhea caused by poisoning until toxins are eliminated, acute bronchial asthma, upper airway obstruction
▶ **Cautions:** head injury, increased intracranial or intraocular pressure, CNS depression or coma, acute asthma, COPD, cor pulmonale, preexisting respiratory depression, hypoxia, hypercapnia, acute abdominal conditions, CV disease, supraventricular tachycardias, myxedema, convulsive disorders, acute alcoholism, delirium tremens, cerebral arteriosclerosis, ulcerative colitis, fever, kyphoscoliosis, hypothyroidism, Addison's disease, prostatic hypertrophy, urethral stricture, gallbladder disease, recent GI or GU surgery, toxic psychosis, renal or hepatic dysfunction, hypovolemia, elderly or debilitated patients

Available forms
▶ *Injection:* 10, 25, 50, 75, 100 mg/mL
▶ *Tablets:* 50, 100 mg
▶ *Syrup:* 50 mg/mL

IV/IM facts
Preparation
▶ *Direct IV injection:* Dilute with D5W; 0.9%NS, or Sterile Water for Injection to a concentration of 10 mg/mL.

Adverse effects in *Italics* are most common; those in **Bold** are life-threatening

▸ *Continuous IV infusion:* Dilute with D5W/LR; D2.5W; D5W; D10W; Dextran 6% in D5W or 0.9%NS; Dextrose-Ringer's Injection combinations; Dextrose-Saline combinations; Fructose 10% in 0.9%NS or water; Ionosol products; LR; 0.45%NS; 0.9%NS; Ringer's Injection; or Sodium Lactate (1/6 Molar) Injection to a concentration of 1 mg/mL.

▸ *IM:* Give undiluted.

Dosage

▸ *Pain relief:* **Direct IV injection:** 10–50 mg IV q2–4h; do not give faster than 25 mg/min. **Patient controlled analgesia system:** Usual intial dosage is 10 mg IV with a 1–5 mg incremental dose. The recommended Lockout Interval is 6–10 min. The minimum recommended Lockout Interval is 5 min. **Continuous IV infusion:** 15–35 mg/h. **IM:** 50–150 mg IM q3–4h as needed. Individualize dosage amount and frequency based on patient's pain level and response to therapy.

▸ *Preoperative use:* 50–100 mg IM 30–90 min before anesthesia.

▸ *Elderly/debilitated patients:* Reduce dosage; use with caution to prevent respiratory depression and adverse reactions.

Compatibility

Meperidine may be given through the same IV line as amifostine, amikacin, ampicillin, ampicillin-sulbactam, atenolol, aztreonam, bumetanide, cefamandole, cefazolin, cefmetazole, cefotaxime, cefotetan, cefoxitin, ceftazidime, ceftizoxime, ceftriaxone, cefuroxime, cephalothin, cephapirin, chloramphenicol, cladribine, clindamycin, dexamethasone, diltiazem, diphenhydramine, dobutamine, dopamine, doxycycline, droperidol, erythromycin, famotidine, filgrastim, fluconazole, fludarabine, gallium, gentamicin, granisetron, heparin, hydrocortisone, insulin (regular), kanamycin, labetalol, lidocaine, magnesium sulfate, melphalan, methyldopate, methylprednisolone, metoclopramide, metoprolol, metronidazole, moxalactam, ondansetron, oxacillin, oxytocin, paclitaxel, penicillin G potassium, piperacillin, piperacillin-tazobactam, potassium chloride, propofol, propranolol, ranitidine, sargramostim, teniposide, thiotepa, ticarcillin, ticarcillin-clavulanate, tobramycin, trimethoprim-sulfamethoxazole, vancomycin, verapamil, vinorelbine.

Incompatibility

Do not administer through the same IV line as allopurinol, cefepime, cefoperazone, idarubicin, imipenem-cilastatin, mezlocillin, minocycline. Do *not* mix meperidine solutions with solutions of aminophylline, barbiturates, heparin, iodide, morphine sulfate, methicillin, phenytoin, sodium bicarbonate, sulfadiazine, sulfisoxazole.

Adverse effects in *Italics* are most common; those in **Bold** are life-threatening

M

Oral dosage

▶ 50–150 mg PO q3–4h as needed. Oral route is less effective than parenteral route. Individualize dosage amount and frequency based on patient's pain level and response to therapy.

> **TREATMENT OF OVERDOSE/ANTIDOTE**
> Discontinue drug or decrease dose. Initiate general supportive and resuscitative measures. Administer the antidote naloxone 0.4––2 mg IV. Repeat at 2- to 3-min intervals if needed to reverse respiratory depression. Gastric lavage or induced emesis may remove oral meperidine.

Pharmacokinetics

Route	Onset	Peak	Duration
IV	Immediate	5–7 min	2–4 h
IM	10–15 min	30–60 min	2–4 h
Oral	15 min	60 min	2–4 h

Metabolism: Hepatic (to activate metabolite); $T_{1/2}$: 3–4 h
Excretion: Urine

Adverse effects

▶ *CNS:* **Convulsions,** *lightheadedness, dizziness, sedation,* euphoria, dysphoria, delirium, insomnia, agitation, anxiety, fear, hallucinations, disorientation, drowsiness, lethargy, impaired mental and physical performance, coma, mood changes, weakness, headache, tremor, miosis, visual disturbances
▶ *CV:* **Circulatory depression, shock, cardiac arrest,** facial flushing, tachycardia, bradycardia, dysrhythmias, palpitations, hypotension, postural hypotension, syncope
▶ *Resp:* **Respiratory depression, apnea, respiratory arrest,** suppressed cough reflex
▶ *GI:* *Nausea, vomiting,* dry mouth, anorexia, constipation, biliary tract spasm, increased colonic motility in patients with chronic ulcerative colitis
▶ *GU:* Ureteral spasm, spasm of vesical sphincters, urinary retention or hesitancy, antidiuretic effect, reduced libido or potency
▶ *Derm:* *Sweating,* injection site irritation and induration (SC injection)
▶ *Allergic:* **Anaphylaxis, laryngospasm, bronchospasm,** pruritus, urticaria, edema
▶ *Dependence:* Tolerance, physical and psychological dependence

Adverse effects in *Italics* are most common; those in **Bold** are life-threatening

Clinically important drug–drug interactions

▸ Increased respiratory depression, hypotension, profound sedation, or coma with barbiturate anesthetics, alcohol, sedatives, antihistamines, phenothiazines, butyrophenones, TCAs
▸ Unpredictable, severe, and fatal reactions (coma, severe respiratory depression, cyanosis, hypotension, hyperexcitability, convulsions, tachycardia, hyperpyrexia, hypertension) with MAO inhibitors; do not give to patients on MAO inhibitors

⬤ NURSING CONSIDERATIONS

Assessment

▸ *History:* Hypersensitivity to narcotics, use of MAO inhibitors, diarrhea caused by poisoning until toxins are eliminated, acute bronchial asthma, upper airway obstruction, head injury, increased intracranial or intraocular pressure, CNS depression or coma, acute asthma, COPD, cor pulmonale, respiratory depression, hypoxia, hypercapnia, acute abdominal conditions, CV disease, myxedema, convulsive disorders, acute alcoholism, delirium tremens, cerebral arteriosclerosis, ulcerative colitis, kyphoscoliosis, hypothyroidism, Addison's disease, prostatic hypertrophy, urethral stricture, gallbladder disease, recent GI or GU surgery, toxic psychosis, renal or hepatic dysfunction, hypovolemia, age, debilitated condition
▸ *Physical:* T, BP, P, R, ECG, SpO_2, ABG, I & O, injection site, weight, neurologic checks, ophthalmic exam, skin assessment, respiratory effort, adventitious lung sounds, pain assessment, orthostatic BP, bowel sounds, hydration status, prostate exam, voiding pattern; thyroid, liver, and kidney function tests

Implementation

▸ Exercise extreme caution when calculating and preparing doses. Meperidine is a potent drug; small dosage errors can cause serious adverse effects. Avoid inadvertent bolus of drug.
▸ Always administer continuous infusion using an IV infusion pump.
▸ Monitor vital signs frequently with IV administration.
▸ Assess for evidence of respiratory depression.
▸ Have emergency equipment (defibrillator, drugs, intubation equipment, oxygen) on standby in case of anaphylaxis or adverse reaction.
▸ Correct hypovolemia before administering drug.
▸ Assess pain status frequently; notify provider if patient does not receive adequate pain relief.

Adverse effects in *Italics* are most common; those in **Bold** are life-threatening

▶ Minimize postural hypotension by helping the patient change positions slowly. Ⓜ

▶ Administer parenteral forms when the patient is lying down.

▶ Use caution when giving IM injections to patients with hypotension or in shock; impaired perfusion may delay absorption; with repeated doses, an excessive amount may be absorbed when circulation is restored.

▶ Reduce dosage of meperidine by 25%–50% in patients receiving phenothiazines or other tranquilizers.

▶ Give each dose of the oral syrup in a half glass of water. If taken undiluted, it may exert a slight local anesthetic effect on mucous membranes.

▶ Reassure patient about addiction liability; most patients who receive opiates for medical reasons do not develop dependence syndromes.

▶ Follow federal, state, and institutional policies for dispensing controlled substances.

⬤ **meropenem** *(mare oh pen' ehm)* Merrem IV
Pregnancy Category B

Drug class
Antibiotic (carbapenem)

Indications
▶ Susceptible intra-abdominal infections caused by viridans group streptococci, *Escherichia coli, Klebsiella pneumoniae, Pseudomonas aeruginosa, Bacteroids fragilis, Bacteroids thetaiotaomicron,* and *Peptostreptococcus* species

Therapeutic actions
▶ Bactericidal, broad-spectrum antibiotic that is effective for gram-positive and gram-negative organisms
▶ Inhibits synthesis of bacterial cell wall and causes cell death in susceptible cells

Contraindications/cautions
▶ **Contraindications:** allergy to meropenem, drugs in the same class, or beta-lactams
▶ **Cautions:** CNS disorders, seizures, renal or hepatic function impairment, bacterial meningitis

Available forms
▶ *Powder for injection:* 500 mg, 1 g

Adverse effects in *Italics* are most common; those in **Bold** are life-threatening

IV facts
Preparation
▸ **ADD-Vantage vials:** Reconstitute only with D5W; 0.45%NS; or 0.9%NS. Activate the ADD-Vantage vial by pulling the inner cap from the drug vial. Allow drug and diluent to mix.
▸ **Other vials:** Reconstitute with D5W; 0.9%NS; or Sterile Water for Injection (add 10 mL diluent to 500-mg vial; 20 mL to 1-g vial). Add contents of vial to 100 mL D2.5W/0.45%NS; D5W/LR; D5W/0.9%NS; D5W/potassium chloride 0.15%; D5W/sodium bicarbonate 0.02%; D5W; D10W; LR; Mannitol 2.5%; 0.9%NS; Normosol M/D5W; Ringer's Injection; Sodium Bicarbonate Injection 5%; Sodium Lactate (1/6 Molar) Injection; or Sterile Water for Injection. Stability of each solution varies depending on solution and temperature. If possible, use freshly reconstituted solution. Consult manufacturer's instructions if not used immediately.

Dosage
▸ 1 g IV q8h over 15–30 min or as an IV bolus injection (5–20 mL) over 3–5 min.
▸ *Renal function impairment:* Reduce dosage (see table below) for patients with creatinine clearance < 50 mL/min.

Creatinine Clearance (mL/min)	Dose
26–50	1 g IV q12h
10–25	500 mg IV q12h
<10	500 mg IV q24h

Compatibility
Meropenem may be given through the same IV line as aminophylline, atenolol, atropine, cimetidine, dexamethasone, digoxin, diphenhydramine, enalaprilat, fluconazole, furosemide, gentamicin, heparin, insulin (regular), metoclopramide, morphine, norepinephrine, phenobarbital, vancomycin.

Incompatibility
Do not administer through the same IV line as amphotericin B, diazepam, metronidazole.

TREATMENT OF OVERDOSE/ANTIDOTE
Discontinue drug or decrease dosage. Initiate general supportive and resuscitative measures. Meropenem and its metabolite are readily removed by hemodialysis.

Adverse effects in *Italics* are most common; those in **Bold** are life-threatening

Pharmacokinetics

Route	Onset	Peak	Duration
IV	Immediate	End of 30-min infusion or 5-min injection	6–8 h

$T_{1/2}$: 1 h
Excretion: Urine

Adverse effects

▶ *CNS:* **Seizures,** *headache,* insomnia, agitation, delirium, confusion, dizziness, paresthesias, nervousness, somnolence, anxiety, depression
▶ *CV:* **Heart failure, cardiac arrest, MI,** bradycardia, hypotension, tachycardia, hypertension, peripheral edema, syncope
▶ *Resp:* **Apnea, pulmonary embolus,** dyspnea, hypoxia
▶ *GI:* **Pseudomembranous colitis, GI hemorrhage, hepatic failure,** *nausea, vomiting, diarrhea,* flatulence, ileus, cholestatic jaundice, oral moniliasis, abdominal enlargement; increased ALT, AST, alkaline phosphatase, LDH, bilirubin
▶ *GU:* **Renal failure,** dysuria, increased BUN and creatinine, RBCs in urine
▶ *Derm:* *Rash, pruritus,* urticaria, sweating; inflammation, phlebitis, pain, edema at injection site
▶ *Allergic:* **Anaphylaxis**
▶ *Hematologic:* Increased platelets and eosinophils, prolonged or shortened PT and PTT, decreased platelets, positive Coombs test, decreased Hgb and Hct, decreased WBC, anemia
▶ *Misc:* **Sepsis, shock,** fever, back pain, epistaxis, superinfections

Clinically important drug–drug interactions
▶ Inhibited renal excretion with probenecid

● NURSING CONSIDERATIONS

Assessment
▶ *History:* Allergy to meropenem, drugs in the same class, or beta-lactams; CNS disorders, seizures, renal or hepatic impairment, bacterial meningitis
▶ *Physical:* T, P, R, BP, ECG, I & O, SpO_2, IV site, neurologic checks, skin assessment, respiratory effort, adventitious lung sounds, edema, JVD, bowel sounds, abdominal exam, renal and liver function tests, CBC, culture and sensitivity of infection site, stool and emesis guaiac, PT, APTT

Adverse effects in *Italics* are most common; those in **Bold** are life-threatening

Implementation
▸ Obtain specimen for culture and sensitivity of infected area before beginning therapy. May begin drug before results are available.
▸ Have emergency equipment (defibrillator, drugs, oxygen, intubation equipment) on standby in case anaphylaxis or adverse reaction occurs.
▸ Assess for evidence of anaphylaxis; if suspected, discontinue drug immediately and notify provider.
▸ Monitor renal, hepatic, and hematopoietic function.
▸ Initiate seizure precautions for patients at increased risk for seizures.
▸ Monitor for occurrence of superinfections; treat as appropriate.
▸ Discontinue drug at any sign of colitis; initiate appropriate supportive treatment.

metaproterenol sulfate *(met a proe ter' e nole)*
Alupent
Pregnancy Category C

Drug classes
Sympathomimetic
Bronchodilator

Indications
▸ Prophylaxis and treatment of bronchial asthma and reversible bronchospasm that may occur with bronchitis and emphysema

Therapeutic actions
▸ In low doses, acts relatively selectively at β_2-adrenergic receptors to cause bronchodilation and vasodilation; bronchodilation may facilitate expectoration
▸ At higher doses, β_2-selectivity is lost, and the drug acts at β_1 receptors, causing increased myocardial contractility and conduction

Contraindications/cautions
▸ **Contraindications:** hypersensitivity to metaproterenol or its components, cardiac dysrhythmias associated with tachycardia
▸ **Caution:** cardiovascular disease, coronary insufficiency, dysrhythmias, hypertension, convulsive disorders, hyperthyroidism, diabetes, patients who are unusually responsive to sympathomimetic amines

Adverse effects in *Italics* are most common; those in **Bold** are life-threatening

M

Available forms
- *Tablets:* 10, 20 mg
- *Syrup:* 10 mg/5 mL
- *Aerosol:* 0.65 mg/dose
- *Solution for inhalation:* 0.4%, 0.6%, 5%

Oral/inhalation dosage
- *Inhalant solutions:* 5–15 inhalations in hand bulb nebulizer using undiluted 5% solution or 0.2–0.3 mL diluted in 2.5 mL saline per IPPB or nebulizer device. One treatment may not relieve acute bronchospasm. If needed, give tid–qid.
- *Metered-dose inhaler:* 2–3 inhalations q3–4h. Allow ≥ 2 min between inhalations. Do not exceed 12 inhalations/d.
- *Oral:* 20 mg PO tablet or two teaspoon (10 mL) syrup PO tid–qid.
- *Elderly:* Patients > 60 y are more likely to develop adverse effects, use caution.

> **TREATMENT OF OVERDOSE/ANTIDOTE**
> Discontinue drug or decrease dosage. Initiate general supportive and resuscitative measures.

Pharmacokinetics

Route	Onset	Peak	Duration
Nebulization	5–30 min	1 h	2–6 h
PO	15 min	1 h	4 h

Metabolism: Hepatic
Excretion: Bile, feces

Adverse effects
- *CNS: Nervousness, headache, shakiness, dizziness,* insomnia, fatigue, drowsiness, syncope, weakness, sensory disturbances, blurred vision
- *CV: Tachycardia, palpitations,* chest pain, edema, hypertension
- *Resp:* **Bronchospasm,** asthma exacerbation, coughing, nasal congestion, hoarseness
- *GI: Nausea, GI distress,* appetite changes, diarrhea, vomiting, dry mouth/throat, bad taste
- *Derm:* Diaphoresis, hives, pruritus
- *Musc/Skel: Tremor,* pain, spasms
- *Misc:* Chills, fever, flu symptoms, facial and finger puffiness, clonus noted on flexing foot

Clinically important drug–drug interactions
- Increased sympathomimetic effects with other beta-adrenergic aerosol bronchodilators
- Enhanced vascular system effects with MAO inhibitors, TCAs

Adverse effects in *Italics* are most common; those in **Bold** are life-threatening

● NURSING CONSIDERATIONS

Assessment
▸ *History:* Hypersensitivity to metaproterenol or its components, cardiovascular disease, coronary insufficiency, hypertension, convulsive disorders, hyperthyroidism, diabetes, unusual responsiveness to sympathomimetic amines
▸ *Physical:* T, P, R, BP, ECG, SpO_2, neurologic checks, vision assessment, skin assessment, respiratory effort, adventitious lung sounds, pain assessment, abdominal assessment, serum electrolytes, serum glucose, ABG, peak flow test, pulmonary function tests, thyroid function tests

Implementation
▸ Use minimal doses for minimal periods of time; drug tolerance can occur with prolonged use.
▸ Before using inhaler the first time, prime the pump. If not used for > 2 wk, reprime the pump.
▸ Do not exceed recommended dosage. Administer aerosol during second half of inspiration, when airways are wider and distribution is more extensive.
▸ Consult manufacturer's instructions for use of aerosol delivery equipment; specifics of administration vary with each product.
▸ Teach patient proper use of inhaler.
▸ Store inhalant solution at < 77°F. Protect solution from light. Do not use if it is darker than slightly yellow or pinkish or if it contains a precipitate.

● **methylene blue** *(meth' i leen)* Methblue 65, Urolene Blue

Pregnancy Category C

Drug class
Antidote

Indications
▸ Treatment of cyanide poisoning and methemoglobinemia
▸ May be useful in managing patients with oxalate urinary tract calculi

Therapeutic actions
▸ Oxidation-reduction agent that, in high concentrations, converts the ferrous iron of reduced hemoglobin into the ferric form, producing methemoglobin, which can bind to cyanide
▸ In low concentrations, hastens the conversion of methemoglobin to hemoglobin

Adverse effects in *Italics* are most common; those in **Bold** are life-threatening

Contraindications/cautions
▶ **Contraindications:** allergy to methylene blue, renal insufficiency, intraspinal injection
▶ **Cautions:** aniline-induced methemoglobulinemia, glucose-6-phosphate dehydrogenase (G-6-PD) deficiency, anemia, cardiovascular disease

Available forms
▶ *Injection:* 10 mg/mL
▶ *Tablets:* 65 mg

IV facts
Preparation
▶ May give undiluted.

Dosage
▶ 1–2 mg/kg IV over several minutes.

Incompatibility
Do not administer through the same IV line as other medications.

Oral dosage
▶ 65–130 mg PO tid after meals with a full glass of water.

TREATMENT OF OVERDOSE/ANTIDOTE
Discontinue drug or decrease dose. Initiate general supportive and resuscitative measures.

Pharmacokinetics

Route	Onset	Duration
IV	Immediate	End of Infusion
Oral	Varies	

Metabolism: Tissue
Excretion: Urine, bile, feces

Adverse effects
▶ *CNS:* Confusion, dizziness, headache
▶ *CV:* Precordial pain
▶ *GI: Blue-green feces,* nausea, vomiting, diarrhea
▶ *GU: Blue-green urine,* bladder irritation
▶ *Misc:* Fever, diaphoresis, cyanosis

⬤ NURSING CONSIDERATIONS

Assessment
▶ *History:* Allergy to methylene blue, renal insufficiency, aniline-induced methemoglobulinemia, G-6-PD deficiency,

Adverse effects in *Italics* are most common; those in **Bold** are life-threatening

anemia, cardiovascular disease, cyanide ingestion, methemoglobinemia
▸ *Physical:* T, P, R, BP, ECG, I & O, IV site, SpO$_2$, neurologic
checks, skin assessment, orthostatic BP, peripheral perfusion,
adventitious lung sounds, cardiac assessment, chest pain assessment, liver evaluation, CBC, ABG, serum lactate level,
cyanide level, methemoglobin level, UA

Implementation
▸ Monitor IV site carefully; SC injection may cause a necrotic
abscess.
▸ Contact with skin will dye the skin blue; remove stain with
hypochlorite solution.
▸ Monitor for evidence of anemia; regularly assess CBC.
▸ Store IV and oral forms in a dry place at room temperature.

⬤ methylprednisolone sodium succinate *(meth ill pred niss' oh lone)* A-Methapred, Solu-Medrol

Pregnancy Category C

Drug classes
Corticosteroid
Glucocorticoid, intermediate-acting
Hormonal agent

Indications
▸ Management of a wide variety of endocrine, rheumatic, collagen, dermatologic, allergic, gastrointestinal, respiratory,
hematologic, neoplastic, and edematous disorders
▸ Unlabeled uses: Treatment of septic shock, acute spinal cord
injury

Therapeutic actions
▸ Suppresses inflammation and normal immune response
▸ Causes profound and varied metabolic effects

> **Contraindications/cautions**
> ▸ **Contraindications:** methylprednisolone allergy; systemic
> infections, especially tuberculosis, fungal infections, amebi-
> asis, vaccinia and varicella, and antibiotic-resistant infections
> ▸ **Cautions:** renal or hepatic disease, cerebral malaria,
> hypothyroidism; ulcerative colitis with impending perfo-
> ration; diverticulitis, active or latent peptic ulcer; inflam-
> matory bowel disease, fresh intestinal anastomoses, psy-
> chotic tendencies, hypertension, metastatic carcinoma,
> *(contraindications continued on next page)*

thromboembolic disorders, osteoporosis, convulsive disorders, myasthenia gravis, diabetes, CHF, Cushing's syndrome, recent AMI, elderly patients

Available forms
▸ *Injection:* 40, 125, 500 mg/vial; 1, 2 g/vial

IV/IM facts
Preparation
▸ Reconstitute vial with 2 mL of Bacteriostatic Water for Injection or Bacteriostatic Sodium Chloride Injection.
▸ If using Act-O-Vial container, press the plastic activator down to force the diluent into the lower chamber. Agitate gently to dissolve drug.
▸ For an intermittent or continuous infusion, further dilute in D5W/0.9%NS; D5W; or 0.9%NS.

Dosage
▸ *Initial dose:* 10–40 mg IV over 1 to several minutes. Give next doses IV or IM.
▸ *High dose therapy:* 30 mg/kg IV over 10–20 min. May repeat q4–6h, not beyond 48–72 h.

Compatibility
Methylprednisolone may be given through the same IV line as acyclovir, amifostine, amrinone, aztreonam, cefepime, cisplatin, cladribine, cyclophosphamide, cytarabine, dopamine, doxorubicin, enalaprilat, famotidine, fludarabine, granisetron, heparin, melphalan, meperidine, methotrexate, metronidazole, midazolam, morphine, piperacillin-tazobactam, sodium bicarbonate, tacrolimus, teniposide, theophylline, thiotepa.

Incompatibility
Do not administer through the same IV line as allopurinol, amsacrine, ciprofloxacin, filgrastim, ondansetron, paclitaxel, propofol, sargramostim, vinorelbine.

TREATMENT OF OVERDOSE/ANTIDOTE
Discontinue drug or decrease dosage. Initiate general supportive and resuscitative measures.

Pharmacokinetics

Route	Onset
IV	Rapid

Metabolism: Hepatic; $T_{1/2}$: 78–188 min
Excretion: Urine

Adverse effects in *Italics* are most common; those in **Bold** are life-threatening

Adverse effects

- Most occur with chronic therapy.
- *CNS:* **Convulsions,** *vertigo, headache,* paresthesias, insomnia, psychosis
- *CV:* **Myocardial rupture after recent AMI, circulatory collapse, lethal dysrhythmias, cardiac arrest, fat embolism,** hypertension, hypotension, CHF secondary to fluid retention, thromboembolism, thrombophlebitis
- *GI:* Peptic ulcer, bowel perforation, pancreatitis, abdominal distention, ulcerative esophagitis, nausea, hiccups, increased appetite, weight gain
- *Derm:* *Impaired wound healing, petechiae, ecchymoses, thin and fragile skin,* acne; burning or tingling after IV injection, increased sweating, allergic dermatitis, urticaria, angioneurotic edema
- *Allergic:* **Anaphylaxis**
- *Fluid/Electrolytes:* *Sodium and fluid retention, hypokalemia,* hypokalemic alkalosis, metabolic alkalosis, hypocalcemia
- *Musc/Skel:* *Muscle weakness,* steroid myopathy, muscle mass loss, osteoporosis, vertebral compression fractures, pathologic fractures, tendon rupture
- *Endocrine:* *Secondary adrenocortical and pituitary unresponsiveness,* decreased carbohydrate tolerance, diabetes mellitus, cushingoid state, menstrual irregularities, negative nitrogen balance, hirsutism
- *Ophthalmic:* Cataracts, increased intraocular pressure, glaucoma
- *Misc:* *Increased susceptibility to infection, masking of signs of infection,* subcutaneous fat atrophy

Clinically important drug–drug interactions

- Decreased clearance with macrolide antibiotics
- Increased blood levels with oral contraceptives, estrogens, ketoconazole
- Decreased blood levels with phenytoin, rifampin
- Decreased serum level of salicylates
- Decreased effectiveness of anticholinesterases (ambenonium, edrophonium, neostigmine, pyridostigmine) in myasthenia gravis
- Increased digitalis toxicity related to hypokalemia
- Altered response to coumarin anticoagulants such as warfarin
- Increased hypokalemia with potassium-depleting diuretics
- Decreased serum concentrations of isoniazid
- Increased cyclosporine toxicity
- Decreased effectiveness with barbiturates

Adverse effects in *Italics* are most common; those in **Bold** are life-threatening

⬤ NURSING CONSIDERATIONS

M

Assessment

❱ *History:* Methylprednisolone allergy; systemic infections, especially tuberculosis, fungal infections, amebiasis, vaccinia and varicella, and antibiotic-resistant infections; renal or hepatic disease, cerebral malaria, hypothyroidism, ulcerative colitis with impending perforation, diverticulitis, active or latent peptic ulcer, inflammatory bowel disease, fresh intestinal anastomoses, psychotic tendencies, hypertension, metastatic carcinoma, thromboembolic disorders, osteoporosis, convulsive disorders, myasthenia gravis, diabetes, CHF, Cushing's syndrome, recent AMI, age

❱ *Physical:* T, P, R, BP, ECG, I & O, IV site, weight, ophthalmologic exam, neurologic checks, skin assessment, muscle strength, peripheral perfusion, adventitious lung sounds, chest x-ray, upper GI x-ray (history or symptoms of peptic ulcer), abdominal assessment, presence of infection, CBC, serum electrolytes, 2-h postprandial blood glucose, serum glucose, UA, adrenal function tests, serum cholesterol, liver and renal function tests

Implementation

❱ Carefully monitor for evidence of fluid overload (I & O, daily weight, edema, lung sounds, JVD).

❱ Evaluate for hypokalemia as evidenced by muscle weakness, fatigue, paralytic ileus, ECG changes, anorexia, nausea, vomiting, abdominal distention, dizziness, or polyuria.

❱ Assess for hypocalcemia as evidenced by Chvostek's or Trousseau's signs, muscle twitching, laryngospasm, or paresthesias.

❱ Have emergency equipment (defibrillator, drugs, oxygen, intubation equipment) on standby in case anaphylaxis or adverse reaction occurs.

❱ Give daily doses before 9:00 AM to mimic normal peak corticosteroid blood levels.

❱ Increase dosage when patient is subject to stress.

❱ Patient is at higher risk of infection; initiate interventions to prevent infection. Drug may mask evidence of infection.

❱ Taper doses when discontinuing high-dose or long-term therapy. Symptoms of adrenal insufficiency from too-rapid withdrawal include nausea, fatigue, anorexia, dyspnea, hypotension, hypoglycemia, myalgia, fever, malaise, arthralgia, dizziness, desquamation of skin, or fainting.

❱ Do not give live virus vaccines with immunosuppressive doses of corticosteroids.

Adverse effects in *Italics* are most common; those in **Bold** are life-threatening

▸ Use minimal doses for minimal duration to minimize adverse effects.

⬤ **metoclopramide** *(met oh kloe pra' mide)*
Apo-Metoclop (CAN), Maxeran (CAN), Maxolon, Nu-Metoclopramide (CAN), Octamide PFS, Reglan

Pregnancy Category B

Drug classes
GI stimulant
Antiemetic

Indications
▸ Relief of symptoms of acute and recurrent diabetic gastroparesis
▸ Short-term therapy (4–12 wk) for adults with symptomatic gastroesophageal reflux who fail to respond to conventional therapy (oral)
▸ Prevention of nausea and vomiting associated with emetogenic cancer chemotherapy (parenteral)
▸ Prophylaxis of postoperative nausea and vomiting when nasogastric suction is undesirable (parenteral)
▸ Facilitation of small bowel intubation when tube does not pass the pylorus with conventional maneuvers (single-dose parenteral use)
▸ Stimulation of gastric emptying and intestinal transit of barium when delayed emptying interferes with radiologic exam of the stomach or small intestine (single-dose parenteral use)
▸ Unlabeled uses: treatment of nausea and vomiting of a variety of etiologies, gastric ulcer, anorexia nervosa, gastric bezoars, diabetic cystoparesis, esophageal variceal bleeding; to improve patient response to ergotamine, analgesics, and sedatives in migraine

Therapeutic actions
▸ Stimulates motility of upper GI tract without stimulating gastric, biliary, or pancreatic secretions
▸ Mode of action unclear; appears to sensitize tissues to action of acetylcholine
▸ Increases the tone and amplitude of gastric contractions; relaxes pyloric sphincter and duodenal bulb; increases peristalsis of duodenum and jejunum, resulting in accelerated gastric emptying and intestinal transit
▸ Raises lower esophageal sphincter pressure for patients with gastroesophageal reflux
▸ Has little or no effect on colon or gallbladder motility

Adverse effects in *Italics* are most common; those in **Bold** are life-threatening

- Produces sedation and may produce extrapyramidal reactions Ⓜ
- Induces release of prolactin and transiently increases circulating aldosterone levels
- Antagonizes central and peripheral dopamine receptors, resulting in antiemetic effects

Contraindications/cautions
- **Contraindications:** metoclopramide allergy, GI hemorrhage, mechanical obstruction or perforation, when stimulation of GI motility might be dangerous, pheochromocytoma, epilepsy, use of other drugs that may cause extrapyramidal reactions, depression (unless expected benefits outweigh risk of severe depression and suicidal ideation)
- **Cautions:** Parkinson's disease, elderly patients, renal or hepatic function impairment, hypertension, diabetes, breast cancer

Available forms
- *Injection:* 5 mg/mL
- *Tablets:* 5, 10 mg
- *Syrup:* 5 mg/5 mL
- *Concentrated solution:* 10 mg/mL

IV/IM facts
Preparation
- May give undiluted by direct IV injection or IM. For doses > 10 mg, dilute in 50 mL of D5W/0.45% NS; D5W; LR; Mannitol 20%; 0.9%NS; or Ringer's Injection.

Dosage
- *Nausea/vomiting (unlabeled use):* 10 mg IV 30 min before each meal and at hs.
- *Facilitation of small bowel intubation:* 10 mg IV over 1–2 min.
- *Prevention of chemotherapy-induced emesis:* 1–2 mg/kg IV over 15 min; give 30 min before beginning chemotherapy. Repeat q2h for 2 doses, then q3h for 3 doses.
- *Radiologic examinations:* 10 mg IV over 1–2 min.
- *Diabetic gastroparesis:* 10 mg IV or IM 30 min before each meal and at hs.
- *Prevention of postoperative nausea and vomiting:* 10–20 mg IM at the end of surgery.
- *Renal/hepatic function impairment:* If creatinine clearance is < 40 mL/min, give about 1/2 the recommended dose. Titrate dose as indicated.

Adverse effects in *Italics* are most common; those in **Bold** are life-threatening

Compatibility

Metoclopramide may be given through the same IV line as acyclovir, aldesleukin, amifostine, aztreonam, bleomycin, ciprofloxacin, cisplatin, cladribine, cyclophosphamide, cytarabine, diltiazem, doxorubicin, droperidol, famotidine, filgrastim, fluconazole, fludarabine, fluorouracil, foscarnet, gallium, granisetron, heparin, idarubicin, leucovorin, melphalan, meperidine, methotrexate, mitomycin, morphine, ondansetron, paclitaxel, piperacillin-tazobactam, propofol, sargramostim, sufentanil, tacrolimus, teniposide, thiotepa, vinblastine, vincristine, vinorelbine, zidovudine.

Incompatibility

Do not administer through the same IV line as allopurinol, amsacrine, cefepime, furosemide.

Oral dosage

▸ *Relief of symptoms of gastroparesis:* 10 mg PO 30 min before each meal and hs for 2–8 wk.
▸ *Symptomatic gastroesophageal reflux:* 10–15 mg PO up to qid 30 min before meals and hs. If symptoms occur only at certain times or in relation to specific stimuli, single doses of 20 mg may be preferable.
▸ *Renal/hepatic function impairment:* If creatinine clearance is < 40 mL/min, give about ½ the recommended dose. Titrate dose as indicated.

> **TREATMENT OF OVERDOSE/ANTIDOTE**
> Discontinue drug or decrease dosage. Initiate general supportive and resuscitative measures. Anticholinergic or antiparkinson drugs (benztropine 1–2 mg IM) or antihistamines with anticholinergic (diphenhydramine 50 mg IM) properties may control extrapyramidal reactions.

Pharmacokinetics

Route	Onset	Peak	Duration
IV	1–3 min		1–2 h
IM	10–15 min		1–2 h
Oral	30–60 min	60–120 min	1–2 h

Metabolism: Hepatic (minimal); $T_{1/2}$: 5–6 h
Excretion: Urine

Adverse effects

▸ *CNS:* **Convulsions,** *restlessness, drowsiness, fatigue, lassitude, extrapyramidal reactions, parkinsonism-like reactions,* akathisia, dystonia, insomnia, myoclonus, dizziness, anxi-

---

Adverse effects in *Italics* are most common; those in **Bold** are life-threatening

ety, tardive dyskinesia, headache, depression with suicidal ideation, hallucinations
- **CV:** Hypertension, hypotension, supraventricular tachycardia, bradycardia
- **GI: Hepatoxicity** (when given with other drugs with known hepatotoxic potential), *nausea, diarrhea*
- **GU:** Urinary frequency, incontinence
- **Allergic: Bronchospasm, angioneurotic edema,** rash, urticaria
- **Hematologic: Neutropenia, leukopenia, agranulocytosis**
- **Endocrine:** Galactorrhea, amenorrhea, gynecomastia, impotence, fluid retention; gynecomastia and nipple tenderness in males
- **Misc: Neuroleptic malignant syndrome** (hyperthermia, altered consciousness, muscular rigidity, autonomic dysfunction, transient flushing of face and upper body)

Clinically important drug–drug interactions
- Increased rate of absorption of alcohol
- Reduced bioavailability of cimetidine related to faster gastric transit time
- Decreased absorption of digoxin from the stomach
- Increased toxic and immunosuppressive effects of cyclosporine
- Increased bioavailability of levodopa and decreased effects of metoclopramide
- Increased marked hypertension with MAO inhibitors
- Increased neuromuscular blocking effects of succinylcholine
- Antagonized by anticholinergics and narcotic analgesics
- Increased gastric emptying could affect absorption of other drugs

● NURSING CONSIDERATIONS
Assessment
- *History:* Metoclopramide allergy, GI hemorrhage, mechanical obstruction or perforation, when stimulation of GI motility might be dangerous, pheochromocytoma, epilepsy, use of other drugs, depression, Parkinson's disease, age, renal or hepatic function impairment, hypertension, diabetes, breast cancer
- *Physical:* T, P, R, BP, I & O, ECG, weight, neurologic checks, mental status, skin assessment, adventitious lung sounds, abdominal assessment, presence of nausea/vomiting, hydration and nutritional status, edema, bowel sounds, renal and liver function tests, CBC, KUB, serum glucose

Adverse effects in *Italics* are most common; those in **Bold** are life-threatening

Implementation

- Monitor BP carefully during IV administration.
- Monitor for extrapyramidal reactions; notify provider if these occur.
- Have emergency equipment (defibrillator, drugs, oxygen, intubation equipment) on standby in case an allergic or adverse reaction occurs.
- Initiate fall precautions; assist patient if he or she is out of bed.
- With gastric stasis, insulin may act before food has left the stomach, leading to hypoglycemia; adjust insulin dose or timing as indicated.
- Keep phentolamine on standby in case of hypertensive crisis (most likely to occur with undiagnosed pheochromocytoma).
- Store solution at room temperature; protect from light during storage; diluted solution is stable for 48 h if protected from light; 24 h if not protected from light.

⬤ **metoprolol tartrate** *(me toe' proe lole)*
Apo-Metoprolol (CAN), Betaloc (CAN), Lopresor (CAN), Lopressor, Novo-Metoprol (CAN), Nu-Metop (CAN), Toprol XL

Pregnancy Category C

Drug classes
Beta-adrenergic blocker (β_1 selective)
Antihypertensive

Indications
- Treatment of angina due to coronary atherosclerosis
- Treatment of hypertension with or without other antihypertensive agents
- Treatment of hemodynamically stable patients with AMI
- Unlabeled uses: ventricular dysrhythmias/tachycardias, atrial dysrhythmias, essential tremors, aggressive behavior, antipsychotic-induced akathisia, enhanced cognitive performance, CHF

Therapeutic actions
- Acts on β_1 (myocardial) receptors to decrease influence of sympathetic nervous system on the heart, excitability of the heart, myocardial contractility, cardiac workload, oxygen consumption, BP, and release of renin
- Acts in CNS to reduce sympathetic outflow and vasoconstrictor tone
- Inhibits β_2 receptors at higher doses

M

Effects on hemodynamic parameters
▶ Decreased BP
▶ Decreased CO
▶ Decreased HR
▶ Decreased or unchanged CVP

Contraindications/cautions
▶ **Contraindications:** beta-blocker allergy, sinus bradycardia (HR < 45 beats/min), second- or third-degree heart block, PRI > 0.24 sec, systolic BP < 100 mmHg, cardiogenic shock, CHF unless secondary to a tachydysrhythmia treatable with beta-blockers
▶ **Cautions:** peripheral or mesenteric vascular disease, chronic bronchitis, emphysema, bronchospastic diseases, diabetes, hepatic or renal dysfunction, thyrotoxicosis, muscle weakness

Available forms
▶ *Injection:* 1 mg/mL
▶ *Tablets:* 50, 100 mg
▶ *Extended release tablets:* 50, 100, 200 mg

IV facts
Preparation
▶ May be given undiluted.

Dosage
▶ Initiate drug as soon as possible after diagnosis.
▶ Give 3 IV bolus doses of 5 mg each at 2-min intervals.
▶ See below for conversion to oral dosing.

Compatibility
Metoprolol may be given through the same IV line as alteplase, meperidine, morphine.

Oral dosage
▶ *HTN:* Initially 100 mg/d PO in single or divided doses; gradually increase dosage at weekly intervals. Usual maintenance dose is 100–450 mg/d.
▶ *Angina pectoris:* Initially 100 mg/d PO in 2 divided doses; gradually increase dosage at weekly intervals. Usual maintenance dose is 100–400 mg/d.
▶ *AMI:* If patient tolerates the IV 15-mg dose, give 50 mg PO 15 min after last IV dose and q6h for 48 h. Thereafter, give a maintenance dose of 100 mg PO bid. Reduce initial PO doses to 25–50 mg q6h or discontinue in patients who do not tolerate the IV doses.

Adverse effects in *Italics* are most common; those in **Bold** are life-threatening

- *AMI, late treatment:* 100 mg PO bid as soon as possible after infarct. Continue at least 3 mo and possibly for 1–3 y.
- *Extended-release HTN:* 50–100 mg/d PO in a single dose. Increase dosage weekly until optimum BP reduction is achieved.
- *Extended-release angina:* 100 mg/d PO as a single dose. Increase dosage weekly until optimum BP reduction is achieved. If treatment is discontinued, reduce dosage gradually over 1–2 wk.

> **TREATMENT OF OVERDOSE/ANTIDOTE**
> Discontinue drug or decrease dosage. Initiate general supportive and resuscitative measures. Initiate gastric lavage or induce emesis to remove drug after oral ingestion. Place patient in supine position with legs elevated. Treat symptomatic bradycardia with atropine, isoproterenol, and/or a pacemaker; cardiac failure with a digitalis glycoside, a diuretic, and/or aminophylline; hypotension with vasopressors, such as dopamine, dobutamine, norepinephrine; hypoglycemia with IV glucose; PVCs with lidocaine or phenytoin; seizures with diazepam; bronchospasm with a β_2-stimulating agent or theophylline derivative. Give glucagon (5–10 mg IV over 30 sec, followed by infusion of 5 mg/h) for severe beta-blocker overdose.

Pharmacokinetics

Route	Onset	Peak	Duration
IV	Immediate	20 min	5–8 h
Oral	Within 1 h		up to 12 h

Metabolism: Hepatic; $T_{1/2}$: 3–7 h
Excretion: Metabolites in urine

Adverse effects

- **CNS:** *Tiredness, dizziness, depression,* mental confusion, headache, nightmares, insomnia, visual disturbances
- **CV: Second- or third-degree heart block, heart failure,** bradycardia, arterial insufficiency, cold extremities, Raynaud's syndrome, CHF, edema, hypotension
- **Resp: Bronchospasm, dyspnea,** wheezing
- **GI:** *Diarrhea,* nausea, dry mouth, gastric pain, constipation, flatulence, heartburn, elevated liver enzymes
- **Allergic: Laryngospasm,** respiratory distress, pruritus, rash, psoriasis, aching, sore throat, fever
- **Hematologic: Agranulocytosis,** nonthrombocytopenic purpura, thrombocytopenic purpura
- **Misc:** Hyperglycemia or hypoglycemia

Adverse effects in *Italics* are most common; those in **Bold** are life-threatening

M

Clinically important drug–drug interactions
‣ Increased marked hypotension and bradycardia with calcium channel-blockers, quinidine, digitalis, oral contraceptives, prazosin, catecholamine-depleting drugs, such as reserpine
‣ Reduced clearance of lidocaine, increasing risk of toxicity
‣ Life-threatening HTN when clonidine is discontinued for patients on beta-blocker therapy or when both drugs discontinued simultaneously
‣ May potentiate, counteract, or have no effect on nondepolarizing muscle relaxants
‣ Increased blood levels with cimetidine
‣ Enhanced effects of either metoprolol and hydralazine or metoprolol and flecainide
‣ Decreased effects with thyroid hormones, nonsteroidal antiinflammatory drugs, rifampin
‣ Increased bradycardia with MAO inhibitors
‣ Hypertension followed by severe bradycardia with epinephrine

◯ NURSING CONSIDERATIONS

Assessment
‣ *History:* Beta-blocker allergy, cardiogenic shock, CHF unless secondary to a tachydysrhythmia treatable with beta-blockers, peripheral or mesenteric vascular disease, chronic bronchitis, emphysema, bronchospastic diseases, diabetes, hepatic or renal dysfunction, thyrotoxicosis, muscle weakness
‣ *Physical:* P, BP, R, ECG, I & O, SpO_2, weight, neurologic checks, vision, cardiac auscultation, JVD, edema, skin condition, adventitious lung sounds, bowel sounds, serum electrolytes, UA, serum glucose, CBC; thyroid, liver, and renal function tests

Implementation
‣ Exercise extreme caution when calculating and preparing doses. Metoprolol is a very potent drug; small dosage errors can cause serious adverse effects.
‣ Carefully monitor P, BP, R, and ECG during IV administration.
‣ Have emergency equipment (defibrillator, drugs, oxygen, intubation equipment) on standby in case anaphylaxis or adverse reaction occurs.
‣ Assess for early evidence of heart failure as evidenced by increased weight, neck vein distention, oliguria, peripheral edema, crackles over lung fields, dyspnea, decreased SpO_2, cough, decreased activity tolerance, increased respiratory

Adverse effects in *Italics* are most common; those in **Bold** are life-threatening

distress when lying flat, S₃ heart sound, tachycardia, hepatomegaly, confusion.

- Patients with history of severe anaphylactic reactions may be more reactive on reexposure to the allergen and may be unresponsive to usual doses of epinephrine.
- Do not discontinue drug abruptly after chronic therapy. Hypersensitivity to catecholamines may have developed, causing exacerbation of angina, MI, and ventricular dysrhythmias. Taper drug gradually over 2 wk with monitoring.
- Consult with physician about withdrawing drug if patient is to undergo surgery (withdrawal is controversial).
- Give oral forms with food to facilitate absorption.

metronidazole *(me troe ni' da zole)*
Apo-Metronidazole (CAN), Flagyl, Metric 21, MetroCream (CAN), MetroGel, Metro I.V., MetroLotion, NidaGel (CAN), Noritate, Novo-Nidazol (CAN), Protostat

Pregnancy Category B

Drug classes
Antibiotic
Amebicide

Indications
- Intra-abdominal infections caused by *Bacteroides* species, *Clostridium* species, *Eubacterium* species, *Peptostreptococcus* species, *Peptococcus* species
- Skin and skin structure infections caused by *Bacteroides* species, *Clostridium* species, *Peptostreptococcus* species, *Peptococcus* species, *Fusobacterium* species
- Gynecologic infections caused by *Bacteroides* species, *Clostridium* species, *Peptostreptococcus* species, *Peptococcus* species
- Bacterial septicemia caused by *Bacteroides* species, *Clostridium* species
- Bone and joint infections caused by *Bacteroides* species, as adjunctive therapy
- CNS infections caused by *Bacteroides* species
- Lower respiratory tract infections caused by *Bacteroides* species
- Endocarditis caused by *Bacteroides* species
- Treatment of amebiasis, trichomoniasis, inflammatory papules, pustules of rosacea, bacterial vaginosis, acne rosacea
- Acute infection with susceptible anaerobic bacteria

Adverse effects in *Italics* are most common; those in **Bold** are life-threatening

M

- Preoperative, intraoperative, and postoperative prophylaxis for patients undergoing colorectal surgery
- Orphan drug use: Grade III and IV anaerobically infected decubitus ulcers; perioral dermatitis
- Unlabeled uses: prophylaxis for patients undergoing gynecologic or abdominal surgery; hepatic encephalopathy, eradication of *Helicobacter pylori*, Crohn's disease, antibiotic-associated pseudomembranous colitis, bacterial vaginosis, giardiasis

Therapeutic actions
- Bactericidal: mode of action not clear; inhibits DNA synthesis in various anaerobic bacteria and protozoa, causing cell death

Contraindications/cautions
- **Contraindications:** hypersensitivity to metronidazole or other nitroimidazole derivatives
- **Cautions:** CNS diseases, hepatic disease, impaired cardiac function, candidiasis (moniliasis), blood dyscrasias, elderly patients

Available forms
- *Powder for injection:* 500 mg
- *Premixed injection:* 500 mg/100 mL
- *Tablets:* 250, 500 mg
- *Extended-release tablets:* 750 mg
- *Capsules:* 375 mg
- *Gel:* 0.75%
- *Cream:* 1%
- *Lotion:* 0.75%

IV facts
Preparation
- If premixed injection is not available, add 4.4 mL of Bacteriostatic 0.9%NS; Bacteriostatic Water for Injection; 0.9%NS; or Sterile Water for Injection to drug vial. Resultant volume is 5 mL with a concentration of 100 mg/mL. Solution will appear clear with a pale yellow to yellow-green color. Add reconstituted drug to D5W; LR; or 0.9%NS. Do not exceed a concentration of 8 mg/mL. Prior to administration, neutralize the IV solution with 5 mEq sodium bicarbonate injection for each 500 mg used. Mix thoroughly. Carbon dioxide gas will be generated and may require venting. Do not refrigerate neutralized solutions.
- Do not use plastic containers in series connections due to risk for air embolism.
- Do not use equipment containing aluminum.

Dosage
- If used with a primary IV fluid system, discontinue the primary solution during infusion.

Adverse effects in *Italics* are most common; those in **Bold** are life-threatening

- *Anaerobic bacterial infection:* **Loading dose:** 15 mg/kg IV infused over 1 h. **Maintenance dose:** Starting 6 h after the loading dose, 7.5 mg/kg IV infused over 1 h q6h for 7–10 d. Do not exceed 4 g/d.
- *Prophylaxis:* 15 mg/kg infused IV over 30–60 min and completed about 1 h before surgery. Then 7.5 mg/kg infused over 30–60 min at 6- and 12-h intervals after initial dose.
- *Hepatic dysfunction:* Reduce dosage; carefully monitor serum drug levels and observe for toxicity.
- *Elderly patients:* Dosage adjustment may be needed; monitor serum drug levels.

Compatibility

Metronidazole may be given through the same IV line as acyclovir, allopurinol, amifostine, amiodarone, cefepime, cyclophosphamide, diltiazem, dopamine, enalaprilat, esmolol, fluconazole, foscarnet, granisetron, heparin, hydromorphone, labetalol, lorazepam, magnesium sulfate, melphalan, meperidine, methylprednisolone, midazolam, morphine, perphenazine, piperacillin-tazobactam, sargramostim, tacrolimus, teniposide, theophylline, thiotepa, vinorelbine.

Incompatibility

Do not administer through the same IV line as aztreonam, filgrastim, meropenem.

Oral/topical/vaginal dosage

- *Anaerobic bacterial infections:* 7.5 mg/kg PO q6h. Do not exceed 4 g/d.
- *Eradication of H. pylori:* 250 mg PO qid in combination with other drugs.
- *Amebiasis:* 750 mg PO tid for 5–10 d.
- *Amebic liver abscess:* 500 or 750 mg PO tid for 5–10 d.
- *Trichomoniasis:* 2 g PO as a single dose or 1 g PO bid for 1 d (1 d treatment) *or* 250 mg PO tid for 7 d.
- *Bacterial vaginosis:* 1 applicatorful intravaginally bid for 5 d. Or 500 mg PO bid for 7 d.
- *Inflammatory papules, pustules of rosacea:* Wash affected area. Then apply and rub gel, lotion, or cream in a thin layer morning and evening to entire affected area.
- *Antibiotic-associated pseudomembranous colitis:* 1–2 g/d PO for 7–10 d.
- *Giardiasis:* 250 mg PO tid for 7 d.

> ### TREATMENT OF OVERDOSE/ANTIDOTE
> Discontinue drug or decrease dosage. Initiate general supportive and resuscitative measures.

Adverse effects in *Italics* are most common; those in **Bold** are life-threatening

Pharmacokinetics

Route	Onset	Peak
IV	Immediate	1–2 h
Oral	Rapid	1–2 h
Topical	Not generally absorbed systemically	

Metabolism: Hepatic; $T_{1/2}$: 8 h
Excretion: Urine, feces

Adverse effects

▸ *CNS:* **Seizures,** *headache, dizziness,* ataxia, vertigo, incoordination, insomnia, peripheral neuropathy, fatigue, syncope, weakness
▸ *CV:* Flattened T wave on ECG
▸ *GI:* **Pseudomembranous colitis,** *unpleasant metallic taste, anorexia, nausea, vomiting, diarrhea,* GI upset, cramps, constipation, stomatitis, furry tongue
▸ *GU:* Dysuria, polyuria, sense of pelvic pressure, incontinence, darkening of the urine
▸ *Derm:* Thrombophlebitis (IV); *redness, burning, dryness, and skin irritation* (topical)
▸ *Allergic:* Urticaria, rash, flushing, nasal congestion, fever; dry mouth, vagina, or vulva
▸ *Misc:* Severe disulfiram-like interaction with alcohol; joint pain, leukopenia, candidiasis, superinfections

Clinically important drug–drug interactions

▸ Decreased effectiveness with barbiturates
▸ Increased serum levels with cimetidine
▸ Prolonged half-life of phenytoin
▸ Lithium toxicity for patients on high lithium doses
▸ Disulfiram-like reaction (flushing, tachycardia, nausea, vomiting) with alcohol
▸ Psychosis with disulfiram
▸ Increased bleeding tendencies with warfarin

⬤ NURSING CONSIDERATIONS

Assessment

▸ *History:* Hypersensitivity to metronidazole or other nitroimidazole derivatives, CNS diseases, hepatic disease, impaired cardiac function, candidiasis (moniliasis), blood dyscrasias, age, alcohol use
▸ *Physical:* T, P, R, BP, IV site, I & O, weight, neurologic checks, skin assessment, abdominal exam, liver palpation, UA, CBC, liver and renal function tests, culture and sensitivity tests of infected area

Adverse effects in *Italics* are most common; those in **Bold** are life-threatening

Implementation
▸ Obtain specimens for culture and sensitivity of infected area before beginning therapy. May begin drug before results are available.
▸ Avoid use unless necessary. Metronidazole is carcinogenic in some rodents.
▸ Administer oral doses with food to decrease GI irritation.
▸ Monitor for occurrence of superinfections; treat as appropriate.
▸ Discontinue drug at any sign of colitis; initiate appropriate supportive treatment.
▸ Reconstituted drug is stable 96 h when stored below 86°F. Use diluted and neutralized IV solutions within 24 h. Store pre-mixed solution at room temperature and protect from light.

◉ **midazolam hydrochloride** (*mid ay' zoe lam*)
Versed

Pregnancy Category D

C-IV controlled substance

Drug classes
Sedative/hypnotic (benzodiazepine)
Amnestic

Indications
▸ Preoperative sedation, anxiolysis, and amnesia (IV and IM)
▸ Sedation, anxiolysis, and amnesia prior to or during short diagnostic, therapeutic, or endoscopic procedures (IV)
▸ Sedation of intubated and mechanically ventilated ICU patients (IV)
▸ Unlabeled uses: treatment of epileptic seizures; alternative for the termination of refractory status epilepticus

Therapeutic actions
▸ Acts at many levels of CNS to produce short-term, generalized CNS depression
▸ Effects dependent on dose administered, route of administration, and use of other drugs
▸ May potentiate GABA, an inhibitory neurotransmitter
▸ Decreases anxiety and promotes sedation, hypnosis, amnesia, and muscle relaxation

Effects on hemodynamic parameters
▸ Decreased MAP
▸ Decreased CO
▸ Decreased SVR
▸ Heart rates < 65/min tend to increase slightly; heart rates > 85/min tend to slow slightly

Adverse effects in *Italics* are most common; those in **Bold** are life-threatening

M

Contraindications/cautions
▶ **Contraindications:** benzodiazepine allergy, acute narrow-angle glaucoma, untreated open-angle glaucoma, shock, coma, acute alcohol intoxication, depressed vital signs
▶ **Cautions:** hypotension; uncompensated acute illness, such as severe fluid and electrolyte imbalances; respiratory depression, higher risk surgical patients, elderly or debilitated patients, COPD, chronic renal failure, CHF; use of other benzodiazepines, alcohol, narcotics, or barbiturates

Available forms
▶ *Injection:* 1, 5 mg/mL

IV/IM facts
Preparation
▶ IV: May be given undiluted or diluted in D5W; D5W/0.9%NS; 0.9%NS. Drug stable in LR for up to 4 h.
▶ IV: Give undiluted.

Dosage and titration
▶ *Conscious sedation for short procedures:* **Healthy adults < 60 y old:** 1–2.5 mg IV over at least 2 min. Wait 2 min to evaluate drug's effect. Administer additional small increments as needed to achieve sedation, waiting 2 min between doses. If narcotic premedication or other CNS depressants are used, patient will require about 30% less midazolam. **Debilitated, chronically ill, or patients > 60 y old:** Give ≤ 1.5 mg IV over ≥ 2 min. Evaluate sedative effect in 2 min. Administer additional 1-mg doses, waiting 2 min between doses. If CNS depressants are used, patient will require about 50% less midazolam than healthy young unpremedicated patients. **Maintenance:** Give by slow titration in increments of 25% of dose used to first reach sedative endpoint.
▶ *Continuous infusion:* **Loading dose:** May give 0.01–0.05 mg/kg (0.5–4 mg for typical adult) IV over several minutes to initiate sedation rapidly. May repeat dose at 10- to 15-min intervals until adequate sedation is achieved. **Maintenance dose:** Usual infusion rate is 0.02–0.1 mg/kg/h (1–7 mg/h). Higher loading or maintenance doses may occasionally be required for some patients. Titrate infusion to desired level of sedation.
▶ *Preoperative sedation anxiolysis and amnesia:* 0.07–0.08 mg/kg IM up to 1 h before surgery. When patient > 60 years old, debilated, chronically ill, or receiving concomitant CNS depressants, reduce and individualize the dosage.

Compatibility
Midazolam may be given through the same IV line as amikacin, amiodarone, atracurium, calcium gluconate, cefazolin, cefmeta-

zole, cefotaxime, cimetidine, ciprofloxacin, clindamycin, digoxin, diltiazem, dopamine, epinephrine, erythromycin, esmolol, etomidate, famotidine, fentanyl, fluconazole, gentamicin, haloperidol, heparin, hydromorphone, insulin (regular), labetalol, lorazepam, methylprednisolone, metronidazole, milrinone, morphine, nicardipine, nitroglycerin, nitroprusside sodium, norepinephrine, pancuronium, piperacillin, potassium chloride, ranitidine, sufentanil, theophylline, tobramycin, vancomycin, vecuronium.

Incompatibility
Do not administer through the same IV line as albumin, amoxicillin, amoxicillin-clavulanate, ampicillin, bumetanide, ceftazidime, cefuroxime, dexamethasone, floxacillin, foscarnet, furosemide, hydrocortisone, imipenem-cilastatin, methotrexate, nafcillin, omeprazole, sodium bicarbonate, thiopental, trimethoprim-sulfamethoxazole.

TREATMENT OF OVERDOSE/ANTIDOTE
Discontinue drug or decrease dosage. Initiate general supportive and resuscitative measures. Maintain a patent airway and support ventilation. Treat hypotension with fluid therapy, repositioning, and vasopressors. Administer flumazenil to reverse sedative effects completely or partially.

Pharmacokinetics

Route	Onset	Peak	Duration
IV	1.5–2.5 min	Rapid	2–6 h

Metabolism: Hepatic; $T_{1/2}$: 1.8–6.4 h
Excretion: Urine

Adverse effects
‣ *CNS: Oversedation, headache, drowsiness,* retrograde amnesia, euphoria, confusion, nervousness, agitation, anxiety, grogginess, restlessness, emergence delirium, dreaming during emergence, insomnia, nightmares, tonic/clonic movements, ataxia, dizziness, dysphoria, slurred speech, paresthesias, dysphonia, blurred vision, nystagmus, pinpoint pupils, visual disturbance, blocked ears, loss of balance, lethargy
‣ *CV:* **Cardiac arrest,** dysrhythmias, vasovagal episode, hypotension
‣ *Resp:* **Respiratory depression, respiratory arrest, apnea, laryngospasm,** *coughing,* bronchospasm, dyspnea, hyperventilation, wheezing, shallow respirations, airway obstruction, tachypnea

Adverse effects in *Italics* are most common; those in **Bold** are life-threatening

M

- ▶ *GI: Hiccoughs, nausea, vomiting,* acid taste, excessive salivation
- ▶ *Derm: Tenderness, pain, induration, phlebitis at IV site, pain during injection,* hives, rash, pruritus, warmth or coldness at injection site
- ▶ *Misc:* Hematoma, yawning, chills, toothache

Clinically important drug–drug interactions
- ▶ Enhanced and prolonged effects with barbiturate anesthetics, tranquilizers, general anesthetics
- ▶ Accentuated hypnotic effects with narcotic analgesics; narcotic premedication depresses ventilatory response to carbon dioxide stimulation
- ▶ Increased hypotension with fentanyl, meperidine
- ▶ Increased effects of propofol
- ▶ Increased and prolonged serum concentration with azole antifungal agents, cimetidine, oral contraceptives, verapamil
- ▶ Decreased sedative effects with theophyllines

● NURSING CONSIDERATIONS

Assessment
- ▶ *History:* Benzodiazepine allergy, acute narrow-angle glaucoma, untreated open-angle glaucoma, shock, coma, acute alcohol intoxication, hypotension, respiratory depression, uncompensated acute illness, high risk for surgery, age, debilitated condition, COPD, chronic renal failure, CHF; benzodiazepine, alcohol, narcotic, or barbiturate use
- ▶ *Physical:* T, P, BP, R, ECG, I & O, SpO_2, IV site, weight, neurologic checks, neurovascular checks, ophthalmic exam, vision, level of sedation, respiratory effort, adventitious lung sounds, pain assessment, renal and liver function studies

Implementation
- ▶ Exercise extreme caution when calculating and preparing doses. Midazolam is a very potent drug; small dosage errors can cause serious adverse effects.
- ▶ Always administer an infusion using an IV infusion pump.
- ▶ Use the smallest dose possible to achieve desired patient response. Perform sedation assessment regularly.
- ▶ Monitor BP, R, and ECG closely during infusion to monitor effectiveness of therapy.
- ▶ Ensure emergency respiratory/cardiac equipment and flumazenil are available to treat respiratory depression or cardiac emergencies.
- ▶ Cautiously administer analgesics as needed for pain.
- ▶ Avoid intra-arterial administration.

Adverse effects in *Italics* are most common; those in **Bold** are life-threatening

396 milrinone lactate ◀

- Half-life is increased in elderly patients and those with CHF, renal or hepatic impairment, or obesity.
- Patients who receive a continuous infusion over an extended period of time may experience withdrawal symptoms if drug is abruptly discontinued.
- Follow federal, state, and institutional policies for dispensing controlled substances.
- Protect from light.

● **milrinone lactate** *(mill' ri none)* Primacor
Pregnancy Category C

Drug classes
Inotropic agent
Vasodilator

Indications
- CHF: short-term IV therapy for patients receiving digoxin and diuretics

Therapeutic actions
- Increases force of ventricular contraction (positive inotropic effect)
- Causes vasodilation by direct relaxant effect on vascular smooth muscle
- Improves diastolic dysfunction through enhanced left ventricular diastolic relaxation

Effects on hemodynamic parameters
- Increased CO
- Decreased PCWP
- Decreased SVR
- Unchanged HR
- Decreased or unchanged CVP
- Decreased BP

Contraindications/cautions
- **Contraindications:** milrinone or bisulfite allergy, severe obstructive aortic or pulmonic valvular disease instead of surgical treatment
- **Cautions:** hypovolemia, hypokalemia, atrial fibrillation or flutter, AMI

Adverse effects in *Italics* are most common; those in **Bold** are life-threatening

M

Available forms
▶ *IV injection:* 1 mg/mL
▶ *Premixed IV infusion:* 200 mcg/mL

IV facts
Preparation
▶ *Loading dose:* May give undiluted.
▶ *Continuous infusion:* Use a premixed solution or dilute as follows: add 20 mg milrinone to 80 mL D5W; 0.45%NS; or 0.9%NS to prepare a solution of 200 mcg/ml; add 20 mg milrinone to 113 mL D5W; 0.45 %NS; or 0.9%NS to prepare a solution of 150 mcg/mL; add 20 mg milrinone to 180 mL D5W; 0.45 %NS; or 0.9%NS to prepare a solution of 100 mcg/mL.

Dosage and titration
▶ *Loading dose:* 50 mcg/kg IV over 10 min.
▶ *Maintenance infusion:* 0.375–0.75 mcg/kg/min IV. Titrate to desired hemodynamic effects. Do not exceed 1.13 mg/kg/d. Duration of therapy depends on patient responsiveness and continues up to 5 d.
▶ *Maintenance infusion for patients with impaired renal function:* Creatinine clearance: 5 (0.2 mcg/kg/min IV), 10 (0.23 mcg/kg/min IV), 20 (0.28 mcg/kg/min IV), 30 (0.33 mcg/kg/min IV), 40 (0.38 mcg/kg/min IV), or 50 (0.43 mcg/kg/min IV).

Titration Guide

milrinone lactate									
add 20 mg to 80 mL									
Body Weight									
lb	88	99	110	121	132	143	154	165	176	187
kg	40	45	50	55	60	65	70	75	80	85
Dose ordered in mcg/kg/min	**Amounts to Infuse in mL/h**									
0.25	3	3	4	4	5	5	5	6	6	6
0.375	5	5	6	6	7	7	8	8	9	10
0.5	6	7	8	8	9	10	11	11	12	13
0.625	8	8	9	10	11	12	13	14	15	16
0.75	9	10	11	12	14	15	16	17	18	19
0.875	11	12	13	14	16	17	18	20	21	22
1.0	12	14	15	17	18	20	21	23	24	26

	Body Weight								
lb	198	209	220	231	242	253	264	275	286
kg	90	95	100	105	110	115	120	125	130
Dose ordered in mcg/kg/min	Amounts to Infuse in mL/h								
0.25	7	7	8	8	8	9	9	9	10
0.375	10	11	11	12	12	13	14	14	15
0.5	14	14	15	16	17	17	18	19	20
0.625	17	18	19	20	21	22	23	23	24
0.75	20	21	23	24	25	26	27	28	29
0.875	24	25	26	28	29	30	32	33	34
1.0	27	29	30	32	33	35	36	38	39

Compatibility

Milrinone may be given through the same IV line as digoxin, diltiazem, dobutamine, dopamine, epinephrine, fentanyl, heparin, hydromorphone, labetalol, lorazepam, midazolam, morphine, nicardipine, nitroglycerin, norepinephrine, propranolol, quinidine, ranitidine, thiopental, vecuronium.

Incompatibility

Do not administer through the same IV line as furosemide or procainamide.

> **TREATMENT OF OVERDOSE/ANTIDOTE**
> Discontinue drug or decrease dosage. Initiate general supportive and resuscitative measures.

Pharmacokinetics

Route	Onset
IV	5–15 min

Metabolism: Hepatic; $T_{1/2}$: 2.3–2.4 h
Excretion: Urine

Adverse effects

▸ *CNS: Headache,* tremor
▸ *CV: **Ventricular dysrhythmias,** hypotension,* SVT, angina, hypertension
▸ *Misc:* **Bronchospasm,** hypokalemia, thrombocytopenia

⬤ NURSING CONSIDERATIONS

Assessment

▸ *History:* Milrinone or bisulfite allergy, severe aortic or pulmonic valvular disease, hypovolemia, AMI

Adverse effects in *Italics* are most common; those in **Bold** are life-threatening

M

▶ *Physical:* T, P, BP, R, SVR, CVP, PCWP, PAP, ECG, I & O, weight, respiratory status, adventitious lung sounds, cardiac auscultation, JVD, edema, hydration status, peripheral pulses, serum electrolytes, platelet count, renal function studies, acid–base balance

Implementation

▶ Exercise extreme caution when calculating and preparing doses. Milrinone is a very potent drug; small dosage errors can cause serious adverse effects.
▶ Always administer an infusion using an IV infusion pump.
▶ Monitor BP, PCWP, CVP, CO, SVR, and ECG closely to monitor effectiveness of therapy.
▶ Administer into large veins of antecubital fossa rather than hand or ankle veins. Use a central line whenever possible.
▶ Correct hypovolemia before administering.
▶ For patients with atrial fibrillation or flutter, consider digitalis treatment prior to starting milrinone to prevent rapid ventricular conduction rates.

● morphine sulfate *(mor' feen)*

Injection: Astramorph PF, Duramorph, Infumorph, RMS
Immediate-release tablets: MSIR
Timed-release: Kadian, MS Contin, M-Eslon (CAN), MS Contin II, Roxanol SR, Oramorph SR
Oral solution: MSIR, OMS Concentrate, Roxanol, Roxanol Rescudose, Roxanol T, Roxanol 100
Rectal suppositories: RMS
Concentrate for microinfusion devices for intraspinal use: Infumorph

Pregnancy Category C

C-II controlled substance

Drug class
Narcotic agonist analgesic

Indications
▶ Relief of moderate to severe acute and chronic pain
▶ Preoperative medication to sedate, allay apprehension, facilitate induction of anesthesia, and reduce anesthetic dosage
▶ Intraspinal use with microinfusion devices for the relief of intractable chronic pain
▶ Dyspnea associated with acute left ventricular failure and pulmonary edema

Adverse effects in *Italics* are most common; those in **Bold** are life-threatening

Therapeutic actions
- Natural opium alkaloid; acts as agonist at specific opioid receptors in the CNS to produce analgesia, euphoria, sedation, and respiratory and physical depression

Contraindications/cautions
- **Contraindications:** hypersensitivity to narcotics, diarrhea caused by poisoning until toxins are eliminated, acute bronchial asthma, upper airway obstruction; epidural and intrathecal routes: infection at injection site, anticoagulant therapy, bleeding diathesis, parenterally administered corticosteroids within previous 2 wk
- **Cautions:** head injury, increased intracranial or intraocular pressure, CNS depression or coma, acute asthma, COPD, cor pulmonale, preexisting respiratory depression, hypoxia, hypercapnia, acute abdominal conditions, CV disease, supraventricular tachycardias, myxedema, convulsive disorders, acute alcoholism, delirium tremens, cerebral arteriosclerosis, ulcerative colitis, fever, kyphoscoliosis, hypothyroidism, Addison's disease, prostatic hypertrophy, urethral stricture, gallbladder disease, recent GI or GU surgery, toxic psychosis, renal or hepatic dysfunction, hypovolemia, elderly or debilitated patients

Available forms
- *Injection:* 0.5, 1, 2, 4, 5, 8, 10, 15, 25, 50 mg/mL
- *Tablets:* 15, 30 mg
- *Soluble tablets:* 10, 15, 30 mg
- *Controlled-release tablets:* 15, 30, 60, 100, 200 mg
- *Capsules:* 15, 30 mg
- *Sustained-release capsules:* 20, 50, 100 mg
- *Solution:* 10 mg/2.5 mL, 10 mg/5 mL, 20 mg/mL, 20 mg/5 mL, 30 mg/1.5 mL, 100 mg/5 mL
- *Suppositories:* 5, 10, 20, 30 mg

IV/SC/IM/Epidural/Intrathecal facts
Preparation
- For IV injection, dilute 2.5–15 mg in 4–5 mL Sterile Water for Injection.
- For IV infusion, add 0.1–1 mg to each mL of D2.5W; D5W; D10W; Dextran 6% in D5W or 0.9%NS; Dextrose-Lactated Ringer's combinations; Dextrose-Ringer's combinations; Dextrose-saline combinations; Fructose 10% in 0.9%NS or water; Invert sugar 5% and 10% in 0.9%NS or water; Ionosol products; LR; 0.45% NS; 0.9%NS; Ringer's injection; or Sodium Lactate (1/6 Molar) Injection.

Adverse effects in *Italics* are most common; those in **Bold** are life-threatening

M

Dosage
- *IV injection:* 2.5–10 mg/70 kg IV over 4–5 min. Individualize dosage and frequency based on patient's pain level and response to therapy.
- *IV infusion:* May give injection dose of up to 15 mg IV. Then begin with 1–10 mg/h IV. Individualize dosage and frequency based on patient's pain level and response to therapy. Doses as high as 150 mg/h have been used.
- *Open-heart surgery:* 0.5–3 mg/kg IV.
- *MI pain:* 8–15 mg IV. For severe pain, give additional smaller doses q3–4h.
- *SC/IM:* 10 mg (range 5–20 mg) IM or SC q4h. Individualize dosage and frequency based on patient's pain level and response to therapy.
- *Epidural:* **Intermittent:** 5 mg in the lumbar region may provide pain relief for up to 24 h. If inadequate pain relief after 1 h, give incremental doses of 1–2 mg at intervals sufficient to assess effectiveness. Avoid > 10 mg/24 h. **Continuous:** 2–4 mg/24 h. Give further doses of 1–2 mg if needed.
- *Intrathecal:* Dosage is usually 1/10 of epidural dosage. 0.2–1 mg may provide pain relief for up to 24 h. Do not inject > 2 mL of the 5 mg/10 mL ampule or > 1 mL of the 1 mg/mL ampule. Use only in the lumbar area. Repeated intrathecal injections are not recommended; use other routes if pain recurs.
- *Elderly/debilitated patients:* Reduce dosage; use with caution to prevent respiratory depression and adverse reactions.

Compatibility
Morphine may be given through the same IV line as allopurinol, amifostine, amikacin, aminophylline, amiodarone, ampicillin, ampicillin-sulbactam, amsacrine, atenolol, atracurium, aztreonam, bumetanide, calcium chloride, cefamandole, cefazolin, cefmetazole, cefoperazone, cefotaxime, cefotetan, cefoxitin, ceftazidime, ceftizoxime, ceftriaxone, cefuroxime, cephalothin, cephapirin, chloramphenicol, cisplatin, cladribine, clindamycin, cyclophosphamide, cytarabine, dexamethasone, digoxin, diltiazem, dobutamine, dopamine, doxorubicin, doxycycline, enalaprilat, epinephrine, erythromycin, esmolol, etomidate, famotidine, fentanyl, filgrastim, fluconazole, fludarabine, foscarnet, gentamicin, granisetron, heparin, hydrocortisone, hydromorphone, IL-2, insulin (regular), kanamycin, labetalol, lidocaine, lorazepam, magnesium, melphalan, meropenem, methotrexate, methyldopa, methylprednisolone, metoclopramide, metoprolol, metronidazole, mezlocillin, midazolam, milrinone, moxalactam, nafcillin, nicardipine, nitroprusside sodium, norepinephrine, ondansetron, oxacillin, oxytocin,

paclitaxel, pancuronium, penicillin G potassium, piperacillin, piperacillin-tazobactam, potassium chloride, propofol, propranolol, ranitidine, sodium bicarbonate, teniposide, ticarcillin, ticarcillin-clavulanate, tobramycin, trimethoprim-sulfamethoxazole, vancomycin, vecuronium, vinorelbine, vitamin B complex with C, warfarin, zidovudine.

Incompatibility
Do not administer through the same IV line as cefepime, gallium, minocycline, sargramostim.

Oral/rectal dosage
‣ *Oral:* **Immediate-release:** 10–30 mg PO q4h or as directed by provider. **Controlled-release:** 30 mg PO q8–12h or as directed by provider. Adjust dosage according to patient's pain and response to therapy.
‣ *Rectal:* 10–20 mg PR q4h or as directed by physician.

TREATMENT OF OVERDOSE/ANTIDOTE
Discontinue drug or decrease dosage. Initiate general supportive and resuscitative measures. Administer the antidote naloxone 0.4–2 mg IV. Repeat at 2- to 3-min intervals if needed to reverse respiratory depression. Gastric lavage or induced emesis may remove oral morphine.

Pharmacokinetics

Route	Onset	Peak	Duration
IV	Immediate	20 min	5–6 h
IM	Rapid	30–60 min	4–6 h
SC	Rapid	50–90 min	4–7 h
Intrathecal/epidural	15–60	30–60 min	3–7 h
Oral	Varies	60 min	5–7 h

Metabolism: Hepatic; $T_{1/2}$: 1.5–2 h
Excretion: Urine, feces

Adverse effects
‣ *CNS:* **Convulsions,** *lightheadedness, dizziness, sedation,* euphoria, dysphoria, delirium, insomnia, agitation, anxiety, fear, hallucinations, disorientation, drowsiness, lethargy, impaired mental and physical performance, coma, mood changes, weakness, headache, tremor, miosis, visual disturbances
‣ *CV:* **Circulatory depression, shock, cardiac arrest,** facial flushing, tachycardia, bradycardia, dysrhythmias, palpitations, chest wall rigidity, hypertension, hypotension, postural hypotension, syncope

Adverse effects in *Italics* are most common; those in **Bold** are life-threatening

M

- **Resp:** **Apnea, respiratory depression, respiratory arrest,** suppressed cough reflex
- **GI:** *Nausea, vomiting,* dry mouth, anorexia, constipation, biliary tract spasm; increased colonic motility in patients with chronic ulcerative colitis
- **GU:** Ureteral spasm, spasm of vesical sphincters, urinary retention or hesitancy, oliguria, antidiuretic effect, reduced libido or potency
- **Derm:** Local tissue irritation and induration (SC injection)
- **Allergic:** **Anaphylaxis, laryngospasm, bronchospasm,** pruritus, urticaria, edema
- **Dependence:** Tolerance, physical and psychological dependence
- **Misc:** *Sweating*

Clinically important drug–drug interactions

- Increased respiratory depression, hypotension, profound sedation or coma with barbiturate anesthetics, alcohol, sedatives, antihistamines, MAO inhibitors, phenothiazines, butyrophenones, TCAs

⬤ NURSING CONSIDERATIONS

Assessment

- *History:* Hypersensitivity to narcotics, diarrhea caused by poisoning until toxins are eliminated, acute bronchial asthma, upper airway obstruction, head injury, increased intracranial or intraocular pressure, CNS depression or coma, acute asthma, COPD, cor pulmonale, preexisting respiratory depression, hypoxia, hypercapnia, acute abdominal conditions, CV disease, supraventricular tachycardias, myxedema, convulsive disorders, acute alcoholism, delirium tremens, cerebral arteriosclerosis, ulcerative colitis, kyphoscoliosis, hypothyroidism, Addison's disease, prostatic hypertrophy, urethral stricture, gallbladder disease, recent GI or GU surgery, toxic psychosis, renal or hepatic dysfunction, hypovolemia, debilitation, age
- *Physical:* T, BP, P, R, ECG, SpO_2, I & O, injection site, weight, neurologic checks, ophthalmic exam, skin assessment, respiratory effort, adventitious lung sounds, pain assessment, orthostatic BP, bowel sounds, hydration status, prostate exam, voiding pattern, ABG, CBC; thyroid, liver, and kidney function tests

Implementation

- Exercise extreme caution when calculating and preparing doses. Morphine is a potent drug; small dosage errors can

cause serious adverse effects. Avoid inadvertent bolus of drug.
▸ Always administer continuous infusion using an IV infusion pump.
▸ Monitor vital signs frequently with IV administration.
▸ Assess for evidence of respiratory depression.
▸ Have emergency equipment (defibrillator, drugs, intubation equipment, oxygen) on standby in case of allergic or adverse reaction.
▸ Correct hypovolemia before administering drug.
▸ Assess pain status frequently; notify physician if patient does not receive adequate pain relief.
▸ Minimize postural hypotension by helping the patient change positions slowly.
▸ Administer parenteral forms when the patient is lying down.
▸ Use caution when giving IM or SC injections to patients with hypotension or in shock; impaired perfusion may delay absorption; with repeated doses, an excessive amount may be absorbed when circulation is restored.
▸ Caution patient not to chew or crush controlled-release preparations.
▸ Reassure patient about addiction liability; most patients who receive opiates for medical reasons do not develop dependence syndromes.
▸ Follow federal, state, and institutional policies for dispensing controlled substances.

N

● **nafcillin sodium** *(naf sill' in)* Nallpen, Unipen
Pregnancy Category B

Drug classes
Antibiotic
Penicillinase-resistant penicillin

Indications
▸ Infections due to penicillinase-producing staphylococci
▸ Initial therapy when penicillin G-resistant staphylococcal infection is suspected
▸ Effective against staphylococcal infections, *Staphylococcus aureus, Streptococcus pneumoniae,* group A beta-hemolytic streptococci, *Streptococcus viridans*

Therapeutic actions
▶ Bactericidal: inhibits cell wall synthesis of sensitive organisms, causing cell death
▶ Most effective during stage of active multiplication

Contraindications
▶ **Contraindications:** allergy to penicillins, cephalosporins, or imipenem

Available forms
▶ *Capsules:* 250 mg
▶ *Powder for injection:* 500 mg; 1, 2, 10 g

IV/IM facts
Preparation
▶ **IV:** Reconstitute by adding 1.7 mL diluent (Bacteriostatic Water for Injection; 0.9%NS; or Sterile Water for Injection) to each 500-mg vial, 3.4 mL diluent to each 1-g vial, or 6.8 mL to each 2-g vial. Shake vigorously to reconstitute. **Direct injection:** Dilute in 15–30 mL 0.9%NS for Injection. **Intermittent infusion:** Dilute in D5W/LR; D5W/0.225%NS; D5W/0.45%NS; D5W/0.9%NS; D5W/1/2Ringer's Injection; D5W/Ringer's Injection; D5W; D10W; D10W/0.9%NS; Ionosol T/D5W; LR; 0.9%NS; Normosol M/D5W; Normosol R; Normosol R/D5W; Ringer's Injection; Sodium Lactate (1/6 Molar) Injection; or Sterile Water for Injection to a final concentration of 2–40 mg/mL. **IM:** Reconstitute with 0.9%NS for Injection or Sterile Water for Injection. See above for diluent amounts.

Dosage
▶ Give by direct IV injection over 5–10 min. Give intermittent infusion over 30–60 min.
▶ Give IM into a large muscle. Aspirate to avoid inadvertent injection into a blood vessel.
▶ *Usual dosage:* 500 mg IV q4h or IM q4–6h.
▶ *Severe infection:* 1 g IV or IM q4h for short-term (24–48 h) therapy only, especially in the elderly. May double this dosage.

Compatibility
Nafcillin may be given through the same IV line as acyclovir, atropine, cyclophosphamide, diazepam, enalaprilat, esmolol, famotidine, fentanyl, fluconazole, foscarnet, hydromorphone, magnesium sulfate, morphine, perphenazine, propofol, theophylline, zidovudine.

Adverse effects in *Italics* are most common; those in **Bold** are life-threatening

Incompatibility

Do not administer through the same IV line as droperidol, fentanyl/droperidol, insulin (regular), labetalol, midazolam, nalbuphine, pentazocine, verapamil.

Oral dosage

▸ *Severe infections:* 1 g PO q4–6h.
▸ *Mild to moderate infections:* 250–500 mg PO q4–6h.

> **TREATMENT OF OVERDOSE/ANTIDOTE**
> Discontinue drug or decrease dosage. Initiate general supportive and resuscitative measures.

Pharmacokinetics

Route	Onset	Peak
IV	Rapid	End of infusion
IM	Rapid	30–60 min
Oral	Varies	1 h

Metabolism: Hepatic; $T_{1/2}$: 1 h
Excretion: Urine, bile

Adverse effects

▸ *CNS:* **Seizures,** lethargy, neuromuscular hyperirritability, hallucinations
▸ *GI:* **Pseudomembranous colitis,** *nausea, vomiting, diarrhea,* glossitis, stomatitis, gastritis, sore mouth, furry tongue, black "hairy" tongue, abdominal pain, bloody diarrhea, enterocolitis, nonspecific hepatitis, anorexia
▸ *GU:* **Renal failure,** impotence, vaginitis, neurogenic bladder, priapism, interstitial nephritis (oliguria, proteinuria, hematuria, hyaline casts, pyuria)
▸ *Derm:* *Pain, phlebitis,* induration, tissue necrosis at injection site; ecchymosis, deep vein thrombosis, hematomas, skin ulcer
▸ *Allergic:* **Anaphylaxis, angioneurotic edema, laryngospasm, bronchospasm, hypotension, vascular collapse, laryngeal edema, Stevens-Johnson syndrome,** dermatitis, vesicular eruptions, erythema multiforme, arthralgia, chills, fever, rash, pain, headache, asthenia
▸ *Hematologic:* **Anemia, thrombocytopenia, leukopenia, granulocytopenia, neutropenia,** decreased Hgb and Hct, bone marrow depression
▸ *Misc:* *Superinfections* (oral and rectal moniliasis, vaginitis); false-positive Coombs' test

Clinically important drug–drug interactions

▸ Increased warfarin resistance
▸ Decreased effectiveness with tetracyclines

Adverse effects in *Italics* are most common; those in **Bold** are life-threatening

N

- Inactivation of parenteral aminoglycosides: amikacin, gentamicin, kanamycin, neomycin, netilmicin, streptomycin, tobramycin
- Increased bleeding with heparin
- Decreased cyclosporine levels
- Prolonged renal excretion with probenecid

⬤ NURSING CONSIDERATIONS

Assessment

- *History:* Allergy to penicillins, cephalosporins, or imipenem
- *Physical:* T, P, R, BP, I & O, IV site, SpO$_2$, neurologic checks, skin assessment, respiratory effort, adventitious lung sounds, edema, bowel sounds, abdominal exam, renal and liver function tests, CBC, culture and sensitivity of infection site, UA

Implementation

- Obtain specimen for culture and sensitivity of infected area before beginning therapy. May begin drug before results are available.
- Have emergency equipment (defibrillator, drugs, oxygen, intubation equipment) on standby in case anaphylaxis or adverse reaction occurs.
- Assess for evidence of anaphylaxis; if suspected, discontinue drug immediately and notify provider.
- Monitor renal, hepatic, and hematopoietic function.
- Initiate seizure precautions for patients at increased risk for seizures.
- Monitor for occurrence of superinfections; treat as appropriate.
- Discontinue drug at any sign of colitis; initiate appropriate supportive treatment.
- Continue therapy for at least 2 d after signs of infection have disappeared, usually 7–10 d.
- Do not give IM injections repeatedly in the same site; atrophy can occur; monitor injection sites.
- Administer oral drug 1 h before or 2 h after meals, with a full glass of water. Do not administer with fruit juices or soft drinks.
- Solution is stable for 24 h at room temperature or 96 h if refrigerated; discard solution after this time.

⬤ **nalbuphine hydrochloride** *(nal' byoo feen)*
   Nubain

Pregnancy Category B

Drug class
Narcotic agonist-antagonist analgesic

Adverse effects in *Italics* are most common; those in **Bold** are life-threatening

Indications
▸ Relief of moderate to severe pain
▸ Preoperative and postoperative analgesia

Therapeutic actions
▸ Acts as an agonist at specific opioid receptors in the CNS to produce analgesia and sedation
▸ Competes with other substances at the mu receptors, which mediate morphine-like supraspinal analgesia, euphoria, and respiratory and physical depression

Contraindications/cautions
▸ **Contraindications:** nalbuphine or sulfite allergy
▸ **Cautions:** emotionally unstable patients, narcotic abuse, head injury, intracranial lesions, increased intracranial pressure, renal or hepatic function impairment, impaired respiration, myocardial infarction with nausea or vomiting, biliary tract surgery, bronchial asthma, COPD, uremia, severe infection, cyanosis, respiratory obstructions

Available forms
▸ *Injection:* 10, 20 mg/mL

IV/IM/SC facts
Preparation
▸ *IV:* Give undiluted or may dilute in D5W/0.9%NS; D10W; or LR.
▸ *IM/SC:* Give undiluted.

Dosage
▸ Individualize dosage.
▸ *Usual dosage:* 10 mg/70 kg IV, IM, or SC q3–6h as needed. Give each 10 mg over 3–5 min.
▸ *Nontolerant individuals:* Maximum single dose of 20 mg IV, IM, or SC. Do not exceed 160/d.
▸ *Patients dependent on narcotics:* These patients may experience withdrawal symptoms when giving nalbuphine. If unduly troublesome, give small increments of morphine IV until relief occurs. If previous analgesic was morphine, meperidine, codeine, or another narcotic with similar duration of activity, give 1/4 the anticipated nalbuphine dose. If no untoward symptoms occur, increase doses at appropriate intervals.
▸ *Renal or hepatic impairment, elderly:* Reduce dosage.

Compatibility
Nalbuphine may be given through the same IV line as amifostine, aztreonam, cefmetazole, cladribine, filgrastim, fludara-

bine, granisetron, melphalan, paclitaxel, propofol, teniposide, thiotepa, vinorelbine.

Incompatibility

Do not administer through the same IV as allopurinol, cefepime, methotrexate, nafcillin, piperacillin-tazobactam, sargramostim, sodium bicarbonate.

> **TREATMENT OF OVERDOSE/ANTIDOTE**
> Discontinue drug or decrease dosage. Initiate general supportive and resuscitative measures. Reverse respiratory depression with naloxone 0.4–2 mg IV.

Pharmacokinetics

Route	Onset	Peak	Duration
IV	2–3 min	30 min	3–6 h
SC/IM	< 15 min	60 min	3–6 h

Metabolism: Hepatic; $T_{1/2}$: 5 h
Excretion: Urine

Adverse effects

- *CNS: Sedation, clamminess, sweating, headache, dizziness, vertigo,* nervousness, restlessness, depression, crying, confusion, faintness, hostility, hallucinations, euphoria, dysphoria, unreality, floating feeling, feeling of heaviness, numbness, tingling, flushing, warmth, blurred vision, speech difficulty
- *CV:* Hypotension, hypertension, bradycardia, tachycardia
- *Resp:* **Respiratory depression, pulmonary edema,** dyspnea, asthma
- *GI: Dry mouth, nausea, vomiting,* cramps, dyspepsia, bitter taste
- *GU:* Urinary urgency
- *Derm:* Itching, burning, urticaria; pain, swelling, redness, and burning at injection site
- *Allergic:* **Anaphylaxis** (shock, respiratory distress or arrest, bradycardia, cardiac arrest, hypotension, laryngeal edema, stridor, bronchospasm, wheezing, edema, rash, pruritus, nausea, vomiting, diaphoresis, weakness, shakiness)
- *Dependence:* Psychological and physical dependence and tolerance

Clinically important drug–drug interactions

- Increased respiratory and CNS depression with other barbiturate anesthetics, narcotic analgesics, tranquilizers, sedatives, hypnotics, CNS depressants, alcohol
- Severe and unpredictable reactions with MAO inhibitors

Adverse effects in *Italics* are most common; those in **Bold** are life-threatening

● NURSING CONSIDERATIONS

Assessment
▸ *History:* Nalbuphine or sulfite allergy, emotional instability, narcotic abuse, head injury, intracranial lesions, increased intracranial pressure, renal or hepatic function impairment, impaired respiration, myocardial infarction with nausea or vomiting, biliary tract surgery, bronchial asthma, COPD, uremia, severe infection, cyanosis, or respiratory obstructions
▸ *Physical:* P, R, BP, I & O, SpO_2, injection site, neurologic checks, vision, skin assessment, adventitious lung sounds, respiratory effort, pain assessment, bowel sounds, liver and kidney function tests

Implementation
▸ Monitor BP, HR, and R closely during IV therapy.
▸ Have emergency equipment (defibrillator, drugs, oxygen, intubation equipment) on standby in case anaphylaxis or adverse reaction occurs.
▸ Assess pain status frequently; notify provider if patient does not receive adequate pain relief.
▸ Assess patient before allowing him or her to ambulate; assist patient as needed to prevent falls.
▸ Drug may produce drug dependence and has the potential for being abused. Psychic dependence, physical dependence, and tolerance may develop with repeated administration.
▸ Reassure patient about drug dependence; most patients who receive opiates for medical reasons do not develop dependence syndromes.

● **nalmefene hydrochloride** *(nal' me feen)*
Revex

Pregnancy Category B

Drug classes
Narcotic antagonist
Antidote

Indications
▸ Complete or partial reversal of opioid drug effects, including respiratory depression, induced by either natural or synthetic opioids
▸ Management of known or suspected opioid overdose

Therapeutic actions
▸ Pure opiate antagonist with no agonist properties
▸ Prevents or reverses effects of opioids, including respiratory depression, sedation, and hypotension
▸ In absence of opioid agonists, nalmefene has essentially no pharmacologic activity

Adverse effects in *Italics* are most common; those in **Bold** are life-threatening

N

Contraindications/cautions
▸ **Contraindications:** nalmefene allergy
▸ **Cautions:** narcotic addiction, cardiac disease, renal or hepatic function impairment

Available forms
▸ *Injection:* 100 mcg/mL, 1 mg/mL

IV/IM/SC facts
Preparation
▸ No further preparation is required.
▸ Ensure that correct concentration is used for indication: blue label, postoperative reversal; green label, overdose.

Dosage
▸ IV administration produces the quickest effect and is recommended in emergency situations.
▸ Titrate nalmefene to reverse undesired opioid effects. Once adequate reversal is achieved, additional administration is not required and may actually be harmful.
▸ *Known or suspected opioid overdose:* Use 1 mg/mL dosage strength (green label). Give 0.5 mg/70 kg IV. If needed, may give second dose of 1 mg/70 kg IV 2–5 min later. If total dose of 1.5 mg/kg produces no clinical effects, additional nalmefene is unlikely to be effective.
▸ *Suspected opioid dependency:* Challenge dose of 0.1 mg/70 kg IV. If no evidence of withdrawal in 2 min, proceed as above.
▸ *Reversal of postoperative opioid depression:* Use 100 mcg/mL strength IV (blue label). Refer to table below for initial doses. 0.25 mcg/kg IV followed by 0.25 mcg/kg incremental doses at 2–5 min intervals until reaching desired reversal; then stop administration. Cumulative doses > 1 mcg/kg do not provide additional therapeutic effects.

Nalmefene Dosage for Reversal of Postoperative Opioid Depression	
Body Weight (kg)	**Amount of Nalmefene 100 mcg/mL Solution (mL)**
50	0.125
60	0.15
70	0.175
80	0.2
90	0.225
100	0.25

Adverse effects in *Italics* are most common; those in **Bold** are life-threatening

- *Loss of IV access:* Give single dose of 1 mg IM or SC. Should be effective within 5–15 min.
- *Patients with renal failure:* Slowly administer incremental doses over 60 s to minimize hypertension and dizziness.
- *Patients with CV risk:* Dilute nalmefene 1:1 with saline or sterile water and use smaller initial and incremental doses of 0.1 mcg/kg.

Compatibility
Information not available. Do not mix or administer with other drugs.

> **TREATMENT OF OVERDOSE/ANTIDOTE**
> Discontinue drug or decrease dosage. Initiate general supportive and resuscitative measures.

Pharmacokinetics

Route	Onset	Peak	Duration
IV	Immediate	5–15 min	Varies
SC/IM	5–15 min	1–3 h	Varies

Metabolism: Hepatic; $T_{1/2}$: 10.8 h
Excretion: Urine

Adverse effects
- ***CNS:*** *Dizziness,* headache, somnolence, depression, agitation, nervousness, tremor, confusion, withdrawal syndrome
- ***CV:*** *Tachycardia, hypertension,* hypotension, bradycardia, dysrhythmias, vasodilation
- ***GI:*** *Nausea, vomiting,* diarrhea, dry mouth, transient increases in AST
- ***Misc:*** *Return of pain, fever,* pharyngitis, pruritus, urinary retention, chills

Clinically important drug–drug interactions
- Use with flumazenil induced seizures in animals

● NURSING CONSIDERATIONS

Assessment
- *History:* Nalmefene allergy, narcotic addiction, cardiac disease, renal or hepatic function impairment, opioid drug use
- *Physical:* P, BP, R, ECG, neurologic checks, skin assessment, edema, adventitious lung sounds, respiratory effort, pain assessment, renal and liver function tests

Implementation
- Nalmefene is not the primary treatment for ventilatory failure. First establish a patent airway, provide ventilatory assistance,

Adverse effects in *Italics* are most common; those in **Bold** are life-threatening

administer oxygen, establish circulatory access, and initiate
cardiac massage.
‣ Carefully monitor P, BP, R, and ECG.
‣ Duration of action is as long as most opioid analgesics; however,
respiratory depression may recur. Continuously monitor patient.
‣ Have emergency equipment (defibrillator, drugs, oxygen, intubation equipment) nearby.
‣ Assess for pain because drug reverses analgesia.
‣ The effects of the drug may last for several days because of
its long half-life.
‣ May cause acute withdrawal symptoms, such as hypertension, tachycardia, and excessive mortality in patients at high
risk for CV complications.
‣ If drug spills on skin or clothing, rinse skin thoroughly with
cool water and remove clothing.

⬤ naloxone hydrochloride *(nal ox' one)* Narcan
Pregnancy Category B

Drug classes
Narcotic antagonist
Antidote

Indications
‣ Complete or partial reversal of the effects of opioids, including respiratory depression induced by opioids, including natural and synthetic narcotics, propoxyphene, methadone, nalbuphine, butorphanol, pentazocine
‣ Diagnosis of suspected acute opioid overdose
‣ Unlabeled uses: improvement of circulation in refractory
shock; Alzheimer-type dementia; schizophrenia; reversal of
alcoholic coma

Therapeutic actions
‣ Pure narcotic antagonist with no agonist properties
‣ Likely competes for same receptor sites as opioids and reverses the respiratory depression, sedation, and hypotension
effects of opioids
‣ Can reverse psychotomimetic and dysphoric effects of ago-
nist-antagonists, such as pentazocine
‣ In absence of narcotics, naloxone has essentially no pharmacologic activity

Contraindications/cautions
‣ **Contraindications:** naloxone allergy
‣ **Cautions:** narcotic addiction, cardiac disease, use of
cardiotoxic drugs

Adverse effects in *Italics* are most common; those in **Bold** are life-threatening

Available forms
▸ *Injection:* 0.4, 1 mg/mL

IV/IM/SC facts
Preparation
▸ *IV bolus:* Give undiluted.
▸ *IV infusion:* Dilute 1 mg in 250 mL D5W or 0.9%NS.

Dosage
▸ IV administration produces the quickest effect and is recommended in emergency situations.
▸ *Known or suspected narcotic overdose:* 0.4–2 mg IV. May repeat IV at 2- to 3-min intervals. If no response after 10 mg, question the diagnosis. May give IM or SC if IV route not available.
▸ *Postoperative narcotic depression:* Titrate dose to patient's response. **Initial dose:** 0.1–0.2 mg IV at 2- to 3-min intervals until reaching desired degree of reversal. **Repeat dose:** May repeat at 1- to 2-h intervals as needed. Supplemental IM doses may have a longer effect.
▸ *Infusion:* Titrate to patient's response. **Narcotic overdose:** 0.4 mg IV followed by an infusion of 0.4 mg/h. **Postoperative opioid depression:** 3.7 mcg/kg/h.

Compatibility
Naloxone may be given through the same IV line as propofol.

Incompatibility
Do not mix naloxone with preparations containing bisulfite, metabisulfite, long-chain or high molecular weight anions, or any alkaline solution.

Pharmacokinetics

Route	Onset	Duration
IV	2 min	45 min
SC/IM	3–5 min	45–60 min

Metabolism: Hepatic; $T_{1/2}$: 30–81 min
Excretion: Urine

Adverse effects
▸ *CNS:* **Seizures,** dizziness, headache
▸ *CV:* **Ventricular tachycardia, ventricular fibrillation,** hypotension, hypertension, pulmonary edema
▸ **Acute narcotic abstinence syndrome:** Reversal of narcotic depression (nausea, vomiting, sweating, tachycardia, hypertension, tremulousness)
▸ *Misc: Return of pain*

Adverse effects in *Italics* are most common; those in **Bold** are life-threatening

● NURSING CONSIDERATIONS

Assessment

▶ *History:* Naloxone allergy, narcotic addiction, cardiac disease, use of cardiotoxic drugs, opioid drug use
▶ *Physical:* P, BP, R, ECG, SpO$_2$, neurologic checks, level of sedation, skin assessment, respiratory effort, adventitious lung sounds, pain assessment

Implementation

▶ Maintain a patent airway and provide artificial ventilation, cardiac massage, and vasopressor therapy when needed to counteract an acute narcotic overdose.
▶ Carefully monitor P, BP, R, and ECG.
▶ Continuously monitor patient because some narcotics have a longer duration of action than naloxone. May need to repeat naloxone dose.
▶ Have emergency equipment (defibrillator, drugs, oxygen, intubation equipment) nearby.
▶ Assess for pain because drug reverses analgesia.
▶ Rapid reversal of postoperative narcotic depression may cause nausea, vomiting, sweating, or circulatory stress.
▶ Use infusion within 24 h.

● **neostigmine methylsulfate**

*(nee oh **stig'** meen)* Prostigmin

Pregnancy Category C

Drug classes

Cholinesterase inhibitor
Antidote
Parasympathomimetic
Urinary tract agent
Antimyasthenic agent

Indications

▶ Symptomatic control of myasthenia gravis
▶ Reversal of nondepolarizing muscle relaxants
▶ Prevention and treatment of postoperative distention and urinary retention after mechanical obstruction is ruled out

Therapeutic actions

▶ Facilitates transmission of impulses across the myoneural junction by inhibiting the destruction of acetylcholine by cholinesterase

▸ Has direct cholinomimetic effect on skeletal muscle and possibly on autonomic ganglion cells and neurons of the central nervous system

Contraindications/cautions
▸ **Contraindications:** anticholinesterase allergy, mechanical intestinal or urinary obstructions, peritonitis, history of reaction to bromides
▸ **Cautions:** bronchial asthma, epilepsy, bradycardia, recent coronary occlusion, vagotonia, hyperthyroidism, dysrhythmias, peptic ulcer

Available forms
▸ *Injection:* 0.25, 0.5, 1 mg/mL
▸ *Tablets:* 15 mg

IV/IM/SC facts
Preparation
▸ Give undiluted.

Dosage
▸ *Antidote for nondepolarizing neuromuscular blocking agents:* Give atropine 0.6–1.2 mg IV several minutes before neostigmine. 0.5–2 mg (1–4 mL of 1:2000 solution) by slow IV injection; repeat as needed. Rarely should total dose exceed 5 mg.
▸ *Symptomatic control of myasthenia gravis:* 0.5 mg (1 mL of 1:2000 solution) SC or IM. Individualize subsequent doses.
▸ *Prevention of postoperative distention and urinary retention:* 0.25 mg (1 mL of 1:4000 solution) SC or IM as soon as possible after operation. Repeat q4–6h for 2–3 d.
▸ *Treatment of postoperative distention:* 0.5 mg (1 mL of 1:2000 solution) SC or IM as needed.
▸ *Treatment of urinary retention:* 0.5 mg (1 mL of 1:2000 solution) SC or IM. If urination does not occur within 1 h, catheterize patient. After patient has voided or bladder emptied, continue the 0.5-mg injections q3h for at least 5 injections.

Compatibility
Neostigmine may be given through the same IV line as heparin, hydrocortisone, potassium chloride, vitamin B complex with C.

Oral dosage
▸ 15–375 mg/d PO. Average dose is 150 mg administered over 24 h.

Adverse effects in *Italics* are most common; those in **Bold** are life-threatening

N

Pharmacokinetics

Route	Onset	Peak	Duration
IV	4–8 min	20–30 min	2–4 h
SC/IM	20–30 min	30 min	2–4 h
PO	45–75 min	1–2 h (varies)	2–4 h

Metabolism: Hepatic, cholinesterases; $T_{1/2}$: 47–60 min (IV), 51–90 min (IM), 42–60 min (PO)
Excretion: Urine

Adverse effects

▶ *CNS:* **Seizures,** *twitch,* dysarthria, dysphonia, dizziness, headache, loss of consciousness, drowsiness, weakness
▶ *CV:* **Cardiac arrest,** dysrhythmias (bradycardia, heart block, nodal rhythm), nonspecific ECG changes, syncope; decreased CO leading to hypotension
▶ *Resp:* **Respiratory arrest; respiratory muscle paralysis, central respiratory paralysis, bronchospasm;** *increased tracheobronchial secretions;* dyspnea, respiratory depression
▶ *GI:* Salivation, nausea, vomiting, flatulence, increased peristalsis, bowel cramps, diarrhea
▶ *GU:* Urinary frequency
▶ *Derm:* Rash, urticaria, diaphoresis, flushing; thrombophlebitis (IV)
▶ *Allergic:* **Anaphylaxis**
▶ *Musc/Skel:* Muscle cramps, spasms, arthralgia

Clinically important drug–drug interactions

▶ Prolongs depolarizing muscle relaxants, such as succinylcholine, decamethonium
▶ Accentuated neuromuscular blockade with antibiotics, such as neomycin, streptomycin, kanamycin
▶ Decreased anticholinesterase effects with corticosteroids; conversely, increased anticholinesterase effects after stopping corticosteroids
▶ Inhibited by magnesium
▶ Local and general anesthetics, antidysrhythmics interfere with neuromuscular transmission and should be used cautiously, if at all, for patients with myasthenia gravis
▶ Additive effects with anticholinesterase muscle stimulants

Adverse effects in *Italics* are most common; those in **Bold** are life-threatening

◉ NURSING CONSIDERATIONS

Assessment

▸ *History:* Anticholinesterase allergy, reaction to bromides, mechanical intestinal or urinary obstructions, peritonitis, bronchial asthma, epilepsy, recent coronary occlusion, vagotonia, hyperthyroidism, dysrhythmias, peptic ulcer
▸ *Physical:* P, BP, R, ECG, I & O, neurologic checks, reflexes, muscle strength, vision, skin assessment, cardiac auscultation, adventitious lung sounds, abdominal percussion, bowel sounds, voiding patterns, serum electrolytes, thyroid function tests, vital capacity

Implementation

▸ Carefully monitor P, BP, R, and ECG.
▸ Have emergency equipment (defibrillator, drugs, oxygen, intubation equipment) on standby in case anaphylaxis or adverse reaction occurs.
▸ When used as an antidote for nondepolarizing neuromuscular blocking agents, keep the patient well ventilated, and maintain a patent airway until complete recovery. Give drug when patient is being hyperventilated and the carbon dioxide level of blood is low. Titrate neostigmine dose using a peripheral nerve stimulator. If patient is bradycardic, use atropine to increase HR to 80/min before giving neostigmine.
▸ Overdosage with anticholinesterase drugs can cause muscle weakness (cholinergic crisis) that is difficult to differentiate from myasthenic weakness. The administration of atropine may mask the parasympathetic effects of anticholinesterase overdose and further confound the diagnosis.
▸ Notify physician if nausea, vomiting, diarrhea, excessive sweating, increased salivation, irregular heartbeat, muscle weakness, severe abdominal pain, or dyspnea occurs.

◉ nicardipine hydrochloride *(nye kar' de peen)*
Cardene, Cardene SR, Cardene IV

Pregnancy Category C

Drug classes
Calcium channel-blocker
Antianginal agent
Antihypertensive

Indications
▸ Short-term treatment of hypertension when oral use is not feasible (IV)

- Chronic stable (effort-associated) angina (immediate-release only)
- Management of essential hypertension alone or with other antihypertensives
- Unlabeled use: treatment of CHF in combination with aminocaproic acid

Therapeutic actions
- Inhibits the movement of calcium ions across cell membranes
- Cardiovascular system effects include depressed myocardial and smooth muscle mechanical contraction, impulse formation, and conduction velocity
- Effective for chronic stable angina because drug dilates peripheral arterioles and reduces afterload, myocardial energy consumption, and oxygen requirements

Effects on hemodynamic parameters
- Increased CO
- Increased HR
- Decreased SVR
- Decreased BP

Contraindications/cautions
- **Contraindications:** nicardipine allergy, advanced aortic stenosis
- **Cautions:** impaired hepatic or renal function, CHF, acute cerebral infarction or hemorrhage

Available forms
- *Injection:* 2.5 mg/mL
- *Capsules:* 20, 30 mg
- *SR capsules:* 30, 45, 60 mg

IV facts
Preparation
- Dilute each 25-mg (10-mL) ampule in 240 mL of D5W/0.45%NS; D5W/0.9%NS; D5W/KCl 40 mEq; D5W; 0.45%NS; or 0.9%NS. Do not mix with LR or sodium bicarbonate.

Dosage
- Individualize dosage based on severity of hypertension and patient's response. Change to oral therapy as soon as possible.
- *Substitute for oral nicardipine:* If oral dose is 20 mg q8h, 0.5 mg/h IV; if oral dose is 30 q8h, 1.2 mg/h IV; if oral dose is 40 mg q8h, 2.2 mg/h IV.
- *Previously untreated patient:* 5 mg/h IV. Increase by 2.5 mg/h q15min, up to a maximum of 15 mg/h, until desired BP is achieved. For more rapid BP reduction, initiate at 5 mg/h IV

Adverse effects in *Italics* are most common; those in **Bold** are life-threatening

and increase by 2.5 mg/h q5min up to maximum of 15 mg/h. Once BP goal is achieved, decrease infusion rate to 3 mg/h. Further adjust dosage as needed.

▸ *Transfer to oral therapy:* If other oral antihypertensive drugs are used, initiate the drug when infusion is discontinued. If oral nicardipine is used, give the first dose 1 h before discontinuing infusion.

Titration Guide

nicardipine hydrochloride

25 mg in 250 mL

mg/h	2.5	3	3.5	4	4.5	5	5.5	6	6.5	7
mL/h	25	30	35	40	45	50	55	60	65	70

mg/h	7.5	8	8.5	9	10	11	12	13	14	15
mL/h	75	80	85	90	100	110	120	130	140	150

Compatibility
Nicardipine may be given through the same IV line as diltiazem, dobutamine, dopamine, epinephrine, fentanyl, hydromorphone, labetalol, lorazepam, midazolam, milrinone, morphine, nitroglycerin, norepinephrine, ranitidine, vecuronium.

Incompatibility
Do not administer through the same line as furosemide, heparin, thiopental.

Oral dosage
▸ *Angina:* Use immediate-release form only. Individualize dosage. Usual initial dose is 20 mg PO tid. Range is 20–40 mg PO tid. Allow at least 3 d before increasing dosage to ensure steady-state plasma levels.
▸ *Hypertension:* **Immediate release:** Initial dose is 20 mg PO tid. Range is 20–40 mg tid. Take BP 1–2 h after dose to assess drug's peak effect; take BP 8 h after dose to assess adequacy of response. Adjust dosage based on BP response, allow at least 3 d before increasing dosage. **Sustained release:** Initial dose is 30 mg PO bid. Range is 30–60 mg bid. Take BP 2–4 h after dose and at end of dosing interval.
▸ *Renal impairment:* Titrate dose beginning with 20 mg PO tid (immediate release) or 30 mg PO bid (sustained release).
▸ *Hepatic impairment:* Titrate dose beginning with 20 mg PO bid (immediate release).

Adverse effects in *Italics* are most common; those in **Bold** are life-threatening

TREATMENT OF OVERDOSE/ANTIDOTE
Discontinue drug or decrease dosage. Initiate general supportive and resuscitative measures. Evacuate gastric contents with oral overdosage. To treat hypotension, elevate the extremities and infuse pressor agents and fluids. IV calcium gluconate may reverse calcium entry blockade.

Pharmacokinetics

Route	Onset	Peak
IV	Minutes	45 min
Oral	20 min	0.5–2 h
Oral SR	20 min	1–4 h

Metabolism: Hepatic; $T_{1/2}$: 8.6 h (oral); 14.4 (long-term IV infusion)
Excretion: Urine, feces

Adverse effects

- *CNS: Dizziness, lightheadedness, headache, asthenia,* fatigue, nervousness, psychiatric disturbances, blurred vision, weakness, paresthesia, somnolence, insomnia, abnormal dreams, confusion, tinnitus, malaise, anxiety
- *CV:* **AMI,** *peripheral edema, palpitations, tachycardia, angina,* hypotension, bradycardia, AV block, syncope, abnormal ECG, atypical chest pain, peripheral vascular disease
- *GI: Nausea,* vomiting, dry mouth, thirst, constipation, abdominal cramps, dyspepsia
- *Derm: Flushing,* rash
- *Misc:* Allergic reaction, sore throat, hyperkinesia, infection, shortness of breath, wheezing, joint stiffness/pain

Clinically important drug–drug interactions

- Increased serum levels and toxicity of cyclosporine
- Increased plasma levels with cimetidine
- Increased digoxin levels
- Increased hypotension with antihypertensives, diuretics, nitrates

◉ NURSING CONSIDERATIONS

Assessment

- *History:* Nicardipine allergy, advanced aortic stenosis, impaired hepatic or renal function, CHF, acute cerebral infarction or hemorrhage
- *Physical:* P, R, BP, ECG, I & O, IV site, neurologic checks, skin assessment, orthostatic BP, peripheral edema, peripheral perfusion, heart murmur, chest pain assessment, adventitious lung sounds, liver evaluation, serum electrolytes, liver and renal function tests, UA

Adverse effects in *Italics* are most common; those in **Bold** are life-threatening

Implementation

- Exercise extreme caution when calculating and preparing IV doses. Nicardipine is a very potent drug; small dosage errors can cause serious adverse effects. Always dilute drug before use; avoid inadvertent bolus of drug.
- Always administer IV nicardipine using an IV infusion pump.
- To minimize peripheral venous irritation, change IV infusion site q12h if administered through peripheral vein.
- Monitor patient carefully (BP, cardiac rhythm, and output) while drug is being titrated to therapeutic dose.
- Minimize postural hypotension by helping the patient change positions slowly.
- Monitor BP very carefully with concurrent doses of antihypertensives, diuretics, or nitrates.
- Nicardipine may increase the QTc on the ECG.
- Monitor cardiac rhythm regularly during stabilization of dosage and long-term therapy.
- Nicardipine does not protect against dangers of abrupt beta-blocker withdrawal.
- Use diluted IV solution within 24 h.
- Store ampules at room temperature and protect from light.

⬤ **nifedipine** (nye fed' i peen) Adalat, Adalat CC, Apo-Nifed (CAN), Gen-Nifedipine (CAN), Novo-Nifedin (CAN), Procardia, Procardia XL

Pregnancy Category C

Drug classes
Calcium channel-blocker
Antianginal agent
Antihypertensive

Indications
- Angina pectoris due to coronary artery spasm (Prinzmetal's or variant angina)
- Chronic stable angina (effort-associated angina) without vasospasm
- Treatment of hypertension (sustained release only)
- Unlabeled uses: hypertensive emergencies; prophylaxis of migraine headaches; treatment of primary pulmonary hypertension, asthma, esophageal disorders, biliary and renal colic, cardiomyopathy, CAD, CHF, and Raynaud's syndrome
- Orphan drug use: treatment of interstitial cystitis

Therapeutic actions
- Inhibits the movement of calcium ions across cell membranes
- Cardiovascular system effects include depressed myocardial and smooth muscle mechanical contraction, impulse formation, and conduction velocity
- Dilates the main coronary arteries and arterioles in both normal and ischemic regions and inhibits coronary artery spasm, thus increasing myocardial oxygen delivery
- Effective for chronic stable angina because drug dilates peripheral arterioles and reduces afterload, myocardial energy consumption, and oxygen requirements

Effects on hemodynamic parameters
- Increased HR
- Increased CO
- Decreased SVR
- Decreased BP

Contraindications/cautions
- **Contraindications:** nifedipine allergy, recent AMI (within 1–2 wk), acute coronary syndrome if infarction may be imminent
- **Cautions:** obstructive CAD, aortic stenosis

Available forms
- *Capsules:* 10, 20 mg
- *SR tablets:* 30, 60, 90 mg

Oral dosage
- *Initial dosage:* 10 mg PO tid. Dose may be increased in 10-mg increments over 4–6 h as required to control pain and dysrhythmias due to ischemia. Do not exceed single dose of 30 mg. **Usual maintenance range:** 10–20 mg PO tid. Higher doses (20–30 mg tid–qid) may be required, depending on patient response. Titrate over 7–14 d. Doses > 180 mg/d not recommended.
- *Sustained release:* 30–60 mg/d PO. Titrate over 7–14 d. Adalat CC doses > 90 mg not recommended. Procardia XL doses > 120 mg not recommended.

TREATMENT OF OVERDOSE/ANTIDOTE
Discontinue drug or decrease dosage. Initiate general supportive and resuscitative measures. To treat hypotension, elevate the extremities, administer calcium judiciously, and infuse pressor agents and fluids. Plasmapheresis may be beneficial.

Adverse effects in *Italics* are most common; those in **Bold** are life-threatening

Pharmacokinetics

Route	Onset	Peak
Oral	20 min	30 min
SR	20 min	6 h

Metabolism: Hepatic; $T_{1/2}$: 2–5 h
Excretion: Urine, feces

Adverse effects

▸ *CNS: Dizziness, lightheadedness, nervousness, headache, weakness, giddiness, shakiness,* asthenia, fatigue, sleep disturbances, blurred vision, depression, amnesia, paranoia, psychosis, hallucinations, somnolence, ataxia, migraine
▸ *CV:* **AMI,** *peripheral edema, pulmonary edema, CHF,* angina, hypotension, palpitations, syncope, dysrhythmias
▸ *Resp: Nasal congestion, cough, shortness of breath,* respiratory infection
▸ *GI: Nausea,* diarrhea, constipation, cramps, flatulence, dry mouth, thirst, dysgeusia, hepatic injury, gastroesophageal reflux, melena
▸ *Derm: Rash, flushing, dermatitis, pruritis, urticaria,* hair loss, sweating
▸ *Hematologic:* **Thrombocytopenia, leukopenia,** anemia, hematoma, petechiae, bruising
▸ *Misc:* Fever, chills, muscle cramps, joint stiffness, sexual difficulties, micturition disorder, weight gain, epistaxis, facial and periorbital edema, hypokalemia, gout

Clinically important drug–drug interactions

▸ Increased bioavailability with cimetidine, ranitidine
▸ Increased CHF, severe hypotension, or exacerbation of angina with beta-adrenergic blockers
▸ Increased hypotension, bradycardia, ventricular tachycardia, AV block, pulmonary edema, and decreased quinidine levels with quinidine
▸ Increased PT with coumarin anticoagulants
▸ Increased severe hypotension or increased fluid volume requirements with fentanyl
▸ Increased neuromuscular blockade and hypotension with parenteral magnesium sulfate
▸ Enhanced effects of theophylline

● NURSING CONSIDERATIONS

Assessment

▸ *History:* Nifedipine allergy, recent AMI, acute coronary syndrome if infarction may be imminent, obstructive CAD, aortic stenosis

Adverse effects in *Italics* are most common; those in **Bold** are life-threatening

▶ *Physical:* P, BP, R, I & O, ECG, neurologic checks, skin assessment, peripheral perfusion, chest pain assessment, heart murmur, adventitious lung sounds, activity tolerance, liver evaluation, abdominal assessment, serum electrolytes, liver function tests, CPK, CPK-MB, cardiac troponin, myoglobin

Implementation

▶ Monitor patient carefully (BP, cardiac rhythm, I & O) while drug is being titrated to therapeutic dose.
▶ Minimize postural hypotension by helping the patient change positions slowly.
▶ May give sublingual nitroglycerin to control angina, especially when titrating nifedipine.
▶ Ensure that patients do not chew or divide sustained-release tablets.
▶ Taper dosage of beta-blockers before nifedipine therapy to prevent increased angina.
▶ Abrupt withdrawal of drug may cause increased frequency and duration of chest pain.
▶ Edema of the lower extremities may occur and is usually associated with arterial vasodilation. Diuretics usually treat edema successfully.
▶ Concomitant ingestion of grapefruit juice may increase plasma levels and risk for hypotension.
▶ Protect drug from light and moisture.

⬤ **nimodipine** *(nye moe' di peen)* Nimotop
Pregnancy Category C

Drug class
Calcium channel-blocker

Indications
▶ Improvement of neurologic deficits due to spasm following SAH from ruptured congenital intracranial aneurysms in patients who are in good neurologic condition postictus (Hunt and Hess Grades I–III)
▶ Unlabeled uses: treatment of common and classic migraines and chronic cluster headaches

Therapeutic actions
▶ Inhibits the movement of calcium ions across the cell membrane
▶ Not clear how drug reduces vasospasm

Contraindications/cautions
▶ **Contraindications:** nimodipine allergy
▶ **Cautions:** impaired hepatic function

Adverse effects in *Italics* are most common; those in **Bold** are life-threatening

Available form
▸ *Capsules, liquid:* 30 mg

Oral dosage
▸ Begin therapy within 96 h of the SAH using 60 mg PO q4h for 21 d.
▸ *Hepatic cirrhosis:* 30 mg PO q4h.

> **TREATMENT OF OVERDOSE/ANTIDOTE**
> Discontinue drug or decrease dosage. Initiate general supportive and resuscitative measures. Treat hypotension with norepinephrine or dopamine.

Pharmacokinetics

Route	Onset	Peak
Oral	Unknown	≤1 h

Metabolism: Hepatic; $T_{1/2}$: 1–2 h
Excretion: Urine

Adverse effects
▸ *CNS: Headache,* dizziness, lightheadedness, asthenia, fatigue, neurologic deterioration, rebound vasospasm, depression, amnesia, paranoia, psychosis, hallucinations
▸ *CV: Hypotension,* CHF, peripheral edema, angina, palpitations, hypertension, abnormal ECG, tachycardia
▸ *GI:* **GI hemorrhage,** *diarrhea,* nausea, abdominal cramps, hepatic injury, vomiting, jaundice
▸ *Derm: Rash,* flushing, urticaria, diaphoresis, acne
▸ *Hematologic:* **Thrombocytopenia, DIC,** anemia, hematoma
▸ *Misc:* Wheezing, hyponatremia, muscle cramps/pain/inflammation, deep vein thrombosis

Clinically important drug–drug interactions
▸ Enhanced cardiovascular action of other calcium channel-blockers

● NURSING CONSIDERATIONS

Assessment
▸ *History:* Nimodipine allergy, impaired hepatic function
▸ *Physical:* P, R, BP, ECG, I & O, neurologic checks, skin assessment, peripheral perfusion, adventitious lung sounds, edema, chest pain assessment, abdominal assessment, liver evaluation, liver function tests, CBC, serum electrolytes

Implementation
▸ Closely monitor BP and HR for patients with hepatic cirrhosis.
▸ Administer on an empty stomach.

Adverse effects in *Italics* are most common; those in **Bold** are life-threatening

- Administer PO. If patient is unable to swallow capsule, make a hole in both ends of the capsule with an 18-gauge needle, and extract the contents into a syringe. Empty the contents into the patient's in-situ nasogastric tube, and flush the tube with 30 mL of normal saline.
- Monitor neurologic effects closely to determine progress and patient response.
- Protect capsules from light and freezing.

⬤ **nitroglycerin** *(nye troe gli' ser in)*

⬤ **nitroglycerin, intravenous** Nitro-Bid IV, Tridil

⬤ **nitroglycerin, sublingual** NitroQuick

⬤ **nitroglycerin, sustained release** Nitroglyn, Nitrong, Nitro-Time

⬤ **nitroglycerin, topical** Nitro-Bid, Nitrol

⬤ **nitroglycerin, transdermal** Deponit, Minitran, Nitrek, Nitro-Dur, Nitrodisc, Transderm-Nitro, Nitro-Derm

⬤ **nitroglycerin, translingual** Nitrolingual

⬤ **nitroglycerin, transmucosal** Nitrogard

Pregnancy Category C

Drug classes
Antianginal
Nitrate
Vasodilator

Indications
- Angina unresponsive to recommended doses of organic nitrates or beta-blockers (IV preparations)
- CHF associated with acute MI (IV preparations)
- Acute angina: sublingual, transmucosal, translingual preparations
- Prophylaxis of angina: oral sustained-release, topical, transdermal, translingual, transmucosal preparations
- Unlabeled uses: reduction of cardiac workload in acute MI and in CHF (sublingual, topical); adjunctive treatment of Raynaud's disease and peripheral vascular disorders (topical); treatment of hypertensive crisis (IV)

Adverse effects in *Italics* are most common; those in **Bold** are life-threatening

Therapeutic actions
▸ Relaxes vascular smooth muscle
▸ Dilates both venous and arterial beds; venous effects predominate
▸ Dilates postcapillary vessels, including large veins
▸ Improves blood flow to ischemic myocardium
▸ Decreases myocardial oxygen consumption

Effects on hemodynamic parameters
▸ Decreased SVR
▸ Decreased LVEDP
▸ Decreased BP
▸ Decreased or unchanged CVP
▸ Decreased PCWP
▸ Possible reflex tachycardia
▸ Unchanged, increased, or decreased CO

Contraindications/cautions
▸ **Contraindications:** allergy to nitrates, severe anemia, closed-angle glaucoma, postural hypotension, head trauma, cerebral hemorrhage, hypotension, uncorrected hypovolemia, inadequate cerebral circulation, increased intracranial pressure, constrictive pericarditis, pericardial tamponade (IV), early MI (sublingual), allergy to adhesives (transdermal)
▸ **Cautions:** hepatic or renal disease, low ventricular filling pressure, low PCWP, hypotension, glaucoma

Available forms
▸ *Injection:* 0.5, 5 mg/mL
▸ *Premixed IV infusion:* 25, 50, 100 mg in 250 mL; 50, 200 mg in 500 mL
▸ *Sublingual tablets:* 0.3, 0.4, 0.6 mg
▸ *Translingual spray:* 0.4 mg/spray
▸ *Transmucosal CR tablets:* 1, 2, 3 mg
▸ *SR tablets:* 2.6, 6.5, 9 mg
▸ *SR capsules:* 2.5, 6.5, 9, 13 mg
▸ *Transdermal:* 0.1, 0.2, 0.3, 0.4, 0.6, 0.8 mg/h
▸ *Topical ointment:* 2%

IV facts
Preparation
▸ Use a premixed solution or dilute 50–100 mg nitroglycerin in 250 mL of D5W or 0.9%NS in a glass bottle. Do not exceed concentration of 400 mcg/mL.

Adverse effects in *Italics* are most common; those in **Bold** are life-threatening

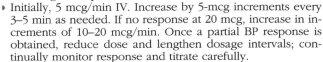

Dosage and titration
▶ Do not give IV push.
▶ Initially, 5 mcg/min IV. Increase by 5-mcg increments every 3–5 min as needed. If no response at 20 mcg, increase in increments of 10–20 mcg/min. Once a partial BP response is obtained, reduce dose and lengthen dosage intervals; continually monitor response and titrate carefully.
▶ When discontinuing the infusion, gradually decrease the dose.

Titration Guide

nitroglycerin

50 mg in 250 mL

mcg/min	3	5	10	20	30	40	50	60	70	80
mL/h	1	2	3	6	9	12	15	18	21	24

mcg/min	90	100	110	120	130	140	150	160	180	200
mL/h	27	30	33	36	39	42	45	48	54	60

Compatibility
Nitroglycerin may be given through the same IV line as amiodarone, amrinone, atracurium, cefmetazole, diltiazem, dobutamine, dopamine, epinephrine, esmolol, famotidine, fentanyl, fluconazole, furosemide, haloperidol, heparin, insulin (regular), labetalol, lidocaine, lorazepam, midazolam, milrinone, morphine, nicardipine, nitroprusside sodium, norepinephrine, pancuronium, propofol, ranitidine, streptokinase, tacrolimus, theophylline, thiopental, vecuronium, warfarin.

Incompatibility
Do not administer through the same IV line as alteplase.

> ### TREATMENT OF OVERDOSE/ANTIDOTE
> Discontinue drug or decrease dosage. Initiate general supportive and resuscitative measures. For ingested nitrates, induce emesis, perform gastric lavage and give activated charcoal. Keep patient warm and recumbent with legs elevated. Passive extremity movement may aid venous return. Monitor methemoglobin levels; treat methemoglobinemia. Treat severe hypotension and reflex tachycardia with IV fluids; consider phenylephrine or methoxamine. Epinephrine is ineffective and contraindicated for hypotension.

Adverse effects in *Italics* are most common; those in **Bold** are life-threatening

Oral/sublingual/topical/transdermal/translingual/transmucosal dosage

▶ *Sublingual:* **Acute attack:** Dissolve 1 tablet under tongue or in buccal pouch at first sign of angina; repeat every 5 min until relief is obtained. Give no more than 3 tablets/15 min. **Prophylaxis:** Use 5–10 min before activities that may precipitate angina.

▶ *Sustained release (oral):* Initially, 2.5–2.6 mg PO tid or qid. Titrate upward by 2.5- or 2.6-mg increments until side effects limit the dose. Doses up to 26 mg qid have been used.

▶ *Topical:* Initially, 1/2-inch q8h. Increase by 1/2 inch with each application to achieve desired results. Usual dose is 1–2 inches q8h; up to 4–5 inches q4h. 1 inch = 15 mg nitroglycerin.

▶ *Transdermal:* Apply one pad each day. Start with 0.2–0.4 mg/h. Titrate to higher doses by using pads that deliver more drug or by applying more than one pad.

▶ *Translingual:* **Acute attack:** At onset of attack, 1–2 metered doses onto or under tongue; use no more than 3 doses/15 min. **Prophylaxis:** Use 5–10 min before activities that may precipitate angina. Spray preparation delivers 0.4 mg/metered dose.

▶ *Transmucosal:* 1 mg q3–5h during waking hours. Place tablet between lip and gum above incisors or between cheek and gum.

▶ When discontinuing nitroglycerin, gradually decrease the dose.

Pharmacokinetics

Route	Onset	Duration
IV	1–2 min	3–5 min
Sublingual	1–3 min	30–60 min
TL spray	2 min	30–60 min
Trans tablet	1–2 min	3–5 min
Oral, SR	20–45 min	3–8 h
Topical ointment	30–60 min	2–12 h
Transdermal	30–60 min	Up to 24 h

Metabolism: Hepatic; $T_{1/2}$: 1–4 min (IV)

Adverse effects

▶ **CNS:** *Headache,* apprehension, restlessness, weakness, vertigo, dizziness, agitation, anxiety, confusion, insomnia, nightmares, malaise

▶ **CV:** **Hypotension, CV collapse,** tachycardia, retrosternal discomfort, palpitations, syncope, postural hypotension, angina, dysrhythmias, edema

▶ **Resp:** Bronchitis, pneumonia, upper respiratory tract infection, wheezing, tracheobronchitis

Adverse effects in *Italics* are most common; those in **Bold** are life-threatening

N

- **GI:** Nausea, vomiting, diarrhea, dyspepsia, incontinence of urine and feces, abdominal pain
- **GU:** Dysuria, impotence, urinary frequency
- **Derm:** Rash, exfoliative dermatitis, cutaneous vasodilation with flushing, pallor, perspiration, cold sweat; contact dermatitis (transdermal preparations); topical allergic reactions (topical nitroglycerin ointment); oral cavity stinging/burning upon dissolution (sublingual preparations)
- **Misc:** **Methemoglobinemia,** alcohol intoxication with large IV doses (alcohol in diluent), arthralgia, muscle twitching, asthenia, blurred vision, diplopia, neck stiffness, rigors, increased appetite

Clinically important drug–drug interactions

- Increased severe hypotension and cardiovascular collapse with alcohol
- Increased serum nitrate concentrations with aspirin
- Increased hypertension and decreased antianginal effect with ergot alkaloids
- Decreased effects of heparin
- Marked symptomatic hypotension with calcium channel-blockers, antihypertensives, beta-blockers, phenothiazines

◉ NURSING CONSIDERATIONS

Assessment

- *History:* Allergy to nitrates, severe anemia, glaucoma, postural hypotension, head trauma, cerebral hemorrhage, hypotension, uncorrected hypovolemia, inadequate cerebral circulation, increased intracranial pressure, constrictive pericarditis, pericardial tamponade, allergy to adhesives, hepatic or renal disease, low ventricular filling pressure, hypotension
- *Physical:* T, BP, R, P, ECG, CO, CVP, SVR, PCWP, I & O, SpO_2, neurologic checks, ophthalmic exam, skin assessment, orthostatic BP, chest pain assessment (type, location, intensity, duration, precipitating events, radiation, quality), hydration status, peripheral perfusion, adventitious lung sounds, liver evaluation, liver and renal function tests, CBC, CPK, CPK-MB, cardiac troponin, myoglobin

Implementation

- Exercise extreme caution when calculating and preparing doses. Nitroglycerin is a very potent drug; small dosage errors can cause serious adverse effects. Always dilute drug before IV use; avoid inadvertent bolus of drug.
- Always administer infusion using an IV pump.
- Monitor patient's response to therapy (vital signs, hemodynamic parameters, ECG, chest pain status).

Adverse effects in *Italics* are most common; those in **Bold** are life-threatening

- Have emergency equipment (defibrillator, drugs, intubation equipment, oxygen) on standby in case adverse reaction occurs.
- Correct hypovolemia before administering drug.
- Minimize postural hypotension by helping the patient change positions slowly.
- The available forms differ in concentration and volume; when switching from one product to another, pay attention to drug, dose, and administration guidelines.
- IV nitroglycerin migrates into many plastics. Use glass bottles and provided administration sets; avoid filters.
- Aspirin or acetaminophen may relieve headaches associated with nitroglycerin therapy.
- Tolerance to vascular and antianginal effects of nitrates may develop. To minimize tolerance, use lowest effective dose, use intermittent dosing, and alternate drug with other coronary vasodilators.
- Give oral nitrates on an empty stomach with water.
- Keep tablets and capsules in original container.
- Give sublingual preparations under the tongue or in the buccal pouch. Encourage patient not to swallow. Ask patient if the tablet "fizzles" or burns. Always check the expiration date on the bottle; store at room temperature, protected from light. Discard unused drug 6 mo after bottle is opened (conventional tablets); stabilized tablets are less subject to loss of potency.
- Give sustained-release preparations with water; tell patient not to chew the tablets or capsules; do not crush these preparations.
- Apply topical ointment in a thin layer on skin using applicator or dose-measuring papers; do not use fingers; do not rub or massage. Cover area with plastic wrap and adhesive tape. Rotate sites of application to decrease the chance of inflammation and sensitization; close tube tightly when finished.
- Administer topical ointment and transdermal systems to skin site free of hair and not subject to much movement. Do not apply to distal extremities or areas with cuts or abrasions. Change sites slightly to decrease local irritation and sensitization. Remove transdermal system before attempting defibrillation or cardioversion; arcing may burn patient.
- Administer transmucosal tablet by placing it between the lip and gum above the incisors or between the cheek and gum. Inform patient not to swallow or chew tablet.
- Administer the translingual spray directly onto the oral mucosa; avoid inhaling preparation.

Adverse effects in *Italics* are most common; those in **Bold** are life-threatening

● **nitroprusside sodium** *(nye troe pruss' ide)*
Nitropress

Pregnancy Category C

Drug classes
Antihypertensive
Vasodilator

Indications
▶ Hypertensive crisis
▶ Acute CHF
▶ Unlabeled uses: AMI with dopamine; left ventricular failure with oxygen, morphine, and a loop diuretic

Therapeutic actions
▶ Acts directly on vascular smooth muscle to cause vasodilation (arterial and venous) and reduce BP

Effects on hemodynamic parameters
▶ Decreased MAP
▶ Decreased or unchanged PCWP
▶ Decreased or unchanged CVP
▶ Decreased SVR
▶ Decreased (slightly) CO
▶ Increased (slightly) HR

> **Contraindications/cautions**
> ▶ **Contraindications:** nitroprusside allergy, compensatory HTN due to aortic coarctation or arteriovenous shunting, congenital optic atrophy, tobacco amblyopia; acute CHF with reduced peripheral vascular resistance, such as high-output failure in endotoxic sepsis
> ▶ **Cautions:** hepatic or renal insufficiency, elderly, high ICP, poor surgical risk patients, hypothyroidism

Available form
▶ *Injection:* 50 mg/vial

IV facts
Preparation
▶ Dissolve contents of a 50-mg vial in 2–3 mL D5W or Sterile Water for Injection. Further dilute in 250–1000 mL D5W.
▶ Promptly wrap container in aluminum foil or other opaque material to protect from light. IV drip chamber and tubing do not need to be covered.

Dosage and titration
▶ Begin infusion at 0.3 mcg/kg/min. Titrate upward every few minutes until desired effect is achieved or maximum recommended infusion rate of 10 mcg/kg/min is reached. Use

Adverse effects in *Italics* are most common; those in **Bold** are life-threatening

smaller doses for patients on antihypertensive drugs. If maximum infusion rate does not reduce BP within 10 min, discontinue drug.

Titration Guide

	nitroprusside sodium									
	50 mg in 250 mL									
	Body Weight									
lb	88	99	110	121	132	143	154	165	176	187
kg	40	45	50	55	60	65	70	75	80	85
Dose ordered in mcg/kg/min	**Amounts to Infuse in mL/h**									
0.1	1	1	2	2	2	2	2	2	2	3
0.3	4	4	5	5	5	6	6	7	7	8
0.5	6	7	8	8	9	10	11	11	12	13
0.7	8	9	11	12	13	14	15	16	17	18
0.9	11	12	14	15	16	18	19	20	22	23
1	12	14	15	17	18	20	21	23	24	26
1.5	18	20	23	25	27	29	32	34	36	38
2	24	27	30	33	36	39	42	45	48	51
2.5	30	34	38	41	45	49	53	56	60	64
3	36	41	45	50	54	59	63	68	72	77
3.5	42	47	53	58	63	68	74	79	84	89
4	48	54	60	66	72	78	84	90	96	102
4.5	54	61	68	74	81	88	95	101	108	115
5	60	68	75	83	90	98	105	113	120	128
5.5	66	74	83	91	99	107	116	124	132	140
6	72	81	90	99	108	117	126	135	144	153
6.5	78	88	98	107	117	127	137	146	156	166
7	84	95	105	116	126	137	147	158	168	179
7.5	90	101	113	124	135	146	158	169	180	191
8	96	108	120	132	144	156	168	180	192	204
8.5	102	115	128	140	153	166	179	191	204	217
9	108	122	135	149	162	176	189	203	216	230
9.5	114	128	143	157	171	185	200	214	228	242
10	120	135	150	165	180	195	210	225	240	255

	Body Weight								
lb	198	209	220	231	242	253	264	275	286
kg	90	95	100	105	110	115	120	125	130
Dose ordered in mcg/kg/min	**Amounts to Infuse in mL/h**								
0.1	3	3	3	3	3	3	4	4	4
0.3	8	9	9	9	10	10	11	11	12
0.5	14	14	15	16	17	17	18	19	20

continued

Adverse effects in *Italics* are most common; those in **Bold** are life-threatening

	nitroprusside sodium *continued*								

50 mg in 250 mL

	Body Weight								
lb	198	209	220	231	242	253	264	275	286
kg	90	95	100	105	110	115	120	125	130

Dose ordered in mcg/kg/min	Amounts to Infuse in mL/h								
0.7	19	20	21	22	23	24	25	26	27
0.9	24	26	27	28	30	31	32	34	35
1	27	29	30	32	33	35	36	38	39
1.5	41	43	45	47	50	52	54	56	59
2	54	57	60	63	66	69	72	75	78
2.5	68	71	75	79	83	86	90	94	98
3	81	86	90	95	99	104	108	113	117
3.5	95	100	105	110	116	121	126	131	137
4	108	114	120	126	132	138	144	150	156
4.5	122	128	135	142	149	155	162	169	176
5	135	143	150	158	165	173	180	188	195
5.5	149	157	165	173	182	190	198	206	215
6	162	171	180	189	198	207	216	225	234
6.5	176	185	195	205	215	224	234	244	254
7	189	200	210	221	231	242	252	263	273
7.5	203	214	225	236	248	259	270	281	293
8	216	228	240	252	264	276	288	300	312
8.5	230	242	255	268	281	293	306	319	332
9	243	257	270	284	297	311	324	338	351
9.5	257	271	285	299	314	328	342	356	371
10	270	285	300	315	330	345	360	375	390

Compatibility

Nitroprusside may be given through the same IV line as amrinone, atracurium, diltiazem, dobutamine, dopamine, enalaprilat, esmolol, famotidine, heparin, indomethacin, insulin (regular), labetalol, lidocaine, midazolam, morphine, nitroglycerin, pancuronium, propofol, tacrolimus, theophylline, vecuronium.

TREATMENT OF OVERDOSE/ANTIDOTE

Discontinue drug or decrease dosage. Initiate general supportive and resuscitative measures. If cyanide toxicity is suspected, discontinue infusion. Do not wait for laboratory confirmation of toxicity. Begin amyl titrate inhalation every 15–30 s until sodium nitrite is prepared. First inject 3%

(treatment continued on next page)

> sodium nitrite (4–6 mg/kg IV over 2–4 min) to convert Hgb
> into methemoglobin. Next inject sodium thiosulfate
> (150–200 mg/kg IV) to convert cyanide into thiocyanate. Af-
> ter 2 h, may repeat the above nitrite-thiosulfate regimen at
> half the original doses. Initiate general supportive and re-
> suscitative measures.

Pharmacokinetics

Route	Onset	Peak	Duration
IV	30–60 s	Rapid	3–5 min

Metabolism: Drug is soluble in blood; cyanide and nitric oxide released; converted to thiocyanate in liver and kidney; $T_{1/2}$: 2 min
Excretion: Thiocyanate eliminated in urine

Adverse effects

▸ *CNS: Headache, apprehension, restlessness, muscle twitching,* dizziness, increased ICP
▸ *CV:* **Hypotension leading to irreversible ischemia or death;** palpitations, bradycardia, ECG changes, tachycardia
▸ *GI: Nausea, vomiting, abdominal pain,* ileus
▸ *Hematologic:* Decreased platelet aggregation, methemoglobinemia
▸ *Endocrine:* Hypothyroidism
▸ *Toxicity:* **Cyanide toxicity (metabolic acidosis, venous hyperoxemia, air hunger, confusion, mental status changes, seizures, pink skin, dysrhythmias, dilated pupils, shallow breathing, death), thiocyanate toxicity**
▸ *Misc:* Venous streaking, skin rash, flushing, irritation at infusion site

Clinically important drug–drug interactions

▸ Increased sensitivity with antihypertensive drugs, ganglionic blocking agents, general anesthetics

● NURSING CONSIDERATIONS

Assessment

▸ *History:* Nitroprusside allergy, compensatory HTN due to aortic coarctation or arteriovenous shunting, congenital optic atrophy, tobacco amblyopia, acute CHF with reduced peripheral vascular resistance, hepatic or renal insufficiency, age, high ICP, surgical risk, hypothyroidism
▸ *Physical:* P, BP, R, ECG, I & O, CVP, PCWP, SVR, CO, SpO_2, IV site, weight, neurologic checks, reflexes, vision, cardiac auscultation, peripheral pulses, peripheral perfusion, hydration status, edema, adventitious lung sounds, abdominal assessment, bowel

Adverse effects in *Italics* are most common; those in **Bold** are life-threatening

sounds, serum electrolytes, acid—base balance, plasma cyanide level, blood thiocyanate level, ABG, serum lactate level, methemoglobin level, UA; liver, thyroid, and renal function tests

Implementation

▸ Exercise extreme caution when calculating and preparing doses. Nitroprusside is a very potent drug; small dosage errors can cause serious adverse effects. Always dilute drug before use; avoid inadvertent bolus of drug.
▸ Always administer using an IV infusion pump.
▸ Carefully monitor P, BP, R, CO, CVP, PCWP, and ECG during administration. Continuous arterial pressure monitoring is preferred. Do not allow BP to drop too rapidly.
▸ Closely monitor injection site for infiltration.
▸ Keep patient supine during drug infusion.
▸ Decrease dose in renal failure.
▸ Keep amyl nitrate inhalation, materials to make 3% sodium nitrite solution, and sodium thiosulfate on standby in case of nitroprusside overdose.
▸ Monitor acid—base balance (metabolic acidosis is an early sign of cyanide toxicity) and serum thiocyanate levels daily during prolonged therapy, especially in patients with renal impairment.
▸ Monitor for rebound hypertension after discontinuing nitroprusside.
▸ Observe solution for color changes. The freshly prepared solution has a faint brown tint; discard it if it is highly colored (blue, green, dark red).
▸ If protected from light, solution is stable for 24 h.

⬤ norepinephrine bitartrate (levarterenol)
(nor ep i nef' rin) Levophed

Pregnancy Category C

Drug classes
Vasopressor
Alpha-adrenergic agonist
Beta-1-selective adrenergic blocker
Cardiac stimulant
Sympathomimetic

Indications
▸ To restore blood pressure in certain hypotensive states (pheochromocytomectomy, sympathectomy, poliomyelitis, spinal anesthesia, AMI, septicemia, blood transfusion, drug reactions)
▸ Adjunct treatment for cardiac arrest and profound hypotension

Adverse effects in *Italics* are most common; those in **Bold** are life-threatening

Therapeutic actions
▸ Powerful arterial and venous vasoconstrictor whose effects are mediated by alpha- or beta-1-adrenergic receptors in target organs
▸ Cardiac stimulant that increases myocardial contraction and increases coronary blood flow

Effects on hemodynamic parameters
▸ Increased MAP
▸ Increased or decreased CO
▸ Increased CVP
▸ Increased SVR
▸ Increased PCWP

Contraindications/cautions
▸ **Contraindications:** norepinephrine or bisulfite allergy, hypovolemia, mesenteric or peripheral vascular thrombosis
▸ **Cautions:** hypoxia, hypercarbia, hypertension, diabetes, elderly patients

Available form
▸ *IV injection:* 1 mg/mL

IV facts
Preparation
▸ For a continuous infusion, add 1–2 mg norepinephrine in 250–500 mL of D5W/0.9%NS or D5W.

Dosage and titration
▸ *Restoration of blood pressure in acute hypotensive states:* Usual dose is 2–4 mcg/min IV. Initially administer 8–12 mcg/min IV. Titrate infusion to maintain a low normal BP (usually 80–100 systolic). Raise the BP no higher than 40 mmHg below the preexisting systolic pressure. Daily doses up to 68 mg may be needed for extreme hypotension.
▸ *Adjunct in cardiac arrest:* Administer IV at 0.5–1 mcg/min to restore and maintain an adequate BP after an effective heartbeat and ventilation have been established.
▸ When discontinuing the infusion, gradually decrease the dose to prevent hypotension.

Titration Guide

norepinephrine bitartrate

2 mg in 250 mL

mcg/min	1	2	3	4	5	6	7	8	9	10
mL/h	8	15	23	30	38	45	53	60	68	75

mcg/min	11	12	14	16	18	20	25	30	35	40
mL/h	83	90	105	120	135	150	188	225	263	300

Adverse effects in *Italics* are most common; those in **Bold** are life-threatening

N

Compatibility

Norepinephrine may be given through the same IV line as amiodarone, amrinone, diltiazem, dobutamine, epinephrine, esmolol, famotidine, fentanyl, furosemide, haloperidol, heparin, hydrocortisone, hydromorphone, labetalol, lorazepam, meropenem, midazolam, milrinone, morphine, nicardipine, nitroglycerin, potassium chloride, propofol, ranitidine, vecuronium, vitamin B complex with C.

Incompatibility

Do not administer through the same IV line as insulin (regular) or thiopental.

> **TREATMENT OF OVERDOSE/ANTIDOTE**
> Discontinue drug or decrease dosage. Initiate general supportive and resuscitative measures, including fluid and electrolyte replacement, as indicated.

Pharmacokinetics

Route	Onset	Peak	Duration
IV	Rapid	Unknown	1–2 min

Metabolism: Sympathetic nerve endings
Excretion: Urine

Adverse effects

▶ *CNS: Headache,* anxiety, tremor, restlessness
▶ *CV: Bradycardia, dysrhythmias,* hypertension
▶ *GU:* Decreased urine output
▶ *Misc:* Ischemic injury due to vasoconstrictor effect and tissue hypoxia; necrosis at injection site, respiratory difficulty

Clinically important drug–drug interactions

▶ Enhanced by bretylium; may cause dysrhythmias
▶ Enhanced pressor response with guanethidine, oxytocic drugs, TCAs, MAO inhibitors

● NURSING CONSIDERATIONS

Assessment

▶ *History:* Norepinephrine or bisulfite allergy, hypovolemia, mesenteric or peripheral vascular thrombosis, hypoxia, hypercarbia, hypertension, diabetes, age
▶ *Physical:* T, P, BP, R, SVR, CVP, PCWP, PAP, CO, ECG, I & O, IV site, neurologic checks, skin assessment, respiratory status, peripheral pulses and perfusion, adventitious lung sounds, acid–base balance, serum electrolytes and glucose

Adverse effects in *Italics* are most common; those in **Bold** are life-threatening

Implementation

▸ Exercise extreme caution when calculating and preparing doses. Norepinephrine is a very potent drug; small dosage errors can cause serious adverse effects.

▸ Always administer an infusion using an IV infusion pump.

▸ Monitor BP every 2 min from start of infusion until desired BP is achieved, then monitor every 5 min if infusion is continued. Adjust dose/rate accordingly. Continuous arterial pressure monitoring is preferred.

▸ Monitor ECG, CO, and SVR closely during infusion.

▸ Correct hypovolemia before administering. Norepinephrine is not a substitute for restoring fluids, plasma, or electrolytes. It should not be used in the presence of blood volume deficits except as an emergency measure to maintain coronary and cerebral perfusion until blood volume replacement is initiated. If administered continuously to maintain BP in the presence of hypovolemia, perfusion of vital organs may be severely compromised and tissue hypoxia may result.

▸ Administer into large veins of antecubital fossa rather than hand or ankle veins. Use a central line whenever possible.

▸ Monitor infusion site closely for evidence of infiltration or phlebitis. If extravasation occurs, prevent sloughing and necrosis by using a fine hypodermic needle to infiltrate area with 5–10 mg phentolamine in 10–15 mL 0.9%NS.

▸ Avoid infusing into femoral or leg veins in elderly patients or those suffering from occlusive vascular disease (atherosclerosis, arteriosclerosis, diabetic endarteritis, Buerger's disease); occlusive disease is more likely to occur in lower extremities.

▸ Avoid catheter tie-in technique, if possible, because stasis around tubing may lead to high local concentrations of drug.

▸ Thrombosis may be reduced if heparin is added to the infusion solution in an amount to supply 100–200 U/h.

▸ Use minimal doses for the shortest time possible.

▸ Do not use if solution is pink or brown or contains a precipitate; solution should be clear and colorless.

⬤ **nystatin** (*nye stat' in*) **Oral, oral suspensions, oral troche:** Candistatin (CAN), Mycostatin, Mycostatin Pastilles, Nadostine (CAN), Nilstat, Nystex, PMS-Nystatin (CAN) **Vaginal preparations:** Mycostatin **Topical application:** Mycostatin, Nadostine (CAN), Nilstat, Nystex, Pedi-Dri

Pregnancy Category A

Drug class
Antifungal

Adverse effects in *Italics* are most common; those in **Bold** are life-threatening

Indications
- Treatment of intestinal candidiasis (oral)
- Treatment of oral candidiasis (oral suspension, troche)
- Local treatment of vaginal candidiasis (moniliasis; vaginal)
- Treatment of cutaneous or mucocutaneous mycotic infections caused by *Candida albicans* and other *Candida* species (topical applications)

Therapeutic actions
- Antifungal antibiotic that is fungistatic and fungicidal against wide variety of yeasts and yeastlike fungi
- Binds to sterols in cell membrane of fungus, which changes membrane permeability, allowing leakage of intracellular components

Contraindications
- **Contraindications:** allergy to nystatin or components used in preparation

Available forms
- *Tablets:* 500,000 U
- *Oral suspension:* 100,000 U/mL
- *Troche:* 200,000 U
- *Vaginal tablets:* 100,000 U
- *Topical cream, ointment, powder:* 100,000 U/g

Oral/vaginal/topical dosage
- *Oral:* 500,000–1,000,000 U PO tid. Continue for at least 48 h after clinical cure.
- *Oral Suspension:* 400,000–600,000 U PO qid (½ of dose in each side of mouth, retaining the drug as long as possible before swallowing).
- *Troche:* Dissolve 1–2 tablets in mouth 4–5 times/d for up to 14 d. Tell patient not to chew or swallow tablet whole.
- *Vaginal preparations:* 1 tablet (100,000 U) intravaginally qd for 2 wk.
- *Topical preparations:* Apply to affected area 2–3 times per d until healing is complete. For fungal infections of the feet, dust powder on feet and in shoes and socks.

TREATMENT OF OVERDOSE/ANTIDOTE
Discontinue drug or decrease dosage. Initiate general supportive and resuscitative measures.

Pharmacokinetics
Not generally absorbed systemically. Excreted unchanged in the feces after oral use.

Adverse effects in *Italics* are most common; those in **Bold** are life-threatening

Adverse effects
Oral Doses
▸ *GI:* Diarrhea, GI distress, nausea, vomiting with large doses

Oral Suspension
▸ *GI:* Nausea, vomiting, diarrhea, GI distress

Vaginal
▸ *Misc:* Irritation, vulvovaginal burning

Topical
▸ *Misc:* Local irritation

⬤ NURSING CONSIDERATIONS

Assessment
▸ *History:* Allergy to nystatin or components used in preparation
▸ *Physical:* Skin color, lesions, area around lesions; bowel sounds, culture of involved area

Implementation
▸ Culture fungus before therapy.
▸ Have patient retain oral suspension in mouth as long as possible before swallowing. Paint suspension on each side of the mouth. Continue local treatment for at least 48 h after clinical improvement is noted.
▸ May prepare nystatin in the form of frozen flavored popsicles to improve oral retention of the drug for local application.
▸ Administer nystatin troche orally for the treatment of oral candidiasis; have patient dissolve 1–2 tablets in mouth.
▸ Insert vaginal suppositories high into the vagina. Have patient remain recumbent for 10–15 min after insertion. Provide sanitary napkin to protect clothing from stains.
▸ Cleanse affected area before topical application, unless otherwise indicated.
▸ Monitor response to drug therapy. If no response is noted, arrange for further cultures to determine causative organism.
▸ Ensure that patient receives the full course of therapy to eradicate the fungus and to prevent recurrence.
▸ Discontinue topical or vaginal administration if rash or sensitivity occurs.

Adverse effects in *Italics* are most common; those in **Bold** are life-threatening

◯ octreotide acetate
(ok trye' oh tide) Sandostatin

Pregnancy Category B

Drug classes
Gastrointestinal hormone
Antidiarrheal

Indications
▸ To reduce blood levels of growth hormone and IGF-I in patients with acromegaly not responsive to other treatment
▸ Symptomatic treatment of severe diarrhea and flushing episodes for patients with metastatic carcinoid tumors
▸ Treatment of profuse watery diarrhea associated with vasoactive intestinal peptide tumors (VIPoma)
▸ Unlabeled uses: to reduce output from GI or pancreatic fistulas, variceal bleeding, other diarrheal states, irritable bowel syndrome, dumping syndrome

Therapeutic actions
▸ Mimics the natural hormone somatostatin
▸ Decreases splanchnic blood flow
▸ Inhibits release of growth hormone, glucagon, insulin, serotonin, gastrin, vasoactive intestinal peptide, secretin, motilin, and pancreatic polypeptide
▸ Inhibits gallbladder contractility and decreases bile secretion

Contraindications/cautions
▸ **Contraindications:** hypersensitivity to any component of octreotide
▸ **Cautions:** renal impairment, elderly, diabetes mellitus, gallbladder disease, thyroid disease, pancreatitis

Available forms
▸ *Injection:* 0.05, 0.1, 0.2, 0.5, 1 mg/mL

IV/SC facts
Preparation
▸ May be given undiluted or diluted in 50–200 mL D5W or 0.9%NS.

Dosage
▸ Give IV injection over 3 min or IV infusion over 15–30 min. In emergency situations, such as carcinoid crisis, may give as a rapid bolus.

Adverse effects in *Italics* are most common; those in **Bold** are life-threatening

- *Acromegaly:* 50 mcg tid IV or SC. Titrate up to 100–500 mcg tid. Withdraw for 4 wk once yearly.
- *Carcinoid tumors:* 100–600 mcg IV or SC qd in 2–4 divided doses for first 2 wk. Mean daily maintenance dose is 450 mcg; dose range is 50–1500 mcg/d.
- *VIPomas:* 200–300 mcg/d IV or SC in 2–4 divided doses for first 2 wk. Dose range is 150–750 mcg.
- *GI fistula:* 50–200 mcg q8h.
- *Variceal bleeding:* 25–50 mcg/h IV for 18 h–5 d.
- *Pancreatic fistulas:* 50–200 mcg q8h.
- *Dumping syndrome:* 50–150 mcg/d.
- *Irritable bowel syndrome:* 100 mcg single dose to 125 mcg SC bid.
- *Elderly or renal impaired patients:* Half-life may be prolonged; adjust dose.

Compatibility

Do not administer through the same IV line as other drugs.

> **TREATMENT OF OVERDOSE/ANTIDOTE**
> Discontinue drug or decrease dosage. Initiate general supportive and resuscitative measures.

Pharmacokinetics

Route	Onset	Peak
IV	Unknown	0.4 h
SC	Rapid	0.4 h

$T_{1/2}$: 1.7 h
Excretion: Urine

Adverse effects

- *CNS:* **Seizures,** *headache, dizziness, fatigue, weakness,* depression, anxiety, syncope, tremor, Bell's palsy, paranoia, increased intraocular pressure, blurred vision
- *CV: Sinus bradycardia, dysrhythmias, and conduction abnormalities in acromegalics;* chest pain; shortness of breath; thrombophlebitis; ischemia; hypertensive reaction; CHF; palpitations; postural hypotension; tachycardia
- *Resp:* Cold symptoms, pneumonia, pulmonary nodule, status asthmaticus
- *GI: Diarrhea, loose stools, nausea, abdominal discomfort, vomiting, flatulence, abnormal stools, abdominal distention, constipation,* hepatitis, jaundice, increase in liver enzymes, GI bleeding, hemorrhoids
- *GU: Pollakiuria, UTI,* nephrolithiasis, hematuria
- *Derm: Injection site pain,* flushing, pruritus, hair loss

Adverse effects in *Italics* are most common; those in **Bold** are life-threatening

▶ *Allergic:* **Anaphylaxis**
▶ *Hematologic: Injection site hematoma, bruise,* anemia, iron deficiency, epistaxis
▶ *Musc/Skel: Backache, joint pain,* arthritis, joint effusion, muscle pain, Raynaud's phenomenon
▶ *Endocrine: Hyperglycemia, hypoglycemia, hypothyroidism,* galactorrhea, hypoadrenalism, diabetes insipidus, gynecomastia, amenorrhea, polymenorrhea, vaginitis
▶ *Misc: Gallbladder abnormalities (stones, biliary sludge),* flu symptoms, edema, fat malabsorption, blurred vision, increased CK

Clinically important drug–drug interactions
▶ Increased bradycardia with beta-blockers
▶ May need to adjust insulin dose related to hypoglycemia or hyperglycemia
▶ Decreased blood levels of cyclosporine, which contributes to transplant rejection

● NURSING CONSIDERATIONS

Assessment
▶ *History:* Hypersensitivity to any component of octreotide, renal impairment, age, diabetes mellitus, gallbladder disease, thyroid disease, pancreatitis
▶ *Physical:* P, BP, R, ECG, I & O, orthostatic BP, neurologic checks, ophthalmic exam, vision, skin assessment, cardiac auscultation, abdominal exam, adventitious lung sounds, presence of bleeding, renal and thyroid function tests, serum glucose, electrolytes, fecal fat and serum carotene determinations, vitamin B_{12} level, growth hormone levels, T_4 level

Implementation
▶ Carefully monitor P, BP, R, and ECG during IV administration.
▶ Have emergency equipment (defibrillator, drugs, oxygen, intubation equipment) on standby in case anaphylaxis or adverse reaction occurs.
▶ Avoid multiple SC injections in the same site within short periods of time.
▶ Monitor patient closely for endocrine reactions: blood glucose alterations, thyroid hormone changes, and growth hormone level.
▶ Monitor serum glucose carefully to detect hypoglycemia or hyperglycemia. Diabetic patients require close monitoring.
▶ Assess frequency and consistency of stools and bowel sounds.
▶ Monitor growth hormone and IGF-I for patients with acromegaly.
▶ Monitor 5-HIAA, plasma serotonin, and plasma substance P for patients with carcinoid tumors.

Adverse effects in *Italics* are most common; those in **Bold** are life-threatening

▸ Monitor VIP for patients with VIPoma.
▸ Perform q72h fecal fat and serum carotene determinations to assess for drug-induced fat malabsorption.
▸ Perform baseline and periodic total or free T_4 measurements during chronic use.
▸ Carefully monitor I & O and weight.
▸ Store ampules in refrigerator and protect from light. Do not warm solution artificially. Open ampules just prior to administration, and discard unused portion.

⬤ omeprazole *(oh me' pray zol)* Losec (CAN), Prilosec
Pregnancy Category C

Drug class
Antisecretory agent

Indications
▸ Short-term treatment of active duodenal ulcer; use with clarithromycin for treatment of active duodenal ulcer associated with *Helicobacter pylori* infection
▸ Short-term treatment of active benign gastric ulcer
▸ Short-term treatment of symptomatic GERD poorly responsive to customary medical treatment
▸ Short-term treatment of erosive esophagitis
▸ Long-term treatment of hypersecretory conditions (Zollinger-Ellison syndrome, multiple endocrine adenomas, systemic mastocytosis)
▸ Unlabeled use: posterior laryngitis, enhanced efficacy of pancreatin (for treatment of steatorrhea in cystic fibrosis)

Therapeutic actions
▸ Suppresses gastric acid secretion by inhibiting the hydrogen/potassium ATPase enzyme system at the secretory surface of the gastric parietal cells, thus blocking the final step in acid production
▸ Effect is dose related and inhibits both basal and stimulated acid secretion regardless of the stimulus
▸ When gastric acid secretion is inhibited, blood flow in the antrum, pylorus, and duodenal bulb decreases
▸ Increases serum pepsinogen levels; decreases pepsin activity
▸ Elevates intragastric pH, which increases nitrate-reducing bacteria and elevates nitrate concentration in gastric juice in patients with gastric ulcer

Contraindications/cautions
▸ **Contraindications:** hypersensitivity to omeprazole or its components
▸ **Cautions:** elderly patients

Adverse effects in *Italics* are most common; those in **Bold** are life-threatening

O

Available forms
▶ *DR capsules:* 10, 20, 40 mg

Oral dosage
▶ *Active duodenal ulcer:* 20 mg/d PO for 4–8 wk. Do not use for maintenance therapy.
▶ *Duodenal ulcer associated with H. pylori:* 40 mg PO q morning plus clarithromycin 500 mg PO tid on days 1–14. Then omeprazole 20 mg/d PO on days 15–28.
▶ *Gastric ulcer:* 40 mg/d PO for 4–8 wk.
▶ *Erosive esophagitis:* 20 mg/d PO for 4–8 wk. Maintenance dose is 20 mg/d PO.
▶ *GERD:* 20 mg/d PO.
▶ *Pathological hypersecretory conditions:* 60 mg/d PO. Doses up to 120 mg tid have been used. Give daily doses > 80 mg in divided doses.

TREATMENT OF OVERDOSE/ANTIDOTE
Discontinue drug or decrease dosage. Initiate general supportive and resuscitative measures.

Pharmacokinetics

Route	Onset	Peak	Duration
Oral	Varies	0.5–3.5 h	≤72 h

Metabolism: Hepatic; $T_{1/2}$: 0.5–1 h
Excretion: Urine, feces

Adverse effects
▶ *CNS:* *Headache,* dizziness, asthenia, vertigo, insomnia, tremors, somnolence, paresthesias, dream abnormalities
▶ *CV:* Tachycardia, bradycardia, peripheral edema
▶ *Resp:* URI symptoms, cough, epistaxis, pharyngeal pain
▶ *GI:* **Pancreatitis, liver necrosis, hepatic failure, hepatic encephalopathy, hepatitis,** *diarrhea, abdominal pain, nausea,* vomiting, constipation, dry mouth, fecal discoloration, flatulence, gastric fundic gland polyps, irritable colon, esophageal candidiasis, mucosal atrophy of tongue, elevated liver enzymes, abdominal swelling
▶ *GU:* Hematuria, glycosuria, gynecomastia, interstitial nephritis, urinary tract infection, microscopic pyuria, urinary frequency, proteinuria, testicular pain
▶ *Derm:* **Stevens-Johnson syndrome, toxic epidermal necrolysis, angioedema,** rash, inflammation, urticaria, pruritus, alopecia, dry skin, erythema multiform, hyperhidrosis

Adverse effects in *Italics* are most common; those in **Bold** are life-threatening

▸ *Hematologic:* **Thrombocytopenia, neutropenia, leuko-cytosis, agranulocytosis, pancytopenia**
▸ *Musc/Skel:* Arthralgia, myalgia, muscle cramps, muscle weakness, leg pain
▸ *Metabolic:* Gout, weight gain, hypoglycemia, hyponatremia
▸ *Misc:* Cancer in preclinical studies, back pain, fever, pain, fatigue

Clinically important drug–drug interactions
▸ Decreased bioavailability with sucralfate
▸ Decreased theophylline clearance
▸ Use with clarithromycin may increase plasma levels of both drugs and 14-hydroxy-clarithromycin
▸ Prolonged elimination of diazepam, flurazepam, triazolam, warfarin, phenytoin, drugs metabolized by oxidation in the liver

● NURSING CONSIDERATIONS

Assessment
▸ *History:* Hypersensitivity to omeprazole or its components, elderly patients
▸ *Physical:* T, P, BP, R, I & O, weight, neurologic checks, skin assessment, adventitious lung sounds, edema, abdominal exam, abdominal pain, liver evaluation, renal and liver function tests, UA, CBC, serum electrolytes, serum glucose

Implementation
▸ Administer before meals. Caution patient to swallow capsules whole and not to open, chew, or crush.
▸ Symptomatic improvement does not rule out gastric cancer, which did occur in preclinical studies.
▸ Administer antacids if needed.

● ondansetron hydrochloride
(on dan' sah tron) Zofran

Pregnancy Category B

Drug class
Antiemetic

Indications
▸ Prevention of postoperative nausea and vomiting when postoperative nausea and vomiting must be avoided
▸ Prevention of nausea and vomiting associated with cancer chemotherapy (parenteral and oral)
▸ Prevention of nausea and vomiting associated with radiotherapy

Adverse effects in *Italics* are most common; those in **Bold** are life-threatening

Therapeutic actions
▶ Blocks specific receptor sites (5-HT$_3$) that are associated with nausea and vomiting in the CTZ (chemoreceptor trigger zone) centrally and peripherally; it is not known whether its antiemetic actions are from actions at the central, peripheral, or combined sites.

Contraindications
▶ **Contraindications:** ondansetron allergy; parabens allergy (injection)

Available forms
▶ *Injection:* 2 mg/mL
▶ *Premixed injection:* 32 mg/50 mL
▶ *Tablets:* 4, 8 mg
▶ *Tablets, orally disintegrating:* 4, 8 mg
▶ *Oral solution:* 4 mg/5 mL

IV facts
Preparation
▶ Give undiluted when used to prevent postoperative nausea and vomiting.
▶ Use premixed injection or dilute in 50 mL of D5W/0.45%NS; D5W/0.9%NS; D5W with potassium chloride 0.3%; D5W; LR; Mannitol 10%; Ringer's Injection; 0.9%NS; 3%NS; or 0.9%NS with potassium chloride 0.3%. Do not mix with alkaline solutions.

Dosage
▶ *Prevention of postoperative nausea and vomiting:* 4 mg IV, preferably over 2–5 min.
▶ *Prevention of nausea and vomiting with chemotherapy:* 0.15 mg/kg IV over 15 min beginning 30 min before starting chemotherapy; repeat 4 and 8 h after the first dose. *Or* infuse a single 32-mg IV dose over 15 min beginning 30 min before starting chemotherapy.
▶ *Hepatic function impairment:* Do not exceed 8 mg/d infused over 15 min beginning 30 min before start of chemotherapy.

Compatibility
Ondansetron may be given through the same IV line as aldesleukin, amifostine, amikacin, aztreonam, bleomycin, carboplatin, carmustine, cefazolin, cefotaxime, cefoxitin, ceftazidime, ceftizoxime, cefuroxime, chlorpromazine, cimetidine, cisplatin, cladribine, clindamycin, cyclophosphamide, cytarabine, dacarbazine, dactinomycin, daunorubicin, dexamethasone, diphenhydramine, dopamine, doxorubicin, doxycycline,

Adverse effects in *Italics* are most common; those in **Bold** are life-threatening

droperidol, etoposide, famotidine, filgrastim, floxuridine, fluconazole, fludarabine, gallium, gentamicin, haloperidol, heparin, hydrocortisone, hydromorphone, hydroxyzine, ifosfamide, imipenem-cilastatin, magnesium sulfate, mannitol, mechlorethamine, melphalan, meperidine, mesna, methotrexate, metoclopramide, miconazole, mitomycin, mitoxantrone, morphine, paclitaxel, pentostatin, piperacillin-tazobactam, potassium chloride, prochlorperazine, promethazine, ranitidine, sodium acetate, streptozocin, teniposide, thiotepa, ticarcillin, ticarcillin-clavulanate, vancomycin, vinblastine, vincristine, vinorelbine, zidovudine.

Incompatibility
Do not administer through the same IV line as acyclovir, allopurinol, aminophylline, amphotericin B, ampicillin, ampicillin-sulbactam, amsacrine, cefepime, cefoperazone, furosemide, ganciclovir, lorazepam, methylprednisolone, mezlocillin, piperacillin, sargramostim, sodium bicarbonate.

Oral dosage
▸ *Prevention of postoperative nausea and vomiting:* 16 mg PO 1 h before anesthesia.
▸ *Prevention of nausea and vomiting with chemotherapy:* 8 mg PO bid. Give the first dose 30 min before starting chemotherapy, with another dose 8 h after the first dose. Give 8 mg PO bid for 1–2 days after completion of chemotherapy.
▸ *Prevention of nausea and vomiting with radiotherapy:* 8 mg PO tid.
▸ *Hepatic impairment:* Do not exceed an 8 mg oral dose.

> ### TREATMENT OF OVERDOSE/ANTIDOTE
> Discontinue drug or decrease dosage. Initiate general supportive and resuscitative measures.

Pharmacokinetics

Route	Onset	Peak
IV	Rapid	15–30 min
Oral	30–60 min	1.7–2.2 h

Metabolism: Hepatic; $T_{1/2}$: 3.5–5.5 h
Excretion: Urine

Adverse effects
▸ **CNS:** *Anxiety, agitation, headache, malaise, fatigue, dizziness, drowsiness, shivers, extrapyramidal syndrome,* cold sensation, weakness, paresthesia
▸ **CV:** *Dysrhythmias,* chest pain, hypotension, angina, hypertension
▸ **Resp:** *Hypoxia*

Adverse effects in *Italics* are most common; those in **Bold** are life-threatening

▸ **GI:** *Constipation, diarrhea,* abdominal pain, xerostomia
▸ **GU:** *Urinary retention*
▸ **Derm:** *Wound problems,* pruritis
▸ **Misc:** *Musculoskeletal pain,* pain at injection site, fever

● NURSING CONSIDERATIONS

Assessment
▸ *History:* Ondansetron or parabens allergy
▸ *Physical:* T, P, R, BP, I & O, IV site, ECG, neurologic checks, skin assessment, abdominal assessment, bowel sounds, presence of nausea or vomiting, hydration status, liver function tests

Implementation
▸ If nausea or vomiting must be avoided postoperatively, IV ondansetron is recommended even if the incidence of postoperative nausea or vomiting is low.
▸ To give orally disintegrating tablets, use dry hands to peel foil backing from 1 blister. Remove tablet and immediately place on top of the patients's tongue. Have the patient swallow. Do not push the tablet through the foil backing. Administration with liquid is not necessary.
▸ Ondansetron does not stimulate gastric or intestinal peristalsis; do not use instead of nasogastric suction. Use after abdominal surgery or for patients receiving chemotherapy may mask a progressive ileus or gastric distention.
▸ Assess for extrapyramidal effects.
▸ Ensure that the timing of drug doses corresponds to that of the chemotherapy or radiation.
▸ Administer oral drug for 1–2 d following completion of chemotherapy or radiation.

● oxycodone hydrochloride (*ox i koe' done*)
Oxycontin, OxyFAST, OxyIR, Percolone, Roxicodone, Roxicodone Intensol, Supeudol (CAN)

Pregnancy Category C

C-II controlled substance

Drug class
Narcotic agonist analgesic

Indications
▸ Relief of moderate to severe pain

Therapeutic actions
▸ Acts as agonist at specific opioid receptors in the CNS to produce analgesia, euphoria, sedation
▸ Produces respiratory depression by direct action on brain stem respiratory centers

Adverse effects in *Italics* are most common; those in **Bold** are life-threatening

- Depresses the cough reflex by direct effect on the cough center in the medulla
- Reduces motility associated with an increase in smooth muscle tone in the antrum of the stomach and duodenum; delays digestion of food; decreases peristalsis
- May produce histamine release with or without peripheral vasodilation

Contraindications/cautions
- **Contraindications:** oxycodone allergy, contraindication for receiving an opioid, significant respiratory depression, acute or severe bronchial asthma, hypercarbia, paralytic ileus
- **Cautions:** COPD, cor pulmonale, decreased respiratory reserve, hypoxia, hypercapnia, acute alcoholism, delirium tremens, toxic psychosis, convulsive disorders, head injury, increased intracranial or ocular pressure, cerebral arteriosclerosis, circulatory shock, CV disease, supraventricular tachycardias, hypotension, acute abdominal conditions, recent GI or GU surgery, gallbladder disease, ulcerative colitis, severe hepatic or renal function impairment, hypothyroidism, Addison's disease, kyphoscoliosis, prostatic hypertrophy, urethral stricture, fever, elderly or debilitated patients

Available forms
- *Tablets:* 5 mg
- *Immediate-release capsules:* 5 mg
- *Controlled-release tablets:* 10, 20, 40, 80 mg
- *Oral solution:* 5 mg/5 mL
- *Solution, concentrate:* 20 mg/mL

Oral dosage
- Adjust dosage to severity of pain and patient's response.
- *Immediate-release forms:* Usual dose is 10–30 mg PO q4h. 5 mg PO q6h as needed (OxyIR and OxyFAST). Give 5–60 mg PO as a rescue dose for patients taking controlled-release forms.
- *Chronic or severe pain:* 10–30 mg PO q4h as needed for pain.
- *Controlled-release forms:* 10–80 mg PO q12h as needed for pain. Use 80-mg tablets only for opioid tolerant patients who require daily oxycodone equivalent dosages of ≥ 160 mg.

TREATMENT OF OVERDOSE/ANTIDOTE
Discontinue drug or decrease dosage. Initiate general supportive and resuscitative measures. Reverse respiratory depression with naloxone 0.4–2 mg IV. Empty the stomach promptly by lavage, or induce emesis with syrup of ipecac. Treat circulatory shock with vasopressors.

Adverse effects in *Italics* are most common; those in **Bold** are life-threatening

Pharmacokinetics

Route	Onset	Peak	Duration
Oral (immediate-release)	15–30 min	1 h	4–6 h

Metabolism: Hepatic; $T_{1/2}$: 3.2 h (immediate-release), 4.5 (controlled-release)
Excretion: Urine

Adverse effects

▸ *CNS: Lightheadedness, dizziness, sedation, somnolence, headache,* euphoria, dysphoria, nervousness, confusion, delirium, insomnia, agitation, anxiety, abnormal dreams, fear, hallucinations, disorientation, drowsiness, malaise, lethargy, impaired mental and physical performance, coma, mood changes, weakness, headache, tremor, convulsions, miosis, visual disturbances, tinnitus
▸ *CV:* **Shock, cardiac arrest, circulatory depression,** hypotension, postural hypotension, syncope, chest pain, ST depression
▸ *Resp:* **Apnea, respiratory arrest, laryngospasm, bronchospasm,** dyspnea, voice alteration, pharyngitis, increased cough
▸ *GI: Nausea, vomiting, constipation, dry mouth,* sweating, anorexia, diarrhea, abdominal pain, dyspepsia, gastritis, hiccups, eructation, flatulence, increased appetite, stomatitis
▸ *GU:* Dysuria, hematuria, impotence, polyuria, urinary retention
▸ *Derm: Pruritus,* urticaria, dry skin, exfoliative dermatitis
▸ *Metabolic:* Dehydration, hyponatremia, peripheral edema, syndrome of inappropriate antidiuretic hormone secretion, thirst
▸ *Dependence:* Tolerance and physical dependence, psychological dependence
▸ *Misc:* Lymphadenopathy

Clinically important drug–drug interactions

▸ Enhanced neuromuscular blocking action of skeletal muscle relaxants; increased respiratory depression
▸ Increased respiratory depression, hypotension, profound sedation or coma in patients receiving CNS depressants, sedatives, hypnotics, general anesthetics, phenothiazines, tranquilizers, alcohol

◉ NURSING CONSIDERATIONS

Assessment

▸ *History:* Oxycodone allergy, contraindication for receiving an opioid, significant respiratory depression, acute or severe

Adverse effects in *Italics* are most common; those in **Bold** are life-threatening

454 pancuronium bromide ◀

bronchial asthma, hypercarbia, decreased respiratory reserve, hypoxia, paralytic ileus, COPD, cor pulmonale, hypercapnia, acute alcoholism, delirium tremens, toxic psychosis, convulsive disorders, head injury, increased intracranial or ocular pressure, cerebral arteriosclerosis, circulatory shock, CV disease, acute abdominal conditions, recent GI or GU surgery, gallbladder disease, ulcerative colitis, severe hepatic or renal function impairment, hypothyroidism, Addison's disease, kyphoscoliosis, prostatic hypertrophy, urethral stricture, age, debilitation

▸ *Physical:* P, BP, R, I & O, SpO$_2$, neurologic assessment, skin assessment, respiratory effort, orthostatic blood pressure, pain assessment, hydration status, abdominal assessment; liver, renal, and thyroid function tests

Implementation
▸ Assess pain status frequently; notify provider if patient does not receive adequate pain relief.
▸ Assess for evidence of respiratory depression.
▸ Have emergency equipment (defibrillator, drugs, naloxone, oxygen, intubation equipment) on standby in case adverse reaction occurs.
▸ Minimize postural hypotension by helping the patient change positions slowly.
▸ Assess patients before allowing him or her to ambulate; assist patient as needed to prevent falls.
▸ Do not crush or allow patient to chew controlled-release preparations.
▸ Follow federal, state, and institutional policies for dispensing controlled substances.
▸ Reassure patient about drug dependence; most patients who receive opiates for medical reasons do not develop dependence syndromes.

P

 pancuronium bromide *(pan cure oh' nee yum)*

Pavulon

Pregnancy Category C

Drug class
Nondepolarizing neuromuscular blocking agent

Indications
▸ Adjunct to general anesthesia to facilitate intubation

Adverse effects in *Italics* are most common; those in **Bold** are life-threatening

P

- To facilitate management of patients undergoing mechanical ventilation
- To facilitate tracheal intubation

Therapeutic actions
- Prevents neuromuscular transmission and produces paralysis by blocking effect of acetylcholine at the myoneural junction

Effects on hemodynamic parameters
- Increased HR
- Increased MAP
- Increased CO
- Decreased CVP

Contraindications/cautions
- **Contraindications:** pancuronium, bromide, or benzyl alcohol allergy
- **Cautions:** neuromuscular disease; myasthenia gravis; pulmonary, liver, or renal disease; cardiovascular disease, old age, edema, severe obesity, electrolyte imbalance, adrenal cortical insufficiency

Available forms
- *IV injection:* 1, 2 mg/mL

IV facts
Preparation
- *Direct IV injection:* May be given undiluted.
- *Continuous IV infusion:* Dilute 50 mg in 250 mL D5W/0.9%NS; D5W; LR; or 0.9%NS to achieve a concentration of 200 mcg/mL.

Dosage and titration
- *Initial adult dose:* 0.04–0.1 mg/kg IV as a bolus dose. Additional doses of 0.01 mg/kg IV may be given q25–60min to maintain paralysis.
- *Skeletal muscle relaxation for endotracheal intubation:* IV bolus dose of 0.06–0.1 mg/kg.

Compatibility
Pancuronium may be given through the same IV line as aminophylline, cefazolin, cefuroxime, cimetidine, dobutamine, dopamine, epinephrine, esmolol, etomidate, fentanyl, fluconazole, gentamicin, heparin, hydrocortisone, isoproterenol, lorazepam, midazolam, morphine, nitroglycerin, nitroprusside sodium, ranitidine, trimethoprim-sulfamethoxazole, vancomycin.

Adverse effects in *Italics* are most common; those in **Bold** are life-threatening

Incompatibility
Do not administer through the same IV line as diazepam or thiopental.

Pharmacokinetics

Route	Onset	Peak	Duration
IV	30–45 s	3–4.5 min	65–100 min

Metabolism: Liver; $T_{1/2}$: 89–161 min
Excretion: Urine, bile

Adverse effects
▸ *CV:* Tachycardia, increased arterial pressure and cardiac output, decreased venous pressure
▸ *Resp:* **Apnea, bronchospasm, laryngospasm**
▸ *Derm:* Rash
▸ *Allergic:* **Anaphylactic reactions** (bronchospasm, flushing, redness, hypotension, tachycardia)
▸ *Musc/Skel:* Inadequate block, prolonged block

Clinically important drug–drug interactions
▸ Intensified neuromuscular blockage with general anesthetics, antibiotics (aminoglycosides, polypeptides), quinidine, magnesium sulfate
▸ Synergistic or antagonist effect with metocurine, tubocurarine
▸ Reversed neuromuscular blockade with acetylcholinesterase inhibitors (neostigmine, edrophonium, pyridostigmine)
▸ Enhanced relaxant effects and duration of action with succinylcholine

● NURSING CONSIDERATIONS

Assessment
▸ *History:* Pancuronium, bromide, or benzyl alcohol allergy; neuromuscular disease; myasthenia gravis; pulmonary, liver, or renal disease; cardiovascular disease, age, edema, severe obesity, adrenal cortical insufficiency
▸ *Physical:* T, P, BP, R, ECG, I & O, IV site, weight, neurologic checks, muscle strength, level of sedation, skin assessment,

respiratory status, method of mechanical ventilation, adventitious lung sounds, peripheral nerve stimulator response, presence of pain, serum electrolytes, acid–base balance

Implementation
▸ Exercise extreme caution when calculating and preparing doses. Pancuronium is a very potent drug; small dosage errors can cause serious adverse effects.
▸ Always administer an infusion using an IV infusion pump.
▸ Do not administer unless equipment for intubation, artifical respiration, oxygen therapy, and reversal agents is readily available. Pancuronium should be administered by people who are skilled in management of critically ill patients, cardiovascular resuscitation, and airway management.
▸ Use the smallest dose possible to achieve desired patient response.
▸ Monitor patient's response to therapy with a peripheral nerve stimulator.
▸ Monitor BP, R, and ECG closely.
▸ Pancuronium does not affect consciousness, pain threshold, or cerebration. Administer adequate sedatives and analgesics before giving pancuronium.
▸ Pancuronium produces paralysis. Provide oral and skin care. Administer artifical tears to protect corneas. May need to tape eyes closed. Position patient appropriately.
▸ Use infusion within 24 h of mixing.

⬤ **pentamidine isethionate** *(pen ta' ma deen)*
Parenteral: Pentacarinat, Pentam 300
Inhalation: NebuPent

Pregnancy Category C

Drug class
Antiprotozoal

Indications
▸ Treatment of *Pneumocystis carinii* pneumonia, especially in patients unresponsive to therapy with the less toxic trimethoprim/sulfamethoxazole combination (injection)
▸ Prevention of *P. carinii* pneumonia in high-risk, HIV-infected patients (inhalation)
▸ Unlabeled uses: treatment of trypanosomiasis, visceral leishmaniasis (injection)

Therapeutic actions
▸ Antiprotozoal activity in susceptible *P. carinii* infections
▸ Mechanism of action is not fully understood, but the drug interferes with nuclear metabolism and inhibits the synthesis of

Adverse effects in *Italics* are most common; those in **Bold** are life-threatening

DNA, RNA, phospholipids, and proteins, which leads to cell death

Contraindications/cautions
▸ If the diagnosis of *P. carinii* pneumonia has been confirmed, there are no absolute contraindications to the use of this drug.
▸ **Contraindications:** history of anaphylactic reaction to inhaled or parenteral pentamidine isethionate (inhalation therapy)
▸ **Cautions:** hypotension, hypertension, hypoglycemia, hyperglycemia, hypocalcemia, leukopenia, thrombocytopenia, anemia, hepatic or renal dysfunction, ventricular tachycardia, pancreatitis, Stevens-Johnson syndrome, history of smoking, asthma

Available forms
▸ *Injection:* 300 mg/vial
▸ *Aerosol:* 300 mg

IV/IM facts
Preparation
▸ *IV:* Dissolve contents of 1 vial in 3–5 mL D5W or Sterile Water for Injection. Further dilute the calculated dose in 50–250 mL D5W.
▸ *IM:* Dissolve contents of 1 vial in 3 mL of Sterile Water for Injection.

Dosage
▸ 4 mg/kg/d IV over 60 min or deep IM for 14 d.
▸ *Renal failure:* Individualize dosage. If needed, reduce dosage, use a longer infusion time, or extend the dosing interval.

Compatibility
Pentamidine may be given through the same IV line as diltiazem or zidovudine.

Incompatibility
Do not administer through the same IV line as aldesleukin, cefazolin, cefoperazone, cefotaxime, cefoxitin, ceftazidime, ceftriaxone, fluconazole, foscarnet.

Aerosol dosage
▸ *Preparation:* Dissolve contents of one vial in 6 mL Sterile Water for Injection. Place entire reconstituted contents into the Respirgard® II nebulizer reservoir for administration. Do not mix with other drugs.

Adverse effects in *Italics* are most common; those in **Bold** are life-threatening

▶ *Administration:* 300 mg q4wk. Deliver dose until nebulizer chamber is empty (about 30–45 min). Set flow rate at 5–7 L/min from a 40–50 lb per square inch (PSI) air or oxygen source. Do not use pressures < 20 PSI.

TREATMENT OF OVERDOSE/ANTIDOTE
Discontinue drug or decrease dosage. Initiate general supportive and resuscitative measures.

Pharmacokinetics

Route	Onset
IM	Slow
Inhalation	Rapid

$T_{1/2}$: 6.4 h
Excretion: Urine

Adverse effects
Parenteral
▶ *CNS:* Confusion, hallucinations, dizziness
▶ *CV: Hypotension,* **ventricular tachycardia,** tachycardia, abnormal ST segment of ECG
▶ *Resp:* **Bronchospasm**
▶ *GI: Nausea, anorexia, elevated liver function tests,* bad taste in mouth, diarrhea
▶ *GU:* **Acute renal failure,** *elevated serum creatinine*
▶ *Hematologic: Leukopenia,* **thrombocytopenia,** anemia
▶ *Metabolic: Hypoglycemia,* **hypocalcemia, hyperkalemia**
▶ *Misc:* **Stevens-Johnson syndrome,** *fever; rash, sterile abscess, pain, or induration at IM injection site;* neuralgia, hyperkalemia

Aerosol
▶ *CNS:* **CVA,** *fatigue, dizziness,* headache, tremors, confusion, anxiety, memory loss, seizure, insomnia, drowsiness
▶ *CV:* Tachycardia, hypotension, hypertension, palpitations, syncope, vasodilatation, vasculitis, edema
▶ *Resp: Bronchospasm,* **laryngospasm,** *shortness of breath, cough, pharyngitis, congestion,* rhinitis, laryngitis, hyperventilation, pneumothorax, hemoptysis, eosinophilic or interstitial pneumonitis, pleuritis, cyanosis, tachypnea, crackles
▶ *GI:* **Pancreatitis,** *metallic taste to mouth, anorexia, nausea, vomiting,* gingivitis, diarrhea, dyspepsia, oral ulcer, gastritis, gastric ulcer, hypersalivation, dry mouth, melena, colitis, abdominal pain, splenomegaly, hepatitis

Adverse effects in *Italics* are most common; those in **Bold** are life-threatening

- *GU:* **Renal failure,** flank pain, nephritis, incontinence
- *Derm:* Pruritis, erythema, dry skin, desquamation, urticaria
- *Hematologic:* **Pancytopenia, neutropenia, eosinophilia, thrombocytopenia**
- *Metabolic:* Hypoglycemia, hyperglycemia, hypocalcemia
- *Misc:* *Rash, night sweats, chills,* anemia, eye discomfort, conjunctivitis, blurred vision, blepharitis, loss of taste and smell, allergic reactions

● NURSING CONSIDERATIONS

Assessment

- *History:* History of anaphylactic reaction to inhaled or parenteral pentamidine isethionate, hypotension, hypertension, leukopenia, thrombocytopenia, anemia, hepatic or renal dysfunction, pancreatitis, Stevens-Johnson syndrome, use of tobacco, asthma
- *Physical:* T, P, BP, R, ECG, SpO_2, I & O, IV/injection site, weight, neurologic checks, skin assessment, respiratory effort, adventitious lung sounds, sputum assessment and culture, BUN, serum creatinine, serum glucose, CBC, platelet count, liver and renal function tests, serum electrolytes (including calcium), CD4+ (T4 helper/inducer) lymphocyte count, UA, ABG, CXR

Implementation

- Monitor patient closely during administration; fatalities have occurred.
- Obtain the following laboratory tests before, during, and after therapy: BUN, serum creatinine, serum glucose, CBC, platelet count, liver function tests, and serum calcium.
- Obtain daily ECG.
- Position patient in supine position before parenteral administration; sudden and severe hypotension may occur.
- Have emergency equipment (defibrillator, drugs, oxygen, intubation equipment) on standby in case an adverse reaction occurs.
- Initiate aggressive pulmonary toilet: incentive spirometer, coughing, deep breathing, suctioning, and hydration.
- Continually assess for evidence of hypotension, dysrhythmias, hypoglycemia, hyperglycemia, nephrotoxicity, and electrolyte abnormalities.
- Inspect injection site regularly; rotate injection sites.

Adverse effects in *Italics* are most common; those in **Bold** are life-threatening

P

phenobarbital *(fee noe bar' bi tal)* *Oral preparation:*
Bellatal, Solfoton

phenobarbital sodium Parenteral: Luminal
Sodium

Pregnancy Category D

C-IV controlled substance

Drug classes
Barbiturate (long acting)
Sedative
Hypnotic
Anticonvulsant
Antiepileptic agent

Indications
▶ Emergency control of acute convulsions (tetanus, eclampsia, epilepticus) (parenteral)
▶ Anticonvulsant treatment of generalized tonic-clonic and cortical focal seizures (parenteral)
▶ Emergency control of certain acute convulsive episodes (eg, those associated with status epilepticus, eclampsia, meningitis, tetanus and toxic reactions to strychnine or local anesthetics) (oral)
▶ Long-term treatment of generalized tonic-clonic and cortical focal seizures (oral)
▶ Preanesthetic (parenteral)
▶ Sedative (oral or parenteral)
▶ Hypnotic, short-term (up to 2 wk) treatment of insomnia (oral or parenteral)

Therapeutic actions
▶ Produces all levels of CNS depression
▶ Depresses sensory cortex; decreases motor activity; alters cerebellar function; produces drowsiness, sedation, and hypnosis
▶ At subhypnotic doses, has anticonvulsant activity, making it suitable for long-term use as an antiepileptic
▶ Induces liver enzymes that metabolize drugs, bilirubin, and other compounds

Contraindications/cautions
▶ **Contraindications:** hypersensitivity to barbiturates; manifest or latent porphyria; marked liver impairment; preexisting CNS depression; nephritis; severe respiratory distress; previous addiction to sedative-hypnotic drugs

(contraindications continued on next page)

Adverse effects in *Italics* are most common; those in **Bold** are life-threatening

> ▸ **Cautions:** acute or chronic pain, seizure disorders, mental depression, suicidal tendencies, fever, hyperthyroidism, diabetes, severe anemia, pulmonary or cardiac disease, status asthmaticus, shock, uremia, impaired liver or kidney function, debilitated or elderly patients

Available forms
▸ *Injection:* 30, 60, 65, 130 mg/mL
▸ *Tablets:* 15, 16, 16.2, 30, 60, 100 mg
▸ *Capsules:* 16 mg
▸ *Elixir:* 15, 20 mg/5 mL

IV/IM facts
Preparation
▸ Reconstitute sterile powder for IV injection with 10 mL Sterile Water for Injection. May be added to D2.5W; D5W; D10W; Dextran 6% in D5W or 0.9%NS; Dextrose-LR combinations; Dextrose-Ringer's combinations; Dextrose-Saline combinations; Fructose 10% in 0.9%NS or Water; Invert Sugar 5% or 10% in 0.9%NS or Water; Ionosol products; LR; 0.45%NS; 0.9%NS; Ringer's injection; or Sodium Lactate (1/6 Molar) Injection.
▸ Prefilled syringes require no further preparation.

Dosage
▸ Use IV route only when other routes are not feasible. Give each 60 mg IV over 1 min. Administer into a large vein if possible; avoid administration into varicose veins.
▸ Administer deep IM into a large muscle or other areas where there is little risk of encountering a nerve or major artery. Do not inject > 5 mL into any one IM injection site.
▸ *Acute convulsions:* 200–320 mg IV or IM. Repeat in 6 h if needed.
▸ *Sedation:* 30–120 mg/d IV or IM in 2–3 divided doses.
▸ *Hypnotic:* 100–320 mg IV or IM.
▸ *Preoperative sedation:* 100–200 IM 60–90 min before surgery.
▸ *Elderly/debilitated patients:* Reduce dosage; monitor patient closely.

Therapeutic serum level
▸ 10–40 mcg/mL

Compatibility
Phenobarbital may be given through the same IV line as enalaprilat, meropenem, propofol, sufentanil.

Incompatibility
Do not administer through the same IV line as hydromorphone.

Adverse effects in *Italics* are most common; those in **Bold** are life-threatening

P

Oral dosage
- *Anticonvulsant:* 60–100 mg/d PO.
- *Sedation:* 30–120 mg/d PO in 2–3 divided doses. Do not give more than 400 mg during a 24-h period.
- *Hypnotic:* 100–200 mg PO.
- *Elderly/debilitated patients:* Reduce dosage; monitor patient closely.

> **TREATMENT OF OVERDOSE/ANTIDOTE**
> Discontinue drug or decrease dosage. Initiate general supportive and resuscitative measures. If patient is conscious and with a gag reflex, induce emesis with ipecac. Then give 30 g activated charcoal. If emesis is contraindicated, perform gastric lavage with a cuffed endotracheal tube in place. Forced diuresis may help eliminate phenobarbital. Alkalinization of urine increases renal excretion. Hemodialysis and hemoperfusion may be used in severe barbiturate intoxication or if the patient is anuric or in shock.

Pharmacokinetics

Route	Onset	Duration
IV	5 min	4–6 h
IM	10–30 min	4–6 h
Oral	30–60 min	10–12 h

Metabolism: Hepatic; $T_{1/2}$: 53–118 h
Excretion: Urine

Adverse effects
- *CNS: Somnolence,* agitation, confusion, hyperkinesia, ataxia, vertigo, CNS depression, nightmares, lethargy, residual sedation (hangover), paradoxical excitement, nervousness, psychiatric disturbance, hallucinations, insomnia, anxiety, dizziness, abnormal thinking
- *CV:* **Circulatory collapse,** bradycardia, hypotension, syncope
- *Resp:* **Apnea, respiratory depression, laryngospasm, bronchospasm,** hypoventilation
- *GI:* Nausea, vomiting, constipation, liver damage
- *Derm: Local pain; tissue necrosis at injection site;* arterial spasm, thrombosis, and gangrene of extremity with inadvertent intra-arterial injection; thrombophlebitis
- *Allergic:* **Angioedema, Stevens-Johnson syndrome, toxic epidermal necrolysis,** skin rashes, urticaria, exfoliative dermatitis

Adverse effects in *Italics* are most common; those in **Bold** are life-threatening

▸ *Dependence:* Tolerance, psychological and physical dependence
▸ *Misc:* **Withdrawal syndrome,** permanent neurologic deficit if injected near a nerve

Clinically important drug–drug interactions

▸ Increased serum levels and therapeutic and toxic effects with sodium valproate, valproic acid
▸ Prolonged barbiturate effects with MAO inhibitors
▸ Increased CNS depression with alcohol, tranquilizers, antihistamines, other CNS depressants, sedatives
▸ Increased nephrotoxicity with methoxyflurane
▸ Increased neuromuscular excitation and hypotension with barbiturate anesthetics
▸ Decreased effects of theophylline, oral anticoagulants, beta-blockers, doxycycline, griseofulvin, corticosteroids, oral contraceptives, estrogens, metronidazole, phenylbutazone, quinidine, verapamil
▸ Increased vitamin D requirements

⬤ NURSING CONSIDERATIONS

Assessment

▸ *History:* Hypersensitivity to barbiturates; manifest or latent porphyria; marked liver impairment; preexisting CNS depression; nephritis, severe respiratory distress, previous addiction to sedative-hypnotic drugs, acute or chronic pain, seizure disorders, mental depression, suicidal tendencies, hyperthyroidism, diabetes, severe anemia, pulmonary or cardiac disease, status asthmaticus, shock, uremia, impaired liver or kidney function, debilitated status, age
▸ *Physical:* T, P, R, BP, ECG, I & O, IV site, weight, neurologic checks, presence of seizure activity, mental status, skin assessment, adventitious lung sounds, pain assessment, bowel sounds, liver evaluation, liver and kidney function tests, serum and urine glucose, BUN, CBC, serum electrolytes

Implementation

▸ Monitor P, BP, R, and ECG carefully during IV administration.
▸ Initiate seizure precautions.
▸ Have emergency equipment (defibrillator, drugs, oxygen, intubation equipment) on standby in case adverse reaction occurs.
▸ Do not administer intra-arterially; may produce arteriospasm, thrombosis, or gangrene.
▸ Monitor injection sites carefully for irritation, extravasation (IV use). Solutions are alkaline and very irritating to the tissues.
▸ Monitor hematopoietic, renal, and hepatic systems during therapy.

Adverse effects in *Italics* are most common; those in **Bold** are life-threatening

- Monitor patient response and blood levels if any of the above interacting drugs are given with phenobarbital.
- Taper dosage gradually after repeated use, especially in epileptic patients. When changing from one antiepileptic drug to another, taper dosage of the drug being discontinued while increasing the dosage of the replacement drug.
- Follow federal, state, and institutional policies for dispensing controlled substances.

⬤ phentolamine mesylate (fen tole' a meen)
Regitine, Rogitine (CAN)

Pregnancy Category C

Drug classes
Alpha-adrenergic blocker

Indications
- Pheochromocytoma: prevention or control of hypertensive episodes that may occur as a result of stress or manipulation during preoperative preparation and surgical excision
- Prevention and treatment of dermal necrosis and sloughing following IV administration or extravasation of norepinephrine or dopamine
- Pharmacologic test for pheochromocytoma (urinary assays of catecholamines, other biochemical tests have largely supplanted the phentolamine test)
- Unlabeled uses: treatment of hypertensive crises secondary to MAO inhibitor/sympathomimetic amine interactions, or rebound hypertension on withdrawal of clonidine, propranolol, or other antihypertensive drugs

Therapeutic actions
- Competitively blocks presynaptic $alpha_2$ and postsynaptic $alpha_1$-adrenergic receptors; acts on arterial tree and venous bed, decreasing sympathetic vasculature tone, dilating blood vessels, and lowering arterial BP
- Has direct positive inotropic and chronotropic effects on cardiac muscle
- When infiltrated locally, reverses vasoconstrictive effects of norepinephrine and dopamine
- Use of phentolamine when testing for pheochromocytoma depends on the premise that a greater BP reduction will occur with pheochromocytoma than with other etiologies of hypertension

Effects on hemodynamic parameters
- Decreased SVR
- Decreased BP

Adverse effects in *Italics* are most common; those in **Bold** are life-threatening

▸ Increased CO
▸ Increased HR
▸ Decreased CVP

Contraindications/cautions
▸ **Contraindications:** hypersensitivity to phentolamine, mannitol, or related compounds; CAD, MI, coronary insufficiency, angina
▸ **Cautions:** tachycardia, dysrhythmias

Available form
▸ *Injection:* 5 mg/vial

IV/IM/SC facts
Preparation
▸ Reconstitute each 5 mg with 1 mL Sterile Water for Injection; results in a 5 mg/mL solution.
▸ To treat a dopamine or norepinephrine extravasation, add 5–10 mg phentolamine to 10 mL 0.9%NS.
▸ To prevent dermal necrosis and sloughing, add 10 mg phentolamine to each liter of norepinephrine.

Dosage
▸ *Prevention or control of hypertensive episodes in pheochromocytoma:* To reduce elevated BP preoperatively, inject 5 mg IV or IM 1–2 h before surgery. Repeat if needed. Administer 5 mg IV during surgery as indicated to control paroxysms of hypertension, tachycardia, respiratory depression, convulsions, or other effects of epinephrine.
▸ *Prevention of dermal necrosis following IV administration or extravasation of norepinephrine:* Add 10 mg to each liter of solution containing norepinephrine. The pressor effect of norepinephrine is not affected.
▸ *Treatment of extravasation by norepinephrine or dopamine:* Inject 5–10 mg in 10 mL saline into the area of extravasation within 12 h.
▸ *Diagnosis of pheochromocytoma:* 2.5–5 mg IV by rapid injection.

Compatibility
Phentolamine may be given through the same IV line as amiodarone.

TREATMENT OF OVERDOSE/ANTIDOTE
Discontinue drug or decrease dosage. Initiate general supportive and resuscitative measures. Treat hypotension vigorously and promptly. Elevate the patient's legs and
(treatment continued on next page)

Adverse effects in *Italics* are most common; those in **Bold** are life-threatening

P

administer a plasma expander. Use norepinephrine to maintain a normal BP. Epinephrine is contraindicated because it stimulates both alpha and beta receptors. Because phentolamine blocks alpha receptors, the net effect of epinephrine is vasodilation and a further drop in BP.

Pharmacokinetics

Route	Onset	Peak	Duration
IV	Immediate	2 min	5–10 min
IM	Rapid	20 min	

$T_{1/2}$: 19 min
Excretion: Urine

Adverse effects

- *CNS:* **Cerebrovascular spasm,** *weakness, dizziness,* cerebrovascular occlusion
- *CV:* **AMI,** *acute and prolonged hypotensive episodes, tachycardia, arrhythmias,* postural hypotension
- *GI:* *Nausea,* vomiting, diarrhea
- *Misc:* Flushing, nasal stuffiness

Clinically important drug–drug interactions

- Severe hypotension with epinephrine
- Decreased vasoconstrictor and hypertensive effects of ephedrine

⬤ NURSING CONSIDERATIONS

Assessment

- *History:* Hypersensitivity to phentolamine, mannitol, or related compounds; CAD, MI, coronary insufficiency, angina
- *Physical:* T, P, R, BP, ECG, I & O, IV site, neurologic checks, orthostatic BP, cardiac assessment, peripheral perfusion, edema, auscultation, bowel sounds, electrolytes, urine catecholamines

Implementation

- Calculate doses carefully. Phentolamine is a very potent drug; small dosage errors can cause serious adverse effects.
- Have emergency equipment (defibrillator, drugs, intubation equipment, oxygen) on standby in case adverse reaction occurs.
- Minimize postural hypotension by helping the patient change positions slowly.
- When using drug to diagnose pheochromocytoma, discontinue sedatives, analgesics, and all other nonessential drugs

Adverse effects in *Italics* are most common; those in **Bold** are life-threatening

for at least 24 h prior to test. Hold antihypertensive drugs until BP returns to untreated, hypertensive level. Do not perform the test on normotensive patients. Place patient in supine position for entire test. Do not perform test until BP is stabilized. After drug injection, take BP immediately, then q30s for 3 min, and then q1min for 7 min. A positive test suggests pheochromocytoma and is indicated by a systolic BP drop of > 35 mmHg and a diastolic drop of > 25 mmHg. Confirm a positive test with measurement of urine catecholamines.

◉ phenylephrine hydrochloride

(feen ill ef' rin) Neo-Synephrine

Pregnancy Category C

Drug classes
Vasopressor
Alpha-adrenergic agonist
Sympathomimetic amine

Indications
▸ To treat vascular failure in shock, shocklike states, drug-induced hypotension, or hypersensitivity
▸ To overcome paroxysmal supraventricular tachycardia

Therapeutic actions
▸ Powerful postsynaptic alpha-adrenergic receptor stimulant that causes vasoconstriction and increased systolic and diastolic BP with little effect on the beta receptors of the heart
▸ Constricts renal, splanchnic, cutaneous, and pulmonary vessels
▸ Increases blood flow to heart; does not produce cardiac irregularities

Effects on hemodynamic parameters
▸ Decreased HR
▸ Increased SVR
▸ Increased BP
▸ Increased PAP
▸ Decreased or increased CO
▸ Increased CVP
▸ Increased PCWP

Contraindications/cautions
▸ **Contraindications:** phenylephrine allergy, severe hypertension, ventricular tachycardia, peripheral or mesenteric ischemia, uncorrected hypovolemia

(contraindications continued on next page)

Adverse effects in *Italics* are most common; those in **Bold** are life-threatening

P

> ▶ **Cautions:** hyperthyroidism, bradycardia, partial heart block, myocardial disease, severe arteriosclerosis, diabetes, prostatic hypertrophy, elderly patients

Available form
▶ *IV injection:* 10 mg/mL

IV facts
Preparation
▶ For a continuous infusion add 10 mg phenylephrine to 250–500 mL of: D5W/LR; D2.5W; D5W; D10W; Dextran 6% in D5W or 0.9%NS; Dextrose-Ringer's combinations; Dextrose-Saline combinations; Fructose 10% in 0.9%NS or Water; Invert Sugar 5% and 10% in 0.9%NS or Water; Ionosol products; LR; 0.45%NS; 0.9%NS; Ringer's Injection; Sodium Bicarbonate 5%; or Sodium Lactate (1/6 Molar) Injection.
▶ Commonly used concentrations are 40 mcg/mL (10 mg in 250 mL) or 20 mcg/mL (10 mg in 500 mL). The 40-mcg/mL concentration is preferred for patients with volume overload.

Dosage and titration
▶ *Mild to moderate hypotension:* 0.1–0.5 mg IV. Do not exceed initial dose of 0.5 mg. Do not repeat injections more often than every 10–15 min.
▶ *Severe hypotension & shock:* Start IV infusion at 100–180 mcg/min. Titrate by 10–100 mcg/min every 10 min as needed to achieve desired BP. Once BP is stabilized, a maintenance rate of 40–60 mcg/min is usually sufficient. If prompt initial pressor response is not obtained, add 10-mg increments of phenylephrine to the bag. Avoid hypertension.
▶ *Paroxysmal supraventricular tachycardia:* Initial dose of not more than 0.5 mg IV given rapidly within 20–30 s. Determine subsequent doses by initial BP response, but do not exceed the preceding dose by more than 0.1–0.2 mg. Never give more than 1 mg.

Titration Guide

phenylephrine hydrochloride

10 mg in 250 mL

mcg/min	20	30	40	50	60	70	80	90	100	110
mL/h	30	45	60	75	90	105	120	135	150	165

mcg/min	120	130	140	150	160	170	180
mL/h	180	195	210	225	240	255	270

Adverse effects in *Italics* are most common; those in **Bold** are life-threatening

Compatibility

Phenylephrine may be given through the same IV line as amiodarone, amrinone, etomidate, famotidine, haloperidol, zidovudine.

Incompatibility

Do not administer through the same IV line as alkaline solutions, thiopental, iron salts.

> **TREATMENT OF OVERDOSE/ANTIDOTE**
> Discontinue drug or decrease dosage. Initiate general supportive and resuscitative measures. Phentolamine may relieve hypertension.

Pharmacokinetics

Route	Onset	Duration
IV	Immediate	15–20 min

Metabolism: Hepatic, tissue

Adverse effects

▸ *CNS: Headache, excitability, restlessness, fear, anxiety, dizziness,* drowsiness, tremor, insomnia, hallucinations, psychological disturbances, convulsions, CNS depression, weakness, blurred vision
▸ *CV: Dysrhythmias, reflex bradycardia,* hypertension, peripheral vasoconstriction
▸ *Resp:* Respiratory difficulty, dyspnea
▸ *GI: Nausea,* vomiting, anorexia
▸ *Misc:* Necrosis and sloughing at infusion site with infiltration

Clinically important drug–drug interactions

▸ Severe headache, hypertension, hyperpyrexia, possibly resulting in hypertensive crisis with MAO inhibitors, oxytocic drugs, guanethidine, vasopressors
▸ Increased or decreased pressor effect with TCAs
▸ Decreased pressor effect or hypotension with adrenergic and ganglionic blocking agents
▸ Increased dysrhythmias with bretylium, digoxin, halogenated hydrocarbon anesthetics

⬤ NURSING CONSIDERATIONS

Assessment

▸ *History:* Phenylephrine allergy, severe hypertension, peripheral or mesenteric ischemia, uncorrected hypovolemia,

Adverse effects in *Italics* are most common; those in **Bold** are life-threatening

hyperthyroidism, myocardial disease, severe arteriosclerosis, diabetes, prostatic hypertrophy, age

▶ *Physical:* T, P, BP, R, CO, SVR, CVP, PCWP, PAP, ECG, I & O, IV site, neurologic checks, skin assessment, adventitious lung sounds; peripheral pulses, perfusion, and sensation; bladder percussion, prostate palpation

Implementation

▶ Exercise extreme caution when calculating and preparing doses. Phenylephrine is a very potent drug; small dosage errors can cause serious adverse effects.
▶ Always administer an infusion using an IV infusion pump.
▶ Correct hypovolemia before administering phenylephrine.
▶ Monitor ECG, CO, PCWP, CVP, PAP, SVR, BP, and urine output closely during infusion. Continuous arterial pressure monitoring is preferred. Adjust dose/rate accordingly.
▶ Administer into large veins of antecubital fossa rather than hand or ankle veins. Use a central line whenever possible.
▶ Monitor infusion site closely for evidence of infiltration or phlebitis. If extravasation occurs, prevent sloughing and necrosis by using a fine hypodermic needle to infiltrate area with 5–10 mg phentolamine in 10–15 mL 0.9%NS.
▶ Maintain an alpha-adrenergic blocking agent on standby in case of severe reaction or overdose.
▶ Protect from light if removed from carton or dispensing bin.

⬤ **phenytoin** *(fen' i toe in)* Dilantin-125, Dilantin Infatab

⬤ **phenytoin sodium** Dilantin, Dilantin Kapseals
Pregnancy Category D

Drug classes
Anticonvulsant agent
Hydantoin

Indications

▶ Control of grand mal (tonic-clonic) and psychomotor seizures
▶ Prevention and treatment of seizures occurring during or following neurosurgery
▶ Control of status epilepticus of the grand mal type (parenteral administration)
▶ Unlabeled uses: antidysrhythmic, particularly in glycoside-induced dysrhythmias (IV preparations); treatment of trigeminal neuralgia (tic douloureux), recessive dystrophic epidermolysis bullosa, and junctional epidermolysis bullosa

Adverse effects in *Italics* are most common; those in **Bold** are life-threatening

Therapeutic

▸ Acts on ~~~~~~~~~~~~~~~~~~ seizure activity;
  may pr~~~~~~~~~~~~~~~~~~s, thus stabilizing
  the thre~~~~~~~~~~~~citability caused by excessive
  stimulati~~~~~~~ironmental changes
▸ Reduces maximal activity of brain stem centers responsible
  for the tonic phase of grand mal seizures
▸ Effective in treating cardiac arrhythmias, especially those induced by digitalis; antiarrhythmic properties are very similar
  to those of lidocaine; both are Class IB antiarrhythmics.

Contraindications/cautions
▸ **Contraindications:** hypersensitivity to hydantoins, sinus
  bradycardia, sinoatrial block, second- or third-degree AV
  block, Adams-Stokes syndrome
▸ **Cautions:** acute intermittent porphyria, hypotension, severe myocardial insufficiency, diabetes, hyperglycemia,
  impaired hepatic function, elderly patients

Available forms
▸ *Injection:* 50 mg/mL
▸ *Capsules:* 30, 100 mg
▸ *Chewable tablets:* 50 mg
▸ *Oral suspension:* 125 mg/5 mL

IV/IM facts
Preparation
▸ Administration by IV infusion is not recommended because
  of low solubility of drug and likelihood of precipitation; however, some studies indicate this may be feasible if proper precautions are observed. Dilute ≤ 100 mg in 25–50 mL 0.9%NS
  or LR, prepare immediately before administration, and use a
  0.22 micron in-line filter.

IM/IV dosage
▸ If possible, avoid IM route due to erratic absorption of phenytoin and pain and muscle damage at injection site.
▸ *Status epilepticus:* 10–15 mg/kg IV at a rate not exceeding 50
  mg/min. Maintenance: 100 mg IV q6–8h. Higher doses may
  be required. Follow each IV injection with an injection of
  0.9%NS through the same needle or IV catheter to avoid local venous irritation by the alkaline solution. Continuous IV
  infusion is not recommended.
▸ *IM therapy in a patient previously stabilized on oral dosage:*
  Increase dosage by 50% over oral dosage. When returning to
  oral dosage, give half the original oral dose for 1 wk to prevent excessive plasma levels due to continued absorption
  from IM tissue sites.

Adverse effects in *Italics* are most common; those in **Bold** are life-threatening

▶ *Neurosurgery (prophylaxis):* 100–200 mg IM q4h during surgery and the postoperative period.

▶ *Antidysrhythmic:* 50–100 mg IV q5min until dysrhythmia is terminated or until 15 mg/kg is given.

Therapeutic serum level
▶ 10–20 mcg/mL

Compatibility
Phenytoin may be given through the same IV line as esmolol, famotidine, fluconazole, foscarnet, tacrolimus.

Incompatibility
Do not administer through the same IV line as ciprofloxacin, diltiazem, enalaprilat, heparin, heparin-hydrocortisone, hydromorphone, potassium chloride, propofol, sufentanil, theophylline, vitamin B complex with C.

Oral dosage
▶ Individualize dosage. Determine serum levels for optimal dosage adjustments.

▶ *Loading dose (hospitalized patients without renal or liver disease):* Initially, 1 g PO of phenytoin capsules (phenytoin sodium, prompt) is divided into 3 doses (400 mg, 300 mg, 300 mg) given q2h. Begin normal maintenance dosage 24 h after the loading dose with frequent serum determinations.

▶ *No previous treatment:* Start with 100 mg (125 mg suspension) PO tid. Maintenance dosage is usually 300–400 mg/d. An increase to 600 mg/d (625 mg/d suspension) may be needed.

▶ *Single daily dosage (phenytoin sodium, extended):* If seizure control is established with divided doses of three 100-mg extended phenytoin sodium capsules per d, consider once-a-day dosage with 300 mg PO.

▶ *Renal or kidney disease, elderly:* Omit loading dose. Use caution; monitor for early signs of toxicity.

> **TREATMENT OF OVERDOSE/ANTIDOTE**
> Discontinue drug or decrease dosage. Initiate general supportive and resuscitative measures. Consider hemodialysis.

Pharmacokinetics

Route	Onset	Peak	Duration
IV	1–2 h		12–24 h
Oral	Slow	2–12 h	6–12 h

Metabolism: Hepatic; $T_{1/2}$: 6–24 h
Excretion: Urine

Adverse effects in *Italics* are most common; those in **Bold** are life-threatening

Adverse effects

Some adverse effects are related to plasma concentrations, as follows:

- 5–10 mcg/mL: Some therapeutic effects
- 10–20 mcg/mL: Usual therapeutic range
- >20 mcg/mL: Far-lateral nystagmus risk
- >30 mcg/mL: Ataxia usually seen
- >40 mcg/mL: Significantly diminished mental capacity
- *CNS: Nystagmus, ataxia, dysarthria, slurred speech, mental confusion, dizziness, drowsiness, insomnia, transient nervousness, motor twitchings, fatigue, irritability, depression, numbness, tremor, headache,* photophobia, diplopia
- *GI:* **Liver damage, toxic hepatitis,** *nausea,* gingival hyperplasia, vomiting, diarrhea, constipation
- *Derm:* **Bullous, exfoliative, or purpuric dermatitis; lupus erythematosus, Stevens-Johnson syndrome, toxic epidermal necrolysis;** scarlatiniform, morbilliform, maculopapular, urticarial and nonspecific rashes; hirsutism, coarsening of the facial features, enlargement of the lips, Peyronie's disease
- *IV use complications:* **Cardiovascular collapse, ventricular fibrillation, severe hypotension, atrial and ventricular conduction depression,** transient hyperkinesia, drowsiness, nystagmus, circumoral tingling, vertigo; IV site irritation and injury
- *Allergic:* Allergic reactions (arthralgias, eosinophilia, fever, lymphadenopathy, rash)
- *Hematologic:* **Aplastic anemia, agranulocytosis, leukopenia, thrombocytopenia, granulocytopenia, pancytopenia,** bone marrow depression; lymphadenopathy, including benign lymph node hyperplasia, pseudolymphoma, lymphoma, and Hodgkin's disease
- *Misc:* Systemic lupus erythematosus, osteomalacia

Clinically important drug–drug interactions

- Severe hypotension and bradycardia when given IV with dopamine
- Increased myocardial depression with beta-blockers, lidocaine
- Increased phenytoin serum levels with acute alcohol intake, amiodarone, chloramphenicol, chlordiazepoxide, diazepam, dicumarol, disulfiram, estrogens, ethosuximide, fluoxetine, H_2-antagonists, halothane, isoniazid, methylphenidate, phenothiazines, phenylbutazone, salicylates, succinimides, sulfonamides, tolbutamide, trazodone
- Decreased phenytoin serum levels with carbamazepine,

Adverse effects in *Italics* are most common; those in **Bold** are life-threatening

chronic alcohol abuse, reserpine, sucralfate, antacids containing calcium if given at same time as phenytoin
‣ Increased or decreased phenytoin serum levels with phenobarbital, sodium valproate, valproic acid; additionally, phenytoin may cause unpredictable effect on these drugs
‣ Increased seizures with TCAs
‣ Impaired efficacy of corticosteroids, coumarin anticoagulants, digitoxin, doxycycline, estrogens, furosemide, oral contraceptives, quinidine, rifampin, theophylline, vitamin D
‣ Reduced therapeutic effects of acetaminophen, but increased potential for hepatotoxicity of acetaminophen, especially with chronic use

⬤ NURSING CONSIDERATIONS

Assessment
‣ *History:* Hypersensitivity to hydantoins, sinoatrial block, Adams-Stokes syndrome, acute intermittent porphyria, hypotension, severe myocardial insufficiency, diabetes, hyperglycemia, impaired hepatic function, age
‣ *Physical:* T, P, R, BP, ECG, EEG, I & O, IV site, weight, neurologic checks, presence and type of seizure activity, skin assessment, lymph node palpation, adventitious lung sounds, bowel sounds, liver evaluation, periodontal exam, liver and thyroid function tests, UA, CBC, blood proteins, serum and urine glucose

Implementation
‣ Exercise extreme caution when calculating and preparing parenteral doses. Phenytoin is a very potent drug; small dosage errors can cause serious adverse effects. Avoid inadvertent bolus of drug.
‣ Always administer an IV infusion using an IV infusion pump.
‣ Continuously monitor HR, BP, and ECG during IV or IM administration.
‣ Initiate seizure precautions.
‣ Use only clear parenteral solutions; a faint yellow color may develop, but this has no effect on potency. If the solution is refrigerated or frozen, a precipitate might form, but this will dissolve if the solution is allowed to stand at room temperature. Do not use solutions that are hazy or contain a precipitate.
‣ Monitor IV and IM injection sites carefully; drug solutions are very alkaline and irritating. Avoid SC administration.
‣ Urine may turn red, reddish brown, or pink.
‣ Provide good oral hygiene.

Adverse effects in *Italics* are most common; those in **Bold** are life-threatening

- Give oral drug with food to enhance absorption and to reduce GI upset. Enteral feedings may decrease phenytoin concentrations; consider giving phenytoin 2 h before and after enteral feedings or stopping enteral therapy for 2 h before and after phenytoin administration.
- Reduce dosage, discontinue phenytoin, or substitute other antiepileptic medication gradually; abrupt discontinuation may precipitate status epilepticus.
- Phenytoin is ineffective in controlling absence (petit mal) seizures. Patients with combined seizures will need other medication for their absence seizures.
- Discontinue drug if skin rash, depression of blood count, enlarged lymph nodes, hypersensitivity reaction, signs of liver damage, or Peyronie's disease (induration of the corpora cavernosa of the penis) occurs. Institute another antiepileptic drug promptly.
- Monitor blood sugar of patients with diabetes mellitus. Adjust dosage of hypoglycemic drug as needed; phenytoin may inhibit insulin release and induce hyperglycemia.
- Evaluate patient for lymph node enlargement. Lymphadenopathy that simulates Hodgkin's disease has occurred. Lymph node hyperplasia may progress to lymphoma.
- Monitor blood proteins to detect early immune system malfunction (eg, multiple myeloma).

● phytonadione (vitamin K₁)

(fye toe nah dye' ohn) AquaMEPHYTON, Mephyton

Pregnancy Category C

Drug class
Vitamin (fat soluble)

Indications
- Coagulation disorders due to faulty formation of Factors II, VII, IX, and X when caused by vitamin K deficiency or interference with vitamin K activity
- Anticoagulant-induced prothrombin deficiency; hypoprthrombinemia secondary to conditions such as obstructive jaundice, biliary fistula, sprue, ulcerative colitis, celiac disease, intestinal resection, cystic fibrosis of pancreas, or regional enteritis, which limit absorption or synthesis of vitamin K; antibiotic or salicylate-induced hypoprothrombinemia due to interference with vitamin K metabolism (parenteral)
- Anticoagulant-induced prothrombin deficiency; hypoprothrombinemia secondary to salicylates or antibacterial therapy; hypoprothrombinemia secondary to obstructive jaundice and

biliary fistulas if bile salts are administered concurrently with phytonadione (oral)

Therapeutic actions
▶ Promotes hepatic synthesis of active prothrombin (Factor II), proconvertin (Factor VII), plasma thromboplastin component (Factor (IX), and Stuart Factor (Factor X)

Contraindications/cautions
▶ **Contraindications:** hypersensitivity to any component of phytonadione
▶ **Cautions:** liver impairment

Available forms
▶ *Injection:* 2, 10 mg/mL
▶ *Tablets:* 5 mg

IV/IM/SC facts
Preparation
▶ May be given undiluted or diluted in D2.5W; D5W; D10W; Dextran 6% in D5W or 0.9%NS; Dextrose-LR combinations; Dextrose-Ringer's combinations; Dextrose-Saline combinations; Fructose 10% in 0.9%NS or Water; Invert Sugar 5% and 10% in 0.9%NS or Water; Ionosol products; LR; 0.45%NS; 0.9%NS; Ringer's Injection; or Sodium Lactate (1/6 Molar) Injection.

Dosage
▶ Give IV only when IM, SC, and PO routes unavoidable.
▶ *Anticoagulant-induced prothrombin deficiency:* 2.5–10 mg IV, SC, or IM. Give each 1 mg IV over 1 min. Do not give infusions faster than 1 mg/min. Up to 25–50 mg may be required. May repeat in 6–8 h if needed.
▶ *Hypoprothrombinemia due to other causes:* 2.5–25 mg IV or more (up to 50 mg). Amount and route depends on severity of condition and patient's response. Give each 1 mg over 1 min. Do not give infusions faster than 1 mg/min.

Compatibility
Phytonadione may be given through the same IV line as ampicillin, epinephrine, famotidine, heparin, hydrocortisone, potassium chloride, tolazoline, vitamin B complex with C.

Incompatibility
Do not administer through the same IV line as dobutamine.

Oral dosage
▶ *Anticoagulant-induced prothrombin deficiency:* 2.5–10 mg PO. Up to 25–50 mg may be required. May repeat in 12–48 h if needed.

▸ *Hypoprothrombinemia due to other causes:* 2.5–25 mg PO or more (up to 50 mg) depending on severity of condition and patient's response.

TREATMENT OF OVERDOSE/ANTIDOTE
Discontinue drug or decrease dosage. Initiate general supportive and resuscitative measures.

Pharmacokinetics

Route	Onset	Peak	Duration
IV	1–2 h	3–6 h	12–14 h
Oral	6–10 h		

Adverse effects

▸ *CV:* **Cardiac arrest and shock (IV use),** hypotension, rapid and weak pulse, dizziness
▸ *Resp:* **Respiratory arrest (IV use),** dyspnea, cyanosis
▸ *GI:* Peculiar taste
▸ *Derm:* Pain, swelling, tenderness at injection site; profuse sweating, "flushing sensation"; erythematous, indurated pruritic plaques at injection site with repeated injections
▸ *Allergic:* **Anaphylaxis (IV use)**

Clinically important drug–drug interactions

▸ Reversed effects of anticoagulants; may need to increase anticoagulant dose when reinstituting therapy
▸ Decreased GI absorption with mineral oil

● NURSING CONSIDERATIONS

Assessment

▸ *History:* Hypersensitivity to any component of phytonadione, liver impairment
▸ *Physical:* P, BP, R, ECG, I & O, neurologic checks, cardiac auscultation, skin condition, adventitious lung sounds, presence of bleeding, PT, PTT, INR, renal function tests

Implementation

▸ Carefully monitor P, BP, R, and ECG during IV administration.
▸ Have emergency equipment (defibrillator, drugs, oxygen, intubation equipment) on standby in case anaphylaxis or adverse reaction occurs.
▸ Initiate bleeding precautions.
▸ Avoid oral route when disease would prevent drug absorption.
▸ Give bile salts with oral phytonadione when endogenous supply of bile to GI tract is deficient.

Adverse effects in *Italics* are most common; those in **Bold** are life-threatening

- Check coagulation tests regularly during therapy.
- If shock or excessive blood loss occurs, transfuse patient with PRBCs or FFP.
- After phytonadione is given, patient is at risk for same clotting hazards present before anticoagulant therapy.
- Protect drug from light.

pindolol *(pin' doe lole)* Apo-Pindol (CAN),
Novo-Pindol (CAN), Nu-Pindol (CAN), Visken

Pregnancy Category B

Drug classes
Nonselective beta-adrenergic blocker
Antihypertensive

Indications
- Management of hypertension, alone or with other drugs, especially thiazide diuretics
- Unlabeled uses: treatment of ventricular dysrhythmias, antipsychotic-induced akathisia, situational anxiety

Therapeutic actions
- Competitively blocks beta-adrenergic receptors, but also has some intrinsic sympathomimetic activity
- Exerts a membrane-stabilizing (local anesthetic) effect that reduces membrane permeability to the fast inward current of sodium ions
- Mechanism of antihypertensive effects not clear

Effects on hemodynamic parameters
- Decreased HR
- Decreased CO
- Decreased BP

Contraindications/cautions
- **Contraindications:** beta-blocker allergy, sinus bradycardia, second- or third-degree heart block, cardiogenic shock, bronchial asthma, bronchospasm, COPD, CHF unless well-compensated
- **Cautions:** peripheral or mesenteric vascular disease, chronic bronchitis, emphysema, bronchospastic diseases, diabetes, hepatic or renal dysfunction, thyrotoxicosis, muscle weakness

Available forms
- *Tablets:* 5, 10 mg

Adverse effects in *Italics* are most common; those in **Bold** are life-threatening

Oral dosage
▸ Initially give 5 mg PO bid. Adjust dose as needed in increments of 10 mg/d at 3- to 4-wk intervals to a maximum of 60 mg/d.

> **TREATMENT OF OVERDOSE/ANTIDOTE**
> Discontinue drug or decrease dosage. Initiate general supportive and resuscitative measures. Initiate gastric lavage or induce emesis to remove drug. Place patient in supine position with legs elevated. Treat symptomatic bradycardia with atropine, isoproterenol, and/or a pacemaker; cardiac failure with a digitalis glycoside, diuretic, and/or aminophylline; hypotension with epinephrine; hypoglycemia with IV glucose; PVCs with lidocaine or phenytoin; seizures with diazepam; bronchospasm with a beta₂-stimulating agent or theophylline derivative. Give glucagon (5–10 mg IV over 30 s, followed by infusion of 5 mg/h) for severe beta-blocker overdose.

Pharmacokinetics

Route	Onset	Peak
Oral	Varies	Varies

$T_{1/2}$: 3–4 h; 7–15 h for elderly hypertensive patients with normal renal function
Excretion: Urine

Adverse effects
▸ *CNS:* **CVA,** dizziness, vertigo, tinnitus, fatigue, depression, paresthesias, sleep disturbances, hallucinations, disorientation, memory loss, slurred speech, headache, confusion, visual disturbances, emotional lability
▸ *CV:* **Ventricular dysrhythmias, cardiac arrest, cardiogenic shock,** *AV block, bradycardia, CHF,* AICD discharge, mitral regurgitation, reinfarction, ventricular septal defect, chest pain, hypertension, hypotension, pallor, peripheral ischemia, peripheral vascular insufficiency, edema, pulmonary edema, palpitations, arterial insufficiency
▸ *Resp:* **Bronchospasm,** dyspnea, cough, bronchial obstruction, nasal stuffiness, rhinitis, pharyngitis, crackles, wheezes
▸ *GI:* **Acute pancreatitis,** *gastric/epigastric pain, flatulence, constipation, diarrhea, nausea, vomiting,* anorexia, ischemic colitis, renal and mesenteric arterial thrombosis, retroperitoneal fibrosis, hepatomegaly, hepatomegaly, elevated liver enzymes
▸ *GU:* **Renal failure,** *impotence, decreased libido,* Peyronie's disease, dysuria, nocturia, frequency, UTI

Adverse effects in *Italics* are most common; those in **Bold** are life-threatening

- *Derm:* Rash, pruritus, sweating, dry skin, increased pigmentation, psoriasis, peripheral skin necrosis
- *Allergic:* **Anaphylaxis, laryngospasm, angioedema,** pharyngitis, rash, fever, sore throat, respiratory distress
- *Hematologic:* **Agranulocytosis,** nonthrombocytopenic purpura, thrombocytopenic purpura
- *Musc/Skel:* Joint pain, arthralgia, muscle cramps, twitching/tremor
- *EENT:* Eye irritation, dry eyes, conjunctivitis, blurred vision
- *Misc: Decreased exercise tolerance,* facial swelling, weight gain or loss, gout, lupus syndrome, hyperglycemia or hypoglycemia, development of antinuclear antibodies

Clinically important drug–drug interactions
- Increased effects with calcium channel-blockers, digitalis, quinidine, oral contraceptives, prazosin
- Reduced clearance of lidocaine
- Life-threatening HTN when clonidine is discontinued for patients on beta-blocker therapy or when both drugs are discontinued simultaneously
- Increased hypoglycemic effect of insulin
- Hypertension followed by severe bradycardia with epinephrine
- May potentiate, counteract, or have no effect on nondepolarizing muscle relaxants
- Decreased effects with nonsteroidal anti-inflammatory drugs, rifampin

◉ NURSING CONSIDERATIONS

Assessment
- *History:* Beta-blocker allergy, cardiogenic shock, bronchial asthma, bronchospasm, COPD, CHF, peripheral or mesenteric vascular disease, chronic bronchitis, emphysema, bronchospastic diseases, diabetes, hepatic or renal dysfunction, thyrotoxicosis, muscle weakness
- *Physical:* P, BP, R, ECG, I & O, weight, neurologic checks, vision, skin assessment, cardiac auscultation, edema, adventitious lung sounds, JVD, abdominal assessment, bowel sounds, UA, serum glucose, serum electrolytes; liver, thyroid, and renal function tests

Implementation
- Carefully monitor P, BP, R, and ECG.
- Have emergency equipment (defibrillator, drugs, oxygen, intubation equipment) on standby in case anaphylaxis or adverse reaction occurs.
- Do not discontinue drug abruptly after chronic therapy. (Hypersensitivity to catecholamines may have developed,

Adverse effects in *Italics* are most common; those in **Bold** are life-threatening

causing exacerbation of angina, MI, and ventricular dysrhythmias). Taper drug gradually over 2 wk with monitoring.
▸ Consult with physician about withdrawing drug if patient is to undergo surgery (withdrawal is controversial).

● piperacillin sodium-tazobactam sodium *(pi per' a sill in-tay zoe back' tam)* Zosyn
Pregnancy Category B

Drug classes
Antibiotic: penicillin

Indications
▸ Moderate to severe infections caused by piperacillin-resistant, piperacillin/tazobactam susceptible, beta-lactamase producing strains of microorganisms listed below
▸ Appendicitis (complicated by rupture or abscess) and peritonitis caused by *Escherichia coli, Bacteroides fragilis, Bacteroides ovatus, Bacteroides thetaiotaomicron, Bacteroides vulgatus*
▸ Uncomplicated and complicated skin and skin structure infections caused by *Staphylococcus aureus*
▸ Postpartum endometritis or pelvic inflammatory disease caused by *E. coli*
▸ Community-acquired pneumonia caused by *Haemophilus influenzae*
▸ Nosocomial pneumonia caused by *S. aureus*

Therapeutic actions
▸ Bactericidal: piperacillin inhibits septum formation and cell wall synthesis, causing cell death; tazobactam component is effective against beta-lactamases that are often associated with drug resistance

Contraindications/cautions
▸ **Contraindications:** allergy to any penicillin, cephalosporin, or beta-lactamase inhibitor
▸ **Cautions:** history of multiple allergies, cystic fibrosis, renal function impairment, hypokalemia, bleeding abnormalities, patients who require sodium restriction

Available forms
▸ *Powder for injection:* 2 g piperacillin/0.25 g tazobactam, 3 g piperacillin/0.375 g tazobactam, 4 g piperacillin/0.5 g tazobactam, 36 g piperacillin/4.5 g tazobactam

---

Adverse effects in *Italics* are most common; those in **Bold** are life-threatening

IV facts
Preparation
- **Vials:** Reconstitute with 5 mL Bacteriostatic Saline/Benzyl Alcohol or Parabens; Bacteriostatic Water/Benzyl Alcohol or Parabens; D5W; 0.9%NS; or Sterile Water for Injection. Shake well until dissolved. Further dilute in 50 mL D5W; Dextran 6% in Saline; 0.9%NS; or Sterile Water for Injection.
- **ADD-Vantage vials:** Reconstitute only with D5W or 0.9%NS. Activate the ADD-Vantage vial by pulling the inner cap from the drug vial. Allow drug and diluent to mix.

Dosage
- *Usual dosage:* 3.375 g (piperacillin 3 g; tazobactam 0.375 g) IV over 30 min q6h.
- *Nosocomial pneumonia:* 3.375 g IV q4h plus an aminoglycoside for 7–14 d.
- *Hemodialysis patients:* Maximum dose of 2.25 g IV q8h. Give one additional 0.75-g dose after each dialysis period.
- *Renal function impairment:* Refer to table below for dosages.

Creatinine Clearance (mL/min)	Dosage
>40–90	3.375 g q6h
20–40	2.25 g q6h
<20	2.25 g q8h

Compatibility
Piperacillin-tazobactam may be given through the same IV line as aminophylline, aztreonam, bleomycin, bumetanide, buprenorphine, butorphanol, calcium gluconate, carboplatin, carmustine, cefepime, cimetidine, clindamycin, cyclophosphamide, cytarabine, dexamethasone, diphenhydramine, dopamine, enalaprilat, etoposide, floxuridine, fluconazole, fludarabine, fluorouracil, furosemide, gallium, granisetron, heparin, hydrocortisone, hydromorphone, ifosfamide, leucovorin, lorazepam, magnesium sulfate, mannitol, meperidine, mesna, methotrexate, methylprednisolone, metoclopramide, metronidazole, morphine, ondansetron, plicamycin, potassium chloride, ranitidine, sargramostim, sodium bicarbonate, thiotepa, trimethoprim-sulfamethoxazole, vinblastine, vincristine, zidovudine.

Incompatibility
Do not administer through the same IV line as acyclovir, aminoglycosides, amphotericin B, chlorpromazine, cisplatin, dacarbazine, daunorubicin, dobutamine, doxorubicin, doxycycline,

Adverse effects in *Italics* are most common; those in **Bold** are life-threatening

droperidol, famotidine, ganciclovir, haloperidol, hydroxyzine, idarubicin, miconazole, minocycline, mitomycin, mitoxantrone, nalbuphine, prochlorperazine, promethazine, streptozocin, vancomycin.

> **TREATMENT OF OVERDOSE/ANTIDOTE**
> Discontinue drug or decrease dosage. Initiate general supportive and resuscitative measures. Hemodialysis and peritoneal dialysis may remove the drug from the circulation.

Pharmacokinetics

Route	Onset	Peak
IV	Rapid	End of infusion

Metabolism: Kidney; $T_{1/2}$: 0.7–1.2 h
Excretion: Urine, bile

Adverse effects
- **CNS:** *Insomnia,* agitation, dizziness, anxiety
- **CV:** Hypertension, chest pain, edema
- **Resp:** Rhinitis, dyspnea
- **GI:** **Pseudomembranous colitis,** *diarrhea, nausea, constipation, vomiting, dyspepsia,* abdominal pain, stool changes; elevated AST, ALT, alkaline phosphatase, and bilirubin
- **GU:** Increased BUN and creatinine; proteinuria, hematuria, pyuria
- **Derm:** *Rash, pruritus*
- **Allergic:** **Anaphylaxis**
- **Hematologic:** **Leukopenia, thrombocytopenia,** prolonged PT and PTT, positive direct Coombs' test, decreased hemoglobin and hematocrit
- **Misc:** Fever, pain, superinfections, thrombophlebitis, hyperkalemia, hypokalemia, hyperglycemia, hypernatremia

Clinically important drug–drug interactions
- Increased and prolonged drug levels related to prolonged half-life with probenecid
- Prolonged neuromuscular blockade of vecuronium
- Inactivated by concurrent administration of aminoglycosides
- Increased risk of bleeding with heparin, oral anticoagulants, other drugs that affect the coagulation system

◉ NURSING CONSIDERATIONS

Assessment
- *History:* Allergy to any penicillin, cephalosporin, or beta-lactamase inhibitor; history of multiple allergies; cystic fibro-

Adverse effects in *Italics* are most common; those in **Bold** are life-threatening

sis, renal function impairment, hypokalemia, bleeding abnormalities, sodium restriction

▶ *Physical:* T, P, R, BP, I & O, IV site, weight, neurologic checks, skin assessment, respiratory status, abdominal assessment, bowel sounds, culture and sensitivity tests of infected area, renal and liver function tests, UA, CBC, serum electrolytes, serum glucose, coagulation studies

Implementation

▶ Obtain specimens for culture and sensitivity of infected area before beginning therapy. May begin drug before results are available.
▶ Have emergency equipment (defibrillator, drugs, oxygen, intubation equipment) on standby in case an anaphylactic reaction occurs.
▶ Assess for evidence of anaphylaxis; if suspected, discontinue drug immediately and notify provider.
▶ Monitor renal, hepatic, and hematopoietic function.
▶ Give aminoglycosides through a separate IV site at least 1 h apart from this drug.
▶ Monitor for occurrence of superinfections; treat as appropriate.
▶ Discontinue drug at any sign of colitis; initiate appropriate supportive treatment.

● **potassium chloride** *(po tass' ee um klor ride)*

Injection: Potassium Chloride
Oral: Apo-K (CAN), Cena-K, Effer-K, Gen-K, Kaochlor 10%, Kaochlor S-F, Kaon-Cl, Kaon Cl–10, Kaon-Cl 20%, Kato, Kay Ciel, K+ Care, K+8, K+10, K-Dur 10, K-Dur (CAN), K-Dur 20, K-Lease, Klor-Con, K-Lor, Klor-Con 8, Klorvess, Klotrix, K-Lyte/Cl, K-Norm, Kolyum, K-Tab, Micro-K LS, Potasalan, Roychlor (CAN), Rum-K, Slow-K, Ten-K

Pregnancy Category C

Drug class
Electrolyte

Indications
▶ Prevention and treatment of moderate or severe potassium deficit when oral replacement therapy is not possible (parenteral)
▶ Treatment of hypokalemia in the following conditions: digitalis toxicity; familial periodic paralysis; diabetic acidosis; diarrhea and vomiting; surgical conditions accompanied by nitrogen loss, vomiting, suction drainage, diarrhea, or increased urinary excretion of potassium; uremia; hyperadrenalism;

starvation and debilitation; corticosteroid or diuretic therapy (oral)
- Prevention of potassium depletion when dietary intake is inadequate for patients on digitalis and diuretics for CHF; patients with dysrhythmias, hepatic cirrhosis with ascites, aldosterone excess with normal renal function, potassium-losing nephropathy, or diarrhea (oral)
- If hypokalemia is associated with alkalosis, use potassium chloride; if patient acidotic, use potassium gluconate, citrate, bicarbonate, or acetate
- Unlabeled use: For patients with mild hypertension, potassium supplements result in long-term reduction of BP

Therapeutic actions
- Principal intracellular cation of most body tissues
- Maintains intracellular tonicity and a proper relationship with sodium across cell membranes
- Maintains cellular metabolism, nerve impulse transmission, acid–base balance, normal renal function; cardiac, skeletal, and smooth muscle contraction
- Participates in carbohydrate use and protein synthesis

Contraindications/cautions
- **Contraindications:** tartrazine or aspirin allergy (tartrazine is found in some preparations marketed as Kaon-Cl, Klor-Con), severe renal impairment with oliguria or azotemia, untreated Addison's disease, hyperkalemia from any cause, use of aldosterone-inhibiting agents, GI disorders that prevent passage of solid forms of potassium, crush syndrome, severe hemolytic reactions, adynamia episodica hereditaria, acute dehydration, heat cramps
- **Cautions:** cardiac disease (especially patients on digitalis drugs), GI lesions, diabetes, esophageal stricture/compression, metabolic acidosis, hyperchloremia, renal disease, adrenal insufficiency, familial periodic paralysis, hyponatremia, fluid overload

Available forms
- *Injection:* 10, 20, 30, 40, 60, 90 mEq; 2 mEq/mL after 90 mEq
- *Liquids:* 20, 30, 40 mEq/15 mL
- *Powders:* 15, 20, 25 mEq/packet
- *Extended-release tablets:* 8, 10 mEq
- *Controlled-release capsules:* 8, 10 mEq
- *Controlled-release tablets:* 6.7, 8, 10, 20 mEq

Adverse effects in *Italics* are most common; those in **Bold** are life-threatening

potassium chloride 487

P

IV facts
Preparation
▸ **Always** dilute before use.
▸ Add 10–80 mEq potassium to 1 L of D2.5W; D5W; D10W; D20W; Dextran 6% in D5W or 0.9%NS; Dextrose-LR combinations; Dextrose-Ringer's combinations; Dextrose-Saline combinations; Fructose 10% in 0.9%NS or Water; Invert Sugar 5% and 10% in 0.9%NS or Water; Ionosol products; LR; 3%NS; 3%NS; 0.45%NS; 0.9%NS; Ringer's Injection; or Sodium Lactate (1/6 Molar) Injection.
▸ In emergencies, add potassium to saline (unless contraindicated) because dextrose may lower serum potassium levels through intravascular shifting.
▸ Do not add potassium to an IV bottle/bag in the hanging position.
▸ Avoid "layering" of potassium by agitating the IV solution.

Dosage
▸ Dosage is determined by serum electrolyte and ECG determinations. Use the following as a guide to administration:

Serum K+	Maximum Infusion Rate	Maximum Infusion Concentration	Maximum 24-h Dose
>2.5 mEq/L	10 mEq/h	40 mEq/L	200 mEq
<2 mEq/L	40 mEq/h	80 mEq/L	400 mEq

Normal potassium level
▸ 3.5–5 mEq/L

Compatibility
Potassium chloride may be given through the same IV line as acyclovir, aldesleukin, allopurinol, amifostine, aminophylline, amiodarone, ampicillin, amrinone, atropine, aztreonam, betamethasone, calcium gluconate, cefmetazole, cephalothin, cephapirin, chlordiazepoxide, chlorpromazine, ciprofloxacin, cladribine, cyanocobalamin, dexamethasone, digoxin, diltiazem, diphenhydramine, dobutamine, dopamine, droperidol, edrophonium, enalaprilat, epinephrine, esmolol, estrogens, ethacrynate, famotidine, fentanyl, filgrastim, fludarabine, fluorouracil, furosemide, gallium, granisetron, heparin, hydralazine, idarubicin, indomethacin, insulin (regular), isoproterenol, kanamycin, labetalol, lidocaine, lorazepam, magnesium sulfate, melphalan, menadiol, meperidine, methicillin, methoxamine, methylergonovine, methylprednisolone, midazolam, minocycline, morphine, neostigmine, norepinephrine, ondansetron, oxacillin, oxytocin, paclitaxel, penicillin G potassium, pentazocine, phytonadione, piperacillin-tazobactam, prednisolone,

*Adverse effects in Italics are most common; those in **Bold** are life-threatening*

procainamide, prochlorperazine, propofol, pyridostigmine, sargramostim, scopolamine, sodium bicarbonate, succinylcholine,
tacrolimus, teniposide, theophylline, thiotepa, trimethaphan,
trimethobenzamide, vinorelbine, zidovudine.

Incompatibility
Do not administer through the same IV line as diazepam, ergotamine, phenytoin.

Oral dosage
▸ Individualize dosage.
▸ *Prevention of hypokalemia:* Usual range is 16–24 mEq/d PO.
▸ *Treatment of potassium depletion:* 40–100 mEq/d PO or
  more.

> TREATMENT OF OVERDOSE/ANTIDOTE
> Discontinue drug or decrease dosage. Initiate general sup-
> portive and resuscitative measures. Infuse dextrose and in-
> sulin in a ratio of 3 g dextrose to 1 U regular insulin to shift
> potassium into cells. Give sodium bicarbonate 50–100 mEq
> IV to reverse acidosis and produce an intracellular shift.
> Give 10–100 mL calcium gluconate or calcium chloride 10%
> to reverse ECG changes. Use sodium polystyrene sulfonate
> resin, hemodialysis, or peritoneal dialysis to remove potas-
> sium from the body.

Pharmacokinetics

Route	Onset
IV	Rapid
Oral	Varies (depending on product)

Excretion: Urine, feces

Adverse effects
▸ *GI:* Nausea, vomiting, diarrhea, abdominal discomfort, GI
  obstruction, GI ulceration or perforation
▸ *Derm:* Tissue sloughing, necrosis, phlebitis at IV site;
  venospasm with injection, rash
▸ *Fluid/electrolytes:* Hyperkalemia—paresthesias of extremities, flaccid paralysis, **muscle or respiratory paralysis,** areflexia, weakness, listlessness, mental confusion,
  weak and heavy legs, hypotension, **dysrhythmias, heart
  block,** disappearance of P waves, spreading and slurring of
  QRS complex with development of biphasic curve, **cardiac
  arrest**

P

Clinically important drug—drug interactions

▸ Elevated serum concentrations with concurrent use of ACE inhibitors, potassium-sparing diuretics, salt substitutes
▸ Hypokalemia may result in digoxin toxicity; use caution if discontinuing potassium in patients maintained on digoxin

● NURSING CONSIDERATIONS

Assessment

▸ *History:* Tartrazine or aspirin allergy, severe renal impairment with oliguria or azotemia, Addison's disease; use of aldosterone-inhibiting agents; GI disorders, crush syndrome, severe hemolytic reactions, adynamia episodica hereditaria, acute dehydration, heat cramps, cardiac disease, diabetes, esophageal stricture/compression, familial periodic paralysis
▸ *Physical:* T, P, BP, R, ECG, I & O, IV site, weight, neurologic checks, reflexes, adventitious lung sounds, bowel sounds, abdominal assessment, acid–base balance, renal function tests, serum electrolytes, digitalis level, UA

Implementation

▸ Always dilute parenteral potassium chloride and infuse using an IV pump.
▸ Carefully monitor patient's HR, BP, ECG, and serum electrolytes during IV therapy.
▸ Regularly assess serum electrolyte levels.
▸ Carefully monitor patient's IV site. Avoid infiltration because it will irritate tissues causing necrosis and sloughing. Use a large peripheral vein and a small bore needle. Use a central line if possible.
▸ ECG: hypokalemia may be evidenced by a flat or inverted T wave, U wave, ST segment depression, or atrial and ventricular dysrhythmias; hyperkalemia may be evidenced by a tall/tented T wave, wide or absent P wave, widened QRS complex, ST segment elevation, shortened QT interval, AV block, or ventricular fibrillation.
▸ Administer oral forms after meals or with food and a full glass of water to decrease GI upset.
▸ Instruct patient not to chew or crush tablets; swallow tablet whole.
▸ Mix or dissolve oral liquids, and soluble powders completely in 3–9 oz cold water, juice, or other beverage; have patient drink slowly.
▸ Further dilute or reduce dosage if GI effects are severe.
▸ Monitor stools for blood.

⬤ **potassium phosphate** *(po tass' ee um foss' fate)*
Neutra-Phos-K

Pregnancy Category C

Drug class
Electrolyte

Indications
▸ Prevents or corrects hypophosphatemia in patients with restricted oral intake
▸ Phosphate salts of potassium may be used in hypokalemic patients with metabolic acidosis or coexisting phosphorus deficiency

Therapeutic actions
▸ Prominent component of all body tissues
▸ Participates in bone deposition, regulation of calcium metabolism, buffering effects on acid–base equilibrium, and various enzyme systems
▸ Phosphate administration lowers urinary calcium levels; increases urinary phosphate levels and urinary pyrophosphate inhibitor

Contraindications/cautions
▸ **Contraindications:** hyperphosphatemia, hypocalcemia, hyperkalemia, untreated Addison's disease, severe renal impairment, infected urolithiasis or struvite stone formation
▸ **Cautions:** cardiac disease (especially patients on digitalis drugs), adrenal insufficiency, electrolyte imbalance, renal or hepatic function impairment, potassium-restricted diet, acute dehydration, extensive tissue breakdown, myotonia congenita, peripheral or pulmonary edema, hypertension, hypoparathyroidism, osteomalacia, acute pancreatitis, rickets

Available forms
▸ *Injection:* 3 mmol phosphorus and 4.4 mEq potassium/mL
▸ *Powder:* 8 mmol phosphorus with 14.25 mEq potassium

IV facts
Preparation
▸ **Always** dilute in a larger volume (250–1000 mL) of D5W/0.45% NS; D5W/0.9%NS; D2.5W; D5W; D10W/LR; D10W/Ringer's; D10W; Dextran 6% in D5W or 0.9%NS; Fructose 10% in 0.9%NS or Water; Invert Sugar 5% and 10% in 0.9%NS or Water; 0.45% NS; 0.9%NS; or Sodium Lactate (1/6 Molar) Injection.

Adverse effects in *Italics* are most common; those in **Bold** are life-threatening

Dosage
▶ Individualize dosage to patient's requirements. Give slowly based on patient's condition.
▶ 10–15 mmol of phosphorus/L of TPN IV daily.

Normal potassium and phosphorus levels
▶ **Potassium:** 3.5–5 mEq/L
▶ **Phosphorus:** 3–4.5 mg/dL

Compatibility
Potassium phosphate may be given through the same IV line as ciprofloxacin, diltiazem, enalaprilat, esmolol, famotidine, labetalol.

Oral dosage
▶ Individualize dosage to patient's requirements.
▶ 1 powder packet reconstituted in 75 mL water qid.

TREATMENT OF OVERDOSE/ANTIDOTE
Discontinue drug or decrease dosage. Initiate general supportive and resuscitative measures. To treat hyperkalemia, infuse dextrose and insulin in a ratio of 3 g dextrose to 1 U regular insulin to shift potassium into cells. Give sodium bicarbonate 50–100 mEq IV to reverse acidosis and produce an intracellular shift. Give 10–100 mL calcium gluconate or calcium chloride 10% to reverse ECG changes and restore decreased calcium levels. Use sodium polystyrene sulfonate resin, hemodialysis, or peritoneal dialysis to remove potassium from the body. Treat hyperphosphatemia with intestinal phosphate-binding agents (such as aluminum hydroxide gel), diuretics, and hemodialysis.

Pharmacokinetics

Route	Onset
IV	Immediate

Excretion: Urine, feces

Adverse effects
▶ *CNS:* **Seizures,** confusion, headache, dizziness, weakness or heaviness of legs and arms, tiredness, paresthesias
▶ *CV:* Fast or irregular heart rate
▶ *Resp:* Shortness of breath
▶ *GI: Nausea, vomiting, diarrhea,* stomach pain, mild laxative effect
▶ *Derm:* Phlebitis at IV site

Adverse effects in *Italics* are most common; those in **Bold** are life-threatening

▶ *Fluid/electrolytes:* Hyperphosphatemia—paresthesias of extremities, flaccid paralysis, **muscle or respiratory paralysis,** areflexia, weakness, listlessness, mental confusion, weak and heavy legs, hypotension, **dysrhythmias,** heart block, disappearance of P waves, spreading and slurring of QRS complex with development of biphasic curve, decreased cardiac output, **cardiac arrest;** hyperkalemia, hypocalcemic tetany, hypomagnesemia

▶ *Misc:* Unusual weight gain, low urine output, bone and joint pain

Clinically important drug–drug interactions

▶ Elevated serum potassium concentrations with ACE inhibitors, potassium-sparing diuretics, salt substitutes

▶ Hypokalemia may result in digoxin toxicity; use caution if discontinuing potassium in patients maintained on digoxin

▶ Antacids containing magnesium, aluminum, or calcium may bind phosphate and prevent its absorption

● NURSING CONSIDERATIONS

Assessment

▶ *History:* Addison's disease, renal or hepatic impairment, infected urolithiasis or struvite stone formation, cardiac disease, use of sodium-retaining medications, adrenal insufficiency, diet, acute dehydration, extensive tissue breakdown, myotonia congenita, peripheral or pulmonary edema, hypertension, hypoparathyroidism, osteomalacia, acute pancreatitis, rickets

▶ *Physical:* T, P, BP, R, ECG, I & O, IV site, weight, neurologic checks, reflexes, adventitious lung sounds, bowel sounds, acid–base balance, renal function tests, serum electrolytes, digitalis level, UA

Implementation

▶ Always dilute parenteral potassium phosphate and infuse using an IV pump.

▶ Carefully monitor patient's HR, BP, ECG, and serum electrolytes during the course of therapy.

▶ Carefully monitor patient's IV site. Avoid infiltration because it will irritate tissues. Use central line if possible.

▶ Hyperphosphatemia may be evidenced on ECG by absent P waves, prolonged QTI, widened or slurred QRS complex, or cardiac arrest.

▶ Hypophosphatemia may be evidenced by irritability, confusion, disorientation, seizures, coma, nystagmus, weakness, paresthesias, ataxia, dysrhythmias, hyperventilation, anorexia,

---

Adverse effects in *Italics* are most common; those in **Bold** are life-threatening

nausea, vomiting, bruising, bone pain, pathological fractures, or arthralgias.
▶ Hyperkalemia may be evidenced by nausea, vomiting, diarrhea, muscle weakness progressing to flaccid paralysis, numbness, increased deep tendon reflexes, fatigue, lethargy, apathy, confusion, dyspnea, oliguria, decreased cardiac output, tall peaked T wave, wide QRS complex, prolonged PRI, flat or absent P wave, bradycardia, or dysrhythmias.
▶ Further dilute or reduce dose if GI effects are severe.

⬤ **prednisone** *(pred' ni sone)* Apo-Prednisone (CAN), Deltasone, Liquid Pred, Meticorten, Orasone, Panasol-S, Prednicen-M, Prednisone Intensol, Sterapred DS, Winpred (CAN)

Pregnancy Category C

Drug classes
Corticosteroid
Glucocorticoid, intermediate-acting
Hormone

Indications
▶ Used to manage a wide variety of endocrine, rheumatic, collagen, dermatologic, allergic, gastrointestinal, respiratory, hematologic, neoplastic, and edematous disorders
▶ Used as replacement therapy in adrenocortical insufficiency

Therapeutic actions
▶ Suppresses inflammation and normal immune response
▶ Causes profound and varied metabolic effects
▶ Is a potent mineralocorticoid that leads to salt retention
▶ Suppresses adrenal function with long-term use

Contraindications/cautions
▶ **Contraindications:** prednisone allergy; infections, especially tuberculosis, fungal infections, amebiasis, vaccinia, and varicella
▶ **Cautions:** renal or hepatic disease, cerebral malaria, hypothyroidism, ulcerative colitis with impending perforation, diverticulitis, active or latent peptic ulcer, inflammatory bowel disease, fresh intestinal anastomoses, psychotic tendencies, hypertension, metastatic carcinoma, thromboembolic disorders, osteoporosis, convulsive disorders, myasthenia gravis, diabetes, CHF, antibiotic-resistant infections, Cushing's syndrome, recent AMI, elderly patients

Adverse effects in *Italics* are most common; those in **Bold** are life-threatening

Available forms
▶ *Tablets:* 1, 2.5, 5, 10, 20, 50 mg
▶ *Oral solution:* 5 mg/mL; 5 mg/5 mL
▶ *Syrup:* 5 mg/5 mL

Oral dosage
▶ Dosage requirements vary and must be individualized on the basis of the disease and the response of the patient. Use smallest effective dose.
▶ *Usual dosage:* 5–60 mg/d PO.
▶ *Maintenance therapy:* Reduce initial dose in small increments at intervals until lowest clinically satisfactory dose is reached.

> **TREATMENT OF OVERDOSE/ANTIDOTE**
> Discontinue drug or decrease dosage. Initiate general supportive and resuscitative measures.

Pharmacokinetics

Route	Onset	Peak	Duration
Oral	Varies	1–2 h	1–1 ½ d

Metabolism: Hepatic; $T_{1/2}$: 60 min
Excretion: Urine

Adverse effects
▶ *CNS:* **Convulsions,** *depression,* mood swings, increased intracranial pressure, vertigo, headache, psychic disturbances
▶ *CV:* **Myocardial rupture after recent AMI, fat embolism,** hypertension, hypotension; CHF secondary to fluid retention; thromboembolism, thrombophlebitis; dysrhythmias secondary to electrolyte imbalances
▶ *GI:* **Pancreatitis,** peptic ulcer, bowel perforation, abdominal distention, ulcerative esophagitis, nausea, hiccups, increased appetite, weight gain
▶ *Derm:* *Impaired wound healing, petechiae, ecchymoses, thin and fragile skin,* acne, increased sweating, allergic dermatitis, urticaria, angioneurotic edema
▶ *Allergic:* **Anaphylaxis**
▶ *Fluid/Electrolytes:* *Sodium and fluid retention, hypokalemia,* hypokalemic alkalosis, metabolic alkalosis, hypocalcemia
▶ *Musc/Skel:* *Muscle weakness,* steroid myopathy, muscle mass loss, osteoporosis, vertebral compression fractures, pathologic fractures, tendon rupture
▶ *Endocrine:* *Secondary adrenocortical and pituitary unresponsiveness,* decreased carbohydrate tolerance, diabetes

Adverse effects in *Italics* are most common; those in **Bold** are life-threatening

mellitus, cushingoid state, menstrual irregularities, negative nitrogen balance, hirsutism

▶ **EENT:** Cataracts, increased intraocular pressure, glaucoma
▶ **Misc:** *Increased susceptibility to infection, masking of signs of infection,* subcutaneous fat atrophy

Clinically important drug–drug interactions

▶ Increased blood levels with oral contraceptives, estrogens, ketoconazole
▶ Decreased blood levels with phenytoin, phenobarbital, rifampin
▶ Decreased serum level of salicylates
▶ Decreased effectiveness of anticholinesterases (ambenonium, edrophonium, neostigmine, pyridostigmine) in myasthenia gravis
▶ Increased digitalis toxicity related to hypokalemia
▶ Altered response to coumarin anticoagulants, such as warfarin
▶ Increased hypokalemia with potassium-depleting diuretics
▶ Increased requirements for insulin, sulfonylurea drugs
▶ Decreased serum concentrations of isoniazid
▶ Increased cyclosporine toxicity
▶ Decreased effectiveness with barbiturates

◯ NURSING CONSIDERATIONS

Assessment

▶ *History:* Prednisone allergy; infections, especially tuberculosis, fungal infections, amebiasis, vaccinia, and varicella; renal or hepatic disease; cerebral malaria, hypothyroidism, ulcerative colitis with impending perforation, diverticulitis, active or latent peptic ulcer, inflammatory bowel disease, fresh intestinal anastomoses, psychotic tendencies, hypertension, metastatic carcinoma, thromboembolic disorders, osteoporosis, convulsive disorders, myasthenia gravis, diabetes, CHF; antibiotic-resistant infections, Cushing's syndrome, recent AMI, age
▶ *Physical:* T, P, R, BP, ECG, I & O, weight, neurologic checks, muscle strength, ophthalmologic exam, skin assessment, peripheral perfusion, adventitious lung sounds, chest x-ray; upper GI x-ray (history or symptoms of peptic ulcer), abdominal assessment, CBC, serum electrolytes, serum glucose, 2-h postprandial blood glucose, UA, adrenal function tests, serum cholesterol, liver and renal function tests

Implementation

▶ Carefully monitor for evidence of fluid overload (I & O, daily weight, edema, lung sounds, JVD).

Adverse effects in *Italics* are most common; those in **Bold** are life-threatening

- Evaluate for hypokalemia as evidenced by muscle weakness, fatigue, paralytic ileus, ECG changes, anorexia, nausea, vomiting, abdominal distention, dizziness, or polyuria.
- Assess for hypocalcemia as evidenced by Chvostek's or Trousseau's signs, muscle twitching, laryngospasm, or paresthesias.
- Have emergency equipment (defibrillator, drugs, oxygen, intubation equipment) on standby in case anaphylaxis or adverse reaction occurs.
- Give daily doses before 9 AM to mimic normal peak corticosteroid blood levels.
- Increase dosage when patient is subject to stress.
- Taper doses when discontinuing high-dose or long-term therapy. Symptoms of adrenal insufficiency from too rapid withdrawal include nausea, fatigue, anorexia, dyspnea, hypotension, hypoglycemia, myalgia, fever, malaise, arthralgia, dizziness, desquamation of skin, or fainting.
- Do not give live virus vaccines with immunosuppressive doses of corticosteroids.
- Use minimal doses for minimal duration to minimize adverse effects.
- Administer with milk or food to minimize GI upset.

● procainamide hydrochloride
(proe kane a' mide) Apo-Procainamide (CAN), Procanbid, Pronestyl, Pronestyl-SR

Pregnancy Category C

Drug class
Antidysrhythmic

Indications
- Treatment of documented ventricular dysrhythmias that are judged to be life threatening

Therapeutic actions
- Type 1A antidysrhythmic: increases the effective refractory period of the atria, bundle of His-Purkinje system, and ventricles
- Reduces impulse conduction velocity in the atria, His-Purkinje fibers, and ventricular muscle
- Reduces myocardial excitability in the atria, Purkinje fibers, papillary muscles, and ventricles by increasing the threshold for excitation and inhibiting ectopic pacemaker activity
- Exerts vagolytic effects
- May decrease cardiac contractility, especially with myocardial damage

Adverse effects in *Italics* are most common; those in **Bold** are life-threatening

Effects on hemodynamic parameters
▸ Increased or decreased HR
▸ May decrease CO slightly
▸ Decreased BP

Contraindications/cautions
▸ **Contraindications:** allergy to procaine, procainamide, or similar drugs; tartrazine or sulfite sensitivity; complete heart block (unless pacemaker operative); SLE; torsades de pointes
▸ **Cautions:** myasthenia gravis, hepatic or renal disease, digitalis toxicity, CHF, acute ischemic heart disease, cardiomyopathy, concurrent use of antidysrhythmics, bone marrow depression, neutropenia, hypoplastic anemia, thrombocytopenia

Available forms
▸ *Injection:* 100, 500 mg/mL
▸ *Tablets:* 250, 375, 500 mg
▸ *Capsules:* 250, 375, 500 mg
▸ *SR tablets:* 250, 500, 750, 1000 mg

IV/IM facts
Preparation
▸ For direct IV injection, dilute drug in at least 10 mL D5W.
▸ For an IV bolus infusion, dilute 1 g in 50 mL D5W.
▸ For an IV maintenance infusion, dilute 1–2 g in 250–500 mL D5W; 0.45%NS; 0.9%NS; or Water for Injection.

Dosage
▸ Use IV or IM route for dysrhythmias that require immediate suppression and for maintenance of antidysrhythmic control. Switch to oral therapy as soon as possible.
▸ Base dosage on patient's response to therapy and procainamide and NAPA levels.
▸ *Loading dose:* Administer in one of two ways. 1) Use prepared bolus injection (see above). 100 mg IV q5min until dysrhythmia is suppressed or 500 mg is given. Wait ≥ 10 min to allow for distribution into tissues, then resume dosing until dysrhythmia is suppressed or total of 1 g is given or patient develops adverse effects (QRS widened by 50% or more, worsened dysrhythmias, hypotension). 2) Use prepared bolus solution (see above). Give 1 mL/min for 25–30 min IV at a constant rate to deliver 500–600 mg. It is unusual to require > 600 mg to achieve satisfactory antidysrhythmic results. Do not give > 1-g loading dose.
▸ *Maintenance dose:* 2–6 mg/min IV.
▸ *IM:* 50 mg/kg/d IM in divided doses q3–6h.

Adverse effects in *Italics* are most common; those in **Bold** are life-threatening

Titration Guide

procainamide hydrochloride

2 g in 250 mL

mg/min	2	3	4	5	6
mL/h	15	23	30	38	45

Therapeutic serum levels
▸ **Procainamide:** 3–10 mcg/mL
▸ **NAPA:** 10–30 mcg/mL

Compatibility
Procainamide may be given through the same IV line as amiodarone, famotidine, heparin, hydrocortisone, potassium chloride, ranitidine, vitamin B complex with C.

Incompatibility
Do not administer through the same IV line as milrinone.

Oral dosage
▸ *Standard preparation:* 50 mg/kg/d PO in divided doses q3h. See table below.
▸ *Sustained-release preparation:* 50 mg/kg/d PO in divided doses q6h, starting 2–3 h after last dose of standard oral preparation. See table below.
▸ *Elderly patients and those with renal, hepatic, or cardiac insufficiency:* Lesser amounts or longer intervals may produce adequate blood levels and decrease occurrence of adverse reactions.

Body Weight	Standard Preparation	Sustained-Release Preparation
40–50 kg	250 mg q3h	500 mg q6h
60–70 kg	375 mg q3h	750 mg q6h
80–90 kg	500 mg q3h	1000 mg q6h
> 100 kg	625 mg q3h	1250 mg q6h

> **TREATMENT OF OVERDOSE/ANTIDOTE**
> Discontinue drug or decrease dosage. Initiate general supportive and resuscitative measures. Treat hypotension with IV pressor agents. Both procainamide and NAPA can be removed from the circulation by hemodialysis.

Adverse effects in *Italics* are most common; those in **Bold** are life-threatening

Pharmacokinetics

Route	Onset	Peak	Duration
IV	Immediate	Minutes	3–4 h
IM	Rapid	15–60 min	3–4 h
Oral	30 min	90–120 min	3–4 h

Metabolism: Metabolized in liver to NAPA, which has significant antidysrhythmic activity; $T_{1/2}$: 2.5–4.7 h
Excretion: Urine

Adverse effects

▶ *CNS:* **Convulsions,** mental depression, giddiness, confusion, psychosis, dizziness, weakness, psychosis with hallucinations
▶ *CV:* **Asystole, ventricular fibrillation, arterial embolization with conversion of atrial fibrillation to sinus rhythm,** *hypotension,* cardiac conduction disturbances, second degree AV block
▶ *GI: Anorexia, nausea, diarrhea,* vomiting, bitter taste, hepatomegaly, elevated liver enzymes
▶ *Derm: Rash,* pruritus, urticaria, flushing
▶ *Hematologic:* **Neutropenia, thrombocytopenia, hemolytic anemia, agranulocytosis**
▶ *Misc:* Lupus syndrome (fever, chills, arthralgia, pleural or abdominal pain, arthritis, pleural effusion, pericarditis, myalgia)

Clinically important drug–drug interactions

▶ Increased levels with amiodarone, beta-blockers, histamine H_2 antagonists, quinidine, trimethoprim; monitor for toxicity
▶ Enhanced effects of succinylcholine
▶ Increased cardiodepressant action and potential for conduction abnormalities with lidocaine, quinidine, disopyramide

⊙ NURSING CONSIDERATIONS

Assessment

▶ *History:* Allergy to procaine, procainamide, or similar drugs; tartrazine or sulfite sensitivity; functioning pacemaker, SLE, myasthenia gravis, hepatic or renal disease, digitalis toxicity, CHF, acute ischemic heart disease, cardiomyopathy, concurrent use of antidysrhythmics, bone marrow depression, neutropenia, hypoplastic anemia, thrombocytopenia
▶ *Physical:* T, P, BP, R, ECG, QTc, I & O, weight, neurologic assessment, skin assessment, adventitious lung sounds, edema, bowel sounds, liver evaluation, UA, renal and liver function tests, digitalis level, serum electrolytes, CBC, procainamide and NAPA levels, serum ANA titer

Adverse effects in *Italics* are most common; those in **Bold** are life-threatening

Implementation

‣ Exercise extreme caution when calculating and preparing doses. Procainamide is a very potent drug; small dosage errors can cause serious adverse effects. Avoid inadvertent bolus of drug.

‣ Always administer IV procainamide infusion using an IV infusion pump.

‣ Continuously monitor BP, HR, and ECG during IV or IM therapy.

‣ Have emergency equipment (defibrillator, drugs, oxygen, intubation equipment) on standby in case an allergic or adverse reaction occurs.

‣ Check to see that patients with atrial flutter or fibrillation have been digitalized before starting procainamide.

‣ Differentiate the sustained-release form from the regular form.

‣ Monitor CBC, serum procainamide and NAPA levels, liver and kidney function tests, and serum electrolytes frequently.

‣ ECG changes associated with procainamide therapy include prolonged PRI, widened QRS, prolonged QTI, prolonged JT interval, decreased QRS and T wave amplitude. Procainamide toxicity may lead to a 50% increase in the QRS complex duration, prolonged QT and PR intervals, lowering of R and T waves, increased AV block; increased ventricular ectopy, including ventricular tachycardia and ventricular fibrillation.

‣ Assess for procainamide toxicity as evidenced by hypotension, CNS depression, tremor, respiratory depression, and ECG changes as above. Discontinue drug immediately if toxicity is suspected or confirmed.

‣ Dosage adjustment may be necessary when procainamide is given with other antidysrhythmics, antihypertensives, cimetidine, or alcohol.

‣ Give dosages at evenly spaced intervals around the clock; determine a schedule that will minimize sleep interruption.

‣ Do not break or crush sustained-release tablets.

‣ IV solution is initially colorless but may turn slightly yellow on standing. Discard solutions darker than a light amber color.

● **prochlorperazine** *(proe klor per' a zeen)*
Rectal suppositories: Compazine, Stemetil Suppositories (CAN)

● **prochlorperazine edisylate** *Oral syrup, injection:* Compazine, Stemetil (CAN), Nu-Prochlor (CAN)

● **prochlorperazine maleate** *Oral tablets and sustained-release capsules:* Compazine, PMS-Prochlorperazine (CAN), Stemetil (CAN)

Pregnancy Category C

Adverse effects in *Italics* are most common; those in **Bold** are life-threatening

P

Drug classes
Phenothiazine
Dopaminergic-blocking agent
Antipsychotic
Antiemetic

Indications
▶ Control of severe nausea and vomiting
▶ Management of manifestations of psychotic disorders
▶ Short-term treatment of nonpsychotic anxiety (not drug of choice)
▶ Unlabeled uses: treatment of patients with severe vascular or tension headaches who present to the emergency department

Therapeutic actions
▶ Mechanism of action not fully understood: blocks postsynaptic dopamine receptors in the brain
▶ Depresses the RAS, including the parts of the brain involved with wakefulness and emesis
▶ Anticholinergic, antihistaminic (H_1), and alpha-adrenergic blocking activity also may contribute to some of its therapeutic (and adverse) actions.

Contraindications/cautions
▶ **Contraindications:** phenothiazine allergy, coma, severe CNS depression, bone marrow depression, blood dyscrasia, circulatory collapse, subcortical brain damage, Parkinson's disease, liver damage, severe hypotension or hypertension
▶ **Cautions:** cardiovascular disease, breast cancer, glaucoma, exposure to extreme heat, seizures, respiratory disorders, GI dysmotility, alcoholism, urinary retention, prostatic hypertrophy, peptic ulcer, thyrotoxicosis, impaired hepatic or renal function, elderly or debilitated patients

Available forms
▶ *Injection:* 5 mg/mL
▶ *Tablets:* 5, 10, 25 mg
▶ *Sustained-release capsules:* 10, 15, 30 mg
▶ *Syrup:* 5 mg/5 mL
▶ *Suppositories:* 2.5, 5, 10, 25 mg

IV/IM facts
Preparation
▶ *Direct IV injection:* Dilute to concentration of 1 mg/mL.
▶ *Intermittent IV infusion:* Dilute 20 mg in 1 L of Dextrose-LR combinations; Dextrose-Ringer's combinations; Dextrose-Saline combinations; D2.5W; D5W; D10W; Fructose 10% in

0.9%NS or Water; Invert Sugar 5% and 10% in 0.9%NS or Water; Ionosol products; LR; 0.45%NS; 0.9%NS; Ringer's injection; or Sodium Lactate (1/6 Molar) Injection.

Dosage

▸ Begin with lowest recommended dosage.
▸ Give IM injections into the upper outer quadrant of the buttock.
▸ *Severe nausea/vomiting:* 5–10 mg IV or IM. Do not give IV faster than 5 mg/min. May repeat IV once if needed. May repeat IM q3–4h. Do not exceed 40 mg IV or IM qd.
▸ *Surgery, to control nausea/vomiting:* 5–10 mg IV 15–30 min before anesthesia or after surgery. Do not give faster than 5 mg/min. Repeat once if needed. Or give IV infusion of 20 mg/L; add to infusion 15–30 min before anesthesia. Or give 5–10 mg IM 1–2 h before anesthesia (may repeat once in 30 min) or after surgery (may repeat once).
▸ *Psychotic disorders:* 10–20 mg IM. May repeat q2–4h (q1h for resistant cases). More than 3–4 doses are seldom needed. For prolonged parenteral therapy, give q4–6h. Switch patient to oral dosing after control is achieved.
▸ *Elderly/debilitated patients:* Decrease dosage; observe patient closely.

Compatibility

Prochlorperazine may be given through the same IV line as amsacrine, calcium gluconate, cisplatin, cladribine, cyclophosphamide, cytarabine, doxorubicin, fluconazole, granisetron, heparin, hydrocortisone, melphalan, methotrexate, ondansetron, paclitaxel, potassium chloride, propofol, sargramostim, sufentanil, teniposide, thiotepa, vinorelbine, vitamin B complex with C.

Incompatibility

Do not administer through the same IV line as aldesleukin, allopurinol, amifostine, aztreonam, cefepime, cefmetazole, fludarabine, foscarnet, filgrastim, gallium, piperacillin-tazobactam.

Oral/rectal dosage

▸ *Severe nausea/vomiting:* 5–10 mg PO tid–qid. Or 15 mg sustained release PO on arising or 10 mg sustained release PO q12h. Or 25 mg PR bid.
▸ *Anxiety:* 5 mg PO tid–qid. Or 15 mg sustained release PO on arising or 10 mg sustained release PO q12h. Do not give > 20 mg/d or for > 12 wk.
▸ *Psychotic disorders:* 5–10 mg tid–qid. Increase dosage gradually. For severe disturbances, optimum dosage is 100–150 mg/d.

Adverse effects in *Italics* are most common; those in **Bold** are life-threatening

▸ *Elderly/debilitated patients:* Decrease dosage; monitor patient closely.

TREATMENT OF OVERDOSE/ANTIDOTE
Discontinue drug or decrease dosage. Initiate general supportive and resuscitative measures. For oral ingestion, initiate early gastric lavage. Do not induce emesis because a dystonic reaction of the head or neck may develop that could lead to aspiration. Treat extrapyramidal symptoms with anti-parkinsonism drugs, barbiturates, or Benadryl. If a stimulant is desirable, give amphetamine, dextroamphetamine, or caffeine with sodium benzoate. Avoid stimulants, such as picrotoxin or pentylenetetrazol, that may cause seizures. Treat hypotension with norepinephrine and phenylephrine. Avoid epinephrine because it may worsen hypotension.

Pharmacokinetics

Route	Onset	Duration
IV	Immediate	3–4 h
IM	10–20 min	3–4 h
Oral	30–40 min	3–4 h (10–12 SR)
PR	60–90 min	3–4 h

Metabolism: Hepatic, GI mucosa
Excretion: Urine

Adverse effects

▸ *CNS:* **Neuroleptic malignant syndrome, cerebral edema, seizures,** *extrapyramidal reactions,* motor restlessness, dystonias, pseudo-parkinsonism, exacerbation of psychotic symptoms, tardive dyskinesia
▸ *CV:* **Cardiac arrest, hypotension,** postural hypotension, tachycardia, ECG changes, edema
▸ *Resp:* **Asphyxia or aspiration due to failure of cough reflex,** dyspnea, nasal congestion
▸ *GI:* *Dry mouth, constipation,* ileus, hepatitis, liver damage, increased appetite
▸ *GU:* Urinary retention, ejaculatory disorders/impotence, priapism, pink or reddish brown urine
▸ *Derm:* Erythema, urticaria, eczema, itching, skin pigmentation
▸ *Allergic:* **Anaphylaxis**
▸ *Hematologic:* **Pancytopenia, thrombocytopenic purpura, leukopenia, agranulocytosis, aplastic anemia, hemolytic anemia, eosinophilia**

Adverse effects in *Italics* are most common; those in **Bold** are life-threatening

▸ **Endocrine:** Hyperglycemia, hypoglycemia, glycosuria, galactorrhea, gynecomastia, menstrual irregularities, false-positive pregnancy test
▸ **EENT:** *Photophobia, blurred vision,* glaucoma, miosis, mydriasis, deposits in the cornea and lens (opacities), pigmentary retinopathy
▸ **Misc:** Hyperthermia, weight gain, systemic lupus erythematosus-like syndrome

Clinically important drug–drug interactions
▸ Diminished effects of oral coagulants
▸ Increased postural hypotension with thiazide diuretics
▸ Counteracted antihypertensive effects of guanethidine, related drugs
▸ Interferes with phenytoin metabolism and thus leads to toxicity
▸ Additive and prolonged CNS depression with alcohol, CNS depressants
▸ Additive anticholinergic effects and possibly decreased antipsychotic efficacy with anticholinergic drugs
▸ Increased tricyclic antidepressant serum concentrations
▸ Use with propranolol may increase plasma levels of both drugs

● NURSING CONSIDERATIONS

Assessment
▸ *History:* Phenothiazine allergy, coma, severe CNS depression, bone marrow depression, blood dyscrasia, circulatory collapse, subcortical brain damage, Parkinson's disease, liver damage, severe hypotension or hypertension, cardiovascular disease, breast cancer, glaucoma, exposure to extreme heat, seizures, respiratory disorders, GI dysmotility, alcoholism, urinary retention, prostatic hypertrophy, peptic ulcer, thyrotoxicosis, impaired hepatic or renal function, age, debilitation
▸ *Physical:* T, P, R, BP, ECG, I & O, weight, neurologic checks, mental status, pain assessment, skin assessment, intraocular pressure, vision, orthostatic BP, respiratory effort, adventitious lung sounds, hydration status, presence of nausea and vomiting, bowel sounds, liver evaluation, prostate size, CBC, UA; thyroid, liver, and kidney function tests

Implementation
▸ Minimize risk for hypotension after injection by having the patient lie down for at least 1/2 h.
▸ Minimize postural hypotension by helping the patient change positions slowly.

Adverse effects in *Italics* are most common; those in **Bold** are life-threatening

- Monitor for evidence of tardive dyskinesia as evidenced by involuntary dyskinetic movements, such as rhythmical involuntary movements of the tongue, face, mouth, or jaw (eg, protrusion of tongue, puffing of cheeks, puckering of mouth, chewing movements). Discontinue drug if above noted.
- Monitor for evidence of extrapyramidal reactions as evidenced by motor restlessness (agitation, jitteriness, insomnia) of the dystonic type (neck muscle spasms, torticollis, extensor rigidity of back muscles, opisthotonos, carpopedal spasm, trismus, swallowing difficulty, oculogyric crisis, tongue protrusion). They may resemble parkinsonism (masklike facies, drooling, tremors, pillrolling motion, cogwheel rigidity, shuffling gait). Report above to the provider.
- Discontinue at least 48 h before myelography because of possible seizures; do not resume therapy for at least 24 h postprocedure. Do not use to control nausea and vomiting before or after myelography.
- Do not change brand names of oral preparations; bioavailability differences have been documented.
- Do not crush or allow patient to chew sustained-release capsules.
- Do not administer SC; may cause local irritation.
- Abrupt withdrawal may cause gastritis, nausea, vomiting, dizziness, headache, tachycardia, insomnia, and tremulousness.
- Avoid skin contact with injection solution; may cause contact dermatitis.
- Discontinue drug if serum creatinine or BUN become abnormal or if WBC count is depressed.
- Monitor elderly patients for dehydration, and institute remedial measures promptly; sedation and decreased sensation of thirst related to the drug's CNS effects may cause severe dehydration.

◖ promethazine hydrochloride

(proe meth' a zeen) Anergan 50, Phenergan,
PMS-Promethazine (CAN)

Pregnancy Category C

Drug classes
Phenothiazine
Antidopaminergic
Antihistamine
Antiemetic
Sedative/hypnotic

Adverse effects in *Italics* are most common; those in **Bold** are life-threatening

Indications
▸ Hypersensitivity reactions: perennial and seasonal allergic rhinitis, vasomotor rhinitis, allergic conjunctivitis; mild, uncomplicated urticaria and angioedema; amelioration of allergic reactions to blood or plasma, dermatographism; adjunctive therapy (with epinephrine and other measures) in anaphylactic reactions
▸ Antiemetic: prevention and treatment of nausea and vomiting associated with anesthesia and surgery
▸ Sedation: preoperative or postoperative sedation; relief of apprehension; production of light sleep
▸ Analgesia: adjunct to analgesics to control postoperative pain

Therapeutic actions
▸ Selectively blocks H_1 receptors, diminishing the effects of histamine on cells of the upper respiratory tract and eyes; decreases sneezing, mucus production, itching, and tearing that accompany allergic reactions in sensitized people exposed to antigens
▸ Blocks cholinergic receptors in the vomiting center that are believed to mediate nausea and vomiting caused by gastric irritation, input from the vestibular apparatus (motion sickness, nausea associated with vestibular neuritis), and input from the chemoreceptor trigger zone (drug- and radiation-induced emesis)
▸ Depresses the RAS, including the parts of the brain involved with wakefulness

Contraindications/cautions
▸ **Contraindications:** hypersensitivity to antihistamines or phenothiazines, coma or severe CNS depression, bone marrow depression, vomiting of unknown cause, concomitant therapy with MAOIs, lower respiratory tract symptoms (asthma, emphysema, chronic bronchitis), sleep apnea
▸ **Cautions:** concurrent use of other CNS depressants, seizure disorder, narrow-angle glaucoma, stenosing peptic ulcer, pyloroduodenal obstruction, urinary bladder obstruction due to prostatic hypertrophy and narrowing of bladder neck, impaired liver function, bone marrow depression, CV disease, hypertension, elderly patients

Available forms
▸ *Injection:* 25, 50 mg/mL
▸ *Tablets:* 12.5, 25, 50 mg
▸ *Syrup:* 6.25, 25 mg/5 mL
▸ *Suppositories:* 12.5, 25, 50 mg

Adverse effects in *Italics* are most common; those in **Bold** are life-threatening

P

IV/IM facts
Preparation
❱ May be given undiluted; do not exceed concentration > 25 mg/mL.

Dosage
❱ *Hypersensitivity reactions:* 25 mg IV or IM. May repeat in 2 h if needed. Convert to oral therapy as soon as possible.
❱ *Nausea/vomiting:* 12.5–25 mg IV or IM. Do not exceed 25 mg/min IV. Repeat q4h as needed. Reduce doses of analgesics, hypnotics, and barbiturates.
❱ *Analgesia:* 25–50 mg IV or IM. Reduce doses of analgesics and hypnotics.
❱ *Sedation:* 25–50 mg IV or IM at hs.

Compatibility
Promethazine may be given through the same IV line as amifostine, amsacrine, aztreonam, ciprofloxacin, cisplatin, cladribine, cyclophosphamide, cytarabine, doxorubicin, filgrastim, fluconazole, fludarabine, granisetron, melphalan, ondansetron, sargramostim, teniposide, thiotepa, vinorelbine.

Incompatibility
Do not administer through the same IV line as aldesleukin, allopurinol, cefepime, cefmetazole, cefoperazone, cefotetan, foscarnet, methotrexate, piperacillin-tazobactam.

Oral/rectal dosage
❱ *Nausea/vomiting:* 25 mg PO or PR; repeat doses of 12.5–25 mg as needed q4–6h.
❱ *Sedation:* 25–50 mg PO or PR at hs.
❱ *Hypersensitivity:* 25 mg PO or PR at hs; 12.5 mg PO or PR before meals and at hs.
❱ *Analgesia:* 50 mg PO or PR with an equal amount of meperidine and appropriate dose of belladonna alkaloid.

TREATMENT OF OVERDOSE/ANTIDOTE
Discontinue drug or decrease dosage. Initiate general supportive and resuscitative measures. If oral forms were used, initiate early gastric lavage; give activated charcoal. Treat convulsions with diazepam. Treat hypotension with norepinephrine or phenylephrine. Avoid analeptics, which may cause convulsions, and epinephrine, which may cause further hypotension. Treat extrapyramidal reactions with anticholinergic antiparkinson agents, diphenhydramine, or barbiturates.

Adverse effects in *Italics* are most common; those in **Bold** are life-threatening

Pharmacokinetics

Route	Onset	Duration
IV	3–5 min	4–6 h
IM	20 min	12 h
Oral	20 min	12 h

Metabolism: Hepatic
Excretion: Urine

Adverse effects

▸ *CNS:* **Convulsions,** *dizziness, drowsiness, poor coordination, confusion,* restlessness, excitation, dizziness, fatigue, euphoria, tremors, headache, blurred vision, diplopia, vertigo, tinnitus, extrapyramidal reactions
▸ *CV:* Hypotension, palpitations, bradycardia, tachycardia, extrasystoles, faintness
▸ *Resp:* *Thickening of bronchial secretions*
▸ *GI:* *Epigastric distress,* nausea, vomiting, dry mouth, jaundice
▸ *Derm:* Urticaria, rash, photosensitivity
▸ *Allergic:* **Angioneurotic edema,** dermatitis, asthma
▸ *Hematologic:* **Leukopenia, thrombocytopenia, agranulocytosis**
▸ *Misc:* Venous thrombosis at injection site

Clinically important drug–drug interactions

▸ Increased extrapyramidal effects with MAO inhibitors
▸ Additive anticholinergic effects with anticholinergic drugs
▸ Enhanced CNS depression with alcohol, narcotics, sedatives, hypnotics, TCAs, tranquilizers, barbiturates

● NURSING CONSIDERATIONS

Assessment

▸ *History:* Hypersensitivity to antihistamines or phenothiazines, coma or severe CNS depression, bone marrow depression, use of MAOIs, lower respiratory tract symptoms, asthma, emphysema, chronic bronchitis, sleep apnea, use of CNS depressants, seizure disorder, narrow-angle glaucoma, stenosing peptic ulcer, pyloroduodenal obstruction, prostatic hypertrophy, narrowing of bladder neck, impaired liver function, bone marrow depression, CV disease, hypertension, age
▸ *Physical:* T, P, BP, R, I & O, IV site, neurologic checks, skin assessment, intraocular pressure, orthostatic BP, adventitious lung sounds, sputum assessment, presence of nausea or vomiting, hydration status, bowel sounds, liver evaluation, prostate size, CBC, UA, liver and kidney function tests

Adverse effects in *Italics* are most common; those in **Bold** are life-threatening

Implementation
‣ Give IM injections deep into muscle.
‣ Do not administer SC; tissue necrosis may occur.
‣ Do not administer intra-arterially; arteriospasm and gangrene of the limb may result.
‣ Assess IV site frequently.
‣ Minimize postural hypotension by helping the patient change positions slowly.
‣ Reduce dosage of barbiturates given concurrently with promethazine by at least half; reduce dosage of narcotic analgesics given concomitantly by one-fourth to one-half.

⬤ propafenone hydrochloride
(*proe paf' a non*) Rythmol

Pregnancy Category C

Drug class
Antidysrhythmic

Indications
‣ Treatment of documented life-threatening ventricular dysrhythmias; reserve use for patients in whom the benefits outweigh the risks
‣ Unlabeled uses: treatment of supraventricular tachycardias, including atrial fibrillation and flutter; dysrhythmias associated with WPW syndrome

Therapeutic actions
‣ Class 1C antidysrhythmic: exerts local anesthetic effects with a direct membrane stabilizing action on the myocardial membranes
‣ Reduces upstroke velocity of the action potential
‣ Reduces fast inward current carried by sodium ions in Purkinje and myocardial fibers
‣ Increases diastolic excitability threshold
‣ Prolongs effective refractory period
‣ Reduces spontaneous automaticity and depresses triggered activity
‣ Exerts beta-adrenergic blocking effects
‣ Prolongs AV conduction but has little or no effect on sinus node function
‣ In patients with WPW, reduces conduction and increases the effective refractory period of the accessory pathway in both directions
‣ Exerts a negative inotropic effect on the myocardium

Adverse effects in *Italics* are most common; those in **Bold** are life-threatening

Effects on hemodynamic parameters
▸ Increased PCWP
▸ Increased SVR/PVR
▸ Decreased CO/CI

Contraindications/cautions
▸ **Contraindications:** propafenone allergy, uncontrolled CHF, cardiogenic shock; cardiac impulse generation or conduction disturbances in the absence of an artificial pacemaker; bradycardia, marked hypotension, bronchospastic disorders, manifest electrolyte imbalance
▸ **Cautions:** hepatic or renal dysfunction, elderly patients

Available forms
▸ *Tablets:* 150, 225, 300 mg

Oral dosage
▸ Initially titrate on the basis of response and tolerance.
▸ *Usual dosage:* Begin with 150 mg PO q8h. May increase at a minimum of 3- to 4-d intervals to 225 mg PO q8h and if needed, to 300 mg PO q8h. Do not exceed 900 mg/d. Decrease dosage with significant widening of the QRS complex or second- or third-degree AV block.
▸ *Elderly patients, previous myocardial damage:* Use with caution; increase dose more gradually during the initial phase of treatment.

Therapeutic serum level
▸ 0.06–1 mcg/mL

TREATMENT OF OVERDOSE/ANTIDOTE
Discontinue drug or decrease dosage. Initiate general supportive and resuscitative measures. Treat hypotension with dopamine; bradydysrhythmias with isoproterenol; convulsions with IV diazepam.

Pharmacokinetics

Route	Onset	Peak
Oral	Varies	3.5 h

Metabolism: Hepatic; $T_{1/2}$: 2–10 h
Excretion: Urine (metabolites)

Adverse effects
▸ *CNS:* **Seizures,** *dizziness,* headache, fatigue, drowsiness, insomnia, tremor, blurred vision, abnormal dreams, speech or vision disturbances, coma, confusion, depression, memory loss, numbness, paresthesias, psychosis/mania, tinnitus

Adverse effects in *Italics* are most common; those in **Bold** are life-threatening

▶ **CV: Cardiac arrest, sinus pause or arrest, ventricular tachycardia,** *first-degree AV block, intraventricular conduction disturbances,* CHF, atrial flutter, AV dissociation, sick sinus syndrome, sinus pause, supraventricular tachycardia, chest pain, bundle branch block, syncope, hypotension, bradycardia, edema

▶ **GI:** *Unusual taste, nausea, vomiting, constipation,* abdominal cramps, diarrhea, dry mouth, flatulence, dyspepsia, cholestasis, gastroenteritis, hepatitis, elevated liver enzymes

▶ **Derm:** Alopecia, pruritus, diaphoresis

▶ **Hematologic: Agranulocytosis, anemia, granulocytopenia, leukopenia, purpura, thrombocytopenia,** positive ANA, bruising

▶ **Musc/Skel:** Muscle weakness, leg cramps, muscle and joint pain

▶ **Misc: Kidney failure,** hyponatremia, nephrotic syndrome, inappropriate ADH secretion, impotence, increased glucose, dyspnea

Clinically important drug–drug interactions

▶ Increased serum levels and increased toxicity with quinidine, cimetidine

▶ Increased clearance with rifampin, resulting in decreased plasma effects and loss of therapeutic effect

▶ Increased serum levels of digoxin, warfarin

▶ Increased plasma levels and effects of beta-blockers metabolized by the liver

▶ Increased whole blood cyclosporine trough levels and decreased renal function

◉ NURSING CONSIDERATIONS

Assessment

▶ *History:* Propafenone allergy, uncontrolled CHF, cardiogenic shock, cardiac impulse generation or conduction disturbances, functioning pacemaker, hypotension, bronchospastic disorders, hepatic or renal dysfunction, age

▶ *Physical:* BP, P, R, ECG, I & O, neurologic checks, skin assessment, respiratory effort, peripheral perfusion, abdominal assessment, renal and liver function tests, CBC, serum electrolytes, ANA, serum glucose, serum propafenone level

Implementation

▶ Monitor patient response carefully, especially when beginning therapy.

▶ Drug may be prodysrhythmic; monitor closely for worsened dysrhythmias.

Adverse effects in *Italics* are most common; those in **Bold** are life-threatening

- Monitor serum drug level; adjust dosage as needed.
- Monitor ECG. May cause these ECG changes: prolonged PR interval, QRS duration, and QT interval.
- Drug may alter pacing and sensing thresholds of artificial pacemakers; monitor and program pacemakers as needed.
- May give with or without food.
- Reduce dosage with renal or liver dysfunction and with marked previous myocardial damage.

⬤ propofol *(proe' poe fol)* Diprivan
Pregnancy Category B

Drug classes
General anesthetic
Sedative-hypnotic agent

Indications
- Induction and maintenance of anesthesia
- Conscious sedation and control of stress responses in intubated or respiratory-controlled patients in ICUs

Therapeutic actions
- Causes hypnosis and amnesia
- Exact mechanism of action unknown

Effects on hemodynamic parameters
- Decreased BP
- Decreased CO
- Decreased RR or apnea

Contraindications/cautions
- **Contraindications:** propofol, soybean oil, glycerol, or egg lecithin allergy
- **Cautions:** elderly or debilitated patients, cardiovascular disease, hypovolemia, primary hyperlipoproteinemia, diabetic hyperlipidemia, pancreatitis, epilepsy, pulmonary edema, hypotension, hyperlipidemia, increased ICP, dysrhythmias

Available forms
- *IV injection:* 10 mg/mL
- *Premixed IV infusion:* 10 mg/mL

IV facts
Preparation
- *Direct IV injection:* Shake well before drawing up dose. Give undiluted.

▶ *Continuous IV infusion:* Use the premixed solution. Shake well before use. If further diluting propofol, dilute only with D5W and do not dilute to a concentration < 2 mg/mL because it is an emulsion.

Dosage and titration

▶ *ICU sedation:* 5 mcg/kg/min for at least 5 min. Administer subsequent increments of 5–10 mcg/kg/min over 5–10 min until desired level of sedation is achieved. Maintenance rates of 5–50 mcg/kg/min or higher may be required.

▶ *MAC sedation:* **Initiation:** Most patients require an infusion of 100–150 mcg/kg/min or a slow injection of 0.5 mg/kg over 3–5 min followed immediately by a maintenance infusion. Elderly, debilitated, or ASA III or IV patients require similar doses but doses must be given slowly. **Maintenance:** Most patients require 25–75 mcg/kg/min or incremental bolus doses of 10–20 mg. Reduce dose by 20% for elderly, debilitated, or ASA III or IV patients. A variable-rate infusion is preferred over intermittent bolus dosing.

▶ *Anesthesia adults < 55 y:* **Induction:** 2.0–2.5 mg/kg given as 40 mg every 10 s until induction onset. **Maintenance:** 100–200 mcg/kg/min. **Maintenance intermittent bolus:** 25–50 mg increments as needed.

▶ *Anesthesia adults > 55 y, debilitated, ASA III or IV:* **Induction:** 1.0–1.5 mg/kg given as 20 mg every 10 s until induction onset. **Maintenance:** 50–100 mcg/kg/min.

▶ *Anesthesia neurosurgical patients:* **Induction:** 1–2 mg/kg given as 20 mg every 10 s until induction onset. **Maintenance:** 100–200 mcg/kg/min.

Titration Guide

propofol									
10 mg/mL vial									

	Body Weight								
lb	88	99	110	121	132	143	154	165	176	187
kg	40	45	50	55	60	65	70	75	80	85
Dose Ordered in mcg/kg/min	**Amounts to Infuse in mL/h**								
5	1	1	2	2	2	2	2	2	2	3
10	2	3	3	3	4	4	4	5	5	5
15	4	4	5	5	5	6	6	7	7	8
20	5	5	6	7	7	8	8	9	10	10

continued

Adverse effects in *Italics* are most common; those in **Bold** are life-threatening

propofol *continued*									
10 mg/mL vial									

	Body Weight									
lb	88	99	110	121	132	143	154	165	176	187
kg	40	45	50	55	60	65	70	75	80	85
Dose Ordered in mcg/kg/min	**Amounts to Infuse in mL/h**									
25	6	7	8	8	9	10	11	11	12	13
30	7	8	9	10	11	12	13	14	14	15
35	8	9	11	12	13	14	15	16	17	18
40	10	11	12	13	14	16	17	18	19	20
45	11	12	14	15	16	18	19	20	22	23
50	12	14	15	17	18	20	21	23	24	26
60	14	16	18	20	22	23	25	27	29	31
70	17	19	21	23	25	27	29	32	34	36
80	19	22	24	26	29	31	34	36	38	41
90	22	24	27	30	32	35	38	41	43	46
100	24	27	30	33	36	39	42	45	48	51
110	26	30	33	36	40	43	46	50	53	56
120	29	32	36	40	43	47	50	54	58	61
130	31	35	39	43	47	51	55	59	62	66
140	34	38	42	46	50	55	59	63	67	71
150	36	41	45	50	54	59	63	68	72	77

	Body Weight								
lb	198	209	220	231	242	253	264	275	286
kg	90	95	100	105	110	115	120	125	130
Dose Ordered in mcg/kg/min	**Amounts to Infuse in mL/h**								
5	3	3	3	3	3	3	4	4	4
10	5	6	6	6	7	7	7	8	8
15	8	9	9	9	10	10	11	11	12
20	11	11	12	13	13	14	14	15	16
25	14	14	15	16	17	17	18	19	20
30	16	17	18	19	20	21	22	23	23
35	19	20	21	22	23	24	25	26	27
40	22	23	24	25	26	28	29	30	31
45	24	26	27	28	30	31	32	34	35
50	27	29	30	32	33	35	36	38	39
60	32	34	36	38	40	41	43	45	47
70	38	40	42	44	46	48	50	53	55
80	43	46	48	50	53	55	58	60	62
90	49	51	54	57	59	62	65	68	70
100	54	57	60	63	66	69	72	75	78

continued

Adverse effects in *Italics* are most common; those in **Bold** are life-threatening

					Body Weight				
lb	198	209	220	231	242	253	264	275	286
kg	90	95	100	105	110	115	120	125	130

propofol *continued*
10 mg/mL vial

Dose Ordered in mcg/kg/min	Amounts to Infuse in mL/h								
110	59	63	66	69	73	76	79	83	86
120	65	68	72	76	79	83	86	90	94
130	70	74	78	82	86	90	94	98	101
140	76	80	84	88	92	97	101	105	109
150	81	86	90	95	99	104	108	113	117

Compatibility

Propofol is may be given through the same IV line as D5LR; D5W/0.45% NS; D5W; LR; acyclovir, alfentanil, aminophylline, ampicillin, amrinone, aztreonam, bumetanide, buprenorphine, butorphanol, calcium gluconate, carboplatin, cefazolin, cefonicid, cefoperazone, cefotaxime, cefotetan, cefoxitin, ceftazidime, ceftizoxime, ceftriaxone, cefuroxime, chlorpromazine, cimetidine, ciprofloxacin, cisplatin, clindamycin, cyclophosphamide, cyclosporine, cytarabine, dexamethasone, digoxin, diphenhydramine, dobutamine, dopamine, doxorubicin, droperidol, enalaprilat, ephedrine, epinephrine, esmolol, famotidine, fentanyl, fluconazole, fluorouracil, furosemide, ganciclovir, glycopyrrolate, granisetron, haloperidol, heparin, hydrocortisone, hydromorphone, hydroxyzine, ifosfamide, imipenem-cilastatin, insulin (regular), isoproterenol, ketamine, labetalol, levorphanol, lidocaine, lorazepam, magnesium sulfate, mannitol, meperidine, metoclopramide, mezlocillin, miconazole, morphine, nafcillin, nalbuphine, naloxone, nitroprusside sodium, nitroglycerin, norepinephrine, ofloxacin, paclitaxel, pentobarbital, phenobarbital, piperacillin, potassium chloride, prochlorperazine, propranolol, ranitidine, scopolamine, sodium bicarbonate, succinylcholine, sufentanil, ticarcillin, ticarcillin-clavulanate, vancomycin, vecuronium, verapamil.

Incompatibility

Do not administer through the same line as amikacin, amphotericin, atracurium, bretylium, calcium chloride, diazepam, gentamicin, methotrexate, methylprednisolone, minocycline, mitoxantrone, netilmicin, phenytoin, tobramycin.

Adverse effects in *Italics* are most common; those in **Bold** are life-threatening

Pharmacokinetics

Route	Onset	Peak	Duration
IV	40 s	Unknown	3–5 min

Metabolism: Hepatic; $T_{1/2}$: 1–3 d
Excretion: Urine

Adverse effects

- *CNS:* **Seizures,** agitation, headache, chills, shivering, intracranial hypertension, somnolence
- *CV:* **AMI,** *hypotension, bradycardia,* dysrhythmias, syncope, edema
- *Resp:* **Apnea,** **bronchospasm,** *respiratory acidosis during weaning,* cough, burning in throat
- *GI:* Hypersalivation, cramping, diarrhea, vomiting, dry mouth, hiccups
- *Derm:* Rash, flushing, pruritus, diaphoresis
- *Metabolic:* *Hyperlipidemia,* dehydration, hyperglycemia; increased BUN, creatinine, and osmolality
- *Misc:* *Burning, stinging, numbness, coolness, or pain at IV site,* hives, itching, abnormal liver function, green urine, ear or eye pain

Clinically important drug–drug interactions

- Increased CNS depression with hypnotics, inhalational anesthetics, narcotics, morphine, meperidine, fentanyl, benzodiazepines, barbiturates, chloral hydrate, droperidol

● NURSING CONSIDERATIONS

Assessment

- *History:* Propofol, soybean oil, glycerol, or egg lecithin allergy; age, cardiovascular disease, hypovolemia, primary hyperlipoproteinemia, diabetic hyperlipidemia, pancreatitis, epilepsy, pulmonary edema, hyperlipidemia
- *Physical:* T, P, BP, R, ECG, SpO₂, I & O, IV site, weight, orientation, mental status, level of sedation, skin assessment, respiratory status, adventitious lung sounds, edema, abdominal assessment, presence of pain, peripheral pulses, serum electrolytes, renal function tests, ABG, serum glucose

Adverse effects in *Italics* are most common; those in **Bold** are life-threatening

Implementation

▸ Exercise extreme caution when calculating and preparing doses. Propofol is a very potent drug; small dosage errors can cause serious adverse effects.

▸ Always administer an infusion using an IV infusion pump.

▸ Use the smallest dose required to achieve desired patient response.

▸ Monitor P, BP, R, and ECG closely during infusion to monitor effectiveness of therapy.

▸ Administer into large veins of antecubital fossa, rather than hand or ankle veins, to prevent burning, pain, or stinging at the site.

▸ Correct hypovolemia before administering propofol.

▸ Propofol should be administered by people who are skilled in management of critically ill patients, cardiovascular resuscitation, and airway management.

▸ Maintain strict aseptic technique during handling because propofol is a single-use parenteral product and contains no antimicrobial preservatives.

▸ Discard solution after 12 h if administered directly from the vial or after 6 h if solution is transferred to a syringe or other container.

▸ Propofol does not affect pain threshold. Administer opioid analgesics as indicated for pain.

▸ Drug may produce apnea or respiratory depression. If patient is not on ventilator, ensure that emergency intubation equipment is readily available. Carefully monitor respiratory status.

▸ When used for ICU sedation, avoid discontinuing drug prior to weaning or for daily wake up assessments, which may result in rapid awakening with associated anxiety, agitation, and resistance to mechanical ventilation. Continue propofol to maintain a light sedation throughout the weaning process.

▸ Do not use solution if there is evidence of separation of the phases of the emulsion.

▸ Store ampules/bottles at room temperature.

● propranolol hydrochloride

(*proe pran' ah lole*) Apo-Propranolol (CAN), Betachron E-R, Inderal, Inderal LA, Novo-Pranol (CAN), PMS-Propranolol (CAN)

Pregnancy Category C

Drug classes
Beta-adrenergic blocker (nonselective)
Antianginal
Antidysrhythmic
Antihypertensive

Adverse effects in *Italics* are most common; those in **Bold** are life-threatening

Indications
▸ Cardiac dysrhythmias: SVT, ventricular tachydysrhythmias related to digitalis toxicity or excessive catecholamine action
▸ Treatment of HTN with or without other antihypertensive agents
▸ Management of exertional or stress-induced angina, palpitations, and syncope for patients with hypertrophic subaortic stenosis
▸ Long-term management of angina
▸ To decrease mortality and risk of reinfarction after AMI
▸ Adjunctive therapy for control of tachycardia related to pheochromocytoma
▸ Prophylaxis of migraine headaches
▸ Treatment of familial or hereditary essential tremor
▸ Unlabeled uses: recurrent rebleeding of esophageal varices, schizophrenia, tardive dyskinesia, acute panic symptoms, parkinsonism tremors, alcohol withdrawal syndrome, situational anxiety, GI bleeding related to portal HTN, thyrotoxicosis symptoms

Therapeutic actions
▸ Acts on β_1-(myocardial) and β_2-adrenergic (lungs, vascular) receptors to decrease the influence of the sympathetic nervous system on these tissues, the excitability of heart, myocardial contractility, cardiac workload, oxygen consumption, BP, and the release of renin
▸ Exerts a membrane-stabilizing (local anesthetic) effect that contributes to its antidysrhythmic action
▸ Acts in the CNS to reduce sympathetic outflow and vasoconstrictor tone

Effects on hemodynamic parameters
▸ Decreased BP
▸ Decreased CO
▸ Decreased HR

Contraindications/cautions
▸ **Contraindications:** beta-blocker allergy, sinus bradycardia, second- or third-degree heart block, cardiogenic shock, CHF unless secondary to a tachydysrhythmia treatable with beta-blockers, bronchial asthma, bronchospasm, COPD
▸ **Cautions:** WPW syndrome, peripheral or mesenteric vascular disease, chronic bronchitis, emphysema, bronchospastic diseases, pheochromocytoma, diabetes, hepatic or renal dysfunction, thyrotoxicosis, muscle weakness

Available forms
▸ *Injection:* 1 mg/mL
▸ *Tablets:* 10, 20, 40, 60, 80, 90 mg
▸ *SR tablets:* 60, 80, 120, 160 mg

Adverse effects in *Italics* are most common; those in **Bold** are life-threatening

- *Extended-release capsules:* 60, 80, 120, 160 mg
- *Oral solution:* 4, 8 mg/mL
- *Concentrated oral solution:* 80 mg/mL

IV facts
Preparation
- Give undiluted or dilute each 1 mg in 10 mL D5W or 0.9%NS.
- For infusion, add 1 mg to 50 mL D5W/0.45%NS; D5W/0.9%NS; D5W; LR; 0.45%NS; or 0.9%NS.

Dosage
- *IV injection:* Use only for life-threatening dysrhythmias. Usual dose is 1–3 mg IV. Do not exceed 1 mg/min to avoid hypotension and cardiac standstill. If needed, give a second dose after 2 min. Do not give another dose for 4 h. Do not give additional doses if desired rate or rhythm is achieved. Transfer to oral therapy as soon as possible.
- *IV infusion:* Infusion not generally recommended. Administer infusion of 1 mg IV over 10–15 min.

Therapeutic serum level
- 50–200 ng/mL

Compatibility
Propranolol may be given through the same IV line as alteplase, amrinone, heparin, hydrocortisone, meperidine, milrinone, morphine, potassium chloride, propofol, tacrolimus, vitamin B complex with C.

Incompatibility
Do not administer through the same IV line as diazoxide.

Oral dosage
- *HTN:* **Initial dose:** 40 mg PO bid or 80 mg PO SR/d. **Usual maintenance dose:** 120–240 mg/d PO given bid–tid or 120–160 mg/d PO SR. Maximum dose 640 mg/d.
- *Angina:* **Initial dose:** 80–320 mg PO daily dose given bid, tid, or qid or 80 mg PO SR/d. **Usual maintenance dose:** 160 mg PO SR/d. Maximum dose 320 mg/d.
- *MI:* 180–240 mg/d PO given tid–qid.
- *Dysrhythmias:* 10–30 mg PO tid–qid given ac and hs.
- *IHSS:* 20–40 mg PO tid–qid ac and hs or 80–160 mg PO SR/d.
- *Pheochromocytoma:* 60 mg/d PO in divided doses for 3 d preoperatively; for inoperable tumor, 30 mg/d in divided doses.
- *Migraines:* **Initial dose:** 80 mg PO SR/d or in divided doses. **Usual maintenance dose:** 160–240 mg/d PO in divided doses.
- *Essential tremor:* **Initial dose:** 40 mg PO bid. **Usual maintenance dose:** 120 mg/d PO. Maximum dose 320 mg/d.

Adverse effects in *Italics* are most common; those in **Bold** are life-threatening

Pharmacokinetics

Route	Onset	Peak	Duration
IV	Immediate	1 min	4–6 h
Oral	20–30 min	60–90 min	6–12 h

Metabolism: Hepatic; $T_{1/2}$: 3–5 h short acting; 8–11 h long acting
Excretion: Urine

Adverse effects

▸ *CNS:* **CVA,** *fatigue,* dizziness, vertigo, tinnitus, depression, paresthesias, sleep disturbances, hallucinations, disorientation, memory loss, slurred speech, peripheral neuropathy, paralysis, mood change, increase in symptoms of myasthenia gravis

▸ *CV:* **Ventricular dysrhythmias, cardiac arrest, cardiogenic shock, reinfarction,** AICD discharge, mitral regurgitation, ventricular septal defect, chest pain, hypertension, hypotension, pallor, peripheral ischemia, peripheral vascular insufficiency, CHF, edema, pulmonary edema, tachycardia, palpitations, arterial insufficiency, atrial dysrhythmias

▸ *Resp:* **Bronchospasm,** dyspnea, cough, bronchial obstruction, nasal stuffiness, rhinitis, pharyngitis, crackles, wheezes

▸ *GI:* **Acute pancreatitis,** *gastric/epigastric pain, flatulence, constipation, diarrhea, nausea, vomiting,* anorexia, ischemic colitis, renal and mesenteric arterial thrombosis, retroperitoneal fibrosis, hepatomegaly, elevated liver enzymes

▸ *GU:* *Impotence, decreased libido,* Peyronie's disease, dysuria, nocturia, frequency, UTI, renal failure

▸ *Derm:* Rash, pruritus, sweating, dry skin, increased pigmentation, psoriasis, peripheral skin necrosis

▸ *Allergic:* **Anaphylaxis, angioedema, laryngospasm,** pharyngitis, rash, fever, sore throat, respiratory distress

Adverse effects in *Italics* are most common; those in **Bold** are life-threatening

▶ *Musc/Skel:* Joint pain, arthralgia, muscle cramps, twitching/tremor
▶ *EENT:* Eye irritation, dry eyes, conjunctivitis, blurred vision
▶ *Misc: Decreased exercise tolerance,* facial swelling, weight gain or loss, Raynaud's phenomenon, gout, lupus syndrome, hyperglycemia or hypoglycemia, development of antinuclear antibodies

Clinically important drug–drug interactions

▶ Increased effects with calcium channel-blockers, quinidine, oral contraceptives, loop diuretics, prazosin
▶ Decreased effects with thyroid hormones, nonsteroidal anti-inflammatory drugs
▶ Hypotension and cardiac arrest with haloperidol
▶ Rate of absorption slowed by ethanol and reduced by aluminum hydroxide gel
▶ Accelerated clearance with phenytoin, phenobarbitone, rifampin
▶ Use with chlorpromazine increases plasma levels of both drugs
▶ Reduced clearance of antipyrine, lidocaine, acetaminophen
▶ Increased blood levels with cimetidine
▶ Increased serum levels and effect with phenothiazines, flecainide
▶ Hypertension followed by severe bradycardia with epinephrine
▶ Life-threatening HTN when clonidine is discontinued for patients on beta-blocker therapy or when both drugs are discontinued simultaneously
▶ Reduced insulin release in response to hyperglycemia
▶ Use with theophylline may reduce theophylline elimination or reduce effectiveness of both drugs
▶ May potentiate, counteract, or have no effect on nondepolarizing muscle relaxants
▶ Increased anticoagulant effects of warfarin

● NURSING CONSIDERATIONS

Assessment

▶ *History:* Beta-blocker allergy, cardiogenic shock, CHF, bronchial asthma, bronchospasm, COPD, WPW syndrome, peripheral or mesenteric vascular disease, chronic bronchitis, emphysema, bronchospastic diseases, pheochromocytoma, diabetes, hepatic or renal dysfunction, thyrotoxicosis, muscle weakness, angina
▶ *Physical:* T, P, BP, R, ECG, I & O, weight, neurologic checks, vision, skin assessment, cardiac auscultation, chest pain assessment, edema, JVD, respiratory effort, adventitious lung sounds, bowel sounds, serum electrolytes, UA, serum glucose, CBC; thyroid, liver, and renal function tests

Adverse effects in *Italics* are most common; those in **Bold** are life-threatening

Implementation

- Exercise extreme caution when calculating and preparing doses. Propranolol is a very potent drug; small dosage errors can cause serious adverse effects.
- Always administer infusion using an IV infusion pump.
- Carefully monitor P, BP, R, ECG, and CVP during IV administration.
- Have emergency equipment (defibrillator, drugs, oxygen, intubation equipment) on standby in case anaphylaxis or adverse reaction occurs.
- Do not discontinue drug abruptly after chronic therapy. (Hypersensitivity to catecholamines may have developed, causing exacerbation of angina, MI, ventricular dysrhythmias.) Taper drug gradually over 2 wk with monitoring.
- Consult with physician about withdrawing drug if patient is to undergo surgery (withdrawal is controversial).
- Give oral forms with food to facilitate absorption.

● protamine sulfate *(proe' ta meen)*

Pregnancy Category C

Drug class
Heparin antagonist

Indication
- Treatment of heparin overdose

Therapeutic actions
- When given alone, has a weak anticoagulant effect
- In the presence of heparin, forms a stable salt that results in loss of anticoagulant activity of both drugs

Contraindications/cautions
- **Contraindications:** protamine sulfate or fish product allergy
- **Cautions:** surgery on cardiopulmonary bypass, previous exposure to protamine, prior use of protamine-containing insulins, infertile or vasectomized men

Available form
- *IV injection:* 10 mg/mL

IV facts
Preparation
- *Ampules:* Drug is ready for use; may be further diluted in D5W or 0.9%NS.
- *Vials:* Reconstitute powder with Bacteriostatic Water or Sterile Water for Injection. Add 5 mL to the 50-mg vial or 25 mL to the 250-mg vial to achieve a concentration of 10 mg/mL. Shake vigorously until dissolved. May be further diluted in D5W or 0.9%NS. Use immediately.

Adverse effects in *Italics* are most common; those in **Bold** are life-threatening

Dosage and titration
▶ Dosage is determined by the amount of heparin in the body and the time that has elapsed since heparin was given; the longer the interval, the smaller the dose required. 1 mg IV neutralizes 90 USP U heparin derived from lung tissue or 115 USP U of heparin derived from intestinal mucosa. Administer each dose IV over 10 min. Because of its anticoagulant effect, avoid giving > 50 mg in 10 min.

Incompatibility
Do not administer through the same IV line as cephalosporins or penicillins.

> **TREATMENT OF OVERDOSE/ANTIDOTE**
> Discontinue drug. Initiate general supportive and resuscitative measures. Replace blood loss with transfusions or FFP. If patient is hypotensive, consider fluids, epinephrine, dobutamine, or dopamine.

Pharmacokinetics

Route	Onset	Duration
IV	Within 5 min	2 h

Metabolism: May be metabolized or degraded

Adverse effects
▶ *CV:* **Circulatory collapse, myocardial failure, *hypotension*,** bradycardia
▶ *Resp:* **Noncardiogenic pulmonary edema, respiratory distress, acute pulmonary HTN**
▶ *Hypersensitivity:* **Anaphylaxis**
▶ *GI:* Nausea, vomiting
▶ *Misc:* Bleeding, flushing, warm feeling, back pain

⬤ NURSING CONSIDERATIONS

Assessment
▶ *History:* Protamine sulfate or fish allergy, surgery on cardiopulmonary bypass, previous protamine exposure, prior use of protamine-containing insulins, infertile or vasectomized males, amount and last time heparin received
▶ *Physical:* T, P, BP, R, ECG, skin assessment, orientation, peripheral perfusion, respiratory effort, adventitious lung sounds, presence of bleeding, CBC, ACT, PTT

Implementation
▶ Discontinue heparin administration.
▶ Correct hypovolemia before administering drug.
▶ Have emergency equipment (defibrillator, drugs, oxygen, in-

Adverse effects in *Italics* are most common; those in **Bold** are life-threatening

tubation equipment) on standby in case anaphylaxis or adverse reaction occurs.
▪ Monitor coagulation studies to adjust dosage and to screen for heparin "rebound" and response to drug.
▪ Monitor patient for bleeding or hemorrhage.
▪ Store drug in refrigerator; do not store diluted solutions; they contain no preservatives.

● pyridostigmine bromide
(peer id oh stig' meen) Mestinon, Regonol

Drug classes
Cholinesterase inhibitor
Antidote
Antimyasthenic agent

Indications
▪ Treatment of myasthenia gravis
▪ Reversal of nondepolarizing muscle relaxants

Therapeutic actions
▪ Facilitates transmission of impulses across the myoneural junction by inhibiting the destruction of acetylcholine by cholinesterase

Contraindications/cautions
▪ **Contraindications:** anticholinesterase allergy, mechanical intestinal or urinary obstructions, history of reaction to bromides
▪ **Cautions:** bronchial asthma, epilepsy, bradycardia, recent coronary occlusion, vagotonia, hyperthyroidism, dysrhythmias, peptic ulcer

Available forms
▪ *Injection:* 5 mg/mL
▪ *Tablets:* 60 mg
▪ *SR tablets:* 180 mg
▪ *Syrup:* 60 mg/5 mL

IV/IM facts
Preparation
▪ Give undiluted.

Dosage
▪ *Antidote for nondepolarizing neuromuscular blocking agents:* Give atropine 0.6–1.2 mg IV several minutes before pyridostigmine. Reversal doses range from 0.1–0.25 mg/kg. Pyridostigmine 10–20 mg IV given slowly usually suffices. Full recovery usually occurs ≤ 15 min but ≥ 30 min may be required.

Adverse effects in *Italics* are most common; those in **Bold** are life-threatening

▸ *Myasthenia gravis:* Give ⅙₀ the oral dose slow IV or IM. Observe for cholinergic reactions.

P

Compatibility

Pyridostigmine may be given through the same IV line as heparin, hydrocortisone, potassium chloride, vitamin B complex with C.

Oral dosage

▸ *Tablets:* 600 mg/d PO spaced to provide maximum relief. Range is 60–1500 mg/d.
▸ *SR tablets:* 180–540 mg PO qd or bid. Use dosage intervals of ≥ 6 h. For optimum control, rapidly acting regular tablets or oral elixir may also be needed.

> **TREATMENT OF OVERDOSE/ANTIDOTE**
> Discontinue drug or decrease dosage. Initiate general supportive and resuscitative measures. Discontinue all cholinergic drugs. Give 0.5–1 mg atropine IV. A total atropine dose of 5–10 mg or more may be required.

Pharmacokinetics

Route	Onset	Duration
IV	2–5 min	2–4 h
IM	< 15 min	2–4 h
PO	20–30 min	3–6 h

Metabolism: Hepatic, cholinesterases; $T_{1/2}$: 1.9 h
Excretion: Urine

Adverse effects

▸ *CNS:* **Seizures,** *twitch,* dysarthria, dysphonia, dizziness, headache, loss of consciousness, drowsiness
▸ *CV:* **Cardiac arrest,** dysrhythmias (bradycardia, heart block, nodal rhythm), nonspecific ECG changes, syncope, decreased CO leading to hypotension
▸ *Resp:* **Respiratory arrest; respiratory muscle paralysis, central respiratory paralysis,** *increased tracheobronchial secretions;* bronchospasm; dyspnea, respiratory depression
▸ *GI:* *Salivation, nausea, vomiting, flatulence, increased peristalsis, bowel cramps, diarrhea*
▸ *Derm:* Rash, urticaria
▸ *Allergic:* **Anaphylaxis**
▸ *Musc/Skel:* Muscle cramps, spasms, arthralgia
▸ *Misc:* Diaphoresis, flushing, weakness; thrombophlebitis (IV)

Clinically important drug–drug interactions

▸ Accentuated neuromuscular blockade with antibiotics, such as neomycin, streptomycin, kanamycin

Adverse effects in *Italics* are most common; those in **Bold** are life-threatening

- Decreased anticholinesterase effects with corticosteroids; increased anticholinesterase effects after stopping corticosteroids
- Inhibited with magnesium
- Additive effects with anticholinesterase muscle stimulants

● NURSING CONSIDERATIONS

Assessment

- *History:* Anticholinesterase or bromide allergy, mechanical intestinal or urinary obstruction, bronchial asthma, epilepsy, recent coronary occlusion, vagotonia, hyperthyroidism, dysrhythmias, peptic ulcer
- *Physical:* P, BP, R, ECG, I & O, neurologic checks, reflexes, muscle strength, vision, skin assessment, cardiac auscultation, respiratory effort, adventitious lung sounds, vital capacity, abdominal percussion, bowel sounds, voiding patterns, serum electrolytes, thyroid function tests

Implementation

- Carefully monitor P, BP, R, and ECG.
- Have emergency equipment (defibrillator, drugs, oxygen, intubation equipment) on standby in case anaphylaxis or adverse reaction occurs.
- When used as an antidote for nondepolarizing neuromuscular blocking agents, keep the patient well ventilated, and maintain a patent airway until complete recovery. Give drug when patient is being hyperventilated and the carbon dioxide level of blood is low. Titrate dose using a peripheral nerve stimulator.
- Overdosage with anticholinesterase drugs can cause muscle weakness (cholinergic crisis) that is difficult to differentiate from myasthenic weakness. The administration of atropine may mask the parasympathetic effects of anticholinesterase overdose and further confound the diagnosis.
- Notify physician if nausea, vomiting, diarrhea, excessive sweating, increased salivation, irregular heartbeat, muscle weakness, severe abdominal pain, or dyspnea occurs.
- Do not crush or allow the patient to chew SR tablets.

● **quinupristin/dalfopristin**
*(kwin you **pris'** tin/dal foh **pris'** tin)* Synercid I.V.

Pregnancy Category B

Drug class
Antibacterial: streptogramin

Indications
▶ Serious or life-threatening infections associated with van-comycin-resistant *Enterococcus faecium* bacteremia
▶ Complicated skin and skin structure infections caused by *Staphylococcus aureus* (methicillin-susceptible) or *Streptococcus pyogenes*

Therapeutic actions
▶ Quinupristin and dalfopristin act synergistically; together their activity is greater than that of the components individually
▶ Bacteriostatic against *E. faecium*
▶ Bactericidal against strains of methicillin-susceptible and me-thicillin-resistant staphylococci
▶ Acts on the bacterial ribosome: quinupristin inhibits the late phase of protein synthesis; dalfopristin inhibits the early phase of protein synthesis

Contraindications/cautions
▶ **Contraindications:** quinupristin or dalfopristin allergy, hypersensitivity to other streptogramins
▶ **Cautions:** hepatic function impairment

Available form
▶ **Powder for injection:** 500 mg (150 mg quinupristin; 350 mg dalfopristin)

IV facts
Preparation
▶ Reconstitute under strict aseptic conditions (eg, Laminar Air Flow Hood).
▶ Slowly add 5 mL of D5W or Sterile Water for Injection. Gently swirl the vial without shaking to ensure dissolution of the contents while limiting foam formation. Allow the solution to sit for a few minutes until all the foam has disappeared. The resulting solution should be clear. Dilute the reconstituted solution within 30 min.
▶ Add the correct dosage of the reconstituted solution to 250 mL of D5W. An infusion volume of 100 mL may be used for central line infusions.

Dosage
▶ *Vancomycin-resistant E. faecium:* 7.5 mg/kg IV q8h. Give over 1 h. Base treatment duration on the site and severity of the infection.
▶ *Complicated skin and skin structure infection:* 7.5 mg/kg IV q12h. Give over 1 h. The minimum recommended treatment duration is 7 d.

Adverse effects in *Italics* are most common; those in **Bold** are life-threatening

Compatibility
Quinupristin/dalfopristin may be given through the same IV line as aztreonam, ciprofloxacin, fluconazole, haloperidol, metoclopramide, potassium chloride 40 mEq/L.

Incompatibility
Do not administer through the same IV line as heparin or saline solutions.

> **TREATMENT OF OVERDOSE/ANTIDOTE**
> Discontinue drug or decrease dosage. Initiate general supportive and resuscitative measures.

Pharmacokinetics

Route	Onset	Peak
IV	Rapid	0.9 h

$T_{1/2}$: 3.07 h (quinupristin); 1.04 h (dalfopristin)
Excretion: Feces, urine

Adverse effects
- *CNS:* Headache, anxiety, confusion, dizziness, hypertonia, insomnia, parasthesia, vasodilation
- *CV:* Chest pain, palpitations
- *Resp:* Dyspnea, pleural effusion
- *GI:* **Pseudomembranous colitis, pancreatitis,** nausea, vomiting, diarrhea, constipation, dyspepsia, oral moniliasis, stomatitis, abdominal pain; elevated bilirubin, AST, ALT, LDH
- *GU:* Hematuria, vaginitis
- *Derm: Inflammation, pain, and edema at infusion site; infusion site reaction, thrombophlebitis,* maculopapular rash, sweating, urticaria, pruritus
- *Allergic:* **Allergic reaction**
- *Musc/Skel:* Arthralgia, myalgia, myasthenia
- *Misc:* Gout, peripheral edema, pain, superinfections, worsening of illness, fever

Clinically important drug–drug interactions
- Increased half-life and levels of cyclosporine
- Increased plasma concentrations of nifedipine, midazolam
- May increase plasma concentrations of antihistamines, such as astemizole, terfenadine; Anti-HIV drugs, such as delavirdine, nevirapine, indinavir, ritonavir; antineoplastic agents, such as vinca alkaloids, docetaxel, paclitaxel; calcium channel-blockers, such as verapamil, diltiazem; HMG-CoA reductase inhibitors, such as lovastatin; GI motility agents, such as cisapride; immunosuppressive agents, such as tacrolimus;

Adverse effects in *Italics* are most common; those in **Bold** are life-threatening

steroids, such as methylprednisolone; carbamazepine, quinidine, lidocaine, and disopyramide
▸ Avoid concomitant use of drugs metabolized by the cytochrome P450 3A4 enzyme system, which may prolong the QTc interval

◉ NURSING CONSIDERATIONS

Assessment
▸ *History:* Quinupristin or dalfopristin allergy, hypersensitivity to other streptogramins, hepatic function impairment
▸ *Physical:* T, P, R, BP, I & O, IV site, neurologic checks, skin assessment, respiratory status, pain assessment, abdominal assessment, bowel sounds, culture and sensitivity tests of infected area, liver function tests, UA, CBC

Implementation
▸ Obtain specimens for culture and sensitivity of infected area before beginning therapy. May begin drug before results are available.
▸ Have emergency equipment (defibrillator, drugs, oxygen, intubation equipment) on standby in case an allergic reaction occurs.
▸ Assess for evidence of an allergic reaction; if suspected, discontinue drug immediately and notify provider.
▸ If moderate-to-severe venous irritation occurs following peripheral administration of the drug diluted in 250 mL of D5W, consider increasing the infusion volume to 500 or 750 mL, changing the infusion site, or infusing by a peripherally inserted central catheter or central venous catheter.
▸ When giving as an intermittent infusion, flush the line before and after administration with D5W. *Do not* flush with heparin or saline solutions.
▸ Monitor renal function tests.
▸ Use caution when giving other drugs that are primarily metabolized by the cytochrome P450 3A4 enzyme system. The potential increased plasma concentrations of these drugs may increase or prolong their therapeutic effect or increase adverse reactions.
▸ Monitor for occurrence of superinfections; treat as appropriate.
▸ Discontinue drug at any sign of colitis; initiate appropriate supportive treatment.
▸ Vials are for single use. Diluted solution is stable for 5 h at room temperature or 54 h if refrigerated. Do not freeze the solution.

Adverse effects in *Italics* are most common; those in **Bold** are life-threatening

R

 ranitidine *(ra nye' te deen)* Alti-Ranitidine (CAN),
Novo-Ranidine (CAN), Nu-Ranit (CAN), Zantac,
Zantac EFFERdose, Zantac GELdose, Zantac 75

Pregnancy Category B

Drug class
Histamine H_2 antagonist

Indications
▸ Short-term and maintenance treatment of duodenal ulcer
▸ Short-term treatment (benign, active) and maintenance therapy of gastric ulcer
▸ Short-term treatment of GERD
▸ Treatment of pathological hypersecretory conditions (eg, Zollinger-Ellison syndrome, systemic mastocytosis, multiple endocrine adenomas)
▸ Treatment of erosive esophagitis; maintenance of healing erosive esophagitis
▸ Symptomatic relief of heartburn
▸ Unlabeled uses: prevention of upper GI bleeding and peptic ulcer, aspiration pneumonitis, and gastric NSAID damage; prophylaxis of stress ulcers

Therapeutic actions
▸ Competitively inhibits the action of histamine at the histamine (H_2) receptors of the parietal cells of the stomach, inhibiting basal gastric acid secretion and gastric acid secretion that is stimulated by food, insulin, histamine, cholinergic agonists, gastrin, and pentagastrin
▸ Reversibly and competitively blocks histamine at the H_2 receptors, especially those in the gastric parietal cells
▸ Inhibits secretions caused by histamine, muscarinic agonists, and gastrin
▸ Inhibits fasting and nocturnal secretions and secretions caused by food, insulin, caffeine, pentagastrin, and betazole
▸ Reduces volume and hydrogen ion concentration of gastric juice
▸ Affects the microsomal enzyme system
▸ Increases gastric nitrate-reducing organisms, increases serum prolactin after IV injections, and may impair vasopressin release

---

Adverse effects in *Italics* are most common; those in **Bold** are life-threatening

R

Contraindications/cautions
▸ **Contraindications:** ranitidine allergy
▸ **Caution:** impaired renal or hepatic function

Available forms
▸ *Injection:* 25 mg/mL
▸ *Premixed injection:* 0.5 mg/mL in 100 mL 0.45%NS
▸ *Tablets:* 75, 150, 300 mg
▸ *Capsules:* 150, 300 mg
▸ *Effervescent tablets and granules:* 150 mg
▸ *Syrup:* 15 mg/mL

IV/IM facts
Preparation
▸ *Direct IV injection:* Dilute 50 mg in D5W/0.45%NS; D5W; D10W; LR; 0.9%NS; or Sodium Bicarbonate 5% to a total volume of 20 mL.
▸ *Intermittent IV infusion:* Use premixed solution or dilute 50 mg in 100 mL of a compatible IV solution (see above).
▸ *Continuous IV infusion:* Dilute 150 mg in 250 mL of a compatible IV fluid (see above). For Zollinger-Ellison patients, use concentration ≤ 2.5 mg/mL.
▸ *IM:* Give undiluted.

Dosage
▸ *Pathological hypersecretory conditions/intractable ulcers/ patients unable to take oral medications:* **Direct injection:** 50 mg q6–8h IV at rate not greater than 4 mL/min. **Intermittent IV infusion:** 50 mg IV solution q6–8h IV. Infuse at a rate no greater than 5–7 mL/min. Do not exceed 400 mg/d. **Continuous IV infusion:** 6.25 mg/h IV. May precede with a 150-mg IV loading dose. For Zollinger-Ellison patients, start infusion at 1 mg/kg/h. After 4 h, measure gastric acid output. If output > 10 mEq/h or if patient is symptomatic, increase dose in 0.5 mg/kg/h increments. Dosages up to 2.5 mg/kg/h have been used. **IM:** 50 mg q6–8h IM.
▸ *Renal impairment:* If creatine clearance < 50 mL/min, give 50 mg IV or IM q18–24h. May increase to q12h with caution. Give scheduled dose at end of hemodialysis.

Compatibility
Ranitidine may be given through the same IV line as acyclovir, aldesleukin, allopurinol, amifostine, aminophylline, amsacrine, atracurium, aztreonam, bretylium, cefepime, cefmetazole,

---

Adverse effects in *Italics* are most common; those in **Bold** are life-threatening

ceftazidime, ciprofloxacin, cisplatin, cladribine, cyclophos-phamide, cytarabine, diltiazem, dobutamine, dopamine, dox-orubicin, enalaprilat, epinephrine, esmolol, filgrastim, flucona-zole, fludarabine, foscarnet, furosemide, gallium, granisetron, heparin, hydromorphone, idarubicin, labetalol, lorazepam, melphalan, meperidine, methotrexate, midazolam, milrinone, morphine, nicardipine, nitroglycerin, norepinephrine, ondan-setron, paclitaxel, pancuronium, piperacillin, piperacillin-tazobactam, procainamide, sargramostim, tacrolimus, tenipo-side, theophylline, thiopental, thiotepa, vecuronium, vin-orelbine, warfarin, zidovudine.

Oral dosage
- *Active duodenal ulcer:* 150 mg PO bid or 300 mg/d PO at hs.
- *Maintenance therapy, duodenal ulcer:* 150 mg PO at hs.
- *Active, benign gastric ulcer:* 150 mg PO bid.
- *Maintenance therapy, gastric ulcer:* 150 mg PO at hs.
- *Pathological hypersecretory syndrome:* 150 mg PO bid. Indi-vidualize dose with patient's response. More frequent doses may be needed. Do not exceed 6 g/d.
- *GERD:* 150 mg PO bid.
- *Treatment, erosive esophagitis:* 150 mg PO qid.
- *Maintenance, erosive esophagitis:* 150 mg PO bid.
- *Treatment of heartburn, acid indigestion:* 75 mg PO as needed.
- *Renal impairment:* If creatine clearance < 50 mL/min, 150 mg PO q24h. May increase to q12h with caution. Give sched-uled dose at end of hemodialysis.

TREATMENT OF OVERDOSE/ANTIDOTE
Discontinue drug or decrease dosage. Initiate general sup-portive and resuscitative measures. Remove unabsorbed drug from GI tract. Hemodialysis reduces levels of circulat-ing ranitidine.

Pharmacokinetics

Route	Onset	Peak	Duration
IV	Immediate	15 min	6–8 h
IM	Rapid	15 min	6–8 h
Oral	Varies	1–3 h	8–12 h

Metabolism: Hepatic; $T_{1/2}$: 2.5–3 h
Excretion: Urine

Adverse effects
- *CNS:* Headache, malaise, dizziness, somnolence, insomnia, vertigo, agitation, anxiety

Adverse effects in *Italics* are most common; those in **Bold** are life-threatening

R

- **CV: Asystole, cardiac arrest,** tachycardia, bradycardia, AV block, PVCs (rapid IV administration)
- **GI:** Constipation, diarrhea, nausea, vomiting, abdominal pain, hepatitis, increased ALT
- **GU:** Gynecomastia, impotence, loss of libido
- **Derm:** *Pain at IM site, local burning or itching at IV site;* rash, alopecia
- **Allergic: Anaphylaxis, bronchospasm,** fever, rash, eosinophilia
- **Hematologic: Leukopenia, granulocytopenia, thrombocytopenia, pancytopenia**
- **Misc:** Arthralgia

Clinically important drug–drug interactions
- Decreased renal clearance of procainamide
- Decreased effectiveness of diazepam
- Increased hypoglycemic effect of glipizide
- Increased plasma ethanol levels
- Decreased absorption with antacids

◉ NURSING CONSIDERATIONS

Assessment
- *History:* Ranitidine allergy, impaired renal or hepatic function
- *Physical:* T, P, BP, R, ECG, I & O, IV site, neurologic checks, skin assessment, adventitious lung sounds, respiratory effort, liver evaluation, abdominal exam, presence of pain, gastric pH, CBC, liver and renal function tests, emesis and stool guaiac

Implementation
- Monitor ECG and BP closely during IV administration.
- Do not administer simultaneously with antacids.
- Administer IM dose undiluted, deep into a large muscle group.

◉ **reteplase** *(ret' ah place)* r-PA
   Retavase

Pregnancy Category C

Drug class
Thrombolytic enzyme

Indication
- Management of AMI to improve ventricular function, reduce CHF, and reduce mortality

Therapeutic actions
- Mutein of tPA produced by recombinant DNA techniques
- Catalyzes cleavage of plasminogen to generate plasmin
- Plasmin degrades the fibrin matrix of thrombus

Adverse effects in *Italics* are most common; those in **Bold** are life-threatening

Contraindications/cautions
▸ **Contraindications:** tPA allergy, active internal bleeding, history of CVA, recent intracranial or intraspinal surgery or trauma; intracranial neoplasm, arteriovenous malformation or aneurysm; bleeding diathesis, severe uncontrolled hypertension
▸ **Cautions:** severe renal or liver dysfunction, advanced age; recent (≤ 10 d) major surgery (CABG, organ biopsy, obstetric delivery); puncture of noncompressible vessels; recent GI or GU bleeding, recent trauma; hypertension (≥ 180 mmHg systolic or ≥ 110 mmHg diastolic); left heart thrombus, acute pericarditis, subacute bacterial endocarditis, hemostatic defects secondary to severe hepatic or renal disease; diabetic hemorrhagic retinopathy or other ophthalmic hemorrhaging; septic thrombophlebitis; occluded AV cannula at seriously infected site; current oral anticoagulant therapy; other conditions in which bleeding is a hazard or would be difficult to manage

Available form
▸ *Powder for injection:* 10.8 IU

IV facts
Preparation
▸ Reconstitute only with provided Sterile Water for Injection (without preservatives) immediately before use.
▸ Slight foaming may occur with reconstitution but should dissipate when left undisturbed for several minutes.
▸ Reconstituted solution is colorless containing 1 U/mL.

Dosage
▸ *AMI:* 10 U + 10 U double-bolus IV injection, each IV over 2 min; give second bolus 30 min after start of first.

Compatibility
Do not mix reteplase with any other drugs or give through an IV line simultaneously with other drugs.

Incompatibility
Reteplase is incompatible with heparin. If IV line contains heparin, flush lines with D5W or 0.9%NS prior to and following reteplase injection.

TREATMENT OF OVERDOSE/ANTIDOTE
Discontinue drug and any other anticoagulant or antiplatelet drugs if severe bleeding, neurologic changes, or
(treatment continued on next page)

Adverse effects in *Italics* are most common; those in **Bold** are life-threatening

severe hypotension occurs. Initiate general supportive and
resuscitative measures. Administer IV fluids, PRBCs, FFP,
platelets, and cryoprecipitate as indicated. Aminocaproic
acid may be given as an antidote.

R

Pharmacokinetics

Route	Onset	Peak
IV	Immediate	End of Infusion

$T_{1/2}$: 13–16 min
Excretion: Cleared by liver and kidneys

Adverse effects

▶ *CNS:* **Intracranial hemorrhage**
▶ *CV:* **Cardiogenic shock, heart failure, cardiac arrest, reinfarction, myocardial rupture, cardiac tamponade,
electromechanical dissociation, cholesterol embolism,
dysrhythmias,** *reperfusion dysrhythmias,* pulmonary
edema, recurrent ischemia, pericarditis, pericardial effusion,
mitral regurgitation, hypotension
▶ *GI:* **GI bleeding,** nausea, vomiting
▶ *GU:* **GU bleeding**
▶ *Allergic:* **Anaphylaxis**
▶ *Hematologic:* **Bleeding** (especially at venous or arterial access sites), anemia
▶ *Misc:* Urticaria, nausea, vomiting, fever

Clinically important drug–drug interactions

▶ Increased hemorrhage with vitamin K antagonists, heparin,
oral anticoagulants, drugs that alter platelet function (aspirin,
dipyridamole, abciximab, tirofiban, eptifibatide, ticlopidine,
clopidogrel)

● NURSING CONSIDERATIONS

Assessment

▶ *History:* tPA allergy; active internal bleeding, history of CVA,
recent intracranial or intraspinal surgery or trauma; intracranial neoplasm, arteriovenous malformation or aneurysm;
bleeding diathesis; severe uncontrolled hypertension; severe
renal or liver dysfunction; age; recent CABG, organ biopsy,
obstetric delivery; recent puncture of noncompressible vessels; recent GI or GU bleeding; recent trauma; left heart
thrombus, acute pericarditis, subacute bacterial endocarditis;
hemostatic defects secondary to severe hepatic or renal disease; diabetic hemorrhagic retinopathy or other ophthalmic

Adverse effects in *Italics* are most common; those in **Bold** are life-threatening

hemorrhaging; septic thrombophlebitis, occluded AV cannula at seriously infected site, current oral anticoagulant therapy; other conditions in which bleeding is a hazard or would be difficult to manage

▸ *Physical:* T, P, R, BP, ECG, I & O, IV site, neurologic checks, skin assessment, peripheral perfusion, presence of bleeding, chest pain assessment, cardiac auscultation, JVD, peripheral perfusion, adventitious lung sounds, liver evaluation, CBC, CPK, cardiac troponin, myoglobin, TT, APTT, PT, INR, FSP, type and crossmatch; urine, stool, and emesis guaiac

Implementation

▸ Administer drug as soon as possible after diagnosis. Initiate within 6 h after onset of AMI symptoms.
▸ Have emergency equipment (defibrillator, drugs, oxygen, intubation equipment) on standby in case anaphylaxis, hemorrhage, or adverse reaction occurs.
▸ Before starting drug, initiate at least 2–3 peripheral IVs.
▸ Assess for chest pain (type, character, location, intensity, radiation). Continuously monitor ECG before, during, and after therapy for evidence of reperfusion (decreased chest pain, decreased ST segment elevation, reperfusion dysrhythmias) and dysrhythmias.
▸ Assess for ST segment changes.
▸ Monitor BP, P, R, and neurologic status continuously.
▸ Initiate other interventions as standard for patients with AMI.
▸ Heparin is often administered with reteplase.
▸ Type and crossmatch blood in case serious blood loss occurs and blood transfusions are required.
▸ Initiate bleeding precautions.
▸ Assess patient for evidence of bleeding and hemorrhage.
▸ Carefully assess recent puncture sites and sites of lines/tubes (catheter insertion sites, cutdown sites, needle puncture sites, recent surgical incisions).
▸ Apply pressure to arterial and venous puncture sites for at least 30 min or until hemostasis is achieved. Apply a pressure dressing to site to prevent bleeding. Assess all puncture sites q15min.
▸ Avoid IM injections before, during, and for 24 h after therapy. Do not attempt central venous access or arterial puncture unless absolutely necessary. If arterial puncture is necessary, use an upper extremity vessel that is accessible to manual pressure.
▸ Guaiac all stools, urine, and emesis for blood.
▸ Handle patient carefully to avoid ecchymosis and bleeding.
▸ If possible, draw blood for laboratory analysis from an existing saline lock.

▸ Take BP with manual BP cuff or ensure that NIBP cuff does not inflate excessively above patient's SBP.
▸ Shave patient with an electric razor.
▸ Use solution within 4 h after reconstitution.
▸ Keep kit sealed prior to use to protect drug from light.

● rocuronium bromide (roh kyou rob' nee um)
Zemuron

Pregnancy Category B

Drug class
Nondepolarizing neuromuscular blocking agent

Indications
▸ Adjunct to general anesthesia to facilitate intubation
▸ To provide skeletal muscle relaxation during surgery or mechanical ventilation

Therapeutic actions
▸ Prevents neuromuscular transmission and produces paralysis by blocking effect of acetylcholine at the myoneural junction

Contraindications/cautions
▸ **Contraindications:** rocuronium or bromide allergy
▸ **Cautions:** myasthenia gravis, cirrhosis, cholestasis, cardiovascular disease, elderly patients, edema, severe obesity, neuromuscular disease, malignant hyperthermia, electrolyte imbalance, respiratory depression, pulmonary disease

Available form
▸ *IV injection:* 10 mg/mL

IV facts
Preparation
▸ *Direction IV injection:* May give undiluted.
▸ *Continuous IV infusion:* Dilute 100 mg in 100 mL D5W/0.9%NS; D5W; LR; 0.9%NS; or Sterile Water for Injection.

Dosage and titration
▸ *Initial adult bolus dose for intubation:* 600–1200 mcg/kg IV.
▸ *Maintenance dose:* Begin IV infusion at 10–12 mcg/kg/min beginning after early evidence of recovery from intubating dose. Dose range is 4–16 mcg/kg/min. Titrate infusion to maintain a 90% suppression of patient's twitch response as determined by peripheral nerve stimulation.

Adverse effects in *Italics* are most common; those in **Bold** are life-threatening

Titration Guide

	rocuronium bromide									
	100 mg in 100 mL									
	Body Weight									
lb	88	99	110	121	132	143	154	165	176	187
kg	40	45	50	55	60	65	70	75	80	85
Dose Ordered in mcg/kg/min	**Amounts to Infuse in mL/h**									
4	10	11	12	13	14	16	17	18	19	20
5	12	14	15	17	18	20	21	23	24	26
6	14	16	18	20	22	23	25	27	29	31
7	17	19	21	23	25	27	29	32	34	36
8	19	22	24	26	29	31	34	36	38	41
9	22	24	27	30	32	35	38	41	43	46
10	24	27	30	33	36	39	42	45	48	51
11	26	30	33	36	40	43	46	50	53	56
12	29	32	36	40	43	47	50	54	58	61
13	31	35	39	43	47	51	55	59	62	66
14	34	38	42	46	50	55	59	63	67	71
15	36	41	45	50	54	59	63	68	72	77
16	38	43	48	53	58	62	67	72	77	82

	Body Weight								
lb	198	209	220	231	242	253	264	275	286
kg	90	95	100	105	110	115	120	125	130
Dose Ordered in mcg/kg/min	**Amounts to Infuse in mL/h**								
4	22	23	24	25	26	28	29	30	31
5	27	29	30	32	33	35	36	38	39
6	32	34	36	38	40	41	43	45	47
7	38	40	42	44	46	48	50	53	55
8	43	46	48	50	53	55	58	60	62
9	49	51	54	57	59	62	65	68	70
10	54	57	60	63	66	69	72	75	78
11	59	63	66	69	73	76	79	83	86
12	65	68	72	76	79	83	86	90	94
13	70	74	78	82	86	90	94	98	101
14	76	80	84	88	92	97	101	105	109
15	81	86	90	95	99	104	108	113	117
16	86	91	96	101	106	110	115	120	125

Incompatibility

Do not administer through the same IV line as alkaline solutions or barbiturates.

Adverse effects in *Italics* are most common; those in **Bold** are life-threatening

TREATMENT OF OVERDOSE/ANTIDOTE
Discontinue drug or decrease dosage. Initiate general supportive and resuscitative measures. Continue to maintain a patent airway and provide mechanical ventilation. Pyridostigmine bromide, neostigmine, or edrophonium in conjunction with atropine or glycopyrrolate will usually reverse skeletal muscle relaxation.

Pharmacokinetics

Route (for 600-mcg/kg dose)	Onset	Peak	Duration
IV	1 min	1.8 min	15–85 min

Metabolism: Hepatic; $T_{1/2}$: 1.4 h
Excretion: Urine

Adverse effects

▸ *CV:* Transient hypotension or hypertension, dysrhythmias, ECG changes, tachycardia
▸ *Resp:* **Bronchospasm,** wheezing, rhonchi, hiccup
▸ *GI:* Nausea, vomiting
▸ *Derm:* Rash, injection site edema, pruritus
▸ *Musc/Skel:* Skeletal muscle weakness, profound and prolonged muscle paralysis

Clinically important drug–drug interactions

▸ Intensified neuromuscular blockage with anesthetics (enflurane, isoflurane, halothane), antibiotics (aminoglycosides, vancomycin, tetracyclines, bacitracin, polymyxin B, colistin, and sodium colistimethate)
▸ Enhanced neuromuscular blockade with magnesium salts
▸ Recurrent paralysis with quinidine given during recovery from use of muscle relaxants
▸ Less effective and a shorter duration with anticonvulsants
▸ Enhanced neuromuscular blocking effect and duration of action with succinylcholine
▸ Counteracted by anticholinesterase, anticholinergic agents

◯ NURSING CONSIDERATIONS

Assessment

▸ *History:* Rocuronium or bromide allergy, myasthenia gravis, cirrhosis, cholestasis, cardiovascular disease, age, edema, severe obesity, neuromuscular disease, malignant hyperthermia, electrolyte imbalance, respiratory depression, pulmonary disease
▸ *Physical:* T, P, BP, R, ECG, I & O, IV site, weight, neurologic checks, level of sedation, muscle strength, skin assessment,

Adverse effects in *Italics* are most common; those in **Bold** are life-threatening

respiratory status, method of mechanical ventilation, adventitious lung sounds, peripheral nerve stimulator response, presence of pain, serum electrolytes, renal and liver function studies, acid–base balance

Implementation

▸ Exercise extreme caution when calculating and preparing doses. Rocuronium is a very potent drug; small dosage errors can cause serious adverse effects.

▸ Always administer an infusion using an IV infusion pump.

▸ Do not administer unless equipment for intubation, artifical respiration, oxygen therapy, and reversal agents is readily available. Rocuronium should be administered by people who are skilled in management of critically ill patients, cardiovascular resuscitation, and airway management.

▸ Monitor BP, R, and ECG closely during infusion.

▸ Use the smallest effective dose to achieve desired patient response.

▸ Monitor patient's response to therapy with a peripheral nerve stimulator.

▸ Rocuronium does not affect consciousness, pain threshold, or cerebration. Administer adequate sedatives and analgesics before giving rocuronium.

▸ Rocuronium produces paralysis. Provide oral and skin care. Administer artifical tears to protect corneas. May need to tape eyes closed. Position patient appropriately.

▸ Store vials in refrigerator.

▸ Use IV solution within 24 h of mixing.

S

⬤ silver sulfadiazine *(sul fah dye' ah zeen)*
SSD Cream, Silvadene, Thermazene, SSD AF Cream

Pregnancy Category B

Drug classes
Burn preparation
Topical antibacterial agent (broad spectrum)

Indications
▸ Adjunct for prevention and treatment of sepsis in second- and third-degree burns

Therapeutic actions
▸ Acts on cell membrane and cell wall to produce a bactericidal effect for many gram-negative and gram-positive bacteria; also effective against yeast

Adverse effects in *Italics* are most common; those in **Bold** are life-threatening

S

▶ Silver is slowly released from drug in concentrations that are selectively toxic to bacteria

Contraindications/cautions
▶ **Contraindications:** hypersensitivity to contents of preparation
▶ **Cautions:** G-6-PD deficiency, leukopenia, renal or hepatic function impairment, sensitivity to other sulfonamides

Available form
▶ *Cream:* 10 mg/g

Topical dosage
▶ Apply under sterile conditions qd–bid to clean and débrided wound so that cream is ⅟₁₆-inch thick. Keep burn covered with cream at all times. When needed, reapply cream to areas where cream has been removed by patient activity. Reapply immediately after hydrotherapy. Continue drug until healing occurs or site is ready for grafting.

TREATMENT OF OVERDOSE/ANTIDOTE
Discontinue drug or decrease dosage. Initiate general supportive and resuscitative measures.

Pharmacokinetics
≤ 1% of silver content is absorbed; up to 10% of sulfadiazine may be absorbed. When treating large burns, serum sulfa concentrations may approach therapeutic levels (8–12 mg/dL).
Excretion: Urine

Adverse effects
▶ *Derm:* Skin necrosis, erythema multiforme, skin discoloration, burning sensation, rashes, interstitial nephritis, fungal superinfection
▶ *Hematologic: Transient leukopenia*
▶ *Sulfonamide reactions (systemic absorption from large burns):* **Agranulocytosis, thrombocytopenia, leukopenia, dermatologic and allergic reactions (Stevens-Johnson syndrome, exfoliative dermatitis), toxic nephrosis,** blood dyscrasias, aplastic anemia, hemolytic anemia, GI reactions, hepatitis, hepatocellular necrosis, CNS reactions

Clinically important drug–drug interactions
▶ Inactivates topical proteolytic enzymes

◉ NURSING CONSIDERATIONS

Assessment
▶ *History:* Hypersensitivity to contents of preparation, G-6-PD deficiency, leukopenia, renal or hepatic function impairment, sensitivity to other sulfonamides

Adverse effects in *Italics* are most common; those in **Bold** are life-threatening

▶ *Physical:* T, P, R, BP, I & O, skin and burn assessment (color, drainage, odor, burn size and depth, pain, itching, rash), edema, pain assessment, liver evaluation, CBC, renal and liver function tests, UA for sulfa crystals, serum sulfa concentration, wound culture of any drainage

Implementation
▶ When possible, bathe patient qd to aid in débridement.
▶ Dressings are not required but may be used.
▶ If indicated, medicate patient for pain before applying cream.

⬤ **simvastatin** *(sim va stah' tin)* Zocor

Pregnancy Category X

Drug classes
Antihyperlipidemic
HMG-coenzyme A (CoA) inhibitor

Indications
▶ Adjunct to diet to reduce elevated total and LDL cholesterol, apoprotein B, and triglyceride levels in patients with primary hypercholesterolemia, mixed dyslipidemia (types IIa and IIb), and homozygous familial hyperlipidemia when diet and other nonpharmacologic therapies alone produced inadequate responses
▶ To reduce risk of mortality, nonfatal MI, need for myocardial revascularization procedures, and stroke or transient ischemic attacks for patients with coronary heart disease and hypercholesterolemia
▶ Unlabeled uses: to lower elevated cholesterol levels in patients with heterozygous familial hypercholesterolemia, familial combined hyperlipidemia, hyperlipidemia secondary to the nephrotic syndrome, diabetic dyslipidemia associated with non–insulin-dependent diabetes, and homozygous familial hypercholesterolemia associated with defective LDL receptors

Therapeutic actions
▶ Inhibits HMG-CoA, the enzyme that catalyses the first step in the cholesterol synthesis pathway
▶ Increases HDL cholesterol; decreases LDL cholesterol, total cholesterol, apolipoprotein B, VLDL cholesterol, and plasma triglycerides

Contraindications/cautions
▶ **Contraindications:** allergy to simvastatin or any product component, active liver disease, unexplained persistent elevated liver function tests
▶ **Cautions:** renal insufficiency, impaired hepatic function, significant alcohol consumption, elderly patients, immunosuppressed patients, cataracts

Adverse effects in *Italics* are most common; those in **Bold** are life-threatening

Available forms
▶ *Tablets:* 5, 10, 20, 40, 80 mg

Oral dosage
▶ *Initial dose:* 5–10 mg/d PO in the evening.
▶ *Maintenance dose:* Dose range is 5–40 PO mg/d. Adjust dose at ≥ 4-wk intervals.
▶ *Patients on immunosuppressants:* 5 mg/d PO; do not exceed 10 mg/d.
▶ *Renal function impairment:* Begin with 5 mg/d PO; monitor patient closely.
▶ *Elderly patients:* Begin with 5 mg/d PO; ≤ 20 mg/d may achieve maximum LDL reductions.

> **TREATMENT OF OVERDOSE/ANTIDOTE**
> Discontinue drug or decrease dosage. Initiate general supportive and resuscitative measures.

Pharmacokinetics

Route	Onset	Peak
Oral	Slow	1.3–2.4 h

Metabolism: Hepatic; $T_{1/2}$: 3 h
Excretion: Urine, feces

Adverse effects
▶ **CNS:** *Headache,* asthenia, taste alteration, impaired extraocular movement, facial paresis, tremor, vertigo, memory loss, peripheral neuropathy
▶ **CV:** Palpitations, vasodilation, syncope, postural hypotension, dysrhythmias, angina pectoris, hypertension
▶ **Resp:** *Upper respiratory tract infection*
▶ **GI:** **Liver dysfunction, pancreatitis,** *abdominal cramps, constipation,* nausea, vomiting, flatulence, dyspepsia, hepatitis, cholestatic jaundice, fatty change in liver; elevated ALT, AST, alkaline phosphatase, bilirubin
▶ **Derm:** Alopecia, pruritus, dry skin and mucous membranes, skin discoloration
▶ **Musc/Skel:** **Rhabdomyolysis,** muscle cramps, myalgia, myopathy, arthralgias
▶ **Misc:** Thyroid function test abnormalities, gynecomastia, loss of libido, erectile dysfunction

Clinically important drug–drug interactions
▶ Increased severe myopathy or rhabdomyolysis with gemfibrozil, cyclosporine, erythromycin, niacin, itraconazole
▶ Reduced maximum effective plasma concentration with propranolol

Adverse effects in *Italics* are most common; those in **Bold** are life-threatening

▸ Elevated PT and bleeding with warfarin
▸ Increased serum digoxin concentrations

● NURSING CONSIDERATIONS

Assessment

▸ *History:* Allergy to simvastatin or any product component, active liver disease, unexplained persistent elevated liver function tests, renal insufficiency, significant alcohol consumption, age, immunosuppression, cataracts

▸ *Physical:* Neurologic checks, skin assessment, muscle pain or weakness, ophthalmic exam, abdominal assessment, liver evaluation, serum lipid studies, liver function tests, serum CPK, thyroid function tests, renal function tests, UA

Implementation

▸ Hold or discontinue drug for patients with acute or serious condition suggestive of a myopathy or those at risk for developing renal failure secondary to rhabdomyolysis (severe acute infection, hypotension, major surgery, trauma, uncontrolled seizures, or severe metabolic, endocrine, or electrolyte disorders).

▸ Provide low-fat, low-cholesterol diet.

▸ Drug decreases cholesterol levels markedly within 2 wk; maximum therapeutic response occurs in 4–6 wk.

● **sodium bicarbonate** *(soe' dee um bye kar' boe nate)*

Neut, Bell/ans

Pregnancy Category C

Drug classes

Electrolyte
Systemic alkalinizer
Urinary alkalinizer
Antacid

Indications

▸ Treatment of metabolic acidosis, with measures to control the cause of the acidosis

▸ Potential adjunctive therapy during advanced cardiac life support (after defibrillation, cardiac compression, intubation, ventilation, and epinephrine) when arrest is associated with preexisting metabolic acidosis, hyperkalemia, or phenobarbital overdose

▸ Treatment of certain drug intoxications (salicylates, lithium) and hemolytic reactions that require alkalinization of the urine to diminish nephrotoxicity of blood pigments

▸ Treatment of severe diarrhea

▸ A gastric, systemic, and urinary alkalinizer

▸ Additive to raise pH in acidic IV solutions; reduces incidence of chemical phlebitis and patient discomfort

Adverse effects in *Italics* are most common; those in **Bold** are life-threatening

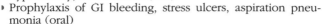

- Symptomatic relief of upset stomach from hyperacidity associated with peptic ulcer, gastritis, peptic esophagitis, gastric hyperacidity, hiatal hernia (oral)
- Prophylaxis of GI bleeding, stress ulcers, aspiration pneumonia (oral)
- Used to correct acidosis in renal tubular disorders and to minimize uric acid crystallization as adjuvants to uricosuric agents in gout

Therapeutic actions

- Increases plasma bicarbonate
- Buffers excess hydrogen ion concentration
- Raises blood pH
- Reverses clinical manifestations of acidosis
- Neutralizes or reduces gastric acidity, resulting in an increase in the gastric pH
- Increases excretion of free base in the urine, effectively raising the urinary pH
- 1 g of sodium bicarbonate provides 11.9 mEq sodium and 11.9 mEq bicarbonate

Contraindications/cautions

- **Contraindications:** allergy to components of preparations; low serum chloride from vomiting, continuous GI suction, or diuretic therapy; metabolic and respiratory alkalosis; hypocalcemia in which alkalosis may produce tetany; hypertension; convulsions or CHF when sodium administration could be dangerous
- **Cautions:** CHF, edematous or sodium-retaining states, renal function impairment, oliguria, anuria, hypokalemia, elderly patients, postoperative patients with renal or cardiovascular insufficiency

Available forms

- *Injection:* 0.5, 0.6, 0.9, 1.0 mEq/mL
- *Neutralizing additive solution:* 0.48, 0.5 mEq/mL
- *Tablets:* 325, 520, 650 mg

IV facts
Preparation

- May be given undiluted or as continuous infusion diluted in D2.5W; D5W; D10W; Dextran 6% in D5W or 0.9%NS; Dextrose-Ringer's combinations; Dextrose-Saline combinations; Fructose 10% in 0.9%NS or Water; Invert Sugar 5% and 10% in 0.9%NS or Water; 0.45%NS; or 0.9%NS.
- Suitable concentrations range from 1.5% (isotonic) to 8.4% (undiluted), depending on patient's condition.

Adverse effects in *Italics* are most common; those in **Bold** are life-threatening

Dosage

▸ *Cardiac arrest:* 1 mEq/kg IV bolus. Repeat with 0.5 mEq/kg IV q10min. Base dose on blood gas analysis.
▸ *Severe metabolic acidosis:* 90–180 mEq/L IV at rate of 1.0–1.5 L during the first h.
▸ *Less urgent metabolic acidosis:* Base dosage on patient's condition and response to therapy. 2–5 mEq/kg IV infused over 4–8 h. Also can estimate sodium bicarbonate dose by either of the following:
  ▸ Bicarbonate dose (mEq) = 0.5 (L/kg) × body weight (kg) × desired increase in serum HCO_3 (mEq/L)
  ▸ Bicarbonate dose (mEq) = 0.5 (L/kg) × body weight (kg) × base deficit (mEq/L)
▸ *Neutralizing additive solution:* Add 1 vial of neutralizing additive solution to 1 L of commonly used parenteral solutions to increase pH.

Normal sodium bicarbonate level by ABG analysis

▸ 22–26 mEq/L

Compatibility

Sodium bicarbonate may be given through the same IV line as acyclovir, amifostine, asparaginase, aztreonam, cefepime, cefmetazole, cladribine, ceftriaxone, cyclophosphamide, cytarabine, daunorubicin, dexamethasone, doxorubicin, etoposide, famotidine, filgrastim, fludarabine, gallium, granisetron, heparin, heparin with hydrocortisone, ifosfamide, indomethacin, insulin (regular Humulin R, beef, pork), melphalan, mesna, methylprednisolone, morphine, paclitaxel, piperacillin-tazobactam, potassium chloride, propofol, tacrolimus, teniposide, thiotepa, tolazoline, vancomycin, vitamin B complex with C.

Incompatibility

Do not administer through the same IV line as allopurinol, amiodarone, amrinone, calcium chloride, idarubicin, imipenem-cilastatin, leucovorin, midazolam, nalbuphine, ondansetron, oxacillin, sargramostim, verapamil, vincristine, vindesine, vinorelbine.

Oral dosage

▸ *Antacid:* 0.3–2 g PO qd–qid.
▸ *Urinary alkalinization:* 325 mg–2 g PO up to qid. Maximum daily dose is 15 g in patients < 60 y; 8 g in those ≥ 60 y.
▸ *Systemic alkalinization:* 325 mg-2 g PO qd-qid. Maximum daily dose is 16 g in patients < 60 y; 8 g in those > 60 y.

Discontinue drug or decrease dosage. Initiate general supportive and resuscitative measures. Control symptoms of alkalosis by rebreathing expired air from paper bag or rebreathing mask. Administer IV calcium gluconate to control tetany and hyperexcitability. Correct severe alkalosis by infusing 2.14% ammonium chloride solution, unless patient has hepatic disease. Infuse sodium chloride or potassium chloride to treat hypokalemia.

Pharmacokinetics

Route	Onset	Peak	Duration
IV	Immediate	Rapid	Unknown
Oral	Rapid	30 min	1–3 h

Excretion: Urine

Adverse effects

▶ *CV:* CHF, edema
▶ *Resp:* Increased CO_2 production
▶ *Fluid/electrolytes:* Alkalosis with headache, nausea, weakness, hyperirritability, tetany, hypernatremia, fluid and water retention, rebound hyperacidity, hypocalcemia; hypokalemia secondary to intracellular shifting of potassium
▶ *Derm:* Cellulitis, tissue necrosis, ulceration or soughing at site of infiltration, local pain with rapid infusion (parenteral)

Clinically important drug–drug interactions

▶ Decreased effect of benzodiazepines, chlorpropamide, iron salts, lithium, methotrexate, salicylates, sulfonylureas, tetracyclines
▶ Increased effect of amphetamines, anorexiants, flecainide, mecamylamine, quinidine, sympathomimetics
▶ Urine alkalinization increases solubility of sulfonamides and the renal elimination of phenobarbital

● NURSING CONSIDERATIONS

Assessment

▶ *History:* Allergy to components of preparations, vomiting, continuous GI suction, diuretic therapy, hypertension, convulsions, CHF, edematous or sodium-retaining states, renal function impairment, oliguria, anuria, age, postoperative patients with renal or cardiovascular insufficiency
▶ *Physical:* T, P, BP, R, I & O, ECG, IV site, weight, neurologic checks, reflexes, adventitious lung sounds, bowel sounds, fluid balance, renal function tests, serum electrolytes, UA, ABG

Implementation

▶ Always administer sodium bicarbonate infusion using an IV pump.

Adverse effects in *Italics* are most common; those in **Bold** are life-threatening

- Monitor arterial blood gases, and calculate base deficit when giving IV sodium bicarbonate. Adjust dosage based on response. Do not attempt to correct total CO_2 content fully during first 24 h because this may lead to systemic alkalosis.
- Continually assess for acidosis (hyperventilation, dyspnea, dysrhythmias, drowsiness, disorientation, headache, weakness, diminished reflexes, tremors) and alkalosis (hypoventilation, dysrhythmias, confusion, irritability, paresthesia, tetany, seizures, dizziness, vomiting, diarrhea) during therapy.
- Continually assess for hypernatremia as evidenced by lethargy, weakness, tremors, increased deep tendon reflexes, seizures, thirst, weight gain, edema, tachycardia, dry/flushed skin, oliguria, and elevated temperature.
- Check serum potassium level before IV administration; risk of metabolic acidosis is increased with hypokalemia; decrease bicarbonate dosage.
- Continually assess for hypokalemia as evidenced by weakness, dizziness, malaise, fatigue, muscle cramps, decreased deep tendon reflexes, respiratory muscle weakness, dyspnea, polyuria, polydipsia, dysrhythmias; ECG with U wave, flattened T waves, wide QRS complex.
- Use only during cardiac arrest, after starting other treatments such as chest compressions, intubation, ventilation, and other drug therapy. CO_2 may not be adequately cleared during CPR. Additionally, sodium bicarbonate induces a left shift of the oxyhemoglobin dissociation curve, which decreases oxygen release from hemoglobin at the tissue level.
- Carefully monitor patient's fluid balance and UA during therapy.
- Monitor ECG carefully during IV administration.
- Carefully monitor patient's IV site. Avoid infiltration because it will irritate tissues, causing necrosis and sloughing. Use largest peripheral vein or, if possible, a central line. If infiltration occurs, immediately stop infusion, elevate extremity, apply warm pack, and inject lidocaine or hyaluronidase to prevent sloughing.
- Replace parenteral administration set q24h.
- Have patient chew oral tablets thoroughly before swallowing, and follow them with a full glass of water.
- Do not give oral sodium bicarbonate within 1–2 h of other oral drugs to reduce risk of drug–drug interactions.

● sodium chloride *(sow' dee um)*
Pregnancy Category C
Drug classes
Electrolyte modifier (replacement solution)

Indications

▸ Parenteral restoration of sodium ion in patients with restricted oral intake
▸ Treatment of hyponatremia or low salt syndrome
▸ May be added to other compatible carbohydrate solutions, such as dextrose in water, to provide electrolytes
▸ Pharmaceutic aid and diluent for the infusion of compatible drug additives
▸ 0.9%NS (isotonic) restores water and sodium chloride losses; also used to dilute or dissolve drugs for IV, IM, or SC injection; flush IV catheters; replace extracellular fluids; treat metabolic alkalosis in the presence of fluid loss and mild sodium depletion; initiate and terminate blood transfusions without hemolyzing RBCs; and prime equipment/catheters during hemodialysis
▸ 0.45%NS (hypotonic) is a hydrating solution; used to assess the status of the kidneys, treat hyperosmolar diabetes when the use of dextrose is inadvisable and there is a need for large amounts of fluid without an excess of sodium ions
▸ 3% or 5%NS (hypertonic) is used to treat hyponatremia and hypochloremia due to electrolyte and fluid loss replaced with sodium-free fluids, drastic dilution of body water following excessive water intake, and emergency treatment of severe salt depletion
▸ Bacteriostatic sodium chloride is used only to dilute or dissolve drugs for IV, IM, or SC injection
▸ Concentrated sodium chloride is used as an additive in parenteral fluid therapy for patients who have special problems of sodium electrolyte intake or excretion

Therapeutic actions

▸ Sodium is the major cation in extracellular fluid and helps maintain water distribution, fluid and electrolyte balance, acid–base equilibrium, and osmotic pressure
▸ Chloride is the major anion in the extracellular fluid and is involved in maintaining acid–base balance
▸ 1 g of sodium chloride provides 17.1 mEq sodium and 17.1 mEq chloride

Contraindications/cautions

▸ **Contraindications:** hypernatremia, fluid retention; whenever the administration of sodium or chloride could be clinically detrimental; 3% and 5% sodium chloride: elevated, normal, or only slightly decreased plasma sodium

(contraindications continued on next page)

Adverse effects in *Italics* are most common; those in **Bold** are life-threatening

and chloride concentrations; Bacteriostatic sodium chloride: for fluid or sodium chloride replacement
- **Cautions:** renal function impairment, surgical or postoperative patients, CHF, circulatory insufficiency, elderly patients, decompensated cardiovascular status, cirrhotic and nephrotic disease, hypoproteinemia, hypervolemia, urinary tract obstruction, edematous states, sodium retention; use of corticosteroids or corticotropin

Available forms
- *Sodium chloride intravenous infusions for admixtures:* 0.45%; 0.9%; 3%; 5%
- *Sodium chloride diluents:* Bacteriostatic sodium chloride injection, 0.9%
- *Concentrated sodium chloride injection:* 14.6%, 23.4%

IV facts
Preparation
- Isotonic, hypotonic, and hypertonic solutions are ready for use.
- Dilute concentrated sodium chloride before use. Determine the mEq of sodium chloride to be given. Divide by 4 to calculate the number of mL to be used. Withdraw this volume and transfer into a compatible IV solution, such as D5W.

Dosage
- Individualize dosage based on laboratory determinations, maintenance or replacement fluid requirements, and clinical evaluation.
- To calculate the amount of sodium that must be administered to raise the serum sodium to the desired level, use the following formula: Sodium deficit (mEq) = TBW (desired − observed plasma sodium). Base the repletion rate on the degree of urgency in the patient. Hypertonic saline will correct the deficit more rapidly.

Normal sodium and chloride levels
- **Sodium:** 135–147 mEq/L
- **Chloride:** 95–110 mEq/L

TREATMENT OF OVERDOSE/ANTIDOTE
Discontinue drug or decrease dosage. Initiate general supportive and resuscitative measures. Diuretics will promote sodium loss.

Adverse effects in *Italics* are most common; those in **Bold** are life-threatening

S

Pharmacokinetics

Route	Onset	Peak
IV	Rapid	End of infusion

Excretion: Urine

Adverse effects

- ◗ *CV:* **CHF, pulmonary edema,** edema
- ◗ *Derm:* Local tenderness, abscess, tissue necrosis or infection at injection site; venous thrombosis or phlebitis extending from the injection site, extravasation
- ◗ *Fluid/electrolytes:* Hypervolemia, hypernatremia, fluid retention, hypokalemia
- ◗ *Postoperative salt intolerance:* cellular dehydration, weakness, disorientation, anorexia, nausea, distention, deep respirations, oliguria, increased BUN
- ◗ *Misc:* Acidosis, fever

Clinically important drug–drug interactions

- ◗ Give cautiously to patients receiving corticosteroids, corticotropin
- ◗ Increased sodium retention with glucocorticoids

● NURSING CONSIDERATIONS

Assessment

- ◗ *History:* Hypernatremia, fluid retention; whenever the administration of sodium or chloride could be clinically detrimental; renal function impairment, surgical or postoperative patients, CHF, circulatory insufficiency, age, decompensated cardiovascular status, cirrhotic and nephrotic disease, hypoproteinemia, hypervolemia, urinary tract obstruction, edematous states, sodium retention; use of corticosteroids or corticotropin
- ◗ *Physical:* T, P, BP, R, I & O, IV site, weight, neurologic checks, skin assessment, respiratory effort, adventitious lung sounds, cardiac auscultation, hydration status, skin turgor, JVD, edema, nutritional status, ABG, serum electrolytes, renal function tests

Implementation

- ◗ Administer using an IV pump to regulate carefully the amount of saline given.
- ◗ Frequently monitor serum electrolytes, I & O, and hydration status.
- ◗ To minimize venous irritation, give hypertonic solutions

Adverse effects in *Italics* are most common; those in **Bold** are life-threatening

slowly through a small-bore IV placed in a large vein. If possible, give through a central line.
- Assess for hyponatremia as evidenced by tachycardia, anorexia, abdominal cramps, nausea, vomiting, weight loss, diarrhea, oliguria, decreased skin turgor, apprehension, headache, weakness, fatigue, lethargy progressing to coma, confusion, disorientation, muscle cramps and twitching, tremors, and seizures.
- Assess for hypernatremia as evidenced by hypertension, tachycardia, edema, weight gain, increased thirst, low-grade fever, dry and sticky tongue and mucous membranes, flushed and dry skin, muscle rigidity and weakness, restlessness, agitation, confusion, disorientation, tremors, seizures, and oliguria.

● sodium phosphate (soe' dee um foss' fate)

Pregnancy Category C

Drug class
Electrolyte

Indications
- To prevent or correct hypophosphatemia in patients with restricted oral intake

Therapeutic actions
- Prominent component of all body tissues
- Participates in bone deposition, regulation of calcium metabolism, buffering effects on acid–base equilibrium, and various enzyme systems
- Phosphate administration lowers urinary calcium levels and increases urinary phosphate levels and urinary pyrophosphate inhibitor

Contraindications/cautions
- **Contraindications:** hyperphosphatemia, hypocalcemia, hypernatremia, untreated Addison's disease, severe renal impairment, infected urolithiasis or struvite stone formation
- **Cautions:** cardiac disease (especially patient on digitalis drugs), use of sodium-retaining medications, adrenal insufficiency, renal or hepatic function impairment, sodium- or potassium-restricted diet, acute dehydration, extensive tissue breakdown, myotonia congenita, peripheral or pulmonary edema, hypertension, hypoparathyroidism, osteomalacia, acute pancreatitis, rickets

Adverse effects in *Italics* are most common; those in **Bold** are life-threatening

Available forms
❯ *Injection:* 3 mmol phosphorus and 4 mEq sodium/mL

IV facts
Preparation
❯ **Always** dilute before use.

Dosage
❯ Individualize dosage to patient's requirements.
❯ 10–15 mM of phosphorus IV daily at a slow rate based on patient's condition.

Normal sodium and phosphorus levels
❯ **Sodium:** 135–145 mEq/L
❯ **Phosphorus:** 3–4.5 mg/dL

Incompatibility
Do not administer through the same IV line as ciprofloxacin.

TREATMENT OF OVERDOSE/ANTIDOTE
Discontinue drug or decrease dosage. Initiate general supportive and resuscitative measures. Treat hypernatremia with diuretics, hemodialysis, and fluid restriction. Treat hyperphosphatemia with phosphate-binding agents, such as aluminum hydroxide gel, diuretics, and hemodialysis.

Pharmacokinetics

Route	Onset
IV	Immediate

Excretion: Urine

Adverse effects
❯ *CNS:* **Seizures,** confusion, headache, dizziness, weakness or heaviness of legs and arms, tiredness, paresthesias
❯ *CV:* Fast or irregular heart rate
❯ *Resp:* Shortness of breath
❯ *GI: Nausea, vomiting, diarrhea,* stomach pain, mild laxative effect
❯ *Derm:* Phlebitis at IV site
❯ *Fluid/electrolytes:* Hyperphosphatemia—paresthesias of extremities, flaccid paralysis, **muscle or respiratory paralysis,** areflexia, weakness, listlessness, mental confusion, weak and heavy legs, hypotension, dysrhythmias, **heart block,** disappearance of P waves, spreading and slurring of QRS complex with development of biphasic curve, decreased cardiac output, **cardiac arrest;** hypernatremia, hypocalcemic tetany, hypomagnesemia

Adverse effects in *Italics* are most common; those in **Bold** are life-threatening

▸ *Misc:* Unusual weight gain, low urine output, bone and joint pain

Clinically important drug–drug interactions
▸ Increased hypernatremia with diazoxide, guanethidine, hydralazine, methyldopa, rauwolfia alkaloid, mineralocorticoids, corticotropin

● NURSING CONSIDERATIONS

Assessment
▸ *History:* Untreated Addison's disease, severe renal impairment, infected urolithiasis or struvite stone formation, cardiac disease, use of sodium-retaining medications, adrenal insufficiency, renal or hepatic function impairment, sodium- or potassium-restricted diet, acute dehydration, extensive tissue breakdown, myotonia congenita, peripheral or pulmonary edema, hypertension, hypoparathyroidism, osteomalacia, acute pancreatitis, rickets
▸ *Physical:* T, P, BP, R, ECG, I & O, IV site, weight, neurologic checks, adventitious lung sounds, hydration status, bowel sounds, acid–base balance, renal function tests, serum electrolytes, digitalis level, UA, liver and thyroid function tests

Implementation
▸ Always dilute sodium phosphate and infuse using an IV pump.
▸ Carefully monitor patient's HR, BP, ECG, and serum electrolytes during the course of therapy.
▸ Carefully monitor patient's IV site. Avoid infiltration because it will irritate tissues. Use central line if possible.
▸ Hyperphosphatemia may be evidenced on ECG by absent P waves, prolonged QTI, widened or slurred QRS complex, or cardiac arrest.
▸ Monitor for hypophosphatemia as evidenced by irritability, confusion, disorientation, seizures, coma, nystagmus, weakness, paresthesias, ataxia, dysrhythmias, hyperventilation, anorexia, nausea, vomiting, bruising, bone pain, pathological fractures, or arthralgias.
▸ Monitor for hypernatremia as evidenced by tachycardia, hypertension, weight gain, edema, thirst, low-grade fever, dry mucous membranes, flushed skin, muscle weakness, restlessness, agitation, confusion, disorientation, muscle cramps, muscle twitching, increased deep tendon reflexes, tremors, seizures, or oliguria.
▸ Further dilute or reduce dose if GI effects are severe.
▸ Monitor stools for blood related to GI bleeding.

Adverse effects in *Italics* are most common; those in **Bold** are life-threatening

● sodium polystyrene sulfonate

(pol ee stye' reen) Kayexalate, K-Exit (CAN), SPS

Pregnancy category C

Drug class
Potassium-removing resin

Indication
▶ Treatment of hyperkalemia

Therapeutic actions
▶ An ion exchange resin that releases sodium ions in exchange for potassium ions as it passes along the intestine after oral administration or is retained in the colon after enema, thus reducing elevated serum potassium levels; action is limited and unpredictable

Contraindications/cautions
▶ **Contraindications:** sodium polystyrene sulfonate allergy, hypokalemia
▶ **Cautions:** severe hypertension, severe CHF, marked edema (risk of sodium overload)

Available forms
▶ *Suspension:* 15 g/60 mL
▶ *Powder:* 4.1 mEq/g

Oral/enema dosage
▶ *Oral:* 15–60 g/d, best given as 15 g qd–qid. May be given as suspension with water or syrup (20–100 mL). Give powder form of resin in an oral suspension with a syrup base to increase palatability. May be mixed with diet or introduced into stomach through a nasogastric tube. Use sorbitol to combat constipation.
▶ *Enema:* Give initial cleansing enema. Suspend the resin in 100 mL D20W or sorbitol at body temperature. Insert a soft, rubber tube about 20 cm with the tip well into the sigmoid colon; tape in place. Introduce suspension of 30–50 g q6h using gravity, keeping the particles in suspension by stirring. Flush with 50–100 mL of fluid and clamp tube. If back leakage occurs, elevate hips or have patient assume the knee–chest position. Retain suspension for several hours if possible, but at least for 30 min. Irrigate colon with a non-sodium-containing solution to remove the resin. Drain the returns constantly through a Y-tube connection.

Adverse effects in *Italics* are most common; those in **Bold** are life-threatening

Pharmacokinetics

Route	Onset
Oral	2–12 h
Rectal	Longer

Excretion: Feces, expelled as enema

Adverse effects

▸ **GI:** *Constipation, gastric irritation, anorexia, nausea, vomiting,* fecal impaction (large doses in elderly), diarrhea, intestinal obstruction
▸ **Fluid/electrolytes:** *Hypokalemia,* hypocalcemia, sodium retention

Clinically important drug–drug interactions

▸ Systemic alkalosis with nonabsorbable cation-donating antacids, laxatives (magnesium hydroxide, aluminum carbonate)

⬤ NURSING CONSIDERATIONS

Assessment

▸ *History:* Sodium polystyrene sulfonate allergy, hypokalemia, severe hypertension, severe CHF, marked edema
▸ *Physical:* P, R, BP, ECG, I & O, neurologic checks, adventitious lung sounds, edema, JVD, abdominal exam, serum electrolytes

Implementation

▸ This drug is not sufficient to correct rapidly severe hyperkalemia associated with rapid tissue breakdown (burns, renal failure) or life-threatening hyperkalemia. In these cases, use IV calcium, sodium bicarbonate, glucose, and/or insulin, and initiate dialysis.
▸ Monitor serum electrolytes (potassium, sodium, calcium, magnesium) regularly; correct imbalances.
▸ Evaluate for hypokalemia as evidenced by muscle weakness, fatigue, paralytic ileus, ECG changes (flat or inverted T wave, U wave, ST segment depression, atrial and ventricular dysrhythmias), anorexia, nausea, vomiting, abdominal distention, dizziness, polyuria.
▸ Monitor for hyperkalemia as evidenced by nausea, vomiting, diarrhea, muscle weakness progressing to flaccid paralysis, numbness, increased deep tendon reflexes, fatigue, lethargy, apathy, confusion, dyspnea, oliguria, decreased cardiac output, or ECG changes (tall peaked T wave, wide QRS complex, prolonged PRI, flat or absent P wave, AV block, bradycardia, ventricular fibrillation).

Adverse effects in *Italics* are most common; those in **Bold** are life-threatening

▸ Treat constipation with 10–20 mL of 70% sorbitol q2h or as needed to produce two watery stools per day. Establish a bowel training program.
▸ Do not heat suspensions; this may alter the exchange properties.
▸ Prepare fresh suspensions for each dose. Do not store beyond 24 h.

● **sodium thiosulfate** *(thigh oh sulf' ate)*
Pregnancy Category C

Drug class
Antidote

Indication
▸ Management of cyanide poisoning; used with or without sodium nitrite or amyl nitrite

Therapeutic actions
▸ Converts cyanide, through the rhodanese enzyme system, to a nontoxic thiocyanate ion

Contraindications
▸ **Contraindications:** none

Available forms
▸ *Powder for injection:* 250 mg/mL

IV facts
Preparation
▸ May be given undiluted.

Dosage
▸ 12.5 g IV over 10 min whether used alone or in combination with other cyanide antidotes.
▸ If clinical response is inadequate 30 min after first dose, may give half the initial dose.

Compatibility
Information not available. Do not administer with other drugs.

Pharmacokinetics

Route	Onset
IV	Rapid

Metabolism: Hepatic, tissues; $T_{1/2}$: .65 h
Excretion: Urine

Adverse effects in *Italics* are most common; those in **Bold** are life-threatening

● NURSING CONSIDERATIONS

Assessment
▸ *History:* Ingestion of cyanide or cyanogenic compounds (route, dose, time since last exposure), smoke inhalation, thyroid disorders, vitamin B_{12} and folate level disorders
▸ *Physical:* P, BP, R, I & O, ECG, neurologic checks, reflexes, skin assessment, heart sounds, respiratory effort, adventitious lung sounds, smell of almonds on breath, cyanosis, abdominal assessment, nausea, vomiting, serum electrolytes, lactate level, thyroid function tests, vitamin B_{12} level, folate level, ABG, UA

Implementation
▸ Death from cyanide poisoning occurs rapidly; avoid delays in administering sodium thiosulfate.
▸ Exposure to some nitrile compounds may result in continued release of cyanide; multiple doses may be needed.
▸ Suspect cyanide poisoning with smoke inhalation injuries.

● **sotalol hydrochloride** *(soh' tal lole)*
Apo-Sotalol (CAN), Betapace, Novo-Sotalol (CAN), Rylosol (CAN), Sotacor (CAN)

Pregnancy Category B

Drug classes
Nonselective beta-adrenergic blocker
Antidysrhythmic

Indications
▸ Treatment of life-threatening ventricular dysrhythmias; because of its prodysrhythmic effects (torsades de pointes, ventricular tachycardia or fibrillation), it is not recommended for use with less than life-threatening dysrhythmias, even if patient is symptomatic

Therapeutic actions
▸ Prolongs cardiac action potential in all cardiac tissues, increases sinus cycle length, decreases AV nodal conduction, increases AV nodal refractoriness
▸ Blocks beta-adrenergic receptors of the sympathetic nervous system in the heart and juxtaglomerular apparatus (kidney), thus decreasing the excitability of the heart, cardiac output, and oxygen consumption

Adverse effects in *Italics* are most common; those in **Bold** are life-threatening

Effects on hemodynamic parameters
▶ Decreased HR
▶ Decreased CI
▶ Increased PCWP
▶ Decreased BP

Contraindications/cautions
▶ **Contraindications:** beta-blocker allergy, sinus brady-cardia, second- or third-degree heart block, cardiogenic shock, CHF unless secondary to a tachydysrhythmia treat-able with beta-blockers, bronchial asthma, bronchospasm, COPD, congenital or acquired long QT syndromes, un-treated hypokalemia or hypomagnesemia
▶ **Cautions:** recent AMI, sick sinus syndrome, peripheral or mesenteric vascular disease, chronic bronchitis, emphy-sema, bronchospastic diseases, diabetes, hepatic or renal dysfunction, thyrotoxicosis, muscle weakness

Available forms
▶ *Tablets:* 80, 120, 160, 240 mg

Oral dosage
▶ Initially give 80 mg PO bid. Adjust gradually every 2–3 d up to 240–320 mg/d. Patients with life-threatening refractory ven-tricular dysrhythmias may require doses as high as 480–640/d.
▶ Modify dosage for patient with renal impairment according to the following table:

Creatinine Clearance (mL/min)	Dosing Intervals
>60	12 h
30–60	24 h
10–30	36–48 h
<10	Individualize dose based on patient's response

TREATMENT OF OVERDOSE/ANTIDOTE
Discontinue drug or decrease dosage. Initiate general sup-portive and resuscitative measures. Initiate gastric lavage or induce emesis to remove drug. Place patient in supine posi-tion with legs elevated. Treat symptomatic bradycardia with atropine, isoproterenol, and/or a pacemaker; torsades de pointes with DC cardioversion, transvenous cardiac pacing,
(treatment continued on next page)

Adverse effects in *Italics* are most common; those in **Bold** are life-threatening

epinephrine, and/or magnesium sulfate; cardiac failure with a digitalis glycoside, diuretic, and/or aminophylline; hypotension with epinephrine; hypoglycemia with IV glucose; PVCs with lidocaine; seizures with diazepam; bronchospasm with a beta₂-stimulating agent or theophylline derivative. Give glucagon (5–10 mg IV over 30 s, followed by infusion of 5 mg/h) for severe overdose. Hemodialysis can reduce sotalol plasma concentrations.

Pharmacokinetics

Route	Onset	Peak
Oral	Varies	2.5–4 h

$T_{1/2}$: 12 h
Excretion: Urine

Adverse effects

▸ *CNS:* **CVA,** dizziness, vertigo, tinnitus, fatigue, depression, paresthesias, sleep disturbances, hallucinations, disorientation, memory loss, slurred speech, headache, confusion, visual disturbances, emotional lability

▸ *CV:* **Ventricular dysrhythmias, cardiac arrest, torsades de pointes, cardiogenic shock,** *AV block, bradycardia, CHF,* AICD discharge, mitral regurgitation, reinfarction, ventricular septal defect, chest pain, hypertension, hypotension, pallor, peripheral ischemia, peripheral vascular insufficiency, edema, pulmonary edema, palpitations, arterial insufficiency

▸ *Resp:* **Bronchospasm,** dyspnea, cough, bronchial obstruction, nasal stuffiness, rhinitis, pharyngitis, crackles, wheezes

▸ *GI: Gastric/epigastric pain, flatulence, constipation, diarrhea, nausea, vomiting,* anorexia, ischemic colitis, renal and mesenteric arterial thrombosis, retroperitoneal fibrosis, hepatomegaly, acute pancreatitis, elevated liver enzymes

▸ *GU: Impotence, decreased libido,* Peyronie's disease, dysuria, nocturia, frequency, UTI, renal failure

▸ *Derm:* Rash, pruritus, sweating, dry skin, increased pigmentation, psoriasis, peripheral skin necrosis

▸ *Allergic:* **Anaphylaxis, angioedema,** pharyngitis, rash, fever, sore throat, laryngospams, respiratory distress

▸ *Hematologic:* **Agranulocytosis,** nonthrombocytopenic purpura, thrombocytopenic purpura

▸ *Musc/Skel:* Joint pain, arthralgia, muscle cramps, twitching/tremor

▸ *EENT:* Eye irritation, dry eyes, conjunctivitis, blurred vision

Adverse effects in *Italics* are most common; those in **Bold** are life-threatening

- *Misc:* *Decreased exercise tolerance,* facial swelling, weight gain or loss, gout, lupus syndrome, hyperglycemia or hypoglycemia, development of antinuclear antibodies

Clinically important drug–drug interactions

- Increased effects with calcium channel-blockers, digitalis, oral contraceptives, prazosin
- Dangerously long refractory periods with phenothiazines, TCAs, astemizole, class Ia antidysrhythmic drugs (disopyramide, quinidine, procainamide), and class III drugs (amiodarone)
- Reduced clearance of lidocaine
- Life-threatening HTN when clonidine is discontinued or when both drugs are discontinued simultaneously
- Increased hypoglycemic effect of insulin
- Increased cardiac arrest with flecainide
- Hypertension followed by severe bradycardia with epinephrine
- Potentiates, counteracts, or has no effect on nondepolarizing muscle relaxants
- Decreased effects with nonsteroidal anti-inflammatory drugs, rifampin

⬤ NURSING CONSIDERATIONS

Assessment

- *History:* Beta-blocker allergy, cardiogenic shock, CHF unless secondary to a tachydysrhythmia treatable with beta-blockers, bronchial asthma, bronchospasm, COPD, congenital or acquired long QT syndromes, recent AMI, sick sinus syndrome, peripheral or mesenteric vascular disease, chronic bronchitis, emphysema, bronchospastic diseases, diabetes, hepatic or renal dysfunction, thyrotoxicosis, muscle weakness
- *Physical:* T, P, BP, R, ECG, I & O, weight, neurologic checks, vision, skin assessment, cardiac auscultation, edema, JVD, adventitious lung sounds, bowel sounds, UA, serum glucose, CBC, serum electrolytes; liver, thyroid, and renal function tests

Implementation

- Do not use unless patient is unresponsive to other antidysrhythmics and has a life-threatening ventricular dysrhythmia.
- Generally withdraw other antidysrhythmics gradually, allowing for 2–3 plasma half-lives of the drug before starting sotalol. After discontinuing amiodarone, do not start sotalol until QT interval has normalized.
- Carefully monitor P, BP, R, ECG, and QTc, PR, and QT intervals. Prodysrhythmic effects can be pronounced.
- Have emergency equipment (defibrillator, drugs, oxygen, intubation equipment) on standby in case anaphylaxis or adverse reaction occurs.

Adverse effects in *Italics* are most common; those in **Bold** are life-threatening

- Consult with provider about withdrawing drug if patient to undergo surgery (withdrawal is controversial).
- Absorption is decreased when taken with a meal.

⬤ **spironolactone** *(speer on oh **lak'** tone)* Aldactone, Novo-Spiroton (CAN)

Pregnancy Category D

Drug class
Potassium-sparing diuretic

Indications
- Diagnosis and treatment of primary hyperaldosteronism
- Adjunctive therapy in edema associated with CHF, nephrotic syndrome, or hepatic cirrhosis
- Treatment of hypokalemia or prevention of hypokalemia in patients taking digitalis
- Treatment of essential hypertension, usually in combination with other drugs
- Unlabeled uses: treatment of hirsutism

Therapeutic actions
- Competitively blocks the effects of aldosterone in the distal renal tubule, causing loss of sodium and water and retention of potassium
- Interferes with testosterone synthesis and may increase peripheral conversion of testosterone to estradiol

Effects on hemodynamic parameters
- Decreased BP

Contraindications/cautions
- **Contraindications:** spironolactone allergy, anuria, acute renal insufficiency, significantly impaired renal function, hyperkalemia; patients receiving amiloride or triamterene
- **Cautions:** hyponatremia, hepatic cirrhosis

Available forms
- *Tablets:* 25, 50, 100 mg

Oral dosage
- *Edema:* 25–200 mg/d PO.
- *Essential hypertension:* 50–100 mg/d PO in single or divided doses. May be combined with other diuretics.
- *Hypokalemia:* 25–100 mg/d PO.
- *Maintenance therapy for hyperaldosteronism:* 100–400 mg/d PO in preparation for surgery. If patient is unable to have

surgery, use the lowest possible dose for long-term mainte-nance therapy.

◗ *Diagnosis of primary hyperaldosteronism:* **Long test:** 400 mg/d PO for 3–4 wk. Correction of hypokalemia and hyper-tension provides presumptive evidence for the diagnosis of primary hyperaldosteronism. **Short test:** 400 mg/d PO for 4 d. If serum potassium increases but decreases when spirono-lactone is discontinued, consider a presumptive diagnosis of primary hyperaldosteronism.

TREATMENT OF OVERDOSE/ANTIDOTE
Discontinue drug or decrease dosage. Initiate general sup-portive and resuscitative measures.

Pharmacokinetics

Route	Onset	Peak	Duration
Oral	24–48 h	48–72 h	48–72 h

Metabolism: Liver; $T_{1/2}$: 20 h
Excretion: Urine, bile, feces

Adverse effects

◗ *CNS:* Drowsiness, lethargy, headache, confusion, ataxia
◗ *GI:* Cramping, diarrhea, gastric bleeding, ulceration, gastritis, vomiting
◗ *Derm:* Maculopapular or erythematous cutaneous eruptions, urticaria
◗ *Fluid/electrolytes:* Hyperkalemia, dehydration, hypona-tremia
◗ *Endocrine:* Hirsutism, deepening of the voice, erectile dys-function, gynecomastia, irregular menses or amenorrhea, postmenopausal bleeding
◗ *Misc:* Drug fever, carcinoma of the breast, agranulocytosis; hyperchloremic metabolic acidosis in decompensated he-patic cirrhosis

Clinically important drug–drug interactions

◗ Decreased hypoprothrombinemic effects of anticoagulants
◗ Unpredictable interactions with digoxin; increased half-life of digoxin, which may lead to increased serum levels and toxi-city; attenuated inotropic action of digoxin; increased or de-creased elimination half-life of digitoxin
◗ Increased hyperkalemia with potassium, increasing risk of dysrhythmias or cardiac arrest
◗ Decreased diuretic effects with salicylates

Adverse effects in *Italics* are most common; those in **Bold** are life-threatening

● NURSING CONSIDERATIONS

Assessment
▸ *History:* Spironolactone allergy, anuria, acute renal insufficiency, significantly impaired renal function; use of amiloride or triamterene; hepatic cirrhosis
▸ *Physical:* T, P, R, BP, ECG, I & O, weight, neurologic checks, skin assessment, adventitious lung sounds, hydration status, edema, JVD, liver assessment, abdominal assessment, menstrual cycle, serum electrolytes, renal and liver function tests, UA

Implementation
▸ Give daily doses early so that increased urination does not interfere with sleep.
▸ Measure and record daily weight to monitor mobilization of edema fluid.
▸ Frequently assess serum electrolytes and renal function tests.
▸ Hyperkalemia may be evidenced by nausea, vomiting, diarrhea, muscle weakness progressing to flaccid paralysis, numbness, increased deep tendon reflexes, fatigue, lethargy, apathy, confusion, dyspnea, oliguria, decreased cardiac output, ECG changes (tall peaked T wave, wide QRS complex, prolonged PRI, flat or absent P wave, bradycardia, or dysrhythmias).
▸ Hyponatremia may be evidenced by lethargy, drowsiness, fatigue, confusion, headache, tremors, hyperreflexia, anorexia, nausea, vomiting, abdominal cramps, diarrhea, oliguria, convulsions, coma.
▸ Food increases the absorption of spironolactone.
▸ Avoid giving a potassium-rich diet.
▸ Drug may falsely elevate serum digoxin levels.

● **streptokinase** *(strep toe kin' ase)* Kabikinase, Streptase

Pregnancy Category C

Drug class
Thrombolytic agent

Indications
▸ Treatment of evolving acute transmural MI to reduce infarct size, reduce congestive heart failure, improve ventricular function, and reduce mortality
▸ Treatment of diagnostically confirmed acute, massive pulmonary embolism where there is obstruction in blood flow to a lobe or multiple segments of the lungs, with or without unstable hemodynamics

▶ Lysis of diagnostically confirmed acute, extensive thrombi of the deep veins
▶ Arterial thrombosis and embolism not originating on the left side of the heart
▶ Clearance of totally or partially occluded arteriovenous cannula

Therapeutic actions
▶ Enzyme isolated from group C β-hemolytic streptococcal bacteria
▶ Acts with plasminogen to produce a complex that converts plasminogen to plasmin
▶ Plasmin degrades fibrin clots, fibrinogen, and other plasma proteins
▶ Increases fibrinolytic activity

Effects on hemodynamic parameters
▶ Decreased BP
▶ Decreased SVR

Contraindications/cautions
▶ **Contraindications:** streptokinase allergy (note: most patients have been exposed to streptococci and to streptokinase and therefore have developed resistance to the drug; allergic reactions are relatively rare); active internal bleeding; recent (within 2 mo) trauma, CVA, intracranial or intraspinal surgery; intracranial neoplasm, arteriovenous malformation, or aneurysm; known bleeding diathesis; severe uncontrolled hypertension
▶ **Cautions:** old age (> 75 y), recent (≤ 10 d) major surgery (CABG, organ biopsy, obstetric delivery, puncture of noncompressible vessels); recent (≤ 10 d) GI or GU bleeding; recent (≤ 10 d) trauma; hypertension (≥ 180 mmHg systolic or ≥ 110 mmHg diastolic); left heart thrombus, acute pericarditis, subacute bacterial endocarditis, hemostatic defects secondary to severe hepatic or renal disease, diabetic hemorrhagic retinopathy or other ophthalmic hemorrhaging, septic thrombophlebitis, occluded AV cannula at seriously infected site, current oral anticoagulant therapy; other conditions in which bleeding is a hazard or would be difficult to manage

Available forms
▶ *Powder for injection:* 250,000; 600,000; 750,000; 1,500,000 IU/vial

Adverse effects in *Italics* are most common; those in **Bold** are life-threatening

IV facts
Preparation
▶ Contains no preservatives; do not reconstitute until immediately before use.
▶ Reconstitute vial with 5 mL of D5W or 0.9%NS; direct diluent at side of the vial, not directly into the streptokinase.
▶ Avoid shaking during reconstitution; gently roll or tilt vial to reconstitute.
▶ If needed, increase total volume to maximum of 500 mL in glass or 50 mL in plastic containers. For ease of administration, dilute to total volume of 45 mL.
▶ Slight flocculation (described as thin translucent fibers) may be noted but does not interfere with safe use of the solution.
▶ Solution may be filtered through 0.8 mcg or larger pore size filter.
▶ For occluded AV cannula, reconstitute the contents of 250,000-IU vial with 2 mL D5W or 0.9%NS.

Dosage
▶ *Acute evolving transmural MI:* **IV infusion:** 1,500,000 IU IV within 60 min. **Intracoronary infusion:** 20,000 IU bolus directly into the coronary artery followed by 2000 IU/min for 60 min for total dose of 140,000 IU.
▶ *Deep vein thrombosis, pulmonary or arterial embolism, arterial thrombosis:* **Loading dose:** 250,000 IU IV infused into a peripheral vein over 30 min. **Maintenance dose: Pulmonary embolism:** 100,000 IU/h IV for 24 h; **DVT:** 100,000 IU/h IV for 72 h; **Arterial thrombosis or embolism:** 100,000 IU/h IV for 24–72 h. If TT, APTT, or PT after 4 h of therapy is < 1½ times baseline, discontinue streptokinase because excessive resistance is present. Initiate heparin therapy (without a bolus) after TT or APTT decreases to < twice the control value.
▶ *AV cannula occlusion:* Slowly instill 250,000 IU in 2 mL D5W or 0.9%NS into the occluded cannula. Clamp cannula for 2 h; then aspirate contents, flush with saline, and reconnect cannula.

Compatibility
Streptokinase may be given through the same IV line as dobutamine, dopamine, heparin, lidocaine, nitroglycerin.

TREATMENT OF OVERDOSE/ANTIDOTE
Discontinue drug and any other anticoagulant or antiplatelet drugs if severe bleeding, neurologic changes, or severe hypotension occur. Intiate general supportive and resuscitative
(treatment continued on next page)

Adverse effects in *Italics* are most common; those in **Bold** are life-threatening

S

measures. Administer IV fluids, PRBCs, FFP, platelets, and cryoprecipitate as indicated. Avoid dextran. Aminocaproic acid may be given as an antidote.

Pharmacokinetics

Route	Onset	Duration
IV	Immediate	4 h (up to 24 h)

Metabolism: Inactivated by antistreptococcal antibodies; $T_{1/2}$: 23 min
Excretion: Cleared by sites in liver

Adverse effects

- *CNS:* **Intracranial bleeding,** Guillain-Barré syndrome, headache
- *CV:* **Dysrhythmias** (with intracoronary artery infusion), **cholesterol embolism,** hypotension
- *Resp:* **Bronchospasm, pulmonary embolism,** noncardiogenic pulmonary edema, minor breathing difficulty, respiratory depression
- *GI:* **GI bleeding,** nausea, vomiting
- *GU:* **GU bleeding**
- *Derm:* Skin rash, urticaria, itching, flushing
- *Allergic:* **Anaphylaxis,** mild allergic reactions
- *Heme: Bleeding* (*minor or surface* to major internal bleeding)
- *Misc: Fever, shivering,* retroperitoneal bleeding, periorbital swelling, musculoskeletal pain, low back pain, facial hematoma, elevated serum transaminases

Clinically important drug–drug interactions

- Increased hemorrhage with vitamin K antagonists, heparin, oral anticoagulants, drugs that alter platelet function (aspirin, dipyridamole, abciximab, tirofiban, eptifibatide, ticlopidine, clopidogrel)

⬤ NURSING CONSIDERATIONS

Assessment

- *History:* Streptokinase allergy; active internal bleeding; recent trauma, CVA, intracranial or intraspinal surgery; intracranial neoplasm, arteriovenous malformation, aneurysm, known bleeding diathesis, severe uncontrolled hypertension, age; recent major surgery (CABG, organ biopsy, obstetric delivery, puncture of noncompressible vessels); recent trauma, GI or GU bleeding; left heart thrombus, acute pericarditis, subacute bacterial endocarditis, hemostatic defects secondary to severe hepatic or renal disease, diabetic hemorrhagic retinopathy or other ophthalmic hemorrhaging, septic thrombophlebitis,

Adverse effects in *Italics* are most common; those in **Bold** are life-threatening

occluded AV cannula at seriously infected site, current oral anticoagulant therapy; other conditions in which bleeding is a hazard or would be difficult to manage

‣ *Physical:* T, P, R, BP, ECG, I & O, IV site, SpO_2, AV cannula patency, neurologic checks, ophthalmic exam, skin assessment, cardiac auscultation, JVD, chest pain assessment, peripheral perfusion, presence of bleeding, respiratory effort, adventitious lung sounds, liver evaluation, CBC, CPK, cardiac troponin, myoglobin, TT, APTT, PT, INR, FSP, ABG, type and crossmatch; urine, stool, and emesis guaiac

Implementation

‣ Administer drug as soon as possible after diagnosis. Most benefit seen if given 4 h after onset of AMI symptoms; however, decreased mortality seen if given up to 24 h after symptom onset. Initiate as soon as possible after onset of other thrombotic events, preferably within 7 d.

‣ Administer infusion using an IV pump.

‣ Have emergency equipment (defibrillator, drugs, oxygen, intubation equipment) on standby in case anaphylaxis, hemorrhage, or adverse reaction occurs.

‣ Before starting drug, initiate at least 2–3 peripheral IVs.

‣ Monitor BP, P, R, and neurologic status continuously.

‣ Do not take blood pressure in lower extremities to avoid dislodging possible deep vein thrombi.

‣ Type and crossmatch blood in case serious blood loss occurs and blood transfusions are required.

‣ When given for AMI, assess for chest pain (type, character, location, intensity, radiation). Assess for ST segment changes before, during, and after therapy.

‣ Continuously monitor for evidence of reperfusion (decreased chest pain, decreased ST segment elevation, reperfusion dysrhythmias).

‣ When given for PE, assess respiratory effort, SpO_2, ABGs, and chest pain.

‣ Initiate other interventions as standard for patients with AMI, DVT, arterial thrombosis or embolism, or PE.

‣ Initiate bleeding precautions.

‣ Assess for evidence of bleeding and hemorrhage.

‣ Carefully assess recent puncture sites and sites of lines/tubes (catheter insertion sites, cutdown sites, needle puncture sites, recent surgical incisions).

‣ Apply pressure to arterial and venous puncture sites for at least 30 min or until hemostasis is achieved. Apply a pressure dressing to site to prevent bleeding. Assess all puncture sites q15min.

- Apply pressure to arterial and venous puncture sites for least 30 min or until hemostasis is achieved.
- Apply pressure or pressure dressings to control superficial bleeding.
- Avoid IM injections before, during, and for 24 h after therapy. Do not attempt central venous access or arterial puncture unless absolutely necessary. If arterial puncture is necessary, use an upper extremity vessel that is accessible to manual pressure.
- Guaiac all stools, urine, and emesis for blood.
- Handle patient carefully to avoid ecchymosis and bleeding.
- If possible, draw blood for laboratory analysis from an existing saline lock.
- Take BP with manual BP cuff or ensure that NIBP cuff does not inflate excessively above patient's SBP.
- Shave patient with an electric razor.
- Drug will clear occluded catheters only if occluded by fibrin clots. Avoid excessive pressure when injecting streptokinase; force could rupture catheter or expel clot into circulation.
- Because of increased likelihood of resistance due to antistreptokinase antibody, drug may not be effective if administered between 5 d and 6 mo of prior anistreplase or streptokinase administration or with streptococcal infections.
- Discard any unused portion of drug.
- Reconstituted solution may be used within 8 h following reconstitution if stored at 36–46°F.

◉ succinylcholine chloride *(sux sin il koe' leen)*
Anectine, Quelicin, Anectine Flo-Pack

Pregnancy Category C

Drug class
Depolarizing neuromuscular blocking agent

Indications
- Adjunct to general anesthesia to facilitate intubation
- Induction of skeletal muscle relaxation during surgery or mechanical ventilation

Therapeutic actions
- Combines with cholinergic receptors of motor endplate to produce depolarization observed as fasciculations
- Subsequent neuromuscular transmission inhibited as long as an adequate amount of succinylcholine remains at the receptor site

Adverse effects in *Italics* are most common; those in **Bold** are life-threatening

Contraindications/cautions

▸ **Contraindications:** allergy to succinylcholine or its components, genetic disorders of plasma pseudocholinesterase, personal or familial history of malignant hyperthermia, myopathies associated with elevated creatine phosphokinase values, acute narrow-angle glaucoma, penetrating eye injuries

▸ **Cautions:** neuromuscular disease, myasthenia gravis; cardiovascular, pulmonary, liver, metabolic, or renal disease; severe burns, electrolyte imbalance, hyperkalemia, hypokalemia, hypocalcemia, concurrent quinidine or digitalis use, severe trauma, paraplegia, spinal cord injury, low plasma pseudocholinesterase, malnutrition, dehydration, cancer, collagen diseases, myxedema, exposure to neurotoxic insecticides, glaucoma, fractures, muscle spasms, elevated ICP

Available forms

▸ *IV injection:* 20, 50, 100 mg/mL
▸ *Powder for infusion:* 500-mg, 1-g vials

IV facts
Preparation

▸ For a continuous infusion, dilute 250–500 mg in 250 mL D5W/LR; D5W/0.9%NS; D2.5W; D5W; D10W; Dextran 6% in D5W or 0.9%NS; Dextrose-LR combinations; Dextrose-Ringer's combinations; Dextrose-Saline combinations; Fructose 10% in 0.9%NS or Water; Invert Sugar 5% and 10% in 0.9%NS or Water; Ionosol products; LR; 0.45% NS; 0.9%NS; Ringer's injection; or Sodium Lactate (1/6 Molar) Injection to achieve a concentration of 1–2 mg/mL (0.1%–0.2% solution).

Dosage and titration

▸ *Test dose for patients with suspected low plasma pseudocholinesterase:* 5–10 mg IV of a 0.1% IV solution.
▸ *Short surgical procedures:* 0.6 mg/kg IV. Range is 0.3–1.1 mg/kg. Give additional doses if relaxation is not complete.
▸ *Long surgical procedures:* 2.5–4.3 mg/min IV. Range is 0.5–10 mg/min.
▸ *Prolonged muscular relaxation:* 0.3–1.1 mg/kg IV. Give subsequent doses of 0.04–0.07 mg/kg to maintain appropriate relaxation.
▸ Patients with hypocalcemia and hypokalemia usually require a reduced dose.

Adverse effects in *Italics* are most common; those in **Bold** are life-threatening

S

Compatibility
Succinylcholine may be given through the same IV line as etomidate, heparin with hydrocortisone, potassium chloride, propofol, vitamin B complex with C.

Incompatibility
Do not administer through the same IV line as alkaline solutions, barbiturates, methohexital, thiopental.

> **TREATMENT OF OVERDOSE/ANTIDOTE**
> Discontinue drug or decrease dosage. Initiate general supportive and resuscitative measures. Continue to maintain a patent airway and provide mechanical ventilation.

Pharmacokinetics

Route	Onset	Peak	Duration
IV	Immediate	30–60 s	4–6 min

Metabolism: Plasma cholinesterase
Excretion: Urine

Adverse effects
▶ *CV:* **Cardiac arrest,** bradycardia, tachycardia, hypertension, hypotension, dysrhythmias
▶ *Resp:* **Apnea, bronchospasm, laryngospasm,** respiratory depression
▶ *GI:* Excessive salivation
▶ *Derm:* Rash
▶ *Allergic:* **Anaphylaxis,** bronchospasm, flushing, redness, hypotension, tachycardia
▶ *Musc/Skel:* Inadequate block, prolonged block, muscle fasciculation, postoperative muscle pain, jaw rigidity
▶ *Misc:* **Malignant hyperthermia,** myoglobinuria, myoglobinemia, hyperkalemia, increased intraocular pressure

Clinically important drug–drug interactions
▶ Intensified neuromuscular blockage with cimetidine, cyclophosphamide, phenelzine, promazine, oxytocin, nonpenicillin antibiotics, quinidine, beta-adrenergic blocking agents, procainamide, lidocaine, trimethaphan, lithium, furosemide, magnesium sulfate, quinine, chloroquine, isoflurane
▶ Increased effects with amphotericin B, thiazide diuretics secondary to electrolyte imbalance
▶ Reduced duration of neuromuscular blockade with diazepam, IV procaine

Adverse effects in *Italics* are most common; those in **Bold** are life-threatening

- Increased bradycardia and sinus arrest with narcotic analgesics
- Synergistic or antagonistic effects with nondepolarizing muscle relaxants
- Muscle cells may lose potassium, leading to ventricular fibrillation or other dysrhythmias in digitalized patients; increased toxicity of both drugs

⬤ NURSING CONSIDERATIONS

Assessment

- *History:* Allergy to succinylcholine or its components, genetic disorders of plasma pseudocholinesterase, personal or familial history of malignant hyperthermia, myopathies associated with elevated creatine phosphokinase values, acute narrow-angle glaucoma, penetrating eye injuries, neuromuscular disease, myasthenia gravis; cardiovascular, pulmonary, liver, metabolic, or renal disease; severe burns, concurrent use of quinidine or digitalis, severe trauma, paraplegia, spinal cord injury, low plasma pseudocholinesterase, malnutrition, dehydration, cancer, collagen diseases, myxedema, exposure to neurotoxic insecticides, glaucoma, fractures, muscle spasms, elevated ICP
- *Physical:* T, P, BP, R, ECG, I & O, SpO_2, IV site, weight, neurologic checks, mental status, ophthalmic exam, level of sedation, respiratory status, method of mechanical ventilation, adventitious lung sounds, muscle strength, peripheral nerve stimulator response, serum electrolytes, acid–base balance, presence of pain, ABG

Implementation

- Exercise extreme caution when calculating and preparing doses. Succinylcholine is a very potent drug; small dosage errors can cause serious adverse effects.
- Always administer an infusion using an IV infusion pump.
- Do not administer unless equipment for intubation, artifical respiration, oxygen therapy, and reversal agents is readily available. Succinylcholine should be administered by people who are skilled in management of critically ill patients, cardiovascular resuscitation, and airway management.
- Use the smallest dose possible to achieve desired patient response.
- Monitor patient's response to therapy with a peripheral nerve stimulator.
- Monitor BP, R, and ECG closely during infusion.
- Throughout the infusion, assess for evidence of malignant hyperthermia.
- Succinylcholine does not affect consciousness, pain thresh-

old, or cerebration. Administer adequate sedatives and analgesics before giving succinylcholine.
▸ Succinylcholine produces paralysis. Provide oral and skin care. Administer artifical tears to protect corneas. May need to tape eyes closed. Position patient appropriately.
▸ Discard unused solutions within 24 h.

⬤ **sucralfate** *(soo kral' fate)* Apo-Sucralfate (CAN), Carafate, Novo-Sucralfate (CAN), Sulcrate (CAN)

Pregnancy Category B

Drug class
Antipeptic agent

Indications
▸ Short-term (up to 8 wk) treatment of duodenal ulcers
▸ Maintenance therapy for duodenal ulcer at reduced dosage after healing
▸ Unlabeled uses: accelerates healing of gastric ulcers, long-term treatment of gastric ulcers, treatment of reflux and peptic esophagitis, treatment of NSAID or aspirin-induced GI symptoms and mucosal damage, prevention of stress ulcers in critically ill patients, treatment of oral and esophageal ulcers due to radiation, chemotherapy, and sclerotherapy
▸ Orphan drug use: treatment of oral mucositis and stomatitis following radiation for head and neck cancer

Therapeutic actions
▸ Forms an ulcer-adherent complex at duodenal ulcer sites, protecting the ulcer against acid, pepsin, and bile salts, thereby promoting ulcer healing
▸ Also inhibits pepsin activity in gastric juices

Contraindications/cautions
▸ **Contraindications:** sucralfate allergy
▸ **Cautions:** chronic renal failure/dialysis (buildup of aluminum may occur with aluminum-containing products)

Available forms
▸ *Tablets:* 1 g
▸ *Suspension:* 1 g/10 mL

Oral dosage
▸ *Active duodenal ulcer:* 1 g PO qid 1 h before meals and hs. Continue treatment for 4–8 wk.
▸ *Maintenance:* 1 g PO bid.

Adverse effects in *Italics* are most common; those in **Bold** are life-threatening

> **TREATMENT OF OVERDOSE/ANTIDOTE**
> Discontinue drug or decrease dosage. Initiate general supportive and resuscitative measures.

Pharmacokinetics

Route	Onset	Duration
Oral	30 min	5 h

Excretion: Feces, urine

Adverse effects

▸ *CNS:* Dizziness, headache, sleepiness, vertigo
▸ *Allergic:* **Laryngospasm, facial swelling, angioedema,** respiratory difficulty, urticaria, rhinitis
▸ *GI: Constipation,* diarrhea, nausea, indigestion, gastric discomfort, dry mouth, flatulence
▸ *Derm:* Rash, pruritus
▸ *Misc:* Back pain

Clinically important drug–drug interactions

▸ Decreased serum levels and effectiveness of cimetidine, digoxin, fluoroquinolone antibiotics, ketoconazole, l-thyroxine, phenytoin, quinidine, ranitidine, tetracycline, theophylline, warfarin; separate administration by 2 h
▸ Aluminum toxicity with aluminum-containing antacids

◯ NURSING CONSIDERATIONS

Assessment

▸ *History:* Sucralfate allergy, chronic renal failure/dialysis
▸ *Physical:* I & O, neurologic checks, skin assessment, respiratory effort, adventitious lung sounds, abdominal assessment, bowel sounds, hydration status, pain assessment, renal function tests, UA, stool and emesis guaiac, gastric pH

Implementation

▸ Monitor pain; use antacids to relieve pain.
▸ Administer antacids between doses of sucralfate, not within 0.5 h before or after sucralfate doses.

T

◯ **terbutaline sulfate** *(ter byoo' ta leen)*
Brethaire, Brethine, Bricanyl
Pregnancy Category B

Drug classes
Sympathomimetic
β_2 selective adrenergic agonist
Bronchodilator
Tocolytic agent

Indications
▶ Prophylaxis and treatment of bronchial asthma and reversible bronchospasm that may occur with bronchitis and emphysema

Therapeutic actions
▶ In low doses, acts relatively selectively at β_2-adrenergic receptors, by formation of c-AMP, to cause bronchodilation; inhibits release of histamine and increases ciliary motility
▶ At higher doses, β_2 selectivity is lost, and the drug acts at β_1 receptors to cause typical sympathomimetic cardiac effects

Contraindications/cautions
▶ **Contraindications:** terbutaline allergy, tocolysis
▶ **Cautions:** CAD, ischemic heart disease, hypertension, dysrhythmias, hyperthyroidism, diabetes, convulsive disorders, patients susceptible to hypokalemia

Available forms
▶ *Injection:* 1 mg/mL
▶ *Tablets:* 2.5, 5 mg
▶ *Aerosol:* 0.2 mg/actuation

SC facts
Preparation
▶ Administer undiluted.

Dosage
▶ 0.25 mg SC into the lateral deltoid area. If no significant improvement in 15–30 min, repeat dose. If no improvement after second dose, consider other therapeutic measures. Do not exceed 0.5 mg in 4 h.

Therapeutic serum level
▶ 0.5–4.1 mg/mL

Oral/inhalation dosage
▶ *Oral:* 5 mg PO at 6-h intervals tid during waking hours. If side effects are pronounced, reduce to 2.5 mg PO tid. Do not exceed 15 mg in 24 h.
▶ *Inhalation:* 2 inhalations separated by 60 s q4–6h. Do not repeat more often than q4–6h.

Adverse effects in *Italics* are most common; those in **Bold** are life-threatening

Pharmacokinetics

Route	Onset	Peak	Duration
SC	5–15 min	30–60 min	1.5–4 h
Oral	30 min	2–3 h	4–8 h
Inhalation	5–30 min	1–2 h	3–6 h

Metabolism: Liver; $T_{1/2}$: 4–14 h
Excretion: Urine

Adverse effects

‣ *CNS:* **Seizures,** *tremors, nervousness, shakiness, headache, drowsiness,* dizziness, weakness, insomnia
‣ *CV: Palpitations, dysrhythmias,* tachycardia, BP changes, chest tightness/pain
‣ *Resp:* **Bronchospasm,** dyspnea, throat dryness/irritation
‣ *GI:* Nausea, vomiting, heartburn, unusual/bad taste, smell change
‣ *Allergic:* **Allergic reaction**
‣ *Misc:* **Death with excessive use of inhaled drug,** flushed feeling, sweating, pain at injection site

Clinically important drug–drug interactions

‣ Enhanced vascular system effects and potential for dysrhythmias and hypertension with MAO inhibitors, TCAs
‣ Pulmonary effects hindered by beta-blockers; may produce severe asthma attacks
‣ Enhanced and potentially deleterious vascular system effects with sympathomimetic bronchodilators, epinephrine

● NURSING CONSIDERATIONS

Assessment

‣ *History:* Terbutaline allergy, tocolysis, CAD, ischemic heart disease, hypertension, dysrhythmias, hyperthyroidism, diabetes, convulsive disorders, susceptibility to hypokalemia
‣ *Physical:* T, P, R, BP, ECG, I & O, SpO_2, weight, neurologic checks, skin color, adventitious lung sounds, respiratory effort, presence of retractions or nasal flaring, use of accessory muscles for breathing, peak flow test, FEV_1, vital capacity, blood and urine glucose, serum electrolytes, thyroid function tests, ABG

Adverse effects in *Italics* are most common; those in **Bold** are life-threatening

Implementation
▸ Shake inhaler well before using.
▸ Do not exceed recommended dosage; administer aerosol during second half of inspiration, because the airways are open wider and distribution is more extensive.
▸ Have emergency equipment (defibrillator, drugs, oxygen, intubation equipment) on standby in case adverse reaction occurs.
▸ Use minimal doses for minimal periods of time; drug tolerance can occur with prolonged use.
▸ Food decreases bioavailability by one third.
▸ Store tablets in tight, light-resistant container; store ampules at room temperature and protect from light.

⬤ **theophylline** *(thee off' i lin)* **Immediate-release** *capsules, tablets:* Bronkodyl, Elixophyllin, Quibron-T Dividose, Slo-Phyllin, Theolair
Timed-release capsules: Slo-bid Gyrocaps, Slo-Phyllin Gyrocaps, Theo-24, Theobid, Theoclear L.A., Theospan-SR, Theovent
Timed-release tablets: Quibron-T/SR Dividose, Respbid, Sustaire, Theochron, Theo-Dur, Theo-Sav, Theolair-SR, T-Phyl, Uni-Dur, Uniphyl
Liquids: Accurbron, Aquaphyllin, Asmalix, Elixomin, Elixophyllin, Lanophyllin, Slo-Phyllin, Theoclear-80, Theolair, Theostat 80

Pregnancy Category C

Drug classes
Bronchodilator
Xanthine

Indications
▸ Symptomatic relief or prevention of bronchial asthma and reversible bronchospasm associated with chronic bronchitis and emphysema
▸ Unlabeled uses: reduction of essential tremor, improvement of pulmonary function and dyspnea in patients with COPD

Therapeutic actions
▸ Relaxes smooth muscle of the bronchi and pulmonary blood vessels, causing bronchodilation and increasing vital capacity that has been impaired by bronchospasm and air trapping
▸ Central respiratory stimulant
▸ Stimulates CNS, induces diuresis, increases gastric acid secretion, reduces lower esophageal sphincter pressure

Adverse effects in *Italics* are most common; those in **Bold** are life-threatening

▸ May inhibit extracellular adenosine, stimulate endogenous catecholamines; antagonize prostaglandins PGE_2 and $FGF_{2\alpha}$; mobilize intracellular calcium, causing smooth muscle relaxation; and exert beta-adrenergic agonist activity on the airways

▸ Actions also may be mediated by phosphodiesterase inhibition, which increases the concentration of c-AMP

Contraindications/cautions
▸ **Contraindications:** hypersensitivity to any xanthines, underlying seizure disorder (unless on anticonvulsant drugs), active peptic ulcer disease or gastritis, status asthmaticus (oral preparations)
▸ **Cautions:** dysrhythmias, cardiac disease, CHF, cor pulmonale, acute pulmonary edema, fever, hypertension, hypoxemia, hepatic disease, hypothyroidism, alcoholism, use of tobacco or marijuana, influenza, multi-organ failure, shock, elderly patients (especially males)

Available forms
▸ *Injection in 5% Dextrose:* 200, 400, 800 mg/container
▸ *Immediate-release tablets:* 100, 125, 200, 250, 300 mg
▸ *Immediate-release capsules:* 100, 200 mg
▸ *Syrup:* 80, 150 mg/15 mL
▸ *Elixir:* 80 mg/15 mL
▸ *Solution:* 80 mg/15 mL
▸ *TR capsules:* 50, 60, 75, 100, 125, 130, 200, 250, 260, 300 mg
▸ *TR tablets:* 100, 200, 250, 300, 400, 450, 500, 600 mg

IV facts
Preparation
▸ Obtain premixed container of theophylline.

Dosage
▸ Individualize dosage to patient's needs, response, and tolerance. Calculate dosages by lean body weight and anhydrous theophylline content. Convert to oral therapy as soon as possible.
▸ *Loading dose:* 4.7 mg/kg over 20–30 min for patients not already receiving theophylline.
▸ *Maintenance dose:* 0.08–0.79 mg/kg/h IV depending on patient's age, condition, and needs. Do not exceed 20–25 mg/min.

Adverse effects in *Italics* are most common; those in **Bold** are life-threatening

Titration Guide

	theophylline								
	800 mg in 250 mL								

	Body Weight								
lb	88	99	110	121	132	143	154	165	176	187
kg	40	45	50	55	60	65	70	75	80	85
Dose Ordered in mg/kg/h	**Amounts to Infuse in mL/h**								
0.08	1	1	1	1	2	2	2	2	2	2
0.1	1	1	2	2	2	2	2	2	3	3
0.15	2	2	2	3	3	3	3	4	4	4
0.2	3	3	3	3	4	4	4	5	5	5
0.25	3	4	4	4	5	5	5	6	6	7
0.3	4	4	5	5	6	6	7	7	8	8
0.35	4	5	5	6	7	7	8	8	9	9
0.4	5	6	6	7	8	8	9	9	10	11
0.45	6	6	7	8	8	9	10	11	11	12
0.5	6	7	8	9	9	10	11	12	13	13
0.55	7	8	9	9	10	11	12	13	14	15
0.6	8	8	9	10	11	12	13	14	15	16
0.65	8	9	10	11	12	13	14	15	16	17
0.7	9	10	11	12	13	14	15	16	18	19
0.75	9	11	12	13	14	15	16	18	19	20
0.79	10	11	12	14	15	16	17	19	20	21

	Body Weight								
lb	198	209	220	231	242	253	264	275	286
kg	90	95	100	105	110	115	120	125	130
Dose Ordered in mg/kg/h	**Amounts to Infuse in mL/h**								
0.08	2	2	3	3	3	3	3	3	3
0.1	3	3	3	3	3	4	4	4	4
0.15	4	4	5	5	5	5	6	6	6
0.2	6	6	6	7	7	7	8	8	8
0.25	7	7	8	8	9	9	9	10	10
0.3	8	9	9	10	10	11	11	12	12
0.35	10	10	11	11	12	13	13	14	14
0.4	11	12	13	13	14	14	15	16	16
0.45	13	13	14	15	15	16	17	18	18
0.5	14	15	16	16	17	18	19	20	20
0.55	15	16	17	18	19	20	21	21	22
0.6	17	18	19	20	21	22	23	23	24
0.65	18	19	20	21	22	23	24	25	26
0.7	20	21	22	23	24	25	26	27	28

continued

Adverse effects in *Italics* are most common; those in **Bold** are life-threatening

theophylline *continued*									
800 mg in 250 mL									
	Body Weight								
lb	198	209	220	231	242	253	264	275	286
kg	90	95	100	105	110	115	120	125	130
Dose Ordered in mg/kg/h	**Amounts to Infuse in mL/h**								
0.75	21	22	23	25	26	27	28	29	30
0.79	22	23	25	26	27	28	30	31	32

Therapeutic serum level
▸ 10–20 mcg/mL; obtain serum sample 1–2 h after giving immediate-release products and 5–9 h after morning dose for sustained-release formulations

Compatibility
Theophylline may be given through the same IV line as acyclovir, ampicillin, ampicillin-sulbactam, aztreonam, cefazolin, cefotetan, ceftazidime, ceftriaxone, cimetidine, clindamycin, dexamethasone, diltiazem, dobutamine, dopamine, doxycycline, erythromycin, famotidine, fluconazole, gentamicin, haloperidol, heparin, hydrocortisone, lidocaine, methyldopa, methylprednisolone, metronidazole, midazolam, nafcillin, nitroglycerin, nitroprusside sodium, penicillin G potassium, piperacillin, potassium chloride, ranitidine, ticarcillin, ticarcillin-clavulanate, tobramycin, vancomycin.

Incompatibility
Do not administer through the same IV line as hetastarch or phenytoin.

Oral dosage
▸ Individualize dosage to patient's needs, response, and tolerance. Calculate dosages by lean body weight and anhydrous theophylline content.
▸ *Acute symptoms requiring rapid theophyllinization in patients not receiving theophylline:* Initial loading dose is required. Dosage recommendations for theophylline anhydrous are:

Patient Group	Oral Loading	Maintenance
Young adult smokers	5 mg/kg	3 mg/kg q6h
Nonsmoking adults, otherwise healthy	5 mg/kg	3 mg/kg q8h
Older patients and patients with cor pulmonale	5 mg/kg	2 mg/kg q8h
Patients with CHF	5 mg/kg	1–2 mg/kg q12h

Adverse effects in *Italics* are most common; those in **Bold** are life-threatening

▸ *Acute symptoms requiring rapid theophyllinization in patients receiving theophylline:* Defer loading dose if serum theophylline concentration can be obtained rapidly. Each 0.5 mg/kg PO administered as a loading dose will increase the serum theophylline concentration 1 mcg/mL. If patient is in respiratory distress to warrant the risk, give 2.5 mg/kg PO of a rapidly absorbed theophylline preparation. This will increase serum theophylline levels by about 5 mcg/mL and is unlikely to cause dangerous adverse effects if the patient is not experiencing theophylline toxicity before this dose. Maintenance doses are as above.

▸ *Chronic therapy:* Initial dose of 16 mg/kg/24 h PO or 400 mg/24 h PO, whichever is less, in divided doses q6–8h for immediate-release preparations or liquids, q8–12h or q24h for timed-release preparations (consult manufacturer's recommendations for specific dosage interval). Increase dosage based on serum theophylline levels. If levels are unavailable, increase in 25% increments at 3-d intervals as long as drug is tolerated or until maximum dose of 13 mg/kg/d or 900 mg, whichever is less, is reached.

▸ *Dosage adjustment based on serum theophylline levels during chronic therapy:*

Serum Theophylline	Directions
Too low	5–10 mcg/mL: Increase dose by 25% at 3-d intervals until either desired clinical response or serum concentration is achieved.
Within normal	10–20 mcg/mL: Maintain dosage if tolerated. Recheck level at 6- to 12-mo intervals.
Too high	20–25 mcg/mL: Decrease dose by 10%. Recheck level after 3 d.
	25–30 mcg/mL: Skip next dose and decrease following doses by 25%. Recheck level after 3 d.
	> 30 mcg/mL: Skip next 2 doses and decrease following doses by 50%. Recheck level after 3 d.

TREATMENT OF OVERDOSE/ANTIDOTE

Discontinue drug or decrease dosage. Initiate general supportive and resuscitative measures. Do not administer stimulants. If a seizure occurs, establish an airway and administer oxygen. Administer diazepam 0.1–0.3 mg/kg, up to 10 mg. Monitor vital signs, maintain blood pressure, and provide adequate hydration. After seizure, perform intubation and gastric lavage instead of inducing emesis. Administer a cathartic and activated charcoal using a large-bore gastric lavage tube. If activated charcoal is not effective or when

(treatment continued on next page)

Adverse effects in *Italics* are most common; those in **Bold** are life-threatening

582 theophylline

serum concentration > 60 mcg/mL, consider charcoal hemoperfusion or hemodialysis. If a seizure *has not* occurred, induce vomiting, preferably with ipecac syrup, even if emesis has occurred spontaneously. Administer a cathartic and activated charcoal. Prophylactic phenobarbital may increase the seizure threshold. Treat atrial dysrhythmias with verapamil; ventricular dysrhythmias with lidocaine or procainamide. Treat dehydration and acid–base imbalance with IV fluids. Treat hypotension with IV fluids and vasopressors.

Pharmacokinetics

Route	Onset	Peak
IV	Rapid	End of infusion
Oral	Varies	2 h

Metabolism: Hepatic, $T_{1/2}$: 3–15 h (nonsmokers) or 4–5 h (smokers, 1–2 packs/d)
Excretion: Urine

Adverse effects

- *Serum theophylline levels < 20 mcg/mL:* Adverse effects uncommon
- *Serum theophylline levels > 20 mcg/mL: Nausea, vomiting, diarrhea, headache, insomnia, irritability* (75% of patients)
- *Serum theophylline levels > 35 mcg/mL:* Hyperglycemia, hypotension, dysrhythmias, tachycardia, **seizures, brain damage, death**
- *CNS:* **Convulsions,** irritability, restlessness, headache, insomnia, reflex hyperexcitability, muscle twitching
- *CV:* **Ventricular dysrhythmias, circulatory failure,** palpitations, tachycardia, hypotension, extrasystoles
- *Resp:* **Respiratory arrest,** tachypnea
- *GI:* Hematemesis, epigastric pain, gastroesophageal reflux during sleep
- *GU:* Proteinuria, increased excretion of renal tubular cells and RBCs; diuresis (dehydration), urinary retention in men with prostate enlargement
- *Misc:* Fever, flushing, hyperglycemia, SIADH, rash, increased AST, alopecia

Clinically important drug–drug interactions

- Increased effects and toxicity with allopurinol, nonselective beta-blockers, calcium channel blockers, cimetidine, corticosteroids, disulfiram, ephedrine, erythromycin, fluoroquinolones interferon, isoniazid, loop diuretics, macrolides, mexiletine, quinolones, ranitidine, thiabendazole, thyroid hormones

Adverse effects in *Italics* are most common; those in **Bold** are life-threatening

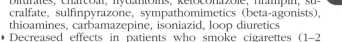

- Decreased theophylline levels with aminoglutethimide, barbiturates, charcoal, hydantoins, ketoconazole, rifampin, sucralfate, sulfinpyrazone, sympathomimetics (beta-agonists), thioamines, carbamazepine, isoniazid, loop diuretics
- Decreased effects in patients who smoke cigarettes (1–2 packs/d)
- Decreased theophylline and phenytoin levels when used concurrently
- Counteracted effects of propofol, benzodiazepines
- Reversed neuromuscular blockade
- Reduced lithium plasma levels
- Enhanced adverse reactions with tetracyclines
- Blocks adenosine receptors and thus decreases effects of adenosine
- Decreased theophylline clearance with alcohol, ticlopidine

Clinically important drug–food interactions
- Increased elimination with a low-carbohydrate/high-protein diet, and by charcoal broiled beef
- Decreased elimination by a high-carbohydrate, low-protein diet
- Bioavailability and absorption of time-released preparations may be altered by food; these may rapidly release their contents with food and cause toxicity

◉ NURSING CONSIDERATIONS

Assessment
- *History:* Hypersensitivity to any xanthines, seizure disorder, active gastritis, status asthmaticus, dysrhythmias, cardiac disease, CHF, cor pulmonale, acute pulmonary edema, hypertension, hypoxemia, hepatic disease, hypothyroidism, peptic ulcer, alcoholism, use of tobacco or marijuana, influenza, multi-organ failure, shock, age, gender
- *Physical:* T, P, BP, R, ECG, I & O, SpO$_2$, weight, neurologic checks, presence of seizures, skin assessment, respiratory effort, retractions, nasal flaring, adventitious lung sounds, bowel sounds, theophylline level, pulmonary function tests, peak flow test, ABG; thyroid, liver, and kidney function tests

Implementation
- Administer IV theophylline using an IV infusion pump.
- Caution patient not to chew or crush enteric-coated timed-release preparations.
- Give immediate-release, liquid dosage forms with food if GI effects occur.
- Give timed-release preparations on an empty stomach, 1 h before or 2 h after meals. May administer capsules whole or

Adverse effects in *Italics* are most common; those in **Bold** are life-threatening

sprinkle beads on spoonful of soft food. Instruct patient not to chew.
- Monitor results of serum theophylline level determinations carefully; reduce dosage if serum levels exceed therapeutic range of 10–20 mcg/mL.
- Monitor carefully for clinical signs of adverse effects, particularly if serum theophylline levels are not available.
- Have emergency equipment (defibrillator, drugs, oxygen, intubation equipment) on standby in case of adverse reaction.
- Maintain diazepam on standby to treat seizures.
- Maintain adequate hydration.
- Theophylline products are not necessarily interchangeable; use caution when switching from one brand to another.

⬤ thiamine (vitamin B₁) *(thye' ah min)*
Thiamilate

Pregnancy Category A (parenteral)

Drug class
Vitamin (water soluble)

Indications
- Treatment or prophylaxis of thiamine deficiency
- Impaired GI absorption in malabsorption syndromes
- Treatment of beriberi

Therapeutic actions
- Combines with ATP to form thiamine pyrophosphate, a coenzyme required for carbohydrate metabolism

Contraindications/cautions
- **Contraindications:** thiamine or chlorobutanol hypersensitivity
- **Cautions:** Wernicke's encephalopathy

Available forms
- *Injection:* 100 mg/mL
- *Tablets:* 50, 100, 250, 500 mg
- *Enteric-coated tablets:* 20 mg

IV/IM facts
Preparation
- *IV:* May be given undiluted or diluted in D5W; D10W; Dextrose-Lactated Ringer's combinations; Dextrose-Ringer's Injection combinations; Dextrose-Saline combinations; Fructose 10% in 0.9%NS or Water; Invert Sugar 5% and 10% in 0.9%NS

or Water; Ionosol products; 0.9%NS; 0.45% NS; Sodium Lactate (1/6 Molar) Injection; LR; or Ringer's injection.
▶ *IM:* Give undiluted.

Dosage
▶ Administer an intradermal test dose for patients with suspected sensitivity.
▶ *Wet beriberi with myocardial failure:* 10–30 mg IV tid. Do not exceed 20 mg/min.
▶ *Beriberi:* 10–20 mg IM tid for 2 wk.
▶ *Wernicke's encephalopathy:* 100 mg IV then 50–100 mg/d IM. Do not exceed 20 mg/min IV.

Compatibility
Thiamine may be given through the same IV line as famotidine.

Oral dosage
▶ *Beriberi:* Give oral vitamin containing 5–10 mg/d thiamine PO for 1 mo after IM dosing.
▶ *Alcoholism:* 100 mg/d PO.

> **TREATMENT OF OVERDOSE/ANTIDOTE**
> Discontinue drug or decrease dosage. Initiate general supportive and resuscitative measures.

Pharmacokinetics
Maximum oral absorption is 3–15 mg qd. Oral absorption may increase if given in divided doses with food. If intake exceeds tissue stores, excess thiamine is excreted in urine.
Metabolism: Liver
Excretion: Urine

Adverse effects
▶ *CNS:* Weakness, restlessness
▶ *CV:* **Cardiovascular collapse, death**
▶ *Resp:* **Pulmonary edema**
▶ *GI:* **GI hemorrhage,** nausea, tightness of throat
▶ *Derm:* Feeling of warmth, pruritus, urticaria, sweating; tenderness and induration (IM use)
▶ *Allergic:* **Anaphylaxis, angioneurotic edema**

Clinically important drug–drug interaction
▶ Enhances neuromuscular blocking agents

● NURSING CONSIDERATIONS
Assessment
▶ *History:* Thiamine or chlorobutanol hypersensitivity, Wernicke's encephalopathy, use of alcohol

Adverse effects in *Italics* are most common; those in **Bold** are life-threatening

> *Physical:* T, P, R, BP, ECG, I & O, weight, neurologic checks, skin assessment, adventitious lung sounds, respiratory effort, edema, nutritional status, serum electrolytes, kidney and liver function tests

Implementation
> Carefully monitor P, BP, R, ECG, and respiratory status during IV administration.
> Have emergency equipment (defibrillator, drugs, oxygen, intubation equipment) on standby in case anaphylaxis or adverse reaction occurs.
> Thiamine-deficient patients may experience a sudden onset or worsening of Wernicke's encephalopathy after receiving glucose; administer thiamine before or along with dextrose-containing fluids.
> Assess for Wernicke's encephalopathy as evidenced by horizontal nystagmus, sixth nerve palsy, ataxia, or confusion.
> When patient is stable, provide diet high in thiamine: asparagus, whole-grain cereal, beef, beans, peanuts, pork, and fresh peas.

● **thiopental sodium** *(thigh oh pen' tal)* Pentothal
Pregnancy Category C

C-III controlled substance

Drug classes
General barbiturate anesthetic
Anticonvulsant

Indications
> Control of convulsive states and in neurosurgical patients with increased ICP if adequate ventilation is provided (parenteral)
> To induce anesthesia; supplement other anesthetic drugs; provide IV anesthesia for short, minimally painful procedures; or induce hypnosis

Therapeutic actions
> Neuroprotective; lowers basal metabolic rate, decreases brain edema, and extends tolerable ischemic time
> Depresses CNS to produce hypnosis and anesthesia with analgesia

Contraindications/cautions
> **Contraindications:** barbiturate hypersensitivity, porphyria
> **Cautions:** impaired respiratory, circulatory, cardiac, renal,
(contraindications continued on next page)

Adverse effects in *Italics* are most common; those in **Bold** are life-threatening

T

hepatic, or endocrine system function; debilitated patients; severe cardiovascular disease, hypotension, shock, excessive premedication, Addison's disease, hepatic or renal dysfunction, myxedema, increased blood urea, severe anemia, increased intracranial pressure, asthma, myasthenia gravis, status asthmaticus

Available forms
◗ *IV injection:* 20, 25 mg/mL

IV facts
Preparation
◗ Dilute drug with D2.5W; D2.5W/0.45%NS; D2.5W/0.9%NS; D5W/0.225%NS; D5W/0.45%NS; D5W; Dextran 6% in D5W or 0.9%NS; Ionosol PSL, 0.45%NS; 0.9%NS; or Sodium Lactate (1/6 Molar) Injection. Do not mix with acid pH drugs or solutions.
◗ **Intermittent injection:** Use a 2%–5% solution (20–50 mg/mL).
◗ **Continuous infusion:** Use a 0.2% or 0.4% solution (200–400 mg/100 mL) in D5W or 0.9%NS.

Dosage and titration
◗ *Test dose:* 25–75 mg IV to assess tolerance and sensitivity. Monitor patient for $\geq$ 60 s.
◗ *Convulsive states:* 75–125 mg IV as soon as possible after convulsion starts. May need up to 250 mg over 10 min.
◗ *Neurosurgical patients with increased ICP:* Intermittent doses of 1.5–3.5 mg/kg IV.
◗ *Narcoanalysis and narcosynthesis:* 100 mg/min IV.
◗ *Anesthesia:* 50–75 mg IV at 20- to 40-s intervals. Once anesthesia is established, additional 25–50 mg IV injections may be given when patient moves. If drug is sole anesthetic agent, may give by continuous drip in a 0.2%–0.4% concentration.

Compatibility
Thiopental may be given through the same IV line as doxacurium, fentanyl, heparin, milrinone, mivacurium, nitroglycerin, ranitidine.

Incompatibility
Do not administer through the same IV line as alfentanil, ascorbic acid, atracurium, atropine, diltiazem, dobutamine, dopamine, ephedrine, furosemide, hydromorphone, labetalol, lidocaine, lorazepam, midazolam, nicardipine, norepinephrine, pancuronium, phenylephrine, succinylcholine, sufentanil, vecuronium.

Adverse effects in *Italics* are most common; those in **Bold** are life-threatening

Pharmacokinetics

Route	Onset	Duration
IV	30–40 s	20–30 min

Metabolism: Hepatic; $T_{1/2}$: 6–46 h
Excretion: Urine (small amts)

Adverse effects

▸ *CNS:* **Seizures,** emergence delirium, headache, restlessness, anxiety, prolonged somnolence and recovery
▸ *CV:* **Cardiac arrest, peripheral vascular collapse,** dysrhythmias, circulatory depression, thrombophlebitis, hypotension, myocardial depression
▸ *Resp:* **Respiratory depression, apnea, laryngospasm, bronchospasm,** coughing, dyspnea, sneezing, rhinitis
▸ *GI:* Nausea, emesis, salivation, abdominal pain
▸ *Derm:* Pain or nerve injury at IV site, rash, extravascular injury (pain, swelling, ulceration, necrosis)
▸ *Allergic:* **Anaphylaxis,** erythema, pruritus, urticaria
▸ *Misc:* Hiccups, skeletal muscle hyperactivity, shivering

Clinically important drug–drug interactions

▸ Enhanced by narcotics; apnea more common
▸ Increased frequency and severity of neuromuscular excitation, hypotension with phenothiazines
▸ Anesthetic effects extended or achieved at lower doses with probenecid
▸ Enhanced anesthetic effects with sulfisoxazole

◉ NURSING CONSIDERATIONS

Assessment

▸ *History:* Barbiturate hypersensitivity; porphyria; impaired respiratory, circulatory, cardiac, renal, hepatic, or endocrine system function; debilitated status; severe cardiovascular disease; hypotension, shock, excessive premedication, Addison's disease, hepatic or renal dysfunction, myxedema, increased blood urea, severe anemia, increased intracranial pressure, asthma, myasthenia gravis, status asthmaticus
▸ *Physical:* T, P, BP, R, ECG, ICP, I & O, IV site, weight, neurologic checks, level of sedation, skin assessment, respiratory sta-

tus, adventitious lung sounds, peripheral perfusion, abdominal assessment, pain assessment, renal and liver function studies

Implementation
▸ Only use if trained in drug's use, airway management, and mechanical ventilation.
▸ Exercise extreme caution when calculating and preparing doses. Thiopental is a very potent drug; small dosage errors can cause serious adverse effects.
▸ Always administer an infusion using an IV infusion pump.
▸ Monitor BP, P, R, ECG, and neurologic status continuously during administration.
▸ Have emergency equipment (defibrillator, drugs, oxygen, intubation equipment) on standby in case anaphylaxis or adverse reaction occurs.
▸ Monitor IV site closely.
▸ Avoid intra-arterial administration, which is dangerous and may produce gangrene of an extremity.
▸ Follow federal, state, and institutional policies for dispensing controlled substances.
▸ Thiopental may be habit forming.
▸ Discard unused drug after 24 h.

⬤ ticlopidine hydrochloride
(tye kloh' pih deen) Ticlid

Pregnancy Category B

Drug classes
ADP receptor antagonist
Antiplatelet agent

Indications
▸ To reduce risk of thrombotic stroke in patients who have experienced stroke precursors and in patients who have a completed thrombotic stroke
▸ Treatment of patients with unstable angina or for patients at risk for platelet aggregation related to turbulent blood flow in a stenotic blood vessel, exposure of an unstable coronary plaque, or abrupt vessel closure associated with cardiac catheterization or angioplasty
▸ Alternative to aspirin for patients with aspirin sensitivity, intolerance, or resistance
▸ Unlabeled uses: intermittent claudication, chronic arterial occlusion, subarachnoid hemorrhage, uremic patients with AV shunts or fistulas, open heart surgery, coronary artery bypass grafts, primary glomerulonephritis, sickle cell disease

Adverse effects in *Italics* are most common; those in **Bold** are life-threatening

590 ticlopidine hydrochloride ◀

Therapeutic actions

▸ Interferes with platelet membrane function by inhibiting ADP-induced platelet fibrinogen binding and platelet–platelet interactions
▸ Inhibits platelet aggregation and prolongs bleeding time
▸ Effect is irreversible for life of the platelet

Contraindications/cautions

▸ **Contraindications:** ticlopidine allergy, neutropenia, thrombocytopenia, TTP, hemostatic disorders, active pathological bleeding (bleeding ulcer, intracranial bleeding), severe liver disease
▸ **Cautions:** renal disorders, elevated cholesterol, recent trauma or surgery

Available form

▸ *Tablets:* 250 mg

Oral dosage

▸ 250 mg PO bid with food.

TREATMENT OF OVERDOSE/ANTIDOTE

Discontinue drug or decrease dosage. Initiate general supportive and resuscitative measures. Methylprednisolone administration of 20 mg IV will normalize bleeding times within 2 h. Platelet transfusions may be used to reverse ticlopidine's effects; however, they may accelerate thrombosis in patients with TTP on ticlopidine.

Pharmacokinetics

Route	Onset	Peak
Oral	Rapid	2 h

Metabolism: Hepatic; $T_{1/2}$: 12.6 h, but 4–5 d with repeated dosing; within 4 d of twice-daily administration of ticlopidine 250 mg, ADP-induced platelet aggregation decreases by over 50%; maximum platelet aggregation inhibition of 60% to 70% occurs after 8–11 d of therapy; after 14–21 d of therapy, ticlopidine reaches steady-state levels; once drug is stopped, bleeding time and platelet function tests return to normal within 2 wk; clearance decreases with age
Excretion: Urine, feces

Adverse effects

▸ *CNS:* Dizziness
▸ *GI:* **GI bleeding,** *diarrhea, nausea, vomiting, abdominal pain,* flatulence, dyspepsia, anorexia, abnormal liver function

Adverse effects in *Italics* are most common; those in **Bold** are life-threatening

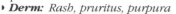

tests, jaundice, anorexia; elevated cholesterol, alkaline phosphatase and transaminases
▶ ***Derm:*** *Rash, pruritus, purpura*
▶ **Hematologic: Neutropenia, thrombocytopenia, TTP, bone marrow depression, eosinophilia, agranulocytosis, aplastic anemia, pancytopenia, ecchymosis, epistaxis, hematuria, conjunctival hemorrhage, bleeding, petechiae**
▶ ***Misc:*** Dark urine

Clinically important drug–drug interactions
▶ Decreased plasma levels of digoxin
▶ Enhanced effects of aspirin on collagen-induced platelet aggregation
▶ Increased half-life and total plasma clearance of theophylline
▶ Reduced clearance of a single dose by 50% with chronic cimetidine use
▶ Decreased absorption with antacids
▶ Elevated plasma phenytoin levels, causing somnolence and lethargy

⬤ NURSING CONSIDERATIONS
Assessment
▶ *History:* Ticlopidine allergy, neutropenia, thrombocytopenia, TTP, hemostatic disorders, active pathological bleeding, severe liver disease, renal disorders, elevated cholesterol, recent trauma or surgery
▶ *Physical:* P, BP, R, ECG, I & O, neurologic checks, skin assessment, presence of bleeding, abdominal assessment, bowel sounds, CBC, liver and renal function tests, serum cholesterol, coagulation studies; urine, stool, and emesis guaiac

Implementation
▶ Monitor CBC before use and frequently while initiating therapy; if neutropenia or TTP is suspected (fever, weakness, difficulty speaking, seizures, yellowing of skin or eyes, dark or bloody urine, pallor, petechiae), discontinue drug immediately.
▶ Administer with food or just after eating to minimize GI irritation and increase absorption.
▶ Maintain IV methylprednisolone (20 mg) on standby in case excessive bleeding occurs.
▶ Monitor patient for any sign of excessive bleeding (eg, bruises, dark urine and stools), and monitor bleeding times.
▶ Provide increased precautions against bleeding during invasive procedures; bleeding will be prolonged.
▶ Mark medical record of patient who receives this drug to alert medical personnel of increased risk of bleeding in cases of surgery or diagnostic procedures.

Adverse effects in *Italics* are most common; those in **Bold** are life-threatening

● tirofiban (tye row feye' ban) Aggrastat
Pregnancy Category B

Drug class
Glycoprotein (GP) IIb/IIIa antagonist
Antiplatelet drug

Indications
▸ Treatment, in conjunction with heparin and aspirin, of acute coronary syndrome, including patients who are to be managed medically or those undergoing PCI

Therapeutic actions
▸ Reversible GP IIb/IIIa antagonist that blocks activation of the GP IIb/IIIa receptor
▸ Prevents fibrinogen from binding to the GP IIb/IIIa receptor, thereby inhibiting platelet aggregation

Contraindications/cautions
▸ **Contraindications:** tirofiban allergy; recent (within 30 d) active internal bleeding, bleeding diathesis, stroke, major surgery, severe trauma; any hemorrhagic stroke; intracranial hemorrhage, neoplasm; arteriovenous malformation, aneurysm, past or present aortic dissection, severe HTN (SBP > 180 mmHg or DBP > 110 mmHg), acute pericarditis, thrombocytopenia after previous tirofiban use, use of another parenteral GP IIb/IIIa inhibitor
▸ **Cautions:** hemorrhagic retinopathy, platelet count < 150,000/mm^3, severe renal function impairment, elderly patients

Available forms
▸ *Injection:* 0.25 mg/mL
▸ *Premixed IV infusion:* 50 mcg/mL

IV facts
Preparation
▸ If premixed bag not available, use concentrated vial to prepare infusion.
▸ Withdraw and discard 50 mL from a 250-mL bag or 100 mL from a 500-mL bag of D5W or 0.9%NS.
▸ Replace the volume removed with an equal volume of tirofiban (using the 0.25 mg/mL vials) to achieve a final concentration of 50 mcg/mL.

Dosage
▸ *Loading dose:* 0.4 mcg/kg/min IV for 30 min. **Maintenance infusion:** 0.1 mcg/kg/min IV.
▸ *Renal insufficiency:* Administer half the dose.

Adverse effects in *Italics* are most common; those in **Bold** are life-threatening

Titration Guide

	tirofiban									
	25 mg in 500 mL									
	Body Weight									
lb	88	99	110	121	132	143	154	165	176	187
kg	40	45	50	55	60	65	70	75	80	85
Dose Ordered in mcg/kg/min	**Amounts to Infuse in mL/h**									
0.1	5	5	6	7	7	8	8	9	10	10
0.4	19	22	24	26	29	31	34	36	38	41

	Body Weight								
lb	198	209	220	231	242	253	264	275	286
kg	90	95	100	105	110	115	120	125	130
Dose Ordered in mcg/kg/min	**Amounts to Infuse in mL/h**								
0.1	11	11	12	13	13	14	14	15	16
0.4	43	46	48	50	53	55	58	60	62

Compatibility

Tirofiban may be administered through the same IV line as heparin.

> **TREATMENT OF OVERDOSE/ANTIDOTE**
> Discontinue drug or decrease dosage. Initiate general and supportive measures. Drug can be removed by hemodialysis.

Pharmacokinetics

Route	Onset	Peak	Duration
IV	Rapid	30 min	4–8 h after infusion is stopped

$T_{1/2}$: 2 h
Excretion: Urine, feces

Adverse effects

- *CNS:* **Hemorrhagic stroke,** *dizziness,* headache
- *CV: Bradycardia, coronary artery dissection,* vasovagal reaction
- *GI:* **GI bleeding,** nausea
- *GU:* **GU bleeding**
- *Hematologic:* **Bleeding (retroperitoneal, venous and arterial access sites), thrombocytopenia**
- *Musc/Skel: Leg pain*
- *Misc: Pelvic pain,* edema, fever, sweating

Adverse effects in *Italics* are most common; those in **Bold** are life-threatening

Clinically important drug–drug interactions
▸ Increased risk of bleeding with anticoagulant, thrombolytic, antithrombotic, aspirin, NSAIDs, other antiplatelet drugs
▸ Increased clearance with levothyroxine, omeprazole; clinical significance not known

● NURSING CONSIDERATIONS

Assessment
▸ *History:* Tirofiban allergy; recent active internal bleeding, bleeding diathesis, stroke, major surgery, severe trauma; hemorrhagic stroke; intracranial hemorrhage, neoplasm; arteriovenous malformation, aneurysm, past or present aortic dissection, severe HTN, acute pericarditis, thrombocytopenia after previous tirofiban use, use of another parenteral GP IIb/IIIa inhibitor, hemorrhagic retinopathy, severe renal function impairment, age
▸ *Physical:* P, BP, R, ECG, I & O, IV site, weight, neurologic checks, skin assessment, arterial and venous access sites, chest pain assessment, peripheral perfusion, pain assessment, bowel sounds, presence of bleeding, CPK, CPK-MB, cardiac troponin, myoglobin, CBC, renal function tests, PT, APTT, ACT; urine, stool, and emesis guaiac

Implementation
▸ Administer infusion using an IV pump.
▸ Frequently assess potential bleeding sites, paying careful attention to arterial and venous puncture sites and femoral access site.
▸ While the arterial and/or venous sheath is in place, maintain patient on bed rest with head of the bed < 30 degrees. Keep affected extremity flat and straight.
▸ Adhere to strict anticoagulation guidelines per hospital protocol. Administer and adjust weight-adjusted heparin as ordered. Discontinue heparin 2–4 h before sheath removal or according to hospital protocol.
▸ Remove sheaths when APTT is ≤ 45–50 s or the ACT is ≤ 175–180 s.
▸ Apply pressure to access site for at least 30 min after sheath removal.
▸ Following initial hemostasis, continue bed rest for 6–8 h or according to hospital policy. Apply a pressure dressing to site.
▸ If bleeding recurs, reapply manual or mechanical compression until hemostasis is achieved.

- Mark and measure the size of any hematoma, and monitor for evidence of enlargement.
- After achieving hemostasis, monitor the patient in hospital for at least 4 h.
- Assess for neurovascular compromise in affected leg. Palpate distal pulses, and note extremity's color and warmth. Assess for pain, numbness, tingling of affected leg.
- Minimize arterial and venous punctures.
- If possible, draw blood from a saline lock.
- Do not insert intravenous access devices into noncompressible sites, such as the subclavian and jugular veins.
- Avoid intramuscular injections, urinary catheter insertion, and nasotracheal and nasogastric intubation whenever possible.
- Continue aspirin therapy.
- Discontinue antiplatelet drug infusions, and determine a bleeding time before surgery if the patient requires CABG or other surgery.
- Check stools, urine, and emesis for occult blood.
- Monitor the patient's WBC, Hgb, Hct, APTT, ACT, platelet, and creatinine values; notify provider of abnormal values. Be prepared to transfuse platelets if platelet count is < 50,000 cells/mcL.
- Have emergency equipment (defibrillator, drugs, oxygen, intubation equipment) on standby in case an adverse reaction occurs.
- Medicate patient for back or groin pain.
- Use a manual blood pressure cuff or ensure that an automatic blood pressure cuff does not apply excessive pressure to the patient's arm.
- Shave patients using an electric razor.
- Protect from light during storage.

tobramycin sulfate *(toe bra mye' sin)*

Parenteral: Nebcin, Scheinpharm Tobramycin (CAN)
Ophthalmic: AKTob, Defy, Tobrex

Pregnancy Category D

Drug class
Aminoglycoside

Indications
Parenteral
- Serious infections caused by susceptible strains of *Pseudomonas aeruginosa, Proteus* species, *Escherichia coli, Providencia* species, *Citrobacter* species, and staphylococci

Adverse effects in *Italics* are most common; those in **Bold** are life-threatening

- Septicemia caused by *P. aeruginosa, E. coli, Klebsiella* species
- Lower respiratory tract infections caused by *P. aeruginosa, Klebsiella* species, *Enterobacter* species, *Serratia* species, *E. coli, Staphylococcus aureus*
- Serious CNS infections (meningitis) caused by susceptible organisms
- Intra-abdominal infections, including peritonitis, caused by *E. coli, Klebsiella* species, and *Enterobacter* species
- Skin, bone, and skin structure infections caused by *P. aeruginosa, Proteus* species, *E. coli, Klebsiella* species, *Enterobacter* species, and *S. aureus*
- Treatment of superficial ocular infections involving the conjunctiva or cornea due to microorganisms susceptible to antibiotics (ophthalmic forms)
- Complicated and recurrent urinary tract infections caused by *P. aeruginosa, Proteus* species, *E. coli, Klebsiella* species, *Enterobacter* species, *Serratia* species, *S. aureus, Providencia* species, *Citrobacter* species
- May be considered in serious staphylococcal infections when penicillin or other potentially less toxic drugs are contraindicated and when bacterial susceptibility testing and clinical judgment indicate its use

Therapeutic actions
- Bactericidal: inhibits protein synthesis in susceptible strains of gram-negative bacteria; binds to the 30S subunit of bacterial ribosomes, blocking the recognition step in protein synthesis, causing misreading of the genetic code; ribosomes separate from messenger RNA, leading to cell death

Contraindications/cautions
- **Contraindications:** allergy to any aminoglycoside; epithelial herpes simplex keratitis, vaccinia, varicella, fungal infections of ocular structures, mycobacterial infections of the eye (ophthalmic preparations)
- **Cautions:** renal dysfunction, sulfite sensitivity, preexisting hearing loss, extensive burns, neuromuscular disorders (myasthenia gravis, parkinsonism), dehydration, elderly patients, concurrent use of other nephrotoxic drugs

Available forms
- *Injection:* 10, 40 mg/mL
- *Powder for injection:* 1.2 g/vial
- *Ophthalmic solution:* 3 mg/mL
- *Ophthalmic ointment:* 3 mg/g

Adverse effects in *Italics* are most common; those in **Bold** are life-threatening

IV/IM facts
Preparation
▶ **IV solution:** Dilute single dose in 50–100 mL of Dextran 40 10% in D5W; D5W/0.9%NS; D5W; D10W; Mannitol 15%; dextrose 5% in 0.45%NS; LR; Mannitol 20%; Normosol M/D5W; Normosol R; Normosol R/D5W; Ringer's Injection; 0.9%NS; Sodium Lactate (1/6 Molar) Injection.
▶ **Powder for injection:** Reconstitute with Sterile Water for Injection.
▶ **ADD-Vantage vials:** Activate the ADD-Vantage vial by pulling the inner cap from the drug vial. Allow drug and diluent to mix.
▶ **IM:** Give undiluted.

Dosage
▶ Base dosage on patient's ideal body weight.
▶ *Serious infections:* 3 mg/kg/d IV over 20–60 min or IM in three equal doses q8h.
▶ *Life-threatening infections:* ≤ 5 mg/kg/d IV over 20–60 min or IM in 3–4 equal doses. Reduce to 3 mg/kg/d as soon as clinically indicated. Do not exceed 5 mg/kg/d unless serum levels are monitored.
▶ *"Once-daily dosing":* 5 or 7 mg/kg (using ideal body weight) IV over 60 min. Obtain serum drug concentration 8–10 h after starting the infusion. Use the 5- or 7-mg nomogram to determine the dosing interval (usually q24h, q36h, or q48h).
▶ *Renal function impairment:* Adjust dosage based on degree of renal impairment, serum creatinine clearance, and peak and trough tobramycin concentrations. Give smaller dosage or adjust the interval between doses.

Therapeutic serum levels
▶ **Trough:** 0.5–2 mcg/mL
▶ **Peak:** 4–8 mcg/mL

Compatibility
Tobramycin may be given through the same IV line as acyclovir, amifostine, amiodarone, amsacrine, aztreonam, ciprofloxacin, cyclophosphamide, diltiazem, enalaprilat, esmolol, filgrastim, fluconazole, fludarabine, foscarnet, furosemide, granisetron, hydromorphone, IL-2, insulin (regular), labetalol, magnesium sulfate, melphalan, meperidine, midazolam, morphine, perphenazine, tacrolimus, teniposide, theophylline, thiotepa, tolazoline, vinorelbine, zidovudine.

Incompatibility
Do not administer through the same IV line as allopurinol, heparin, hetastarch, indomethacin, propofol, sargramostim.

Adverse effects in *Italics* are most common; those in **Bold** are life-threatening

Ophthalmic dosage

▶ *Mild to moderate disease:* 1–2 drops into affected eye(s) q4h or 1/2-in ribbon of ointment bid–tid.
▶ *Severe disease:* 2 drops into affected eye(s) hourly until improvement occurs or 1/2-in ribbon ointment q3–4h.

> ### TREATMENT OF OVERDOSE/ANTIDOTE
> Discontinue drug or decrease dosage. Initiate general supportive and resuscitative measures. Support respiration as neuromuscular blockade or respiratory paralysis may occur. Adequately hydrate patient and carefully monitor fluid balance, creatinine clearance, and drug levels. Peritoneal dialysis and hemodialysis will remove the drug from the blood. Complexation with ticarcillin or carbenicillin may lower high serum concentrations.

Pharmacokinetics

Route	Onset	Peak
IV	Immediate	End of infusion
Opthalmologic	Rapid	

$T_{1/2}$: 2–3 h
Excretion: Urine

Adverse effects

▶ *CNS:* Headache, confusion, lethargy, disorientation, delirium
▶ *Resp:* **Apnea**
▶ *GI:* Vomiting, nausea, diarrhea; increased AST/ALT, bilirubin, LDH
▶ *GU:* Oliguria, cylindruria, proteinuria; increased serum creatinine, BUN, NPN
▶ *Derm:* Pain/irritation at injection site
▶ *Allergic:* Rash, urticaria, itching
▶ *Hematologic:* **Thrombocytopenia, granulocytopenia, leukopenia, eosinophilia,** anemia, leukocytosis
▶ *EENT:* Tinnitus, roaring in ears, dizziness, hearing loss/deafness
▶ *Misc:* Fever; decreased serum calcium, sodium, potassium, magnesium

Ophthalmic Preparations

▶ *Derm:* Local transient irritation, burning, stinging, itching, angioneurotic edema, urticaria, vesicular and maculopapular dermatitis

Adverse effects in *Italics* are most common; those in **Bold** are life-threatening

Clinically important drug–drug interactions

▸ Increased ototoxic, nephrotoxic, and neurotoxic effects with aminoglycosides, cephalosporins, loop diuretics, enflurane, methoxyflurane, vancomycin
▸ Increased neuromuscular blockade and muscular paralysis with depolarizing and nondepolarizing blocking agents
▸ Inactivation of both drugs if mixed with beta-lactam-type antibiotics (space doses with concomitant therapy)
▸ Increased bactericidal effect with penicillins, cephalosporins, carbenicillin, ticarcillin
▸ Increased respiratory paralysis and renal dysfunction with polypeptide antibiotics

● NURSING CONSIDERATIONS

Assessment

▸ *History:* Allergy to any aminoglycoside; epithelial herpes simplex keratitis, vaccinia, varicella, fungal infections of ocular structures, mycobacterial infections of the eye, renal dysfunction, sulfite sensitivity, preexisting hearing loss, extensive burns, neuromuscular disorders (myasthenia gravis, parkinsonism), dehydration, age, use of other nephrotoxic drugs
▸ *Physical:* T, P, R, BP, I & O, weight, neurologic checks, eighth cranial nerve function, skin assessment, respiratory effort, adventitious lung sounds, bowel sounds, UA, serum electrolytes, renal and liver function tests, CBC, culture and sensitivity tests of infected area

Implementation

▸ Obtain specimens for culture and sensitivity of infected area before beginning therapy. May begin drug before results are available.
▸ Monitor for occurrence of superinfections; treat as appropriate.
▸ Separate administration of other antibiotics by at least 1 h.
▸ Ensure adequate hydration of patient before and during therapy.
▸ Monitor renal function tests and complete blood counts during therapy. Adjust dosage as indicated.
▸ Monitor serum concentrations in patients with renal dysfunction to reduce risk of toxicity.
▸ Febrile and anemic patients may have shorter drug half-life. Severely burned patients may have a significantly decreased half-life and lower serum drug concentrations.
▸ Use ophthalmologic tobramycin only when indicated by sensitivity tests; use of ophthalmologic tobramycin may cause

Adverse effects in *Italics* are most common; those in **Bold** are life-threatening

sensitization that will contraindicate the systemic use of tobramycin or other aminoglycosides in serious infections.

▸ Store in refrigerator; however, may be stored at room temperature for ≤ 28 d. The solution in the ampule may darken with age if not refrigerated; however, the quality will not be affected if it is stored under the recommended storage conditions.

U

⬤ **urokinase** *(yoor oh kin' ase)* Abbokinase, Abbokinase Open-Cath

Pregnancy Category B

Drug class
Thrombolytic agent

Indications
▸ Lysis of diagnostically confirmed acute massive pulmonary emboli where there is obstruction in blood flow to a lobe or multiple segments of the lungs or where embolis is accompanied by unstable hemodynamics; initiate within 7 d of onset
▸ Lysis of coronary artery thrombosis with evolving transmural MI within 6 h of onset of symptoms
▸ To restore patency to IV catheters, including central venous catheters

Therapeutic actions
▸ Obtained from human kidney cells by tissue culture techniques
▸ Converts plasminogen to the enzyme plasmin
▸ Plasmin degrades fibrin clots, fibrinogen, and other plasma proteins

Contraindications/cautions
▸ **Contraindications:** urokinase allergy; active internal bleeding; recent (within 2 mo) trauma, CVA, intracranial or intraspinal surgery; intracranial neoplasm, arteriovenous malformation, or aneurysm; known bleeding diathesis; severe uncontrolled hypertension
▸ **Cautions:** old age (> 75 y), recent (≤ 10 d) major surgery (CABG, organ biopsy, obstetrical delivery, puncture of noncompressible vessels); recent (≤ 10 d) GI or GU bleeding; recent (≤ 10 d) trauma; hypertension (≥ 180 mmHg systolic or ≥ 110 mmHg diastolic); left heart thrombus, acute pericarditis, subacute bacterial endocarditis, hemostatic defects secondary to severe hepatic or
(contraindications continued on next page)

T

renal disease; diabetic hemorrhagic retinopathy or other
ophthalmic hemorrhaging; septic thrombophlebitis, occluded AV cannula at seriously infected site, current oral
anticoagulant therapy, other conditions in which bleeding
is a hazard or would be difficult to manage

Available forms:
▶ *Powder for injection:* 250,000 IU/vial
▶ *Powder for catheter clearance:* 1, 1.8 mL unidose vials

IV facts
Preparation
▶ Contains no preservatives; do not reconstitute until immedi-
ately before use.
▶ Reconstitute three 250,000 IU vials with 5 mL Sterile Water for
Injection without preservatives. Solution will appear slightly
straw-colored.
▶ Avoid shaking during reconstitution; gently roll or tilt vial to
reconstitute.
▶ Consult manufacturer's directions for further dilution.
▶ Solution may be terminally filtered through ≤ 0.45 micron
cellulose membrane filter administration set.

Dosage
▶ *Lysis of coronary artery thrombi:* Before therapy, administer
heparin bolus of 2,500–10,000 IU IV. Infuse urokinase into
occluded artery at rate of 6,000 IU/min for up to 2 h. Continue infusion until the artery is maximally opened, usually
15–30 min after initial opening.
▶ *Pulmonary embolism:* Give through constant infusion pump.
Give a priming dose of 4400 IU/kg as an admixture with D5W
or 0.9%NS at a rate of 90 ml/h IV over 10 min. Then give continuous infusion of 4400 IU/kg/h at a rate of 15 mL/h for 12
h. At end of infusion, flush the tubing with D5W or 0.9%NS
(equal to the volume of the tubing) at 15 mL/h. At the end of
the infusion, treat with continuous heparin IV infusion; begin
heparin when the thrombin time has decreased to < twice
the normal control.
▶ *IV catheter clearance:* When clearing a central venous
catheter, have patient exhale and hold his or her breath any
time catheter is not connected to IV tubing. Disconnect
catheter, attach an empty 10-mL syringe, and determine occlusion by gently attempting to aspirate blood from the
catheter. If aspiration is not possible, remove syringe and attach tuberculin syringe with urokinase solution. Slowly and
gently inject an amount equal to volume of catheter. Remove
tuberculin syringe and connect an empty 5-mL syringe to the

Adverse effects in *Italics* are most common; those in **Bold** are life-threatening

catheter. Wait 5 min and attempt to aspirate. Repeat aspirations every 5 min for up to 30 min. If catheter is not open within 30 min, cap catheter and allow urokinase to remain in catheter 30–60 min before attempting to aspirate again. A repeat infusion of urokinase may be necessary in resistant cases. When patency is restored, aspirate 4–5 mL of blood to ensure removal of drug and residual clot. Irrigate gently with 0.9%NS and reconnect IV tubing.

Compatibility
Do not give through the same line as other drugs; may infuse through D5W or 0.9%NS.

> ### TREATMENT OF OVERDOSE/ANTIDOTE
> Discontinue infusion and any other anticoagulant or antiplatelet drugs for severe bleeding, neurologic changes, or severe hypotension. Initiate general supportive and resuscitative measures. Administer IV fluids, PRBCs, FFP, platelets, and cryoprecipitate as indicated. Avoid dextran. Aminocaproic acid may be given as an antidote.

Pharmacokinetics

Route	Onset	Duration
IV	Immediate	12–24 h

Metabolism: Liver; $T_{1/2}$: $\leq$ 20 min
Excretion: Urine, bile

Adverse effects
- *CNS:* **Intracranial bleeding**
- *CV:* **Dysrhythmias** (with intracoronary artery infusion), **cholesterol embolism,** transient hypotension or hypertension, tachycardia, cyanosis
- *Resp:* **Bronchospasm,** dyspnea
- *GI:* **GI bleeding,** nausea, vomiting
- *GU:* **GU bleeding,** vaginal bleeding
- *Derm:* Skin rash, urticaria, itching, flushing
- *Allergic:* **Anaphylaxis,** mild allergic reactions
- *Hematologic:* ***Bleeding*** (*minor or surface* to major internal bleeding)
- *Misc:* *Fever,* retroperitoneal bleeding, chills, rigors, back pain

Clinically important drug–drug interactions
- Increased hemorrhage with vitamin K antagonists, heparin, oral anticoagulants, drugs that alter platelet function (aspirin, dipyridamole, abciximab, tirofiban, eptifibatide, ticlopidine, clopidogrel)

Adverse effects in *Italics* are most common; those in **Bold** are life-threatening

U

● NURSING CONSIDERATIONS

Assessment

▶ *History:* Urokinase allergy; active internal bleeding, recent trauma, CVA, intracranial or intraspinal surgery; intracranial neoplasm, arteriovenous malformation, or aneurysm; known bleeding diathesis, severe uncontrolled hypertension, age; recent major surgery (CABG, organ biopsy, obstetrical delivery; puncture of noncompressible vessels); recent GI or GU bleeding; left heart thrombus, acute pericarditis, subacute bacterial endocarditis, hemostatic defects secondary to severe hepatic or renal disease; diabetic hemorrhagic retinopathy or other ophthalmic hemorrhaging; septic thrombophlebitis, occluded AV cannula at seriously infected site, current oral anticoagulant therapy, other conditions in which bleeding is a hazard or would be difficult to manage

▶ *Physical:* T, P, R, BP, ECG, I & O, SpO_2, IV site, IV catheter patency, neurologic checks, skin assessment, chest pain evaluation, heart sounds, JVD, peripheral perfusion, adventitious lung sounds, evidence of bleeding, liver evaluation, CBC, CPK, CPK-MB, cardiac troponin, myoglobin, TT, APTT, PT, INR, FSP, ABG, type and crossmatch; urine, stool, and emesis guaiac

Implementation

▶ Use only in critical cases because of the risk of transmitting infectious agents.
▶ Administer drug as soon as possible after diagnosis. Initiate within 6 h after onset of AMI symptoms.
▶ Administer infusion using an IV pump.
▶ Have emergency equipment (defibrillator, drugs, oxygen, intubation equipment) on standby in case anaphylaxis, hemorrhage, or adverse reaction occurs.
▶ Before starting drug, initiate at least 2–3 peripheral IVs.
▶ Discontinue heparin unless to be used with intracoronary administration.
▶ Monitor BP, P, R, and neurologic status continuously.
▶ Do not take BP in lower extremities to avoid dislodging possible deep vein thrombi.
▶ Type and crossmatch blood in case serious blood loss occurs and blood transfusions are required.
▶ When given for AMI, assess for chest pain (type, character, location, intensity, radiation). Monitor ECG before, during, and after therapy. Assess for ST segment changes and reperfusion dysrhythmias.
▶ When given for PE, assess respiratory effort, SpO_2, ABGs, and chest pain.

Adverse effects in *Italics* are most common; those in **Bold** are life-threatening

- Initiate other interventions as standard for patients with AMI or PE.
- Drug will clear occluded catheters only if occluded by fibrin clots. Avoid excessive pressure when injecting urokinase; force could rupture catheter or expel clot into circulation.
- Initiate bleeding precautions.
- Assess patient for evidence of bleeding and hemorrhage.
- Carefully assess recent puncture sites and sites of lines/tubes (catheter insertion sites, cutdown sites, needle puncture sites, recent surgical incisions).
- Apply pressure to arterial and venous puncture sites for at least 30 min or until hemostasis achieved. Apply a pressure dressing to site to prevent bleeding. Assess all puncture sites q15min.
- Apply pressure or pressure dressings to control superficial bleeding.
- Avoid IM injections before, during, and for 24 h after therapy. Do not attempt central venous access or arterial puncture unless absolutely necessary. If arterial puncture is necessary, use an upper extremity vessel that is accessible to manual pressure.
- Guaiac all stools, urine, and emesis for blood.
- Handle patient carefully to avoid ecchymosis and bleeding.
- If possible, draw blood for laboratory analysis from an existing saline lock.
- Take BP with manual BP cuff or ensure that NIBP cuff does not inflate excessively above patient's SBP.
- Shave patient with an electric razor.
- Discard any unused portion of drug.

V

⬤ **valproic acid** *(val proe' ik)* Alti-Valproic (CAN), Depakene, Deproic (CAN)

⬤ **valproate sodium** Depacon, Depakene

⬤ **divalproex sodium** Depakote, Epival (CAN)
Pregnancy Category D

Drug class
Anticonvulsant

Indications
- Sole and adjunctive therapy in simple (petit mal) and complex absence seizures

- Adjunctive therapy with multiple seizure types, including absence seizures
- Monotherapy and adjunctive therapy for complex partial seizures that occur either in isolation or in association with other types of seizures (divalproex sodium, valproate injection)
- Treatment of manic episodes associated with bipolar disorder (divalproex-DR tablets)
- Prophylaxis of migraine headaches (divalproex-DR tablets)
- Unlabeled uses: sole and adjunctive therapy in atypical absence, myoclonic, and grand mal seizures; possibly effective therapy in atonic, elementary partial, and infantile spasm seizures; may be effective for intractable status epilepticus unresponsive to other therapies; management of anxiety disorders/panic attacks; treatment of minor incontinence after ileoanal anastomosis

Therapeutic actions
- Mechanism of action not established; antiepileptic activity may be related to increased brain levels of the inhibitory neurotransmitter, GABA
- May exert prolactin-lowering effects, inhibit the enzyme that catabolizes GABA, potentiate postsynaptic GABA responses, affect the potassium channel, and have a direct membrane-stabilizing effect

Contraindications/cautions
- **Contraindications:** valproic acid allergy, hepatic disease/dysfunction
- **Cautions:** acute head injury, thrombocytopenia, coagulation disorders, psychiatric disorders

Available forms
- *Injection:* 5 mL
- *Capsules:* 250 mg
- *Syrup:* 250 mg/5 mL
- *Delayed-release tablets:* 125, 250, 500 mg
- *Sprinkle capsules:* 125 mg

IV facts
Preparation
- Dilute each dose in at least 50 mL D5W; LR; or 0.9%NS.

Dosage
- Maximum dosage is 60 mg/kg/d. If total daily dose > 250 mg, give in divided doses. Infuse as a 60-min infusion (≤ 20 mg/min). Use IV route for ≤ 14 d. Switch to oral therapy as soon as possible.

Adverse effects in *Italics* are most common; those in **Bold** are life-threatening

- *Complex partial seizures:* 10–15 mg/kg/d IV. Increase by 5–10 mg/kg/wk.
- *Simple and complex absence seizures:* 15 mg/kg/d IV. Increase at 1-wk intervals by 5–10 mg/kg/d.
- *Conversion of oral therapy to IV therapy:* Use the same IV dose as oral dose. Give dose q6h to maintain drug levels. Closely monitor drug levels.
- *Elderly patients:* Reduce starting dose; base dose on patient response.

Therapeutic serum level
- 50–100 mcg/mL

Compatibility
Do not administer through the same IV line as other drugs.

Oral dosage
- *Complex partial seizures:* 10–15 mg/kg/d PO. Increase by 5–10 mg/kg/wk.
- *Simple and complex absence seizures:* 15 mg/kg/d PO. Increase at 1-wk intervals by 5–10 mg/kg/d.
- *Conversion from valproic acid to divalproex sodium:* Start divalproex sodium at same total daily dose and dosing schedule. Once stabilized, may administer bid–tid.
- *Mania (divalproex sodium delayed release tablets):* 750 mg/d PO in divided doses. Do not exceed 60 mg/kg/d.
- *Migraine (divalproex sodium delayed release tablets):* 250 mg PO bid; up to 1000 mg/d has been used.
- *Elderly patients:* Reduce starting dose; base dose on patient response.

TREATMENT OF OVERDOSE/ANTIDOTE
Discontinue drug or decrease dosage. Initiate general supportive and resuscitative measures. Maintain adequate urinary output. Naloxone may reverse both CNS depression and anticonvulsant effects. Hemodialysis and hemoperfusion have been used.

Pharmacokinetics

Route	Onset	Peak
IV	Rapid	1 h
Oral	Varies	1–4 h

Metabolism: Hepatic; $T_{1/2}$: 6–16 h
Excretion: Urine, feces

Adverse effects
- *CNS: Sedation, somnolence,* tremor (may be dose related), hallucinations, ataxia, headache, nystagmus, diplopia, emo-

Adverse effects in *Italics* are most common; those in **Bold** are life-threatening

tional upset, depression, psychosis, aggression, weakness, hyperactivity, behavioral deterioration, weakness, fecal incontinence, flatulence, hearing loss, neck pain and rigidity
▶ *CV:* Hypertension, hypotension, palpitations, postural hypotension, tachycardia, edema
▶ *Resp:* Dyspnea, rhinitis, cough, pneumonia
▶ *GI:* **Hepatic failure, pancreatitis,** *nausea, vomiting, indigestion;* minor ALT, AST, LDH, bilirubin elevations; jaundice, diarrhea, abdominal cramps, constipation, anorexia with weight loss, increased appetite with weight gain
▶ *Derm:* Alopecia, rash, petechiae, dry skin
▶ *Hematologic:* **Thrombocytopenia, hemorrhage, leukopenia, eosinophilia,** bruising, hematoma formation, relative lymphocytosis, hypofibrinogenemia, eosinophilia, anemia, bone marrow suppression, altered bleeding time
▶ *Endocrine:* Irregular menses, secondary amenorrhea, abnormal thyroid function tests, breast enlargement, galactorrhea, parotid gland swelling
▶ *Misc:* Fever, urinary tract infection, otitis media, pain at injection site, arthralgia, leg cramps, arthrosis

Clinically important drug–drug interactions
▶ Increased serum levels of phenobarbital, lamotrigine, primidone, ethosuximide, diazepam, zidovudine
▶ Complex interactions with phenytoin; breakthrough seizures have occurred with phenytoin
▶ Increased serum levels and toxicity with salicylates, cimetidine, chlorpromazine, erythromycin, felbamate
▶ Decreased effects with carbamazepine, rifampin, lamotrigine
▶ Decreased absorption with charcoal
▶ Increased CNS effects of CNS depressants

◉ NURSING CONSIDERATIONS
Assessment
▶ *History:* Valproic acid allergy, hepatic disease/dysfunction, acute head injury, thrombocytopenia, coagulation disorders, psychiatric disorders
▶ *Physical:* T, P, BP, R, ECG, EEG, I & O, IV site, weight, neurologic checks, presence of seizure activity, presence of bleeding, bowel sounds, CBC, coagulation tests, liver and thyroid function tests, exocrine pancreatic function tests, serum ammonia level

Implementation
▶ Initiate seizure precautions.
▶ Administration at hs minimizes CNS depression.

Adverse effects in *Italics* are most common; those in **Bold** are life-threatening

- Minimize GI irritation by giving drug with food, slowly increasing dosage, or using delayed-release divalproex sodium.
- Patient may swallow sprinkle capsules whole, or open capsule and sprinkle entire contents on soft food. Do not chew.
- Reduce dosage, discontinue, or substitute other antiepileptic medications gradually; abrupt discontinuation of all antiepileptic medication may precipitate absence status.
- Frequently monitor liver function tests. Discontinue drug immediately with suspected or apparent hepatic dysfunction. Hepatic dysfunction may progress in spite of drug discontinuation.
- Monitor platelet counts and coagulation tests before therapy, periodically during therapy, and prior to surgery. Monitor patient carefully for clotting defects (bruising, blood-tinged toothbrush). Discontinue with evidence of hemorrhage, bruising, or hemostasis disorders.
- Monitor ammonia levels; discontinue if elevated.
- Monitor serum levels of valproic acid and other antiepileptic drugs given concomitantly, especially during the first few weeks of therapy. Adjust dosage based on drug levels and clinical response.

● vancomycin hydrochloride

(van koe mye' sin) Vancocin, Vancoled

Pregnancy Category C

Drug class
Antibiotic

Indications
- Serious or severe infections not treatable with other antimicrobials (parenteral)
- Severe staphylococci infections in patients who cannot receive or have failed to respond to penicillins and cephalosporins (parenteral)
- Severe infections with resistant staphylococci, such as endocarditis, septicemia, or bone, lower respiratory tract, or skin/skin-structure infections (parenteral)
- Prevention of bacterial endocarditis in penicillin-allergic patients undergoing dental procedures or surgical procedures of the GU, GI, or upper respiratory tract (parenteral)
- Staphylococcal enterocolitis and antibiotic-associated pseudomembranous colitis caused by *Clostridium difficile* (oral)

Therapeutic actions
- Bactericidal: inhibits cell wall synthesis and alters bacterial-cell membrane permeability and RNA synthesis of susceptible organisms, causing cell death

Adverse effects in *Italics* are most common; those in **Bold** are life-threatening

Contraindications/cautions
- **Contraindications:** vancomycin allergy
- **Cautions:** hearing loss, renal dysfunction, elderly patients

Available forms
- *Pulvules:* 125, 250 mg
- *Powder for injection:* 1, 5, 10 g
- *Powder for oral solution:* 1, 10 g

IV facts
Preparation
- Reconstitute 500-mg vial with 10 mL or 1-g vial with 20 mL Sterile Water for Injection. Further dilute 500 mg in 100 mL or 1 g in 200 mL of Acetated Ringer's Injection; D5W/LR; D5W/0.9%NS; D5W; D10W; Dextran 6% in D5W or 0.9%NS; Isolyte E; Normosol-M/D5W; LR; 0.9%NS; Sodium Bicarbonate 3.75%; Sodium Lactate (1/6 Molar) Injection; or Sterile Water for Injection.

Dosage
- Give each IV dose over at least 60 min.
- 500 mg IV q6h or 1 g q12h.
- *Prevention of bacterial endocarditis (high-risk penicillin-allergic patients):* 1 g IV over 1–2 h. Also give gentamicin as ordered. Complete infusion within 30 min of starting the procedure.
- *Prevention of bacterial endocarditis (moderate-risk penicillin-allergic patients):* 1 g IV over 1–2 h. Complete infusion within 30 min of starting the procedure.
- *Renal function impairment:* Calculate the dose using the following table:

Creatinine Clearance (mL/min)	Dose (mg/24 h)
100	1545
90	1390
80	1235
70	1080
60	925
50	770
40	620
30	465
20	310
10	155

Therapeutic serum level
- **Trough:** 5–15 mg/mL
- **Peak:** 20–40 mcg/mL

Adverse effects in *Italics* are most common; those in **Bold** are life-threatening

Compatibility

Vancomycin may be given through the same IV line as acyclovir, allopurinol, amifostine, amiodarone, amsacrine, atracurium, cyclophosphamide, diltiazem, enalaprilat, esmolol, filgrastim, fluconazole, fludarabine, gallium, granisetron, hydromorphone, insulin (regular), labetalol, lorazepam, magnesium sulfate, melphalan, meperidine, meropenem, morphine, midazolam, ondansetron, paclitaxel, pancuronium, perphenazine, propofol, sodium bicarbonate, tacrolimus, teniposide, theophylline, thiotepa, tolazoline, vecuronium, vinorelbine, zidovudine.

Incompatibility

Do not administer through the same IV line as albumin, cefepime, heparin, idarubicin, piperacillin-tazobactam.

Oral dosage

▸ 500–2000 mg/d PO given tid–qid for 7–10 d.
▸ *C. difficile:* 125 mg PO tid–qid may be as effective as the 500-mg dose regimen.

TREATMENT OF OVERDOSE/ANTIDOTE
Discontinue drug or decrease dosage. Initiate general supportive and resuscitative measures. Maintain glomerular filtration. Hemofiltration and hemoperfusion with polysulfone resin may increase vancomycin clearance.

Pharmacokinetics

Route	Onset	Peak
IV	Rapid	End of infusion
Oral	Varies	

$T_{1/2}$: 4–6 h
Excretion: Urine

Adverse effects

▸ *CNS:* Ototoxicity
▸ *CV:* Hypotension (IV administration)
▸ *Resp:* Wheezing
▸ *GI:* Nausea
▸ *GU:* Nephrotoxicity
▸ *Derm: Urticaria,* macular rashes, pruritus, inflammation at IV site
▸ *Allergic:* **Anaphylaxis**
▸ *Hematologic:* Eosinophilia, neutropenia
▸ *Misc:* **"Red neck or red man syndrome"** (sudden and profound fall in BP; erythema of the face, neck, and back), superinfections, fever

Adverse effects in *Italics* are most common; those in **Bold** are life-threatening

Clinically important drug–drug interactions

▸ Enhanced neuromuscular blockade of nondepolarizing muscle relaxants
▸ Increased toxicity with other neurotoxic and nephrotoxic agents; monitor carefully
▸ Increased nephrotoxicity with aminoglycosides

⬤ NURSING CONSIDERATIONS

Assessment

▸ *History:* Vancomycin allergy, hearing loss, renal dysfunction, age
▸ *Physical:* T, P, R, BP, I & O, neurologic checks, eighth cranial nerve function, skin assessment, adventitious lung sounds, liver evaluation, UA, serum electrolytes, renal function tests, CBC, culture and sensitivity tests of infected area

Implementation

▸ Obtain specimens for culture and sensitivity of infected area before beginning therapy. May begin drug before results are available.
▸ Have emergency equipment (defibrillator, drugs, oxygen, intubation equipment) on standby in case anaphylactic reaction occurs.
▸ Assess for evidence of anaphylaxis; if suspected, discontinue drug immediately and notify provider.
▸ Monitor for occurrence of superinfections; treat as appropriate.
▸ Monitor renal function tests, CBC, and serum drug levels during therapy. Adjust dosage as indicated.
▸ Observe the patient very closely when giving IV doses, particularly the first dose. "Red neck" syndrome can occur (see adverse effects). Slower administration decreases the risk of adverse effects.
▸ Do not give IM.
▸ Oral solution: Add 20 mL distilled water to the contents of the 1-g bottle to obtain 250 mg/5 mL. Add 115 mL distilled water to the contents of the 10-g bottle to obtain 500 mg/6 mL.
▸ IV and oral solutions are stable for 14 d if refrigerated after initial reconstitution. After further dilution, the IV solution is stable for 24 h at room temperature and for 2 mo under refrigeration.

⬤ **vasopressin** *(vay soe press' in)* (8-arginine vasopressin)
   Pitressin Synthetic, Pressyn (CAN)

Pregnancy Category C

Drug class
Hormone

Adverse effects in *Italics* are most common; those in **Bold** are life-threatening

Indications
▸ Neurogenic diabetes insipidus
▸ Prevention and treatment of postoperative abdominal distention
▸ Dispelling of gas interfering with abdominal roentgenography
▸ Unlabeled use: Management of esophageal varices

Therapeutic actions
▸ Purified form of the posterior pituitary that possesses vasopressor and ADH activity
▸ Promotes water resorption in the renal tubular epithelium
▸ Promotes smooth muscle contraction throughout the vascular bed
▸ Enhances GI motility and tone

Contraindications/cautions
▸ **Contraindications:** allergy or anaphylaxis to vasopressin or its components, chronic nephritis until nitrogen blood levels are reasonable
▸ **Cautions:** vascular disease, coronary artery disease, water intoxication, epilepsy, migraine, asthma, heart failure, any state in which a rapid increase in extracellular water may harm patient

Available form
▸ *Injection:* 20 U/mL

IV/IM/SC facts
Preparation
▸ For an IV infusion, dilute drug to a concentration of 0.1–1 U/mL in D5W or 0.9%NS.

Dosage
▸ *Esophageal varices (IV):* Initially 0.2 U/min IV. Increase to 0.4 U/min if bleeding continues. Maximum dose is 0.9 U/min.
▸ *Esophageal varices (intra-arterial infusion):* 0.1–0.5 U/min.
▸ *Diabetes insipidus:* 5–10 U IM or SC bid or tid. May also give intranasally on cotton pledgets, by nasal spray, or by nasal dropper. Individualize dosage.
▸ *Abdominal distention:* Initially 5 U IM; increase to 10 U IM at subsequent injections given q3–4h.
▸ *Abdominal roentgenography:* Administer 2 IM injections of 10 U each. Give 2 h and ½ h before films are exposed. An enema may be given prior to first dose.

Adverse effects in *Italics* are most common; those in **Bold** are life-threatening

Titration Guide

vasopressin

100 U in 100 mL

U/min	0.1	0.2	0.3	0.4	0.5	0.6	0.7	0.8	0.9
mL/h	6	12	18	24	30	36	42	48	54

Compatibility
Do not mix or give with other drugs.

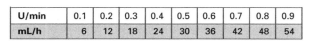

TREATMENT OF OVERDOSE/ANTIDOTE
Discontinue drug or decrease dosage. Initiate general supportive and resuscitative measures. Treat water intoxication with water restriction. Severe water intoxication may require osmotic diuresis with mannitol, hypertonic dextrose, or urea with or without furosemide.

Pharmacokinetics

Route	Onset	Duration
IV	Rapid	10–20 min
IM/SC	10–15 min	2–8 h

Metabolism: Hepatic, renal; $T_{1/2}$: 10–20 min
Excretion: Urine

Adverse effects
▶ *CNS: Tremor, vertigo, sweating,* "pounding" in head
▶ *CV:* **Cardiac arrest, MI, dysrhythmias,** angina, circumoral pallor, hypertension
▶ *Resp:* Bronchial constriction
▶ *GI:* Abdominal cramps, nausea, vomiting, flatulence, ischemic colitis
▶ *Allergic:* **Anaphylaxis**
▶ *Misc:* **Water intoxication (drowsiness, lightheadedness, headache, coma, convulsions),** local tissue necrosis, gangrene of extremities, tongue necrosis

Clinically important drug–drug interactions
▶ Increased effects with carbamazepine, chlorpropamide

○ NURSING CONSIDERATIONS

Assessment
▶ *History:* Allergy to vasopressin acetate or its components, chronic nephritis, vascular disease, coronary artery disease, water intoxication, epilepsy, migraine, asthma, heart failure,

any state in which a rapid increase in extracellular water may harm patient
▸ *Physical:* P, BP, R, ECG, I & O, IV site, daily weight, neurologic checks, skin assessment, cardiac auscultation, edema, JVD, respiratory effort, adventitious lung sounds, abdominal exam, bowel sounds, presence of bleeding, serum electrolytes, renal and liver function tests, UA, BUN, creatinine

Implementation

▸ Exercise extreme caution when calculating and preparing IV doses. Always dilute drug before use; avoid inadvertent bolus of drug.
▸ Administer IV or intra-arterial infusion using an IV infusion pump.
▸ Carefully monitor P, BP, ECG, and fluid and electrolyte status during administration.
▸ Have emergency equipment (defibrillator, drugs, oxygen, intubation equipment) on standby in case anaphylaxis occurs.
▸ Administer by IM injection if possible; SC may be used if needed.
▸ Monitor patients with CV disease very carefully for cardiac reactions. May infuse IV nitroglycerin simultaneously to prevent coronary artery vasoconstriction and chest pain.
▸ Monitor fluid volume for signs of water intoxication and excess fluid load; decrease dosage if this occurs.
▸ Monitor the infusion site closely for evidence of infiltration or phlebitis. Infuse into a central line if possible. May treat infiltration with phentolamine.
▸ If patient can tolerate oral intake, give patient 1–2 glasses of water with dose to minimize skin blanching, abdominal cramps, and nausea.
▸ Monitor condition of nasal passages during long-term intranasal therapy; inappropriate administration may lead to nasal ulceration.

⬤ **vecuronium bromide** *(ve kure oh' nee um)*

Norcuron

Pregnancy Category C

Drug class

Nondepolarizing neuromuscular blocking agent

Indications

▸ Provides skeletal muscle relaxation during surgery or mechanical ventilation
▸ Adjunct to general anesthesia to facilitate intubation

Adverse effects in *Italics* are most common; those in **Bold** are life-threatening

Therapeutic actions
▶ Prevents neuromuscular transmission and produces paralysis by blocking effect of acetylcholine at the myoneural junction

Contraindications/cautions
▶ **Contraindications:** vecuronium or bromide allergy
▶ **Caution:** myasthenia gravis, cirrhosis, cholestasis, cardiovascular disease, elderly patients, edema, severe obesity, neuromuscular disease, malignant hyperthermia, electrolyte imbalance, respiratory depression, pulmonary disease

Available forms
▶ *IV injection:* 10-mg vials with or without diluent, 20-mg vials without diluent

IV facts
▶ Reconstitute drug with Bacteriostatic Water for Injection; D5W/ 0.9%NS; D5W; LR; or 0.9%NS.
▶ For a continuous infusion, dilute 10–20 mg in 100 mL D5W/ 0.9%NS; D5W; LR; or 0.9%NS to achieve a concentration of 100–200 mcg/mL.

Dosage and titration
▶ *Initial adult dose:* **Intubation:** 80–100 mcg/kg as an IV bolus. **With succinylcholine:** 40–60 mcg/kg by IV.
▶ *Maintenance dose:* Usual dose is 1 mcg/kg/min by continous IV infusion. Dose range is 0.8–1.2 mcg/kg/min.
▶ Titrate infusion by 0.1–0.2 mcg/kg/min to maintain a 90% suppression of patient's twitch response as determined by peripheral nerve stimulation.

Titration Guide

vecuronium bromide									
100 mg in 250 mL									
Body Weight									
lb	88	99	110	121	132	143	154	165	176	187
kg	40	45	50	55	60	65	70	75	80	85
Dose Ordered in mcg/kg/min	**Amounts to Infuse in mL/h**								
0.7	4	5	5	6	6	7	7	8	8	9
0.8	5	5	6	7	7	8	8	9	10	10
0.9	5	6	7	7	8	9	9	10	11	11
1	6	7	8	8	9	10	11	11	12	13
1.1	7	7	8	9	10	11	12	12	13	14

continued

Adverse effects in *Italics* are most common; those in **Bold** are life-threatening

vecuronium bromide									
100 mg in 250 mL									
Body Weight									
lb	88	99	110	121	132	143	154	165	176	187
kg	40	45	50	55	60	65	70	75	80	85

Dose Ordered in mcg/kg/min	Amounts to Infuse in mL/h									
1.2	7	8	9	10	11	12	13	14	14	15
1.3	8	9	10	11	12	13	14	15	16	17

	Body Weight								
lb	198	209	220	231	242	253	264	275	286
kg	90	95	100	105	110	115	120	125	130

Dose Ordered in mcg/kg/min	Amounts to Infuse in mL/h								
0.7	9	10	11	11	12	12	13	13	14
0.8	11	11	12	13	13	14	14	15	16
0.9	12	13	14	14	15	16	16	17	18
1	14	14	15	16	17	17	18	19	20
1.1	15	16	17	17	18	19	20	21	21
1.2	16	17	18	19	20	21	22	23	23
1.3	18	19	20	20	21	22	23	24	25

Compatibility
Vecuronium may be given through the same IV line as aminophylline, cefazolin, cefuroxime, cimetidine, diltiazem, dobutamine, dopamine, epinephrine, esmolol, fentanyl, fluconazole, gentamicin, heparin, hydrocortisone, hydromorphone, isoproterenol, labetalol, lorazepam, midazolam, milrinone, morphine, nicardipine, nitroglycerin, nitroprusside sodium, norepinephrine, propofol, ranitidine, trimethoprim-sulfamethoxazole, vancomycin.

Incompatibility
Do not administer through the same IV line as diazepam, etomidate, furosemide, thiopental.

TREATMENT OF OVERDOSE/ANTIDOTE
Discontinue drug or decrease dosage. Initiate general supportive and resuscitative measures. Continue to maintain a patent airway and provide mechanical ventilation. Pyridostigmine bromide, neostigmine, or edrophonium in conjunction with atropine or glycopyrrolate will usually reverse skeletal muscle relaxation.

Adverse effects in *Italics* are most common; those in **Bold** are life-threatening

Pharmacokinetics

Route	Onset	Peak	Duration
IV	1 min	3–5 min	25–65 min

Metabolism: Hepatic with conversion to active metabolite; $T_{1/2}$: 65–75 min
Excretion: Urine, bile

Adverse effects

▶ *Resp: **Apnea**, respiratory insufficiency, respiratory acidosis during weaning,* cough, burning in throat
▶ *Allergic:* **Anaphylactic reactions, bronchospasm,** flushing, redness, hypotension, tachycardia
▶ *Musc/Skel:* Skeletal muscle weakness, profound and prolonged muscle paralysis

Clinically important drug–drug interactions

▶ Intensified neuromuscular blockage with antibiotics (aminoglycosides, tetracyclines, bacitracin, polymyxin B, colistin, sodium colistimethate)
▶ Enhanced neuromuscular blockade with magnesium salts
▶ Recurrent paralysis with quinidine given during recovery from use of muscle relaxants
▶ Enhanced neuromuscular blocking effect and duration of action with succinylcholine
▶ Counteracted by anticholinesterase, anticholinergic agents

◉ NURSING CONSIDERATIONS

Assessment

▶ *History:* Vecuronium or bromide allergy, myasthenia gravis, liver or kidney disease, cardiovascular disease, age, edema, neuromuscular disease, malignant hyperthermia, respiratory depression, pulmonary disease
▶ *Physical:* T, P, BP, R, ECG, SpO_2, I & O, IV site, weight, neurologic checks, level of sedation, skin assessment, respiratory status, method of mechanical ventilation, adventitious lung sounds, muscle strength, presence of pain, peripheral nerve stimulator response, serum electrolytes, renal and liver function studies, ABG

Implementation

▶ Exercise extreme caution when calculating and preparing doses. Vecuronium is a very potent drug; small dosage errors can cause serious adverse effects.
▶ Always administer an infusion using an IV infusion pump.

Adverse effects in *Italics* are most common; those in **Bold** are life-threatening

- Do not administer unless equipment for intubation, artifical respiration, oxygen therapy, and reversal agents is readily available. Vecuronium should be administered by people who are skilled in management of critically ill patients, cardiovascular resuscitation, and airway management.
- Use the smallest dose possible to achieve desired patient response.
- Monitor patient's response to therapy with a peripheral nerve stimulator.
- Monitor BP, R, and ECG closely during infusion.
- Vecuronium does not affect consciousness, pain threshold, or cerebration. Administer adequate sedatives and analgesics before giving vecuronium.
- Vecuronium produces paralysis. Provide oral and skin care. Administer artifical tears to protect corneas. May need to tape eyes closed. Position patient appropriately.
- Protect vials from light.
- When vial is reconstituted with supplied Bacteriostatic Water for Injection, solution is good for 5 d. When reconstituted with other solutions, use within 24 h.

⬤ verapamil hydrochloride *(ver ap' a mill)*
Calan, Calan SR, Isoptin, Isoptin SR, Verelan, Verelan PM
Pregnancy Category C

Drug classes
Calcium channel-blocker
Antianginal agent
Antidysrhthmic
Antihypertensive

Indications
- Treatment of supraventricular tachydysrhythmias (parenteral)
- Temporary control of rapid ventricular rate in atrial flutter or atrial fibrillation (parenteral)
- Treatment of vasospastic (Prinzmetal's variant), chronic stable (effort-associated), and unstable (crescendo, preinfarction) angina (oral)
- Used with digitalis to control ventricular rate with chronic atrial fibrillation and flutter (oral)
- For prevention of repetitive paroxysmal supraventricular tachycardia
- Treatment of essential hypertension
- Unlabeled oral uses: prophylaxis of migraine headache, cluster headache, and exercise-induced asthma; treatment of hy-

pertrophic cardiomyopathy, manic depression, recumbent
nocturnal leg cramps

Therapeutic actions
▶ Inhibits the movement of calcium ions across cell membranes
▶ Cardiovascular system effects include depressed myocardial
and smooth muscle mechanical contraction, impulse formation, and conduction velocity
▶ Dilates the main coronary arteries and arterioles both in normal and ischemic regions and inhibits coronary artery spasm,
thus increasing myocardial oxygen delivery
▶ Effective for chronic stable angina as drug dilates peripheral
arterioles and reduces afterload, myocardial energy consumption, and oxygen requirements
▶ Slows AV conduction and prolongs the refractory period
within the AV node in a rate-related manner, thus reducing
ventricular rate due to atrial flutter and fibrillation
▶ Interrupts reentry at the AV node, thus converting supraventricular tachycardia to normal sinus rhythm
▶ Interferes with sinus node impulse generation; depresses amplitude and velocity of depolarization and conduction in depressed atrial fibers

Effects on hemodynamic parameters
▶ Decreased SVR
▶ Decreased HR
▶ Decreased or unchanged CVP
▶ Increased or decreased CO
▶ Decreased BP

Contraindications/cautions
▶ **Contraindications:** verapamil allergy, sick sinus syndrome (except in presence of ventricular pacemaker),
heart block (second or third degree), hypotension (SBP
< 90), severe left ventricular dysfunction, cardiogenic
shock, CHF (unless related to supraventricular tachycardia
amenable to verapamil therapy), atrial fibrillation or atrial
flutter with an accessory bypass tract (WPW, Lown-
Ganong-Levine syndromes), concomitant use of beta-
blockers, ventricular tachycardia
▶ **Cautions:** idiopathic hypertrophic subaortic stenosis, impaired renal or hepatic function, increased intracranial
pressure, Duchenne's muscular dystrophy, elderly patients

Available forms
▶ *Injection:* 5 mg/2 mL
▶ *Tablets:* 40, 80, 120 mg

Adverse effects in *Italics* are most common; those in **Bold** are life-threatening

- *SR tablets:* 120, 180, 240 mg
- *SR capsules:* 100, 120, 180, 200, 240, 300 mg

IV facts
Preparation
- May be given undiluted.
- For IV infusion, dilute drug in D5W/LR; D5W/0.45%NS; D5W/0.9%NS; D5W/Ringer's Injection; D5W; LR; 0.45%NS; 0.9%NS; or Ringer's Injection.

Dosage
- *Supraventricular tachycardia:* 5–10 mg IV over 2 min (over 3 min for elderly patients). Repeat dose of 10 mg IV 30 min after first dose if initial response is not adequate.
- *IV infusion:* IV infusion of 5 mg/h IV has been used. Give IV loading dose first.

Therapeutic serum level
- 0.08–0.3 mcg/mL

Compatibility
Verapamil may be given through the same IV line as amrinone, ciprofloxacin, dobutamine, dopamine, famotidine, hydralazine, meperidine, methicillin, milrinone, penicillin G potassium, piperacillin, propofol, ticarcillin.

Incompatibility
Do not administer through the same IV line as albumin, ampicillin, mezlocillin, nafcillin, oxacillin, sodium bicarbonate, solutions/drugs with a pH > 6.

TREATMENT OF OVERDOSE/ANTIDOTE
Discontinue drug or decrease dosage. Initiate general supportive and resuscitative measures. Beta-adrenergic stimulation or IV calcium administration may reverse drug's effects. Treat symptomatic hypotension with calcium chloride, isoproterenol, and vasopressors such as dopamine. Treat bradycardia, AV block, and asystole with isoproterenol, calcium chloride, cardiac pacing, and atropine. Treat rapid ventricular rates due to antegrade conduction with DC-cardioversion, procainamide, or lidocaine.

Pharmacokinetics

Route	Onset	Peak	Duration
IV	1–5 min	3–5 min	30–60 min
Oral	30 min	1–2.2 h	3–7 h

Metabolism: Hepatic; $T_{1/2}$: 3–7 h; 4.5–12 h with multiple doses
Excretion: Urine, feces

Adverse effects in *Italics* are most common; those in **Bold** are life-threatening

Oral dosage

◗ *Angina at rest and chronic stable angina:* Initial dose of 80–120 mg PO tid; titrate dose to achieve optimum therapeutic effects. Give 40 mg PO tid to elderly and patients with decreased hepatic function.

◗ *Dysrhythmias:* 240–320 mg/d PO in 3–4 divided doses. Dosage range for prophylaxis of PSVT (non-digitalized patients) is 240–480 mg/d in 3–4 divided doses.

◗ *Essential hypertension:* Initial dose of 80 mg PO tid. Daily doses of 360–480 mg have been used, but there is no evidence that doses > 360 mg provide added effect. Give 40 mg PO tid to elderly and patients with decreased hepatic function. Titrate dose to desired effects.

◗ *Essential hypertension, sustained release:* 240 mg/d PO in the morning with food. If response is not adequate, give 240 mg in the morning and 120 mg in the evening. If needed, may give 240 mg PO q12h. Give 120 mg/d PO to elderly and patients with decreased hepatic function. Titrate dose to desired effects.

◗ Do not exceed 480 mg/d.

Adverse effects

◗ *CNS: Dizziness, headache,* vertigo, emotional depression, sleepiness, nystagmus, fatigue

◗ *CV:* **Sinus arrest, asystole, dysrhythmias (ventricular tachycardia, ventricular fibrillation),** *peripheral edema, hypotension,* CHF, pulmonary edema, bradycardia, AV heart block

◗ *Resp:* **Respiratory failure,** dyspnea

◗ *GI: Nausea, constipation,* abdominal discomfort, elevated liver enzymes

◗ *Misc:* Muscle fatigue, diaphoresis, rash, flushing

Clinically important drug–drug interactions

◗ Depressed myocardial contractility and AV conduction with beta-adrenergic blocking agents; do not give verapamil and IV beta-blockers within a few hours of each other

◗ Slow AV conduction, heart block, and bradycardia with digitalis

◗ Increased serum levels of carbamazepine

◗ Increased hypotension, bradycardia, ventricular tachycardia, AV block, and pulmonary edema with quinidine

◗ Increased clearance with sulfinpyrazone

◗ Additive negative inotropic effects and prolonged AV conduction with flecainide, verapamil

◗ Do not administer disopyramide within 48 h before or 24 h after verapamil

◗ Enhanced activity of neuromuscular blocking agents

◗ Increased cardiovascular collapse, hyperkalemia, and myocardial depression with dantrolene

Adverse effects in *Italics* are most common; those in **Bold** are life-threatening

▸ Decreased effects with calcium, rifampin, vitamin D
▸ Increased clearance with phenobarbital
▸ Decreased bioavailability with barbiturates
▸ Decreased levels with hydantoins
▸ Increased cyclosporine levels and toxicity
▸ Prolonged anesthetic effect of etomidate, increasing respiratory depression, apnea
▸ Increased serum concentrations of prazosin and postural hypotension

● NURSING CONSIDERATIONS

Assessment
▸ *History:* Verapamil allergy, sick sinus syndrome, functioning pacemaker, hypotension, severe left ventricular dysfunction, cardiogenic shock, CHF, idiopathic hypertrophic subaortic stenosis, impaired renal or hepatic function, increased intracranial pressure, Duchenne's muscular dystrophy, age
▸ *Physical:* P, BP, R, ECG, I & O, neurologic checks, skin assessment, chest pain assessment, edema, orthostatic BP, peripheral perfusion, adventitious lung sounds, liver evaluation, liver and renal function tests, serum electrolytes, UA

Implementation
▸ Monitor BP and ECG continuously when giving IV verapamil.
▸ Monitor patient carefully (BP, cardiac rhythm, output) while drug is being titrated to therapeutic dose.
▸ Monitor BP very carefully with concurrent doses of antihypertensives.
▸ Have emergency equipment (defibrillator, drugs, oxygen, intubation equipment) on standby in case adverse reaction occurs.
▸ Minimize postural hypotension by helping the patient change positions slowly.
▸ Monitor elderly patients and those with renal or hepatic impairment carefully for possible drug accumulation and adverse reactions.
▸ Ensure that patient does not chew or divide sustained-release forms.
▸ Protect IV solution from light.

W

 warfarin sodium *(war' far in)* Coumadin,
Warfilone (CAN)

Pregnancy Category X

W

Drug classes
Anticoagulant
Coumarin derivative

Indications
▶ Prevention and treatment of venous thrombosis and its extension
▶ Prevention and treatment of thromboembolic complications associated with atrial fibrillation and cardiac valve replacement
▶ Prevention and treatment of pulmonary embolism
▶ Prophylaxis of systemic embolization after AMI and with valvular disease
▶ Unlabeled uses: prevention of recurrent TIAs, prevention of recurrent MI, adjunct to therapy in small-cell carcinoma of the lung

Therapeutic actions
▶ Interferes with the hepatic synthesis of vitamin K-dependent clotting factors (Factors II [prothrombin] VII, IX, and X), resulting in their eventual depletion and prolongation of clotting times
▶ Has no direct effect on existing thrombus and does not reverse ischemic tissue damage; may prevent further extension of formed clot

Contraindications/cautions
▶ **Contraindications:** warfarin allergy, SBE, hemophilia, thrombocytopenic purpura, hemorrhagic disorders, bleeding diathesis, blood dyscrasias, severe uncontrolled or malignant HTN, pericarditis, pericardial effusion, severe hepatic or renal disease, GI or GU bleeding, spinal puncture, cerebral or dissecting aortic aneurysm, visceral carcinoma, severe trauma, recent diagnostic procedures with potential for uncontrollable bleeding, prostatectomy, continuous tube drainage of small intestine, polyarthritis, diverticulitis, emaciation, malnutrition, ascorbic acid deficiency, menometrorrhagia, history of warfarin-induced necrosis; recent or contemplated CNS or eye surgery, major regional or lumbar block anesthesia, or surgery resulting in large, open surfaces
▶ **Cautions:** CHF, trauma, infection, edema, severe to moderate HTN, active TB, polycythemia vera, vasculitis, diarrhea, renal and hepatic function impairment, obstructive jaundice, biliary fistula, recent surgery, x-ray therapy, vitamin K deficiency, steatorrhea, collagen disease, severe diabetes, initial hypoprothrombinemia, vascular damage,
(contraindications continued on next page)

Adverse effects in *Italics* are most common; those in **Bold** are life-threatening

indwelling catheters, dietary insufficiencies, fever, thyrotoxicosis, hypothyroidism, hypercholesterolemia, hereditary resistance to oral anticoagulants, severe allergic disorders, anaphylactic disorders; female, elderly, debilitated, senile, psychotic, or depressed patients

Available forms
▸ *Tablets:* 1, 2, 2.5, 3, 4, 5, 6, 7.5, 10 mg
▸ *Powder for injection:* 2 mg/mL once reconstituted

IV facts
Preparation
▸ Reconstitute vial with 2.7 mL Sterile Water for Injection.

Dosage
▸ Use for patients who cannot receive PO drugs.
▸ Give IV over 1–2 min.
▸ *Induction:* 5–10 mg/d IV for 2–4 d. Adjust daily dosage according to PT or INR values.
▸ *Maintenance:* 2–10 mg IV qd based on PT or INR.
▸ *Elderly/debilitated patients or those with increased sensitivity:* Use lower dose.
▸ Adjust dosage to maintain PT of 1.3–2 or INR of 2–4.5, depending on treated condition.

Compatibility
Warfarin may be given through the same IV line as amikacin, ascorbic acid, cefazolin, cephapirin, dopamine, epinephrine, heparin, lidocaine, metaraminol, morphine, nitroglycerin, oxytocin, ranitidine.

Incompatibility
Do not administer through the same IV line as bretylium, cimetidine, ciprofloxacin, dobutamine, esmolol, gentamicin, labetalol, promazine, Ringer's Injection.

Oral dosage
▸ *Induction:* 5–10 mg/d PO for 2–4 d. Adjust daily dosage according to PT or INR values.
▸ *Maintenance:* 2–10 mg PO qd based on PT or INR.
▸ *Elderly/debilitated patients or those with increased sensitivity:* Use lower dose.
▸ Adjust dosage to maintain PT of 1.3–2 or INR of 2–4.5, depending on treated condition.

Adverse effects in *Italics* are most common; those in **Bold** are life-threatening

W

Pharmacokinetics

Route	Onset	Peak	Duration
IV	24 h	72–96 h	2–5 d
Oral		3–4 d	2–5 d

Metabolism: Hepatic, T$_{1/2}$: 1–2.5 d
Excretion: Urine

Adverse effects

▶ *GI: Nausea,* vomiting, anorexia, abdominal cramping, diarrhea, retroperitoneal hematoma, hepatitis, jaundice, mouth ulcers
▶ *GU:* Priapism, nephropathy, red-orange urine
▶ *Hematologic:* Granulocytosis, leukopenia, eosinophilia
▶ *Derm: Alopecia, urticaria, dermatitis*
▶ *Bleeding:* **Hemorrhage;** GI or GU bleeding (hematuria, dark stools, paralytic ileus, intestinal obstruction from hemorrhage into GI tract), petechiae and purpura, bleeding from mucous membranes, hemorrhagic infarction, vasculitis, skin necrosis or gangrene; adrenal hemorrhage with resultant adrenal insufficiency; ovarian hemorrhage, compressive neuropathy secondary to hemorrhage near a nerve; hemorrhage may present as paralysis, headache, shortness of breath, difficulty swallowing, unexplained swelling, shock; chest, abdomen, joint, or other pain
▶ **Misc:** Fever, "purple toes" syndrome

Clinically important drug–drug interactions

▶ Increased bleeding tendencies with acetaminophen, aminoglycosides, amiodarone, androgens, beta blockers, cephalosporins, chloral hydrate, chloramphenicol, chlorpropamide, cimetidine, corticosteroids, danazol, erythromycin, famotidine, fluconazole, gemfibrozil, glucagon, heparin, hydantoins, loop diuretics, lovastatin, metronidazole quinidine, nalidixic acid, nizatidine, NSAIDs, penicillins, quinine, quinolones,

streptokinase, sulfonamides, tetracyclines, thyroid hormones, urokinase, vitamin E, and others
- Decreased anticoagulation effects with adrenal cortical steroid inhibitors, aminoglutethimide, antacids, anticonvulsants, antidysrhythmics, ascorbic acid, barbiturates, carbamazepine, cholestyramine, dicloxacillin, estrogens, ethchlorvynol, glutethimide, griseofulvin, oral contraceptives, phenytoin, rifampin, thiazide diuretics, vitamin K, and others
- Altered effects with methimazole, propylthiouracil
- Increased activity and toxicity of phenytoin

⬤ NURSING CONSIDERATIONS
Assessment
- *History:* Warfarin allergy, SBE, bleeding/hemostatic disorders, HTN, pericarditis, pericardial effusion, hepatic or renal disease, spinal puncture, cerebral or dissecting aortic aneurysm, visceral carcinoma, recent diagnostic procedures, prostatectomy, continuous tube drainage of small intestine, polyarthritis, diverticulitis, emaciation, malnutrition, ascorbic acid deficiency, menometrorrhagia, warfarin-induced necrosis, CHF, trauma, infection, edema, active TB, polycythemia vera, vasculitis, diarrhea, obstructive jaundice, biliary fistula, x-ray therapy, vitamin K deficiency, steatorrhea, collagen disease, severe diabetes, initial hypoprothrombinemia, vascular damage, indwelling catheters, dietary insufficiencies, thyrotoxicosis, hypothyroidism, hypercholesterolemia, hereditary resistance to oral anticoagulants, severe allergic disorders, anaphylactic disorders, age, debilitated status; senility, depression, psychosis; recent or contemplated CNS or eye surgery, major regional or lumbar block anesthesia, or surgery resulting in large, open surfaces
- *Physical:* T, P, BP, R, ECG, I & O, neurologic checks, skin assessment, adventitious lung sounds, peripheral perfusion, presence of bleeding, liver evaluation, bowel sounds, CBC, UA, PT, INR, renal and hepatic function tests, stool and emesis guaiac

Implementation
- Monitor PT or INR regularly; adjust dosage accordingly.
- Administer IV form to patients stabilized on Coumadin who are not able to take oral drug. Return to oral form as soon as feasible.
- Give oral dose same time qd to maintain steady drug levels.
- Because there is a delayed onset of oral anticoagulant effects, give heparin and warfarin simultaneously until PT or INR is therapeutic.

- Maintain consistent amount of vitamin K in foods.
- Do not change brand names once stabilized; bioavailability problems exist.
- Evaluate patient regularly for signs of blood loss (petechiae, bleeding gums, bruises, dark stools, dark urine).
- Do not give patient IM injections unless absolutely needed; give to upper extremities for manual compression; apply pressure dressing.
- Double check all drugs ordered for potential drug–drug interaction; dosage of both drugs may need to be adjusted.
- Use caution when discontinuing other medications; warfarin dosage may need to be adjusted; carefully monitor PT values.
- Maintain vitamin K_1 on standby in case of overdose.
- Use reconstituted IV drug within 4 h; discard unused solution.

Adverse effects in *Italics* are most common; those in **Bold** are life-threatening

APPENDICES

▶ APPENDIX A

Conversions

Weight
- 1 kilogram (kg) = 2.2 pounds (lb)
- 1 kilogram (kg) = 1000 grams (g)
- 1 g = 1000 milligrams (mg)
- 1 mg = 1000 micrograms (mcg)
- 1 grain (gr) = 60 mg
- 5 grains = 324 mg

Volume
- 1 liter (L) = 1000 milliliters (mL)
- 500 mL = 1 pint (pt)
- 30 mL = 1 ounce (oz)
- 15 mL = 1 tablespoon (tbsp)
- 5 mL = 1 teaspoon (tsp)

Temperature
- Celsius temperature = (F − 32) × 5 ÷ 9
- Fahrenheit temperature = (C × 9 ÷ 5) + 32

Length
- 1 inch (in) = 2.54 cm
- 1 m = 100 cm
- 1 cm = 10 mm

Pressure
- 1 mm mercury (Hg) = 1.36 cm water (H_2O)

▶ APPENDIX B

Formulae For Calculation of IV Doses

To calculate rate in mL/h if you know the dose in mcg/kg/min

$$\frac{(dose\ in\ mcg/kg/min) \times (kg\ of\ body\ weight) \times (60\ min/h)}{(mg/mL\ of\ the\ solution) \times (1000\ mcg/mg)}$$

To calculate mcg/kg/min if you know the rate of infusion

$$\frac{(mg/mL\ of\ the\ solution) \times (1000\ mcg/mg) \times (mL/h)}{(kg\ of\ body\ weight) \times (60\ min/h)}$$

To calculate rate in mL/h if you know the dose in mcg/min

$$\frac{(dose\ in\ mcg/min) \times (60\ min/h)}{(mg/mL\ of\ the\ solution) \times (1000\ mcg/mg)}$$

To calculate mcg/min if you know the rate of infusion

$$\frac{(mg/mL\ of\ the\ solution) \times (1000\ mcg/mg) \times (mL/h)}{(60\ min/h)}$$

To calculate rate in mL/h if you know the dose in mg/min

$$\frac{(dose\ in\ mg/min) \times (60\ min/h)}{(mg/mL\ of\ the\ solution)}$$

To calculate mg/min if you know the rate of infusion

$$\frac{(mg/mL\ of\ the\ solution) \times (mL/h)}{(60\ min/h)}$$

To calculate rate in mL/h if you know the dose in U/h

$$\frac{(dose\ in\ U/h)}{(U/mL\ of\ the\ solution)}$$

To calculate U/h if you know the rate of infusion

$$(U/mL\ of\ the\ solution) \times (mL/h)$$

To calculate rate in mL/h if you know the dose in mg/h

$$\frac{(dose\ in\ mg/h)}{(mg/mL\ of\ the\ solution)}$$

To calculate mg/h if you know the rate of infusion

$$\text{(mg/mL of the solution)} \times \text{(mL/h)}$$

To calculate rate in mL/h if you know the dose in U/min

$$\frac{\text{(dose in U/min)} \times \text{(60 min/h)}}{\text{(U/mL of the solution)}}$$

To calculate U/min if you know the rate of infusion

$$\frac{\text{(U/mL of the solution)} \times \text{(mL/h)}}{\text{(60 min/h)}}$$

To calculate rate in mL/h if you know the dose in mg/kg/h

$$\frac{\text{(dose in mg/kg/h)} \times \text{(kg of body weight)}}{\text{(mg/mL of the solution)}}$$

To calculate mg/kg/h if you know the rate of infusion

$$\frac{\text{(mg/mL of the solution)} \times \text{(mL/h)}}{\text{(kg of body weight)}}$$

To calculate rate in mL/h if you know the dose in g/h

$$\frac{\text{(dose in g/h)}}{\text{(g/mL of the solution)}}$$

To calculate g/h if you know the rate of infusion

$$\text{(g/mL of the solution)} \times \text{(mL/h)}$$

▶ APPENDIX C

Hemodynamic Formulae and Values Relevant to Drug Administration

Parameter	Formula	Normal
Mean arterial pressure (MAP)	$\dfrac{(DBP \times 2) + SBP}{3}$	70–115 mmHg
Pulmonary artery mean (PAM)	$\dfrac{(PAD \times 2) + PAS}{3}$	7–18 mmHg
Cardiac output (CO)	$HR \times SV$	4–8 L/min
Cardiac index (CI)	$\dfrac{CO}{BSA}$	2.2–4 L/min/m^2
Stroke volume (SV)	$\dfrac{CO \times 1000}{HR}$	60–135 mL/beat
Stroke volume index (SVI)	$\dfrac{CI \times 1000}{HR}$	35–70 mL/beat/m^2
Pulmonary vascular resistance (PVR)	$\dfrac{(PAM - PCWP) \times 80}{CO}$	< 250 dynes/s/cm^{-5}
Pulmonary vascular resistance indexed (PVRI)	$\dfrac{(PAM - PCWP) \times 80}{CI}$	160–280 dynes/s/cm^{-5}/m^2
Systemic vascular resistance (SVR)	$\dfrac{(MAP - CVP) \times 80}{CO}$	800–1200 dynes/s/cm^{-5}
Systemic vascular resistance indexed (SVRI)	$\dfrac{(MAP - CVP) \times 80}{CI}$	1970–2390 dynes/s/cm^{-5}/m^2
Central venous pressure (CVP)		2–6 mmHg
Pulmonary artery systolic (PAS)		15–25 mmHg
Pulmonary artery distolic (PAD)		6–12 mmHg
Pulmonary capillary wedge pressure (PCWP)		4–12 mmHg
Right ventricular stroke work index (RVSWI)	SVI (PAM − CVP) × 0.0136	5–12 g–m/m^2/beat
Left ventricular stroke work index (LVSWI)	SVI (MAP − PCWP) × 0.0137	45–65 g–m/m^2/beat
Left ventricular ejection fraction (EF)		60%–70%
Coronary artery perfusion pressure (CAPP)	DBP − PCWP	60–80 mmHg
Intracranial pressure (ICP)		0–15 mmHg

Cerbral perfusion pressure (CPP)	MAP − ICP	60–100 mmHg
Serum osmolality	$(NA \times 2) + \dfrac{BUN}{3} + \dfrac{glucose}{18}$	280–295 Osm/L
Creatinine clearance (Ccr) from serum creatinine (male)	$\dfrac{weight\ (kg) \times (140 - age)}{72 \times serum\ creatinine\ (mg/dl)}$	120 ± 25 mL/min
Creatinine clearance (Ccr) from serum creatinine (female)	0.85 × calculation for males	95 ± 20 mL/min
Ideal body weight (kg) Male		50 kg + 2.3 kg (each inch > 5 ft)
Female		45.5 kg + 2.3 kg (each inch > 5 ft)

▶ APPENDIX D
DEA Schedules of Controlled Substances

The Controlled Substances Act of 1970 regulates the manufacturing, distribution, and dispensing of drugs that have abuse potential. The Drug Enforcement Administration (DEA) within the United States Department of Justice is the chief federal agency responsible for enforcement. The controlled drugs are divided into five DEA schedules based on their potential for abuse and physical and psychological dependence.

- **Schedule I** (*c-I*): High abuse potential and no accepted medical use (eg, heroin, LSD).
- **Schedule II** (*c-II*): High abuse potential with severe dependence liability (eg, narcotics, amphetamines, barbiturates).
- **Schedule III** (*c-III*): Less abuse potential than schedule II drugs and moderate dependence liability (eg, nonbarbiturate sedatives, nonamphetamine stimulants, limited amounts of certain narcotics).
- **Schedule IV** (*c-IV*): Less abuse potential than schedule III drugs and limited dependence liability (eg, some sedatives, antianxiety agents, nonnarcotic analgesics).
- **Schedule V** (*c-V*): Limited abuse potential. Primarily small amounts of narcotics (codeine) used as antitussives or antidiarrheals. Under federal law, limited quantities of certain Schedule V drugs may be purchased without a prescription directly from a pharmacist if allowed under state statues. The purchaser must be at least 18 years old and must furnish suitable identification. All such transactions must be recorded by the dispensing pharmacist.

Prescribing physicians and dispensing pharmacists must be registered with the DEA. In many cases, state laws are more restrictive than federal laws and therefore impose additional requirements. In any given situation, the more stringent law applies.

▶ APPENDIX E

FDA Pregnancy Categories

The Food and Drug Administration (FDA) has established five categories to indicate the potential of a systemically absorbed drug for causing birth defects. The key differentiation among the categories rests on the degree (reliability) of documentation and the risk-versus-benefit ratio.

- **Category A:** Adequate studies in pregnant women have not demonstrated a risk to the fetus in the first trimester of pregnancy, and there is no evidence of risk in later trimesters.
- **Category B:** Animal studies have not demonstrated a risk to the fetus, but there are no adequate studies in pregnant women . . . or . . . Animal studies have shown an adverse effect, but adequate studies in pregnant women have not demonstrated a risk to the fetus during the first trimester of pregnancy, and there is no evidence of risk in later trimesters.
- **Category C:** Animal studies have shown an adverse effect on the fetus, but there are no adequate studies in humans; the benefits from the use of the drug in pregnant women may be acceptable despite its potential risks . . . or . . . There are no animal reproduction studies and no adequate studies in humans.
- **Category D:** There is evidence of human fetal risk, but the potential benefits from the use of the drug in pregnant women may be acceptable despite its potential risks.
- **Category X:** Studies in animals or humans demonstrate fetal abnormalities or adverse reaction; reports indicate evidence of fetal risk. The risk of use in a pregnant woman clearly outweighs any possible benefit.

Regardless of the designated pregnancy category or presumed safety, no drug should be administered during pregnancy unless it is clearly needed and potential benefits outweigh potential hazards to the fetus.

▶ APPENDIX F

Peripheral Nerve Stimulator Estimates of Neuromuscular Blockade

Number of Twitches	Percent Blockade
Four	75%
Three	80%
Two	85%
One	90%
Zero	100%

▶ APPENDIX G

Emergency Treatment of an Acute Drug Overdose, Poisoning, or Exposure

1. Discontinue administration of the drug. For external contamination, remove the causative agent, and initiate individualized decontamination procedures as determined by the agent.
2. Establish and maintain a patent airway. Initiate CPR/ACLS protocols if the patient is without respirations or a pulse.
3. Assess the patient. If possible, identify the ingested drug and determine the amount of the drug received. Attempt to find out when the drug was taken. Obtain specimens for toxicology screening.
4. If unsure how to manage the patient, consult the Poison Control Center for advice.
5. Establish IV access and administer 0.45%NS; 0.9%NS; LR; or other IV solution as ordered. Plasma, plasma protein fractions, blood, or plasma expanders may be required.
6. Administer the drug's antidote if one exists.
7. Treat severe hypotension with vasoconstrictors, such as dopamine and norepinephrine. Treat severe hypertension with vasodilators, such as nitroprusside and diazoxide.
8. Treat dysrhythmias as dictated by the offending drug.
9. Treat seizures with IV diazepam or lorazepam followed by phenobarbital or fosphenytoin.
10. Unless contraindicated after an oral overdose, empty gastric contents to reduce drug absorption.
    a. Give 30 mL syrup of ipecac followed by a glass of water to induce vomiting. Emesis may not occur for 20–30 min. Give syrup of ipecac only to alert patients who have a gag reflex. Give a second dose if no emesis occurs in 20–30 min.
    b. For faster effects and for comatose patients or patients unable to protect their airway, begin gastric lavage. Endotracheal intubation is often initiated for comatose patients or for patients without a gag reflex. Insert a large-bore nasogastric or orogastric tube. Instill at least 1000 mL normal saline or water, and continue lavage until the solution is clear.
11. Administer activated charcoal alone or after emesis or lavage to adsorb the drug. Give 50–100 g mixed in 240 mL of water.
12. Cathartics increase the elimination of the charcoal–poison

complex. Sorbitol is usually added to charcoal to improve its palatability and hasten its elimination. Magnesium sulfate and magnesium citrate are also commonly used.

13. Whole bowel irrigation may be initiated to remove controlled-release drugs, cocaine-containing condoms or balloons, or iron.

14. Forced diuresis with furosemide or mannitol, alkaline diuresis with sodium bicarbonate, or acid diuresis with ascorbic acid or ammonium chloride may be used to promote the drug's elimination.

15. Hemodialysis, peritoneal dialysis, or charcoal hemoperfusion may be initiated to eliminate the drug; however, these are not indicated for most overdoses.

16. Document all drug administration and other interventions.

17. Assess and document the patient's response to drugs and other interventions.

▶ APPENDIX H

Emergency Treatment of Anaphylaxis Reactions

1. Discontinue administration of the drug. For a sting or bite, apply a tourniquet to the patient's extremity above the sting or bite.

2. Establish and maintain a patent airway. Initiate CPR/ACLS protocols if the patient is without respirations or a pulse. Severe respiratory distress may respond to IV aminophylline or other bronchodilators.

3. Assess the patient. If possible, identify the ingested drug or antigen. For drug reactions, determine the amount of drug received. Ascertain when the exposure occurred.

4. Administer oxygen to maintain the desired SpO_2 and acid–base balance.

5. Administer epinephrine 1:1000, 0.2–0.5 mg (0.2–0.5 mL) SC or 1:10,000 0.3–0.5 mg IV over 5 min. Repeat q5–15min if needed. If needed, give an epinephrine IV infusion at a rate of 1–4 mcg/min. Epinephrine may be given through an endotracheal tube (see Appendix Q). Finally, epinephrine 0.1 mg may be given into an injection site where the offending drug was administered.

6. Establish IV access and administer 0.45%NS; 0.9%NS; LR; or other IV solution as ordered.

7. Treat severe hypotension by elevating the patient's feet and giving IV fluids, plasma expanders, and vasoconstrictors, such as dopamine, dobutamine, phenylephrine, and norepinephrine.

8. Adjunctive therapies may modify the process or shorten the course of the reaction.
   a. Antihistamines: Diphenhydramine 50–100 mg IV or IM. Then 5 mg/kg/d or 50 mg PO q6h for 1–2 d. Chlorpheniramine 10–20 mg IV or IM. Hydroxyzine 25–50 mg IM tid–qid or 10–20 mg PO tid–qid.
   b. Corticosteroids: Hydrocortisone 100–1000 mg IV. Then 7 mg/kg/d IV or PO for 1–2 d.
   c. H_2 antagonists: Cimetidine 300 mg IV q6h. Ranitidine 50 mg IV over 3–5 min.

9. Document drug administration and other interventions.

10. Assess and document the patient's response to drugs and other interventions.

▶ APPENDIX I

Commonly Used Blood Products

Product	Contents	Approximate Volume	Comments
Cryoprecipitate	Fibrinogen, von Willebrand factor, factor VIII	10 mL/bag	10 U or more are often pooled together. Must be thawed before use; then use immediately. Give 10 mL/min. Restores clotting factors.
Fresh frozen plasma	Clotting factors, plasma proteins, plasma	200–250 mL/U	Give 10 mL/min. Restores clotting factors and expands blood volume.
Platelets	Platelets, WBCs, plasma	50–60 mL/pack	Four to eight packs are often pooled together. Give as rapidly as tolerated. Controls bleeding due to thrombocytopenia. Each unit should raise the platelet count 5,000–10,000/mm³.
PRBCs	RBCs, plasma	250–300 mL/U	Ideally, give each unit over 2–4 h. Each unit should increase Hgb 1 g/dL and Hct 3%. Increases oxygen-carrying capacity. If giving large amounts, also give FFP to prevent dilutional coagulopathy. If unable to obtain a type and crossmatch during an emergency, administer group O negative blood.
Whole blood	RBCs, WBCs, platelets, plasma, clotting factors	500 mL	Ideally, give each unit over 2–4 h. Increases oxygen-carrying capacity and intravascular volume. Not available at many institutions.

▶ APPENDIX J

Blood Product Compatibility

Blood is typed to determine its ABO group and the presence or absence of Rh factors. Except in life-threatening emergencies, obtain a type and crossmatch before administering a blood transfusion. Transfusing incompatible blood may lead to a life-threatening transfusion reaction

The following lists ABO compatibility:

Recipient's Blood Group	Compatible Red Blood Cells
O	O
A	A or O
B	B or O
AB	AB, A, B, or O

▶ APPENDIX K

Components of Common Intravenous Solutions

Solution	Sodium (mEq/L)	Potassium (mEq/L)	Calcium (mEq/L)	Magnesium (mEq/L)	Chloride (mEq/L)	Acetate (mEq/L)	Osmolarity (mOsm/L)	Calories (Cal/L)
D5W/LR	130	4	3	—	109–112	—	525–530	170–180
D5W/0.2%NS	34–38.5	—	—	—	34–38.5	—	320–330	170
D5W/0.45%NS	77	—	—	—	77	—	405	170
D5W/0.9%NS	154	—	—	—	154	—	560	170
D10W/0.9%NS	154	—	—	—	154	—	813	340
D5W/Ringer's	147	4	4.5	—	156	—	560	170
D5W	—	—	—	—	—	—	170	253
D10W	—	—	—	—	—	—	340	505
Isolyte E	140	10	5	3	103	49	310	—
Isolyte M/D5W	38	35	—	—	44	20	400	170
Isolyte S	140	5	—	3	98	27	295	—
LR	130	4	3	—	109	—	273	—
0.45%NS	77	—	—	—	77	—	155	—
0.9%NS	154	—	—	—	154	—	310	—
3%NS	513	—	—	—	513	—	1030	—
5%NS	855	—	—	—	855	—	1710	—

(continued)

Components of Common Intravenous Solutions

Solution	Sodium (mEq/L)	Potassium (mEq/L)	Calcium (mEq/L)	Magnesium (mEq/L)	Chloride (mEq/L)	Acetate (mEq/L)	Osmolarity (mOsm/L)	Calories (Cal/L)
Normosol M/D5W	40	13	—	3	40	16	363	170
Normosol R/D5W	140	5	—	3	98	27	552	185
Plasma-Lyte 56	40	13	—	3	40	16	111	—
0.075% potassium chloride in D5W/0.45%NS	77	10	—	—	87	—	425	170
0.15% potassium chloride in D5W/0.45%NS	77	20	—	—	97	—	445	170
0.22% potassium chloride in D5W/0.45%NS	77	30	—	—	107	—	465	170
0.3% potassium chloride in D5W/0.45%NS	77	40	—	—	117	—	490	170
0.22% potassium chloride in D5W/0.9%NS	154	30	—	—	184	—	620	170
0.3% potassium chloride in D5W/0.9%NS	154	40	—	—	194	—	640	170
0.15% potassium chloride in D10W/0.2%NS	34	20	—	—	54	—	615	340
0.15% potassium chloride in 0.9%NS	154	20	—	—	174	—	350	—
0.22% potassium chloride in 0.9%NS	154	30	—	—	184	—	365	—
0.3% potassium chloride in 0.9%NS	154	40	—	—	194	—	390	—
Ringer's	147	4	4	—	156	—	310	—

▶ APPENDIX L

Procedure for Adding Drugs to an Intravenous Solution

1. Wash your hands.
2. Confirm the order for the drug according to your facility's policies.
3. Obtain the ordered drug and IV solution.
4. Ensure that the drug and solution are compatible.
5. Remove any covering from the IV bag/bottle.
6. **Prefilled syringe, solution in a vial, or ampule:** ready for use. **Powder for injection in a vial:** follow the manufacturer's directions for reconstituting the drug. Using a sterile needle or needleless device, withdraw the correct amount of drug from an ampule or vial. If the prefilled syringe contains more drug than needed, discard the excess drug.
7. Cleanse the injection port on the bag or bottle with an alcohol swab.
8. Insert a needle or needleless device connected to an empty sterile syringe into the solution's injection port.
9. Withdraw the volume of fluid that equals the volume of drug that will be added to the solution.
10. Remove the syringe and discard according to your facility's policies.
11. Insert the needle or needleless device connected to the syringe that contains the drug.
12. Inject the drug into the bag/bottle.
13. Tilt the bag/bottle back and forth to ensure that the drug and solution mix.
14. Label the bag/bottle with the patient's name, date, time, drug, amount of drug, and your initials.

▶ APPENDIX M

Procedure for Administering Multiple Solutions or Drugs Through the Same IV Line

1. Wash your hands.
2. Confirm the order for the solutions or drugs according to your facility's policies.
3. Verify that the solutions or drugs are compatible.
4. Obtain the required solutions or drugs.
5. Attach the correct IV tubing to the bags; prime the tubings to remove the air. Follow your facility's policies for labeling IV tubings.
6. Connect the solutions or drugs by inserting the needle or needleless device from one tubing to the correct port of the other solution or drug.
7. Verify the patient's identity and allergies before giving the solutions or drugs.
8. Inform the patient about the procedure or drug.
9. Assess the IV site for patency. Aspirate for a blood return to confirm that the catheter is positioned in the vein. Sometimes there is not a positive blood return; in these cases, carefully assess the site for infiltration.
10. Insert the IV tubing into the IV pump according to your facility's policies.
11. Label the IV pump with the appropriate solution or drug.
12. Connect the solutions or drugs to the IV catheter, or insert the needle or needleless device into the saline port.
13. Program the IV pump's primary infusion feature for each solution or drug. Ensure that each solution or drug is set for the correct rate. *Do not* use the secondary infusion feature, because one of the solutions or drugs will not infuse.
14. Open the clamps on the IV tubings and start the IV pumps.
15. Document the drug administration according to your facility's policies.
16. Record the fluid volume as intake.
17. Assess and document the patient's response to the drug.
18. Frequently assess the patient's IV site.

▶ APPENDIX N

Procedure for Administering an IV Bolus Dose

1. Wash your hands.
2. Confirm the order for the drug.
3. Use a prefilled preparation or use a sterile syringe with needle or needleless device to withdraw the correct amount of drug from an ampule or vial.
4. Verify the patient's identity and allergies before giving the drug.
5. Inform the patient about the procedure and drug.
6. If an IV solution or drugs are infusing, verify that the solution or drugs are compatible with the drug that you plan to administer.
7. Cleanse the injection port with an alcohol swab.
8. If a solution or drug is infusing, pinch the tubing above the port to stop infusion.
9. Insert the needleless device or needle into the appropriate IV tubing injection port or saline lock.
10. Aspirate for a blood return to confirm that the catheter is positioned in the vein. Sometimes there is not a positive blood return; in these cases, carefully assess the site for infiltration.
11. Inject the drug at the prescribed rate.
12. Remove the needle and dispose of it according to your facility's policies.
13. Document the drug administration according to your facility's policies.
14. Assess and document the patient's response to the drug.

▶ APPENDIX O

Procedure for Administering IV Piggyback Drugs

1. Wash your hands.
2. Confirm the order for the drug according to your facility's policies.
3. Use a premixed preparation, activate the provided delivery system, or prepare the drug (see appendix L).
4. Attach the correct IV tubing to the bag; prime the tubing to remove the air. (If reusing a piggyback tubing, allow the tubing to fill from the primary solution during step 14.)
5. Verify the patient's identity and allergies before giving the drug.
6. Inform the patient about the procedure and drug.
7. Verify that the hanging solution or drugs are compatible with the drug that you plan to administer.
8. Assess the IV site for patency. Aspirate for a blood return to confirm that the catheter is positioned in the vein. Sometimes there is not a positive blood return; in these cases, carefully assess the site for infiltration.
9. Cleanse the injection port with an alcohol swab.
10. Lower the primary solution bag to 6–8 in below the piggyback bag.
11. Stop the IV pump.
12. Insert the needle or needleless device into the appropriate IV tubing injection port or saline lock.
13. Program the secondary infusion feature on the IV pump to deliver the drug at the correct rate.
14. Open the piggyback tubing's clamp and start the IV pump.
15. Document the drug administration according to your facility's policies.
16. Record the fluid volume as intake.
17. When the infusion is completed, disconnect the piggyback tubing from primary IV line. Discard or save for future use, according to your facility's policies.
18. Assess and document the patient's response to the drug.

▶ APPENDIX P

Procedure for Administering IM or SC Drugs

1. Wash your hands.
2. Confirm the order for the drug according to your facility's policies.
3. Obtain the correct drug and dosage.
4. Use a syringe to draw up the drug. If giving > 1 drug per injection, ensure that the drugs are compatible in a syringe. **SC:** use a 25- to 27-guage, $\frac{1}{2}$- to $\frac{5}{8}$-in needle. Unless contraindicated, add 0.1–0.2 mL air to the syringe. Do not give > 2 mL at a time. **IM:** use an 18- to 23-guage, 1- to 3-in needle. Unless contraindicated, add 0.2 mL air to the syringe. Do not give > 3 mL at a time.
5. Verify the patient's identity and allergies before giving the drug.
6. Inform the patient about the procedure and drug.
7. Don a clean pair of gloves.
8. Assist the patient into a position that will facilitate drug administration.
9. Select an appropriate site (see figures). **SC:** the preferred sites are the abdomen, upper thigh, and upper arm. **IM:** the preferred site is the ventrogluteal muscle.
10. Cleanse the site with an alcohol swab and allow to dry.
11. Remove the needle cap. **SC:** use thumb and forefinger to create a skin fold. Insert the needle at a 45-degree angle for $\frac{5}{8}$-in needle or 90-degree angle for $\frac{1}{2}$-in needle. Pull back the plunger, and observe for a blood return. If no blood returns, inject the drug. Withdraw the needle and dispose of it according to your facility's policies. Unless contraindicated, gently massage the site. Do not use this method for patients with shock, hypotension, or poor perfusion because the drug may not be absorbed predictably. **IM:** spread the skin taut. Quickly insert the needle at a 90-degree angle. Pull back the plunger and observe for a blood return. If no blood returns, inject the drug. Withdraw the needle and dispose of it according to your facility's policies. Unless contraindicated, gently massage the site.
12. Place the patient in his or her desired position.
13. Remove gloves and wash your hands.
14. Document the drug administration according to your facility's policies.
15. Assess and document the patient's response to the drug.

APPENDIX P-1

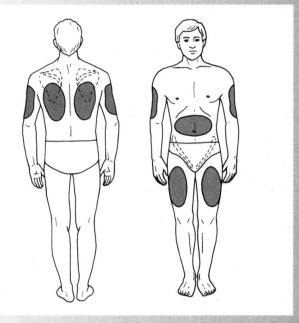

Subcutaneous injection sites.

▶ APPENDIX P-2

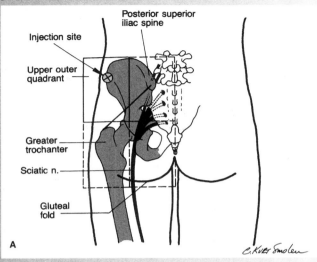

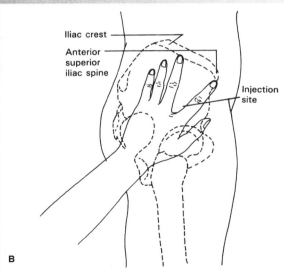

Intramuscular injection sites. **(A)** Landmarks for the dorsogluteal injection site. **(B)** Landmarks for the ventrogluteal injection site.

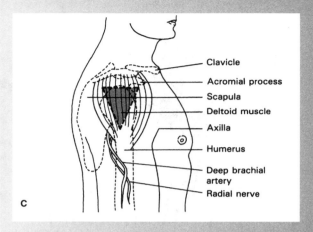

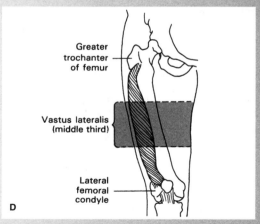

Intramuscular injection sites *(continued)*. **(C)** Landmarks for the deltoid injection site. **(D)** Landmarks for the vastus lateralis injection site. *(continued)*.

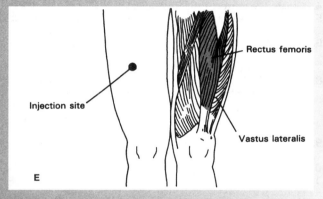

Intramuscular injection sites *(continued)*. **(E)** Landmarks for the rectus femoris injection site.

▶ APPENDIX Q

Procedure for Administering Drugs Through an Endotracheal Tube

1. This is used during emergencies for emergency drugs, such as atropine, epinephrine, lidocaine, naloxone, or diazepam, when IV access is not available.
2. Wash your hands.
3. Confirm the order for the drug according to your facility's policies.
4. Obtain the correct drug and dosage.
5. Verify the patient's identity and allergies before giving the drug.
6. Insert a sterile catheter through the endotracheal tube just past the tip of the endotracheal tube.
7. Stop any ongoing chest compressions.
8. Dilute 2–2.5 times the normal dose of the drug in 10 mL of normal saline. Inject the diluted drug through the catheter. *Or* first inject 2–2.5 times the normal dose of the drug through the catheter; follow with 10 mL of normal saline.
9. Attach the ventilation bag and forcefully ventilate 3–4 times.
10. If indicated, resume chest compressions.
11. Document the drug administration according to your facility's policies.
12. Assess and document the patient's response to the drug.

▶ APPENDIX R

Procedure for Administering Drugs Through a Nasogastric/Orogastric Tube

1. Wash your hands.
2. Confirm the order for the drug according to your facility's policies.
3. Assess the type of tube. Small-bore feeding tubes may easily obstruct if crushed tablets are not completed dissolved; use elixirs whenever possible.
4. Prepare the drugs. If possible, use suspensions or elixirs. Crush drugs and dissolve in water. *Never* crush controlled-release drugs.
5. Verify the patient's identity and allergies before giving the drug.
6. Inform the patient about the procedure and drug.
7. Assess for positive bowel sounds.
8. Ensure that the head of the patient's bed is elevated at least 30 degrees.
9. Don clean gloves.
10. Stop the infusion of any continuous tube feedings.
11. Verify tube placement. The preferred method is to assess the gastric pH of aspirated gastric contents. Other methods include aspirating gastric contents or injecting air into the stomach while auscultating the epigastric area.
12. Using a syringe that will connect to the tube, draw up the dissolved drugs.
13. Connect the syringe to the tube; gently apply pressure to the plunger or bulb to move the drug down the tube.
14. Flush the tube with at least 30 mL water or according to your institution's policies.
15. Restart continuous tube feedings if the drug and formula are compatible. Clamp the tube for at least 30–60 min before returning the tube to suction.
16. Keep the head of the patient's bed elevated 30 degrees for at least 30 min.
17. Remove gloves and wash your hands.
18. Document the drug administration according to your facility's policies.
19. Record the fluid volume as intake.
20. Assess and document the patient's response to the drug.

▶ APPENDIX S

Procedure for Administering Inhaler Drugs

1. Wash your hands.
2. Confirm the order for the drug according to your facility's policies.
3. Obtain the correct drug and dosage.
4. Verify the patient's identity and allergies before giving the drug.
5. Inform the patient about the procedure and drug.
6. Elevate the head of the patient's bed or help the patient sit up.
7. Assess the patient's breath sounds, respiratory effort, respirations, and pulse.
8. Shake the inhaler well.
9. If using an inhaler for the first time or if it has not recently been used, prime the inhaler according to the manufacturer's directions.
10. Instruct the patient to take a deep breath and exhale completely.
11. Holding the inhaler upright, place the entire mouthpiece into the patient's mouth and instruct the patient to close his or her mouth around the mouthpiece. Alternatively, may be given through the ventilator circuit during inspiration.
12. As the patient inhales slowly and deeply, press down on the inhaler to give the patient a dose.
13. Instruct the patient to hold his or her breath for 10 s and then to slowly exhale.
14. If > 1 puff is ordered, wait 2–5 min and repeat the procedure.
15. Assess the patient's breath sounds, respiratory effort, respirations, and pulse.
16. Place the patient in his or her desired position.
17. Document the drug administration according to your facility's policies.
18. Assess and document the patient's response to the drug.

▶ APPENDIX T

Procedure for Administering Nebulized Drugs

1. Wash your hands.
2. Confirm the order for the drug according to your facility's policies.
3. Obtain the nebulizer tubing and correct drug and dosage.
4. Fill the nebulizer cup with the correct dosage and diluent.
5. Verify the patient's identity and allergies before giving the drug.
6. Inform the patient about the procedure and drug.
7. Elevate the head of the patient's bed or help the patient sit up.
8. Assess the patient's breath sounds, respiratory effort, respirations, and pulse.
9. Connect the tubing to oxygen or medical air as prescribed.
10. Turn on the oxygen or air at the ordered flow rate.
11. Instruct the patient to close his or her lips around the entire mouthpiece. Alternatively, connect the device to a face mask or ventilator circuit.
12. Continue the treatment until the dosage is completed and no mist is being generated.
13. Assess the patient's breath sounds, respiratory effort, respirations, and pulse.
14. Clean the nebulizer cup and mouthpiece according to your facility's procedures.
15. Place the patient in his or her desired position.
16. Document the drug administration according to your facility's policies.
17. Assess and document the patient's response to the drug.

▶ APPENDIX U

Procedure for Administering Transdermal Drugs

1. Wash your hands.
2. Confirm the order for the drug according to your facility's policies.
3. Obtain the correct drug and dosage. Do not cut or alter transdermal systems.
4. Verify the patient's identity and allergies before giving the drug.
5. Inform the patient about the procedure and drug.
6. Remove any previously placed transdermal system. Fold the system so that the adhesive adheres to itself. Flush down the toilet.
7. Select a new site of intact skin over the upper chest or upper arm.
8. Prepare site by clipping (not shaving) hair at site. Do not use soap, oils, lotions, or alcohol. Allow skin to dry completely before application.
9. Apply the system immediately after removal from package. Firmly press the system in place with palm of hand. Ensure that contact is complete.
10. Document the drug administration according to your facility's policies.
11. Assess and document the patient's response to the drug.

▶ APPENDIX V

Procedure for Administering Sublingual Drugs

1. Wash your hands.
2. Confirm the order for the drug according to your facility's policies.
3. Obtain the correct drug and dosage.
4. Verify the patient's identity and allergies before giving the drug.
5. Inform the patient about the procedure and drug.
6. Place the drug under the patient's tongue.
7. Instruct the patient not to chew or swallow the drug and to keep the drug under the tongue until it has dissolved.
8. Document the drug administration according to your facility's policies.
9. Assess and document the patient's response to the drug.

▶ APPENDIX W

Management of IV Extravasation

1. Immediately stop the infusion or injection if the site is swollen or if the patient complains of burning or pain at the site.
2. Assess the site for redness, swelling, tenderness, difficulty injecting solution, and inability to aspirate blood.
3. Aspirate any drug that remains in the IV catheter.
4. Inform the provider about the extravasation.
5. Remove the IV catheter unless needed to administer the antidote.
6. If indicated, administer an antidote to minimize complications of extravasation. Common antidotes are hyaluronidase and phentolamine.
7. Elevate the extremity to minimize swelling.
8. Apply cool or warm compresses to the site, depending on the infiltrated drug and according to your facility's protocols.
9. Frequently assess the site for redness, swelling, tenderness, skin breakdown, and tissue necrosis.
10. Thoroughly document the IV site assessment, all interventions, and the patient's response.
11. Severe tissue necrosis may require surgical débridement and skin grafting.

▶ APPENDIX X

Selected Pharmaceutical Web Sites

1. **Food and Drug Administration:** http://www.fda.gov/
2. **DrugDB:** http://pharminfo.com/drugdb/db_mnu.html
3. **Centers for Disease Control and Prevention:**
   http://www.cdc.gov/
4. **Internet Self-Assessment in Pharmacology:**
   http://www.horsetooth.com/ISAP/welcome.html
5. **Pharmaceutical Companies:**
   http://www.pharmacy.org/company.html
6. **Pharmaceutical Information Network:**
   http://pharminfo.com/pin_hp.html
7. **Pharmacokinetic and Pharmacodynamic Resources:**
   http://www.boomer.org/pkin/
8. **PharmPC:**
   http://www.pharmacy.org/lists.html#PharmPC
9. **PharmPK:**
   http://www.pharmacy.org/lists.html#PharmPK
10. **PharmWeb:** http://www.pharmweb.net/
11. **Rinfocan:** http://www.islandnet.com/~rinfocan/
12. **RxList—The Internet Drug Index:**
    http://www.rxlist.com/
13. **The *"Virtual"* Pharmacy Center:** http://www-
    sci.lib.uci.edu/~martindale/Pharmacy.html

NOTE: This is a list of selected web sites. The authors do not
endorse these sites but provides them for the reader's use. Web
site addresses are subject to change.

▶ APPENDIX Y

Bibliography

Alspach, J. G. (Ed.). (1998). *Core curriculum for critical care nursing* (5th ed.). Philadelphia: W.B. Saunders.

Darovic, G. O. (1995). *Hemodynamic monitoring* (2nd ed.). Philadelphia: W.B. Saunders.

Drug facts and comparisons. (1999). St. Louis: Facts and Comparisons.

Karch, A. M. (2000). *Lippincott's nursing drug guide.* Philadelphia: J. B. Lippincott.

Kinney, M. R., Dunbar, S. B., Brooks-Brunn, J. A., Molter, N., & Vitello-Cicciu, J. M. (1998). *AACN Clinical reference for critical care nursing* (4th ed.). St. Louis: C. V. Mosby.

Physician's desk reference (44th ed.) (1999). Oradell, NJ: Medical Economics Company.

Rosdahl, C. B. (1999). *Textbook of basic nursing* (7th ed.). Philadelphia: J. B. Lippincott.

Thelan, L. A., Urden, L. D., Lough, M. E., & Stacy, K. M. (1998). *Critical care nursing* (3rd ed.). St. Louis: C. V. Mosby.

Trissel, L. A. (1998). *Handbook on injectable drugs* (10th ed.). Bethesda, MD: American Society of Health-System Pharmacists.

Woods, S. L., Froelicher, E. S. S., Halpenny, C. J., & Motzer, S. U. (1995). *Cardiac nursing* (3rd ed.). Philadelphia: J. B. Lippincott.

▶ APPENDIX Z

Common Abbreviations

α = alpha
$\geq$ = greater than or equal to
$\leq$ = less than or equal to
$<$ = less than
$>$ = greater than
ABG = arterial blood gas
ACE = angiotensin-converting enzyme
ACLS = Advanced Cardiac Life Support
ACT = activated clotting time
ADH = antidiuretic hormone
ADP = adenosine diphosphate
AICD = automatic implantable cardioverter defibrillator
AIDS = acquired immunodeficiency syndrome
ALT = alanine aminotransferase
AMI = acute myocardial infarction
ANA = antinuclear antibodies
ANC = absolute neutrophil count
APTT = activated partial thromboplastin time
ASA = American Society of Anesthesiologists
ASAP = as soon as possible
AST = aspartate aminotransferase
ATP = adenosine triphosphate
AV = atrioventricular
β = beta
bid = twice a day
BMT = bone marrow transplant
BP = blood pressure
BUN = blood urea nitrogen
C = Celsius, centigrade
Ca^{2+} = calcium
CABG = coronary artery bypass grafting
CAD = coronary artery disease
c-AMP = cyclic adenosine monophosphate
CAN = Canada
CAPP = coronary artery perfusion pressure
CBC = complete blood count
Ccr = creatinine clearance
CHF = congestive heart failure
CI = cardiac index
CLL = chronic lymphocytic leukemia
cm = centimeter
CMV = cytomegalovirus
CNS = central nervous system
CO = cardiac output

CO_2 = carbon dioxide
COPD = chronic obstructive pulmonary disease
CPK = creatine phosphokinase
CPP = cerebral perfusion pressure
CPR = cardiopulmonary resuscitation
CR = controlled release
CSF = cerebrospinal fluid
CTZ = chemoreceptor trigger zone
CV = cardiovascular
CVA = cerebrovascular accident
CVP = central venous pressure
CXR = chest x-ray
d = day
D10W = 10% Dextrose in Water
D20W = 20% Dextrose in Water
D2.5W = 2.5% Dextrose in Water
D5W = 5% Dextrose in Water
DBP = diastolic blood pressure
DC = direct current
DEA = Drug Enforcement Administration
Derm = dermatologic
dL = deciliter
DNA = deoxyribonucleic acid
DR = delayed release
DVT = deep vein thrombosis
ECG = electrocardiogram
EEG = electroencephalogram
EENT = eye, ear, nose, throat
EF = ejection fraction
ETOH = alcohol
F = Fahrenheit
FDA = Food and Drug Administration
FEV_1 = forced expiratory volume in 1 second
FFP = fresh frozen plasma
FSP = fibrin split products
g = gram
G-6-PD = glucose-6-phosphate dehydrogenase
GABA = gamma-aminobutyric acid
GERD = gastroesophageal reflux disease
GI = gastrointestinal
GP = glycoprotein
gr = grain
GU = genitourinary
h = hour
H_2O = water

HCl = hydrochloride
Hct = hematocrit
HDL = high density lipoproteins
Hg = mercury
Hgb = hemoglobin
HR = heart rate
hs = at bedtime
HSV = herpes simplex virus
HTN = hypertension
I & O = intake and output
ICP = intracranial pressure
ICU = Intensive Care Unit
IgA = anti-immunoglobulin A
IGF-I = insulin-like growth factor-I
IgG = immunoglobulin G
IgM = immunoglobulin M
IHSS = idiopathic hypertrophic subaortic stenosis
IM = intramuscular
in = inch
INR = international normalized ratio
IPPB = intermittent positive pressure breathing
IU = international units
IV = intravenous
IVPB = intravenous piggyback
JVD = jugular venous distention
K^+ = potassium
KCl = potassium chloride
kg = kilogram
KUB = kidney, ureter, bladder x-ray
L = liter
lb = pound
LDH = lactate dehydrogenase
LDL = low-density lipoproteins
LE = lupus erythematosus
LMW = low-molecular-weight
LR = Lactated Ringer's
LVEDP = left ventricular end diastolic pressure
LVSWI = left ventricular stroke work index
m = meter
MAO = monoamine oxidase
MAP = mean arterial pressure
mcg = microgram
mcm = micrometer
mEq = milliequivalent
mg = milligram
MI = myocardial infarction
min = minute

Misc = miscellaneous
mL = milliliter
mm = millimeter
mmol = millimole
mo = month
Musc/Skel = musculoskeletal
Na^+ = sodium
NAPA = N-acetylprocainamide
ng = nanogram
NG = nasogastric
NIBP = noninvasive blood pressure
NPN = nonprotein nitrogen
NS = Normal Saline
NSAID = nonsteroidal anti-inflammatory drug
NSR = normal sinus rhythm
OG = orogastric
OTC = over the counter
oz= ounce
P = pulse
PAD = pulmonary artery diastolic
PAM = pulmonary artery mean
PAP = pulmonary artery pressure
PAS = pulmonary artery systolic
PCI = percutaneous coronary intervention
PCWP = pulmonary capillary wedge pressure
PE = pulmonary embolus
pH = hydrogen ion concentration
PID = pelvic inflammatory disease
PO = orally, by mouth
PR = per rectum
PRBCs = packed red blood cells
PRI = PR interval
PRN = when required
PSI = per square inch
PSVT = paroxysmal supraventricular tachycardia
pt = pint
PT = prothrombin time
PTCA = percutaneous transluminal coronary angioplasty
PVC = polyvinyl chloride
PVCs = premature ventricular contractions
PVR = pulmonary vascular resistance
PVRI = pulmonary vascular resistance indexed
q = every
qd = every day
qid = four times a day
QTc = corrected QT interval

QTI = QT interval
R = respirations
RAS = reticular activating system
RBC = red blood cell
Resp = respiratory
RNA = ribonucleic acid
RR = respiratory rate
RVSWI = right ventricular stroke work index
SA = sinoatrial
SAH = subarachnoid hemorrhage
SBE = subacute bacterial endocarditis
SBP = systolic blood pressure
SC = subcutaneous
SIADH = syndrome of inappropriate antidiuretic hormone secretion
SL = sublingual
SLE = systemic lupus erythematosus
SpO_2 = oxygen saturation by pulse oximetry
SR = sustained release
STAT = immediately
SV = stroke volume
SVI = stroke volume index
SVR = systemic vascular resistance
SVRI = systemic vascular resistance indexed
SVT = supraventricular tachycardia
T = temperature
$T_{1/2}$ = half-life
T_3 = triiodothyronine
T_4 = thyroxine
TB = tuberculosis
tbsp = tablespoon
TBW = total body weight
TCA = tricyclic antidepressant
TIA = transient ischemic attack
tid = three times a day
tPA = tissue plasminogen activator
TPN = total parenteral nutrition
TSH = thyroid stimulating hormone
tsp = teaspoon
TT = thrombin time
TTP = thrombotic thrombocytopenic purpura
U = unit
UA = urinalysis
UD = unit dose
USA = unstable angina
USP = United States Pharmacopeia

UTI = urinary tract infection
VIP = vasoactive intestinal polypeptide
VLDL = very low-density lipoproteins
WBC = white blood cell
wk = week
WPW = Wolff-Parkinson-White
y = year

INDEX

CRITICAL CARE DRUG GUIDE

Generic drugs appear in **boldface** type; trade names in plain print; Canadian trade names are followed by (CAN).